McMinn's
Functional
& Clinical
Anatomy

Robert M H McMinn MD, PhD, FRCS
Emeritus Professor of Anatomy
Royal College of Surgeons of England and
University of London
London, England

Penelope Gaddum–Rosse PhD
Associate Professor, Department of Biological Structure
University of Washington; Formerly Coordinator of courses in
Anatomy and Physiology for students of Nursing and Pharmacy
University of Washington
Seattle, USA

Ralph T Hutchings
Freelance Photographer
Formerly Chief Medical Laboratory Scientific Officer
Royal College of Surgeons of England
London, England

Bari M Logan MA, FMA, Hon MBIE
University Prosector, Department of Anatomy
University of Cambridge
Cambridge, England

M Mosby

London Baltimore Bogotá Boston Buenos Aires Caracas Carlsbad, CA Chicago Madrid Mexico City Milan Naples, FL New York Philadelphia St. Louis Sydney Tokyo Toronto Wiesbaden

Copyright © 1995 Times Mirror International Publishers Limited

Published in 1995 by Mosby, an imprint of Times Mirror International Publishers Limited

Printed by Grafos, S.A. Arte sobre papel, Barcelona, Spain

ISBN 0 7234 0967 6

For full details of all Times Mirror International Publishers Limited titles, please write to Times Mirror International Publishers Limited, Lynton House, 7–12 Tavistock Square, London WC1H 9LB, England.

A CIP catalogue record for this book is available from the British Library.

Library of Congress Cataloging-in-Publication Data Applied For

Project Manager:	Roderick Craig
Developmental Editor:	Lucy Hamilton
Layout:	Ian Spick
Cover design:	Lara Last
Illustration:	Lynda Payne Marion Tasker Lee Smith
Production:	Mike Heath
Index:	Jill Halliday
Publisher:	Geoff Greenwood
Cover photography:	Mark Howard *Twenty-Five Educational* *London NW1*

CONTENTS

PREFACE

The object of this book is to provide an account of body structure and function for those who are entering the health care professions. The account of body anatomy and physiology is enlivened by reference to common diseases and injuries that are so often seen as part of the daily routine by those involved in health care. The purpose of bringing clinical material to this early stage of learning is not to teach clinical details, but simply to introduce to students commonly used medical terms and to explain their anatomical and physiological backgrounds, in order to emphasize how necessary a knowledge of normal form and function is for understanding what happens when things go wrong. Heart transplants may hit the headlines, but varicose veins and hernias, coronary artery disease and diabetes, gallstones and fractures of the wrist are the stuff of everyday medical practice with which all medical and paramedical attendants must become familiar, and this is why we have used such common conditions for illustrating the application of basic science to clinical problems. Our aim has been to be informative but concise, and we make no apology for having been selective and for not trying to drag in every possible detail. The background to many standard procedures commonly carried out by nurses and doctors is also included to add interest and relevance to learning, by showing how knowledge of what often appear to be dull facts is put to practical use in patient care.

The first part of the book summarizes the tissues and the various body systems, and this is followed by adding further details on a regional basis. This plan has been chosen because, although the function of body systems as a whole has to be appreciated, patients usually have something wrong with a particular organ or area, or need attention to a particular organ or area, and this is what has to be tackled by their attendants. This may not be the usual approach to basic science teaching but we believe it is a practical one that will add to student understanding and interest (and to stimulate interest instead of boring the pants off readers is always one of the problems of teaching basic sciences, which often seem remote from practical problems). We hope our presentation will be just such a stimulus and will lead to a desire for further study.

Despite the need for a sound background in basic sciences, those responsible for looking after patients should remember that there will always be times when a kind word, and the gentle touch that says 'I care', are more important than all the latest technological advances.

R M H McMinn
Penelope Gaddum–Rosse
R T Hutchings
B M Logan

ACKNOWLEDGEMENTS

We are grateful to many friends and colleagues for help with illustrations. In particular we wish to thank Rosemary Watts and Philip Ball for original artwork; Dr Oscar Craig, Dr Paul Grech and Dr Peter Abrahams for radiographs and scans; and our models for surface anatomy. We are also indebted to Christopher Brett for assistance with the Index, and to the following for the use of pictures from their own Mosby–Wolfe publications:

- Prof W F Walker for 8.6, 19.7 (from *A Colour Atlas of Peripheral Vascular Diseases*) and 19.9 (from *A Colour Atlas of General Surgical Diagnosis*)
- Prof M B L Craigmyle for 8.8a–f (from *A Colour Atlas of Histology*)
- Prof R Hall and Dr D Evered for 16.40 (from *A Colour Atlas of Endocrinology*)
- Mr G Page, Mr K Mills and Mr R Morton for 16.39a (from *A Colour Atlas of Cardio-Pulmonary Resuscitation Techniques*)
- Dr R E Pounder, Dr M C Allison and Dr A P Dhillon for 19.12 (from *A Colour Atlas of the Digestive System*)
- Dr W Guthrie and Mr R Fawkes for 19.20b, 19.29 and 19.42 (from *A Colour Atlas of Surgical Pathology*)
- Mr C Vaughan Ruckley for 20.15d (from *A Colour Atlas of Surgical Management of Venous Disease*)

We would also like to thank Roddy Craig of Mosby, who was left holding many editorial babies and reared them successfully.

CHAPTER 1

ANATOMICAL TERMS AND DESCRIPTIONS

PARTS OF THE BODY

The **body** (**1.1a**) is made up of the head, trunk and limbs. The **trunk** consists of the **neck**, the **thorax** (i.e. the chest), and the **abdomen** (the belly). The lower part of the abdomen is the **pelvis**, but this word is also used to refer to the bones of the pelvis. The lowest part of the pelvis – and hence the lowest part of the trunk – is the **perineum**. The central axis of the trunk is the **vertebral column** (the spinal column or spine), and the upper part of it (the cervical part or cervical spine) supports the **head**.

The main parts of the **upper limb** are the **arm**, **forearm** and **hand**. Note that in strict anatomical terms the word 'arm' means the upper arm, between the shoulder and elbow, although the word is commonly used to mean the whole of the upper limb.

The main parts of the **lower limb** are the **thigh**, **leg** and **foot**. The word 'leg' strictly means the part between the knee and foot, but is commonly used to mean the whole of the lower limb.

DESCRIPTIVE TERMS

For the description of the positions of structures, the body is assumed to be standing upright with the feet together and the head and eyes looking to the front, with the arms straight by the sides and the palms of the hands facing forwards (**1.1a**). This is the *anatomical position*, and structures are always described relative to one another using this standard position, even when the body is, for example, lying in bed or on a dissecting room table (or even when standing on its head!).

To the student who is new to the subject, many of the anatomical terms described below will seem strange at first sight, but every subject has its own jargon, and anatomy is no exception. When necessary, reference should be made back to the following paragraphs when reading the later text; there is no need to memorize every definition at this stage, since continued use will soon make the meanings clear and familiar.

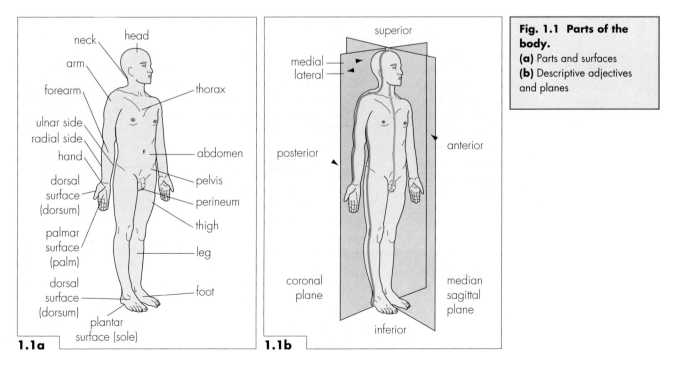

1.1a

1.1b

Fig. 1.1 Parts of the body.
(a) Parts and surfaces
(b) Descriptive adjectives and planes

The *median sagittal plane* is an imaginary vertical, longitudinal plane through the middle of the body from front to back, dividing the body into the right and left halves (**1.1b**). The adjective *medial* means nearer the median plane, and *lateral* means farther from it. Thus, in the anatomical position, the little finger is on the medial side of the hand and the thumb is on the lateral side; the great toe is on the medial side of the foot and the little toe on the lateral side.

In the forearm, where there are two bones, with the radius on the lateral (thumb) side and the ulna on the medial side, the adjectives *radial* and *ulnar* can be used instead of lateral and medial. Similarly, in the lower leg, where there are two bones, with the fibula on the lateral side and the tibia on the medial side, the adjectives *fibular* and *tibial* are sometimes used.

Anterior and *posterior* mean 'nearer the front' and 'nearer the back' of the body respectively (**1.1b**). Thus, on the face, the nose is anterior to the ears (more strictly, anteromedial) and the ears are posterior to the nose (more strictly, posterolateral). Sometimes *ventral* is used instead of anterior, and *dorsal* instead of posterior; these are terms from comparative anatomy that are appropriate for four-footed animals.

The hand and foot have special terms applied to them. The anterior or ventral surface of the hand is usually called the **palm** or palmar surface, and the posterior or dorsal surface is the **dorsum**. In the foot, however, the upper surface is the dorsal surface or dorsum and the under surface, or **sole**, is the plantar surface.

Superior and *inferior* mean nearer the upper or lower end of the body respectively (**1.1b**); the nose is superior to the mouth and inferior to the forehead (even if the body is upside down; the upright anatomical position is always the reference position).

Superficial means near the skin surface, and *deep* means farther away from the surface.

Proximal and *distal* mean nearer to and further from the root of the structure respectively; in the upper limb, the forearm is distal to the elbow and proximal to the hand.

The words *sagittal* and *coronal* describe certain planes of section, most often used in the head and brain. The *sagittal plane* is any front-to-back plane that is parallel to the median plane, and the *coronal plane*, sometimes called the *frontal plane*, is a vertical plane at right angles to the median plane (**1.1b**).

MOVEMENTS

Other terms are used to describe movements. They are defined below and many are illustrated in **1.2a**–r.

Flexion means bending or decreasing the angle between bones, as in bending the elbow; this can also be described as 'flexion of the elbow', 'flexion of the elbow joint', or 'flexion

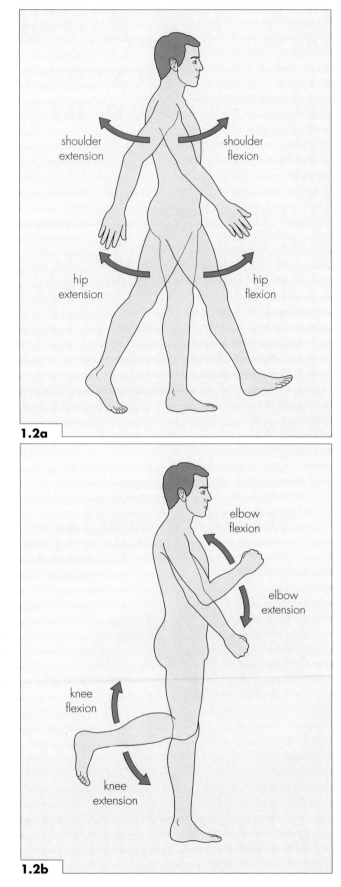

1.2a

1.2b

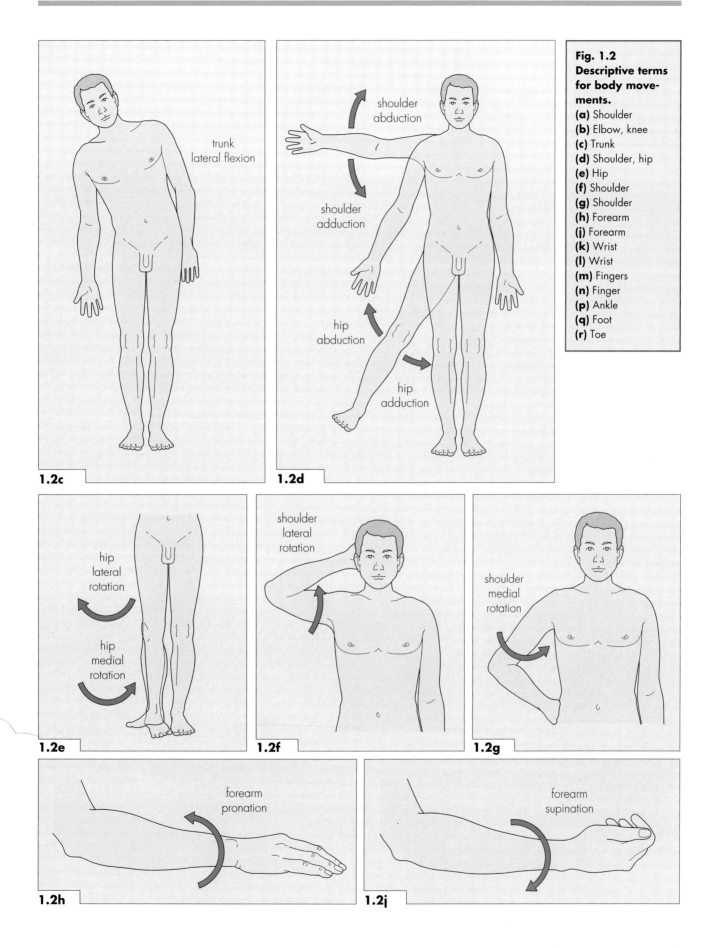

Fig. 1.2
Descriptive terms for body movements.
(a) Shoulder
(b) Elbow, knee
(c) Trunk
(d) Shoulder, hip
(e) Hip
(f) Shoulder
(g) Shoulder
(h) Forearm
(j) Forearm
(k) Wrist
(l) Wrist
(m) Fingers
(n) Finger
(p) Ankle
(q) Foot
(r) Toe

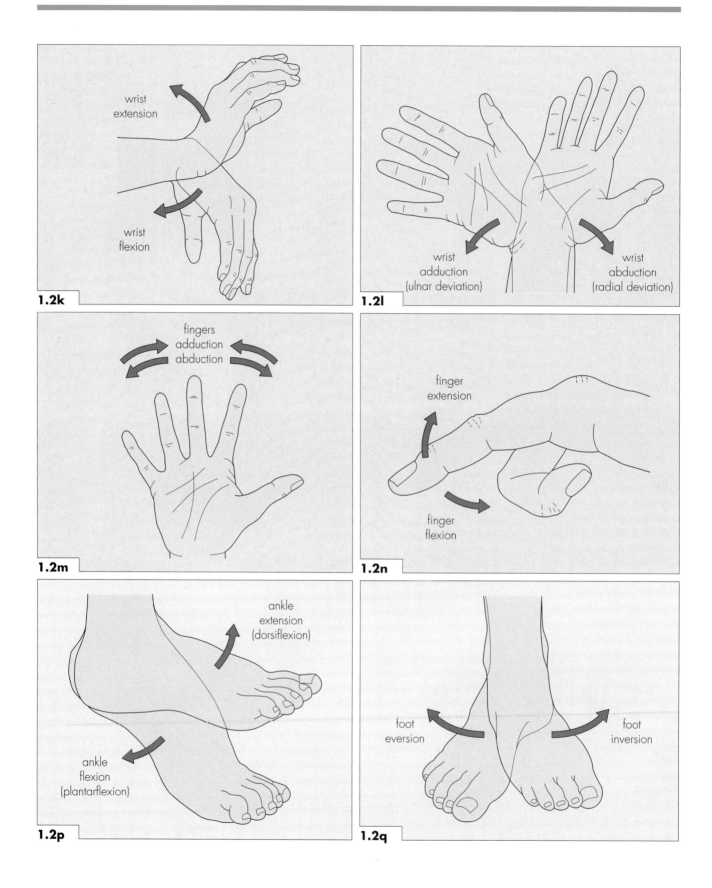

1.2k wrist extension / wrist flexion

1.2l wrist adduction (ulnar deviation) / wrist abduction (radial deviation)

1.2m fingers adduction abduction

1.2n finger extension / finger flexion

1.2p ankle extension (dorsiflexion) / ankle flexion (plantarflexion)

1.2q foot eversion / foot inversion

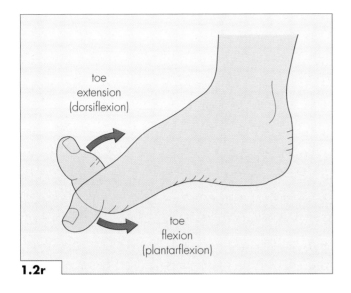

toe
extension
(dorsiflexion)

toe
flexion
(plantarflexion)

1.2r

of the forearm at the elbow joint'. Flexion can be applied to the trunk of the body as well as to the limbs; bending the trunk forwards is 'flexion of the spine or vertebral column'. Bending sideways (but still facing forwards, without twisting sideways or rotation) is 'lateral flexion'.

Extension means straightening out or increasing the angle between bones (the opposite of flexion), such as in straightening the flexed elbow, or, equivalently, 'extension of the elbow or elbow joint', or 'extension of the forearm at the elbow'. Straightening up the trunk from the flexed position, or bending backwards from the upright position, is 'extension of the spine'.

Abduction is movement away from the midline of the body, as in lifting the arm away from the side at the shoulder, which is described as 'abduction of the shoulder or shoulder joint', or 'abduction of the arm at the shoulder joint'.

Adduction is the opposite of abduction, or movement towards the midline, as when bringing the abducted arm back to the side.

Circumduction is not a term commonly used, but is a combination of the above four movements carried out in sequence, as at the shoulder or hip. In circumduction of the shoulder the hand is made to go round in a wide circle.

Rotation is a twisting movement in the long axis of a bone, applied particularly to the humerus and femur, and can occur in lateral (outward) and medial (inward) directions. Lateral rotation of the humerus, often called 'lateral rotation of the shoulder or shoulder joint', is best illustrated by putting the hand behind the head (which also of course involves abduction of the shoulder and flexion of the elbow). The humerus is medially rotated in putting the hand behind the back.

Pronation and *supination* are terms applied to the forearm. The anatomical position is one of supination, with the radius and ulna parallel; in pronation the lower end of the radius rotates across the lower end of the ulna, turning the palm over. Supination from the pronated position 'untwists' the radius, making it parallel to the ulna again. Many actions of everyday life are carried out with the forearm in the 'midprone position' – halfway between full pronation and full supination, as when holding a cup or pencil.

Inversion and *eversion* are terms applied to the foot. In inversion, the inner (medial) border of the foot is raised so that the sole is tilted to face medially. In eversion, the lateral border is raised so that the sole is tilted laterally. These movements are illustrated when walking transversely across a slope: one foot will be inverted and the other everted.

CHAPTER 2

CELLS AND TISSUES

Cells, tissues, organs and systems – these are the units from which all vertebrate animal bodies are composed, and the human body is no exception. Many thousands of millions of **cells** become grouped together to form **tissues**, and tissues combine in varied ways to form structures such as bones, muscles and **organs**. (The stomach, kidneys, lungs, etc., are often collectively called **viscera**, from the plural of the Latin *viscus*, meaning an internal organ.) Organs, in turn, become grouped together into **systems**, each with a particular role to play in keeping the body alive.

Human life depends upon taking in oxygen and food, which can be broken down into the substances that the body must use in order to provide the necessary chemical energy for maintaining bodily structure and function.

CELL STRUCTURE

The fundamental unit of life is the **cell** (**2.1**). All cells have a **cell membrane** (i.e. a **boundary membrane**) that serves to contain the **cytoplasm**, which is the internal material in which the **nucleus** and the other components – the **organelles** – of the cell lie. Certain organelles are common to most cells, and each organelle has a specific role to play within the cell.

In the very earliest developing embryos, where one original cell becomes two, then four, eight, sixteen etc., all of the cells are similar. Soon, however, they develop into different kinds; some become muscle cells, others become nerve cells, epithelial cells or connective tissue cells – these are the cells that make up the four basic tissue types (see below).

Each type of cell differs from others in function because certain kinds of organelles are predominant; in muscle cells there are masses of filaments that cause contraction, in secretory cells there is a predominance of the organelles concerned with manufacturing the secretory product, and so on. The chemical influences that determine cell type are derived from the cell's genetic material, which is contained in the nucleus; the nucleus is the most obvious structural feature of most cells when they are examined microscopically. The 'messages' that the nucleus sends out to the cytoplasm determine which kind of cell it is going to be. Although the total genetic mate-

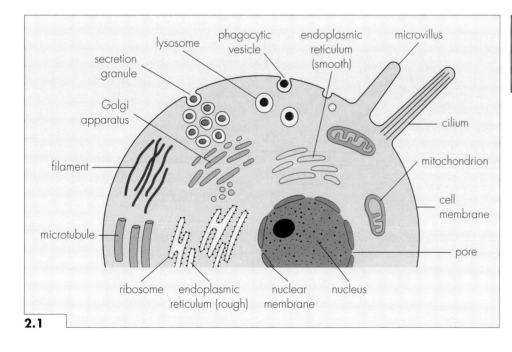

Fig. 2.1 Diagrammatic representation of parts of the cell, as seen with the electron microscope.

2.1

rial is identical in every cell of any one individual, only a small part of the vast number of possible messages becomes effective in any one cell, and the message depends upon which **genes** become *expressed* (i.e. activated). The control of gene expression is one of the major fields of research in cell biology today.

CELL MEMBRANE

The **cell membrane** – also known as the **plasma membrane** or **plasmalemma** – controls what enters or leaves the cytoplasm. Cell membranes contain lipids, protein and carbohydrate components, with lipid molecules being particularly numerous.

Certain substances can pass into (or out of) cells, either through minute pores (also called *channels*) in the membrane, or by becoming attached to some of the membrane's 'carrier' molecules which transport the substance across the membrane. Larger particles, such as bacteria, can be 'taken into' some cells through their becoming engulfed in a pocket of membrane which then breaks away from the surface to lie free within the cell as a membrane-bound package called a **vesicle**; this is the process of *phagocytosis* (from the Greek meaning 'cell eating'). *Exocytosis* is phagocytosis 'in reverse'; it is the process of cell secretion, allowing the liberation from the cell of substances manufactured within it.

NUCLEUS

The **nucleus** is a membrane-bound structure, with the enclosed material being called the **nucleoplasm**. The **nuclear membrane**, which is the boundary of the nucleus, is double-layered, with numerous pores that allow substances to pass between the nucleoplasm (inside) and the cytoplasm (outside).

In most cells, the genetic material, which is called DNA (deoxyribonucleic acid), is in the form of extremely fine, tangled **chromatin threads**; if stretched out, the total length of the threads in each nucleus would be about 2 m (7 ft), which seems unbelievable, but is true. Short lengths of the threads constitute the genes, each of which acts as an instruction (i.e. a genetic code) to the chemical machinery of the cell and causes the production of a particular product. The thread-like nature of the chromatin cannot be appreciated by light microscopy, where the nucleus usually appears as a rather darkly staining mass. Only as the cell is preparing for division – called *mitosis* – does the chromatin become separated out into recognizable clumps; these are the **chromosomes**, which are bunched-up versions of the original threads.

In human cells there are 46 chromosomes, which can be arranged into 23 pairs; one pair are the sex chromosomes, designated X and Y; females have two X chromosomes, and males have one X and one Y. To examine chromosomes it is necessary to grow some cells in tissue culture, to make them divide, and then to stop the cell division (with the drug colchicine) to 'capture' the chromosomes while they are still

condensed and, therefore, visible microscopically. The tissue is then examined under the microscope and the chromosomes photographed for identification; the process is known as *karyotyping*. Each pair of chromosomes has a characteristic size and shape, and has been given an identification number (1–22); the twenty-third pair are the sex chromosomes. Certain inherited diseases are known to be associated with defects in particular chromosomes (e.g. cystic fibrosis, where there is a defect in chromosome 7), and the total numbers of chromosomes may also be abnormal (as in most cases of Down's syndrome, with three of chromosome 21, known as trisomy 21).

So-called 'DNA fingerprinting' depends on the sequence of amino acids that make up an individual's DNA and, although not quite as unique as a fingerprint, has forensic use for identification from cells in mere fragments of tissue or secretions such as saliva or semen. The discovery that there is some DNA in mitochondria which is inherited only by females is of great interest for long-term genealogical studies.

ORGANELLES

Apart from the nucleus, various other structural components of the cell are found in the cytoplasm. The most important are considered below; many have membranes as part of their structure.

Mitochondria are rounded or sausage-shaped structures which, because of their capacity to generate ATP (adenosine triphosphate, p.83), are responsible for meeting the energy requirements of the cell. When ATP is broken down, a large amount of energy is made available, thus enabling the cell to undertake many other chemical reactions. Mitochondria have therefore been called the 'powerhouses' of the cell.

Lysosomes are membrane-bound packages of enzymes that can join up with phagocytic vesicles so that the enzymes can break down (i.e. digest) the engulfed material into smaller and harmless molecules that are then allowed to enter the cell cytoplasm.

The **endoplasmic reticulum** (**ER**) is a closed-membrane system which, in electron microscope sections, appears as groups of interconnecting channels or flattened sacs that are called **cisternae**. It serves to segregate substances from the rest of the cytoplasm, and is particularly prominent in those cells that are manufacturing substances for export, i.e. secretion. Such substances must be collected together in a membrane-bound system and not become mixed up and lost in the general cytoplasm of the cell.

Some ER has ribosomes (small particles that are the sites of protein synthesis) attached to its outer surface, and is called **rough ER**; newly synthesized proteins can pass through the membrane of the ER and become collected in its internal cavity. Large amounts of rough ER are characteristic of cells engaged in protein secretion, such as the digestive cells of the pancreas and salivary glands. ER without ribosomes attached is **smooth ER**, and is characteristic of cells engaged in the secretion of steroid hormones, such as those of the adrenal cortex.

While ribosomes occur frequently in association with the ER (as mentioned above), they also occur in an 'unattached' form; these are **free ribosomes**. In this case, they function in the synthesis of proteins to be used inside the cell, rather than to be exported.

The **Golgi apparatus** (also called the **Golgi complex**) is another membrane system, appearing as a collection of elongated sacs and vesicles. It is prominent especially in many secretory cells, for it receives substances from the rough ER, perhaps concentrating them or modifying them chemically, and then forming membrane-bound vesicles of secretory product – called **secretion granules** – that migrate to the apex of the cell and fuse with the boundary membrane, so liberating the secretory material from the cell.

On the surfaces of many cells are numerous small, rod-like projections of the cell membrane; they have an internal core of cytoplasm. These **microvilli** increase the surface area of the cell, and are particularly numerous in cells whose main function is absorption, such as the epithelial cells of the small intestine and in certain kidney tubules.

In the respiratory tract there are many cells whose surfaces bear numerous hair-like processes or **cilia**. They are larger than microvilli and are quite different in structure, for their internal cores contain a regular arrangement of rod-like proteins that are responsible for a rhythmic beating of the cilia. Waves of ciliary movement help to clear the surface of adherent mucus and dust particles. The tail of a spermatozoon is like an extremely long cilium with the internal structure discussed above.

Minute **filaments** and **microtubules** in the cytoplasm act as a kind of internal scaffolding for cells, helping them to preserve their usual shape. Tubules, as in certain nerve cells, may act as transport channels to conduct materials from one region of the cell to another. In muscle cells, the filaments (myofilaments) are composed of special proteins which can 'latch on' to one another to cause contraction.

TISSUES

There are four basic **tissues**: epithelium (epithelial tissue), connective tissue, muscle (muscular tissue) and nerve (nervous tissue). Every structure in the body is made up of varying combinations of these tissues.

EPITHELIUM

Epithelial tissues form sheets of cells that cover surfaces, line cavities, and form glands. As a covering tissue, epithelium forms the outer part of the skin and the thin layer of cells on the outer surface of many organs in the thorax and abdomen (e.g. the lungs, stomach and intestine). As an internal lining, it is found as the innermost layer of cells in hollow viscera

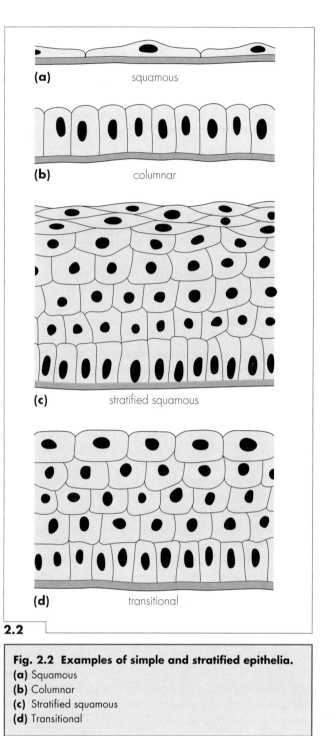

2.2

Fig. 2.2 Examples of simple and stratified epithelia.
(a) Squamous
(b) Columnar
(c) Stratified squamous
(d) Transitional

(such as the stomach), and as the main component of organs made up of tubular structures, such as the kidney and testis.

Epithelial tissues are classified as **simple epithelia** if they consist of a single layer of cells, or **stratified epithelia** if they consist of several layers. Among the simple epithelia are the extremely flattened, *squamous* cells (**2.2a**) ('squamous' meaning 'leaf-like') that form the lining of the alveoli (the air sacs) of the lungs (p.75), and the taller (*columnar*) cells (**2.2b**) that line the intestines (p.81). Organs such as the mouth (p.147), the oesophagus (p.103) and the vagina (p.301) are lined by thicker epithelia called **stratified squamous epithelia** (**2.2c**) – 'stratified' because there are several layers, and 'squamous' because the uppermost layers of cells are flattened. The parts of the kidneys that collect urine, as well as the rest of the urinary tract (ureters, urinary bladder and urethra), are lined by a special kind of stratified epithelium called *transitional* epithelium (**2.2d**); here the cells of the uppermost layer are not flattened but remain rather bulbous, to allow for stretching when the organ becomes distended (p.293), a feature of particular importance in the bladder which is subject to frequent distension and collapse.

The term **mucous membrane** (or **mucosa**) is used to refer to the internal lining of hollow organs that communicate, whether directly or indirectly, with the exterior. It includes not only the epithelium, but also some underlying connective tissue, and, in most of the digestive tract, some smooth muscle too (p.81).

Despite the adjective 'mucous', not all mucous membranes secrete mucus; they usually do, but those of the urinary tract, for example, do not. **Serous membranes**, on the other hand, line body cavities that do not communicate with the exterior (such as the thoracic cavity), and are reflected over the organs in those cavities. The pleura (in the thorax), the peritoneum (in the abdomen and pelvis) and the pericardium (surrounding the heart) are the major serous membranes. Like mucous membranes they consist of epithelium and connective tissue, with the epithelium being a simple squamous type that secretes a watery (**serous**) fluid for lubrication of the surfaces.

Epithelia in certain localities are given special names: in serous membranes, the epithelium is called **mesothelium**, and when lining blood and lymph vessels it is **endothelium**. The epithelium of the skin has the special name of **epidermis**, and is a stratified squamous keratinizing epithelium, where the uppermost layers of cells have become converted into keratin (p.17).

CONNECTIVE TISSUE

Connective tissue is a supporting tissue that helps to bind other tissues together. Unlike epithelial tissue, which consists almost entirely of cells, connective tissue contains not only cells but a considerable amount of material around and between the cells – the **extracellular matrix** (ECM). The matrix consists of **fibres** and a 'ground' substance containing a variety of macromolecules. Both of these components of the matrix are manufactured by the principal kind of connective tissue cell – the **fibroblasts**. Other common connective tissue cells are the **macrophages**, the 'scavengers' of the body, which help to get rid of unwanted material (such as dead and dying cells and invading organisms). The fibres of connective tissue may be *collagenous* or *elastic*; collagenous fibres are tough and unyielding, while elastic fibres are thin and stretchable. Both are widely distributed throughout the body, but sometimes collagen fibres are aggregated together to form such structures as ligaments and tendons.

There are several different types of connective tissue, ranging from **areolar tissue**, which is loose, such as is found under some areas of the skin, allowing a fold to be pinched up (as on the back of the hand), to **dense connective tissue**, as in tendons, where there are many fibres and very little ground substance. In **adipose tissue**, which is fatty, many of the cells contain large globules of lipid in their cytoplasm. In **cartilage** and **bone** the matrix contains many fibres and is firm (in cartilage) and impregnated with calcium salts (in bone). At the other extreme is **blood**, which is a connective tissue where the matrix is fluid (i.e. **blood plasma**) with red and white blood cells suspended in it and with no fibres – however, when it clots, even blood has fibres.

Bone

If a **bone** is sawn open (**2.3**), it can be seen to consist of an outer shell of **compact bone**, which appears as a dense mass, as in the shaft of a long limb bone, and **cancellous** or **spongy bone**, which partly or completely fills the inside of the bone and consists of a network of fine bone **spicules** (also called **trabeculae**, from the Latin meaning little beams). The bone trabeculae are not randomly arranged, but develop in such a way as to resist the stress to which the bone is usually subjected.

Microscopically (**2.3d**), both types of bone consist of masses of bone cells, the **osteocytes**, and **collagen fibres** embedded in the **calcified matrix**. Despite the solid appearance of much of it, bone is a very vascular tissue and bleeds when cut; in compact bone, for example, there are many capillary blood vessels (with lymphatics and nerve fibres) running in minute tunnels through the matrix (the **Haversian** and **Volkmann's canals**). Many of the osteocytes lie in concentric rings (*lamellae*) of matrix arranged around a capillary; the combination of vessel, cells and matrix (with its embedded collagen fibres) forms a **Haversian system**. The spaces, or *lacunae*, in the matrix in which the bone cells lie are connected to adjacent lacunae by minute channels – called **canaliculi** – so that tissue fluid from nearby capillaries can diffuse through the canaliculi and so reach every bone cell.

All internal bone surfaces are lined by a single layer of cells that is called the **endosteum**. Unless covered by cartilage at the joints, the outer surfaces of bones are ensheathed in **periosteum**, which is a kind of fibrous tissue 'stocking' consisting of several layers of cells, the deepest of which are osteoblasts. **Osteoblasts** form the **osteogenic** layer and lie against the bone surface; they are capable of multiplying and forming new bone, as at a fracture site or at the surface of a bone during development; osteocytes, in contrast, are not capable of cell division. Periosteum is vascular, and also has a good nerve supply; any bruised bone, where the periosteum becomes raised from the surface and stretched by escaped blood, is very painful.

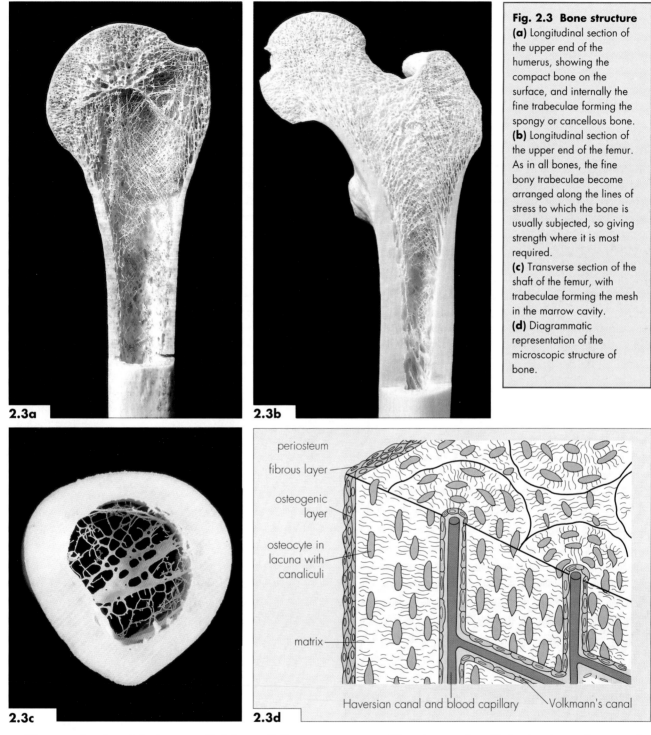

2.3a

2.3b

2.3c

2.3d

Fig. 2.3 Bone structure
(a) Longitudinal section of the upper end of the humerus, showing the compact bone on the surface, and internally the fine trabeculae forming the spongy or cancellous bone.
(b) Longitudinal section of the upper end of the femur. As in all bones, the fine bony trabeculae become arranged along the lines of stress to which the bone is usually subjected, so giving strength where it is most required.
(c) Transverse section of the shaft of the femur, with trabeculae forming the mesh in the marrow cavity.
(d) Diagrammatic representation of the microscopic structure of bone.

periosteum
fibrous layer
osteogenic layer
osteocyte in lacuna with canaliculi
matrix
Haversian canal and blood capillary
Volkmann's canal

The central cavity of the bone – called the **medullary** or **marrow cavity** – and the small spaces between the spicules of spongy bone are both filled by **bone marrow**, which is described as red or yellow in colour. **Red marrow** is a mass of loose connective tissue with many dilated blood capillaries containing developing blood cells; it is thus the site of *haemopoiesis* (from the Greek meaning 'forming blood'). **Yellow marrow** is not a site of blood formation, being largely a mass of fatty tissue and capillaries, but it can change to the red variety if there is a need for increased blood cell formation. In young children all marrow is red, but as adulthood is approached, red marrow normally becomes confined mostly to the ends of long limb bones, the sternum, vertebrae and hip bones.

In the developing fetus, most bones are first formed of cartilage which then becomes replaced by bone – a process known as *endochondral ossification*, meaning 'bone formation in cartilage'. It is important to appreciate that the cartilage is not converted into bone; it is destroyed (by cellular and chemical activity) and then replaced by the formation of new bone. The site of the first bone formation (which is detectable on a radiograph) is a **centre of ossification**, and in typical long bones is in the middle of the shaft – in which case it is a **primary centre of ossification**. The ends of long bones develop similar sites, called **epiphyses**, but not until much later (usually after birth) – these are **secondary centres of ossification**. The ends eventually fuse with the shaft (usually between puberty and about 18 years of age), but until then there is a region filled with cartilage between the shaft and the epiphysis – the **epiphyseal plate** or **epiphyseal cartilage** (see **5.2b**) – which is detectable in a radiograph. It is the presence of growth in these epiphyseal cartilage plates which enables a bone to grow in length; when the epiphyseal cartilage disappears, growth stops. Some of the smaller bones (such as those of the wrist and skull) have no secondary centres (i.e. no epiphyses). Radiologists and surgeons must be aware of the normal positions for epiphyseal cartilages in order to distinguish them from suspected fracture lines.

A few bones, in particular some skull bones and the clavicle, do not begin their life as a preformed cartilage model but develop from centres of ossification in fibrous tissue; this type of bone development is *intramembranous ossification*.

The growth of bone during development is an interplay between new bone formation – *osteogenesis* by osteoblasts – and bone destruction or resorption, associated with the cells called osteoclasts, with the whole process often being called *bone remodelling*; bone may be laid down in one area and taken away at another. This is how, for example, long bones grow in width without the dense bone of the shaft itself getting thicker and thicker; bone is added to the outer surface at the same time as it is taken away from the inner surface.

When a bone is broken or fractured, osteoblasts from the endosteum and periosteum multiply, and manufacture new bone fibres and matrix. The mass of new tissue is called **callus**, and eventually forms new bone that unites the broken ends – provided the ends are reasonably apposed to one another and are held immobile (usually in a plaster cast) during the healing period of several weeks. The bone ends often have to be manipulated into position under anaesthesia but, if badly displaced, surgical operation may be required to screw metal plates on to the broken pieces to hold them together in the correct position. Inadequate immobilization results in nonunion, with the new tissue failing to become ossified; it may simply persist as fibrous tissue or cartilage, and leads to permanent instability.

In later life, a decrease in the amount of calcium and bone matrix in limb bones and vertebrae is common – this is called *osteoporosis*. No specific cause has been found, but complications such as fractures of the neck of the femur and collapse of the bodies of vertebrae are particularly common in females after child-bearing age, suggesting a hormonal link; oestrogen therapy (p.300) decreases the incidence of these complications.

Cartilage

Cartilage is a type of connective tissue where the cells (the **chondrocytes**) and fibres are embedded in a firm gel-like material or matrix (**2.4**). There are three kinds: hyaline cartilage, elastic cartilage and fibrocartilage.

Hyaline cartilage is the commonest type; it covers the ends of the bones – taking part in synovial joints (p.31) – and forms the costal cartilages of the thorax (p.97) and the cartilages of the trachea (p.74).

Elastic cartilage has a high content of elastic fibres, and is found in the epiglottis of the larynx (p.186) and in the pinna (i.e. the auricle) of the ear (p.169).

Fibrocartilage has a high collagen fibre content, and is found in intervertebral discs (p.27) and other joint cartilages, such as the menisci of the knee joint (p.325).

Apart from being free of calcium salts, cartilage differs from bone in having no internal blood vessels; the cells obtain their nutrition by diffusion of substances through the matrix. (Bone matrix, being calcified, does not allow diffusion, hence the need for bone matrix to have a vascular system and canaliculi, p.10). A further difference from bone is that, during body growth, cartilage can grow by the multiplication of chondrocytes within the cartilage mass as well as at the surface; the osteocytes of bone are not capable of doing this – only osteoblasts can multiply.

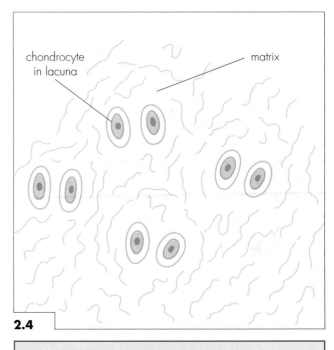

2.4

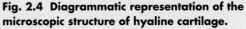

Fig. 2.4 Diagrammatic representation of the microscopic structure of hyaline cartilage.

MUSCLE

Contractility – the ability to generate force and movement – is present to some degree in virtually all cells, but is especially well developed in **muscle cells**. The contractile proteins, **actin** and **myosin**, whose interaction is responsible for contraction, are abundant in muscle cells and occur in the form of long filaments that are called **myofilaments**. Muscle cells themselves are also long and thin as a rule, and are therefore often called **muscle fibres**. There are three types of muscle fibres: *skeletal*, *cardiac* and *smooth* (**2.5**).

Skeletal Muscle

Skeletal muscle is often called **striated** or **striped muscle** because the myofilaments are arranged in regular overlapping groups (**2.5d**) that give a transversely striped appearance to the fibres in well-prepared microscope sections.

All skeletal muscle fibres have many nuclei (**2.5a**). These nuclei do not lie in the centre of the fibre, but rather are scattered at the periphery just underneath the cell membrane; in the longer muscle fibres (which may be many centimeters long), there are thousands of nuclei in any one fibre.

Every single muscle fibre must receive its own branch of a motor nerve fibre (at the neuromuscular junction, p.49) in order to contract.

Skeletal muscle fibres are collected together to form the individually named muscles (p.35) that move the skeleton, and that are found in certain other sites such as the tongue, the pharynx (throat) and the larynx (voicebox), and in sphincters at the lower ends of the digestive and urinary tracts. Skeletal muscles are often called *voluntary muscles* because they are under the control of the will. They can contract only when they have an intact motor nerve supply.

Cardiac Muscle

The cells or fibres of **cardiac muscle**, which is present only in the heart, have the same kind of filamentous arrangement, with striations, as skeletal muscle. (Strictly speaking, cardiac muscle is also classified as striated muscle, but this term is usually taken to mean the skeletal variety.)

Cardiac muscle fibres (**2.5b**) are more like conventional cells, having usually only one nucleus in the centre of each cell. They are never as long as skeletal muscle fibres, and are

Fig. 2.5 Diagrammatic representation of the microscopic structure of muscle.
(a) Skeletal muscle: long cells with many nuclei just under the cell membrane.
(b) Cardiac muscle: short branching cells.
(c) Smooth muscle: slender cells.
(d) Arrangement of myofilaments in skeletal and cardiac muscle. (Upper) Relaxed. (Lower) Contraction, caused by the actin filaments sliding between the myosin filaments. The distance between the Z-lines, to which the actin filaments are attached, decreases.

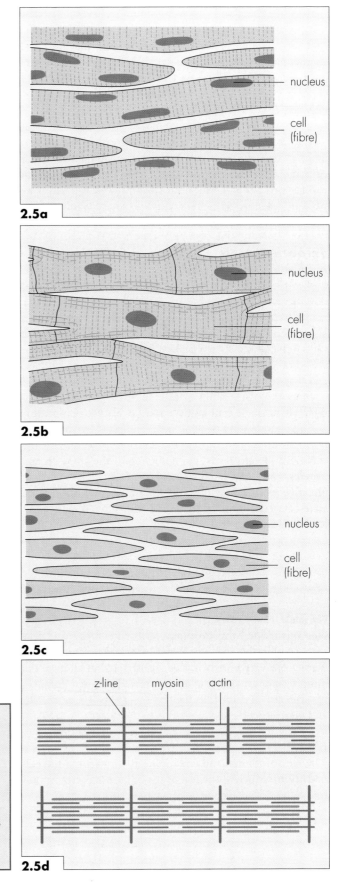

2.5a

nucleus

cell (fibre)

2.5b

nucleus

cell (fibre)

2.5c

nucleus

cell (fibre)

z-line   myosin   actin

2.5d

shaped like short and sometimes branched cylinders; they become attached to one another end-on, where their adjacent cell membranes become elaborately folded against one another like pieces in a complicated jigsaw puzzle. This interdigitation serves to increase the surface area for the rapid conduction of the electrical impulse; unlike skeletal muscle, only very few of the cells receive nerve fibres, hence the need for the spread of the impulse from one cell to another.

Cardiac muscle has the unique property of having its own inherent *rhythmicity* – regularly beating or contraction – from early in embryonic life until death. The rate of contraction is controlled by autonomic nerves (sympathetic and parasympathetic nerves, p.46) and certain hormones. Cardiac muscle is considered to be *involuntary*.

Smooth Muscle

In **smooth muscle**, the same kinds of filaments are present as in the other two types, but they are arranged differently and do not give the striated appearance, hence its alternative names: *non-striated* or *unstriped muscle*. Smooth muscle, often also called **visceral** or **involuntary muscle**, is found in the walls of blood vessels and hollow organs (the hollow viscera) such as the stomach, intestine, uterus and urinary bladder, and in part of the eye.

Smooth muscle fibres or cells (**2.5c**) are rather narrow, each with a single central nucleus. Like cardiac muscle, it is not under voluntary control, but is supplied by autonomic nerve fibres (p.46) that help to control such features as the calibre of blood vessels, the emptying of the stomach and bladder, and the size of the pupil. In many sites, such as in blood vessels and the intestine, the fibres are normally in a state of partial contraction, so that the nerve impulses can lead to either further contraction or lengthening. As with cardiac muscle, most smooth muscle fibres do not receive nerve fibres, and impulse conduction spreads from one cell to another via special intercellular junctions that permit the flow of ions between adjacent cells (**gap junctions**, **nexuses**).

NERVE

Nervous tissue consists of nerve cells – neurons – and cells with a supportive role – Schwann cells and neuroglial cells. Nerve cells vary greatly in size and shape, but all have the unique property of being able to transmit nerve impulses (p.47) between nerve cells themselves or between nerve cells and muscles or glands.

Neurons

The part of the **neuron** containing the nucleus is the **cell body** (**2.6**). Much of the rest of the cell is usually drawn out into long, thread-like cytoplasmic processes. (Although the term *nerve cell* should mean, strictly speaking, the entire nerve cell or neuron, including all its processes, in practice, *nerve cell* or even *neuron* are often used interchangeably with *cell body*. However, it is usually clear from the context whether

the entire cell or only its cell body is meant.) In most neurons, the processes include a number of **dendrites** and a single **axon**. The function of the dendrites is to enlarge the surface area for receiving stimuli; the dendrites, together with the cell body, constitute the 'receptive zone' of the neuron, which receives and integrates input from other neurons. The axon, on the other hand, is the 'conducting zone' – it carries the response of the neuron to the input it has received. The response is in the form of an electrical signal (the nerve impulse, p.47) which travels down the axon and can, in its turn, provide input to other neurons or to muscle or gland cells. The term *nerve fibre* is often used synonymously with the word *axon*.

Most nerve cell bodies are within the central nervous system (the brain and spinal cord, p.39), collectively forming the **gray matter**, but some are situated outside it (in the peripheral nervous system, p.39), collected into small groups called **ganglia** (such as the dorsal root ganglia of spinal

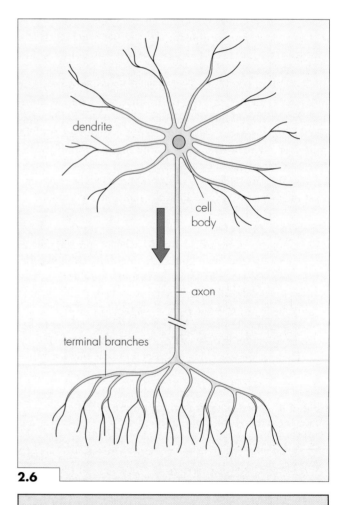

2.6

Fig. 2.6 Diagrammatic representation of the microscopic structure of a neuron.
The arrow indicates the direction of nerve impulses in the axon.

nerves, p.40, or the ganglia of the sympathetic trunk, p.47). Within the central nervous system, groups of cell bodies of similar function are usually called **nuclei** (such as the caudate nucleus within the cerebral hemisphere, and the thalamus, the largest of all the cerebral nuclei, p.193). Do not confuse the word *nucleus* used in this sense with the more common use of the word referring to the darkly staining part of the cell that contains its genetic material.

The **white matter** of the nervous system contains nerve fibres rather than cell bodies. In the brain and spinal cord, fibres of similar function are collected together to form **tracts** (p.40), while in the peripheral nervous system bundles of fibres form the **peripheral nerves** (p.40). Note that in the spinal cord the gray matter is centrally situated with the white matter surrounding it, while in the cerebral hemispheres of the brain the surface layer (the cerebral cortex) consists of gray matter and the white matter is internal (although some nuclei of gray matter are embedded within it).

Supporting Cells

Neurons are by no means the only cells within the nervous system. An even larger category of cells are the non-neuronal cells with *supporting* or *insulating functions*: the **neuroglial cells** within the central nervous system and the **Schwann cells** (or the **neurilemmal cells**) in the peripheral nervous system.

Support cells do not conduct nerve impulses but rather assume a variety of functions for the benefit of neurons. **Oligodendrocytes** (a type of neuroglial cell) and Schwann cells, for example, provide nerve fibres with insulation and, in some cases, a layer (of variable thickness) of fatty tissue, called **myelin**.

Myelin is formed by the condensation of layers of cell membrane that appear to have spiralled round the nerve fibre (**2.7**). Fibres are said to be *myelinated* or *unmyelinated*, depending on whether or not they are surrounded by myelin.

A second type of neuroglial cell, the **astrocyte**, is thought to influence the environment of neurons in the central nervous system by virtue of its purported role in the establishment of the blood–brain barrier (p.199). A third type, the **microgial cell**, is the phagocytic cell of the central nervous system which removes cellular debris or invading microorganisms. Tumours of the nervous system are growths of neuroglial cells, not of neurons.

Like most other tissues, nervous tissue contains blood vessels but, perhaps surprisingly, there are no lymphatics (p.67). Ordinary connective tissue cells and fibres are also found in nervous structures, forming such features as the boundary layer of the brain (the pia mater, p.132). Connective tissue is also needed to bind nerve fibres together as peripheral nerves, or cell bodies together as peripheral nerve ganglia.

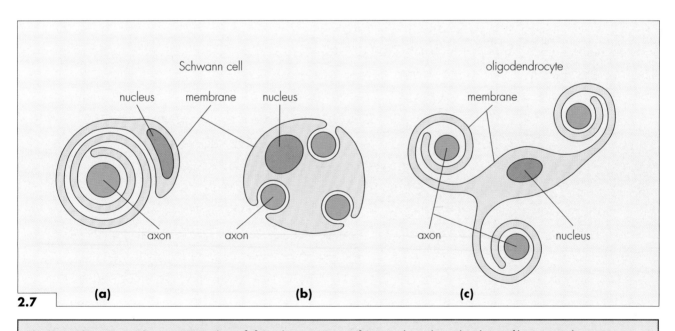

2.7

(a)   (b)   (c)

Fig. 2.7 Diagrammatic representation of the microscopic structure of myelinated and unmyelinated nerve fibres.
(a) Myelinated peripheral nerve fibre: the axon is surrounded by several layers of Schwann cell membrane (widely separated here and in **(c)** for clarity but in reality closely applied to one another).

(b) Unmyelinated peripheral nerve fibres: several axons are surrounded by a single layer of Schwann cell membrane.
(c) Myelinated fibres of the central nervous system: several axons are surrounded by several layers of membrane from a single oligodendrocyte.

CHAPTER 3

SKIN

Skin is the surface covering for the body, and has a number of functions (summarized later), among which the most important are protection, temperature control and providing an acceptable personal appearance. It consists of two layers of tissue (**3.1**): an outer epithelium with the special name of epidermis, and an inner connective tissue layer called the dermis. The epidermis gives rise to the skin appendages, which are the sweat glands, sebaceous glands, hair and nails.

EPIDERMIS

The **epidermis** is a *stratified squamous keratinizing epithelium*; it is called *stratified* because there are many layers of cells, *squamous* because the upper layers of cells are flattened, and *keratinizing* because the uppermost cells have lost their nuclei

and become converted into flakes of **keratin**, the protein which forms the protective and waterproof outer covering. This keratin is called *soft keratin*, to distinguish it from the hard keratin of hair and nails.

The epidermis undergoes continual renewal; cells are constantly being shed from the surface and replaced by those moving upwards from below. The basal layer of epithelial cells is immediately above the dermis; it is here that the cell division occurs. As new cells are formed, older ones are gradually displaced towards the surface. As they are displaced, they synthesize the protein keratin, which accumulates in the cytoplasm. Eventually, keratin replaces virtually all of the cytoplasmic components, even the nucleus. This process (called *keratinization*) gives rise to the dead, superficial layer of the epidermis – the **keratinized** or **cornified layer**. The keratinized layer is particularly thick on

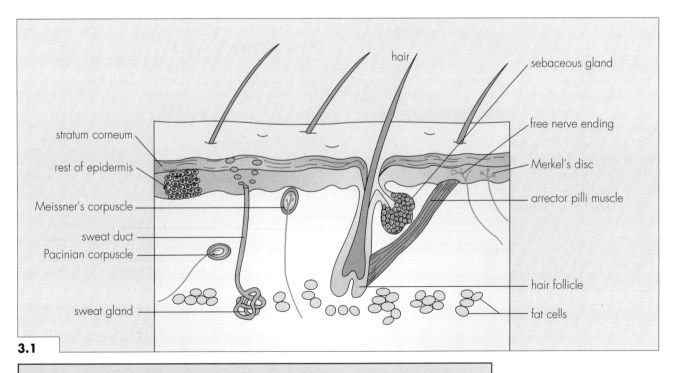

3.1

Fig. 3.1 Diagrammatic representation of the microscopic structure of skin, including several kinds of nerve endings; only free nerve endings and Merkel's discs penetrate into the epidermis.

the palms and soles, which are subject to considerable wear-and-tear. The constant shedding and renewal of cells does not depend upon them being rubbed off by the friction of clothes or other contacts; it is an inherent property of epidermis. The loss of epidermal cells is not normally noticed, but dandruff of the scalp is a condition in which the keratin flakes off in larger clumps than usual, and is thus noticeable.

Although the majority of cells in the epidermis undergo keratinization (and are commonly called **keratinocytes**), two other cell types are scattered among them: **melanocytes** and **Langerhans cells** (also called **granular dendrocytes**). Melanocytes are responsible for manufacturing melanin, the pigment that gives skin (and hair) its colour. There are several types of melanin giving rise to various colours (i.e. blacks, browns and yellows) that are racially characteristic. The darker-skinned races have the same number of melanocytes as those of lighter hue; the difference is in the type and quantity of melanin produced. The melanin granules formed by melanocytes are transferred to neighbouring keratinocytes; most of the cells that contain melanin have not themselves manufactured it. Suntanning is due to the ultraviolet rays of sunlight, which darken existing melanin and stimulate further melanin synthesis in melanocytes. Undue exposure to sunlight can cause sunburn, with redness, pain and perhaps blistering (collections of tissue fluid between layers of the epidermis); this is especially likely to occur in those with light skin and hair (i.e. blondes and redheads). The so-called 'healthy tan' often so admired in the western world is not without danger, since fair skin exposed to excessive sunlight shows a much greater incidence of cancerous change than darker skin.

A further effect of ultraviolet light on skin is to cause the synthesis (from some of the derivatives of cholesterol) of vitamin D, one of the factors that is necessary for normal bone formation. Insufficient exposure to sunlight is a possible cause of childhood rickets, in which there is an inadequate calcification of bone; this is manifested by bowing of the tibia and femur and enlarged painful epiphyses. Decades ago, when more children lived in overcrowded slum conditions than at present, the condition was commoner.

The **Langerhans cells of skin** (not to be confused with the islets of Langerhans of the pancreas that are named after the same German pathologist) are now known to be part of the immune system (p.69).

Epidermis does not contain blood vessels or lymphatics; it gets its nutrition by diffusion from the underlying dermis. A few nerve fibres (concerned with pain sensation) *do* penetrate into the lower part of the epidermis but most do not. Any break in the continuity of the surface, however small, is a possible portal of entry for invading organisms. Complete coverage is also important for preventing the loss of body fluids; in extensive burns, which destroy this cover, the loss of fluid may be dangerous to life.

DERMIS

The **dermis** is the connective tissue component of skin, and contains all of the usual connective tissue elements (p.10), such as fibroblasts and macrophages, collagen and elastic fibres, and ground substance. Blood vessels, lymphatics, and nerves are also present, including specialized nerve endings concerned with touch, pain, pressure and temperature differences. The junction between the dermis and epidermis is not flat, being irregular, with the dermis forming numerous upward projections into the epidermis – these are called **dermal papillae**. In certain areas, such as the pads of the fingertips, this arrangement results in the ridges that lead to the characteristic pattern of fingerprints, which are, of course, unique to each individual. The directions in which the bundles of dermal collagen are arranged give rise to tension lines; these determine the directions in which skin will gape when cut, and also the directions of certain creases that appear with age, such as the 'crow's foot' creases at the outer edges of the eyes. Despite the blandishments of the cosmetic industry, there is no miracle substance that can prevent aging, whether in skin or any other tissue.

Below the dermis is **subcutaneous tissue** – the **superficial fascia** – which connects the skin to underlying structures. The subcutaneous tissue varies in density in different areas; on the back of the hand, for example, it is very loose, so that a fold of skin can be pinched up easily, but on the sole of the foot or scalp it is dense. It is the subcutaneous tissue, not the dermis of skin, which contains much of the body's fat.

SKIN APPENDAGES

During development, certain down-growths of epidermis become specialized as sweat glands, sebaceous glands, hair follicles and nails.

SWEAT GLANDS

Sweat glands, of which there are about three million on each body, are formed from groups of epidermal cells which have dipped down into the dermis and become modified to secrete sweat, a fluid containing salt (sodium chloride). Under the microscope, the glands look like coiled test-tubes; they often extend beyond the dermis into subcutaneous tissue, and their ducts pierce the epidermis like a corkscrew to open on the skin surface, forming the pores of the skin. Their purpose is to deliver water to the body surface so that it can evaporate and, in so doing, cause the body to lose heat. About 900 ml of sweat is lost imperceptibly every day, even on the coldest day, by evaporation and absorption by clothes. In hot weather, and on other occasions when body temperature rises, as with exercise, sweat secretion is increased to increase the evaporation rate (urine production is decreased simultaneously, to compensate for the fluid and salt lost in sweat, p.285). Some sweat glands, such as those on the forehead and palms, are under emotional control – as is well known to students in oral examinations and at other times of stress!

SEBACEOUS GLANDS

Sebaceous glands are modified clusters of epidermal cells that lie adjacent to hair follicles (see below); they discharge their oily secretion (**sebum**) usually into the top of the follicle. The purpose of sebum is to keep the skin surface slightly moist; in so doing the skin and hair may appear greasy – this is something that varies greatly between individuals, and depends upon the amount of sebum produced. If the secretion exit gets blocked, the gland swells to form a sebaceous cyst (also called a 'wen'); they are most common in the scalp, where hair and sebaceous glands are commonest.

HAIR FOLLICLES

Hair follicles are slanting, tubular down-growths of epidermis; the cells at the base of the tube (called the hair matrix) produce the special type of hard keratin called **hair**. Most hair follicles have a few smooth muscle cells attached to one side, forming the **arrector pili muscle**. The sebaceous glands are often situated between the muscle and the follicle, meaning that when the muscle contracts a little secretion is squeezed out. The 'goose pimples' of a cold day are due to these tiny muscles pulling the hair follicles upright and causing slight dimples in the skin beside the follicles. Boils are septic infections of hair follicles; when several adjacent follicles are affected they form a carbuncle. Hair follicles do not produce hair continually, and the growth period varies in different sites (see Scalp, p.129).

Natural hair colour is due to various melanins, and the changes with age are caused by changes in melanin production. Hair is a dead structure, with only the matrix at the bottom of the follicle containing the living cells that divide to cause hair growth; all kinds of physical and chemical agents are used to alter the colour and shape of scalp hair.

The hair follicles and sebaceous glands are often known as *pilosebaceous units*, because the sebaceous glands open into the follicles, and are the site of one of the commonest of all skin conditions – acne (p.20).

NAILS

Nails, like hair, are composed of a hard type of keratin which grows up from a specialized epidermal area, the **nail matrix**. The **nail bed**, over which the nail grows, appears pinkish because the blood capillaries show through it; here, the nail really takes the place of the keratinized layer of the epidermis. At the nail base there is a crescentic whitish area, the *lunule* (usually best seen in the thumb), where the capillaries are less prominent. Nail growth is quicker on the fingers than on the toes.

FUNCTIONS OF SKIN

Following the above description of the structure of skin, its functions may now be summarized:

- It is a protective layer that is not only waterproof but also prevents the escape of fluid from the body. An intact skin surface keeps bacteria and other organisms from gaining entry into the body.
- It helps to control body temperature by the amount of bloodflow within it and the evaporation of sweat secreted by sweat glands.
- Sebaceous glands secrete sebum, an oily substance which helps to keep the surface slightly moist and lubricates it, as well as lubricating the hairs which grow from hair follicles.
- The body is made aware of its environment by the nerves of the skin which allow the appreciation of touch, pain, pressure and temperature.
- Melanocytes control skin pigmentation which, in turn, helps to prevent the harmful effects of the ultraviolet rays of sunlight.
- Vitamin D, which is necessary for normal bone formation, is synthesized in skin from a cholesterol derivative under the influence of ultraviolet light.
- Langerhans cells are part of the body's immune system (p.69).
- Fine ridges on the surface of the palms of the hands and soles of the feet provide slight friction to assist in gripping.
- The appearance of the skin that covers the parts of the body that are normally exposed is an important element in personal relationships.

SKIN WOUNDS AND GRAFTS

Clean cuts of the skin, with the edges taped or stitched together (sutured), whether accidental or carefully planned surgical incisions, heal by the formation of new epidermis and connective tissue. Dilated blood vessels of the injured area bring in polymorphs and macrophages (p.10) to break down and remove cellular debris and invading organisms, and fibroblasts manufacture new collagen fibres and ground substance to fill the gap. Increased cell division in the epidermis produces new cells that migrate to cover the new connective tissue. A **scar** is the name given to the fibrous tissue that replaces original tissue destroyed by disease or injury. At first it is reddish due to the vascularity of the underlying tissue shining through the new epidermis, but it later becomes pale due to a decrease in the vascularity, and not to thickening of the epidermis. Scarring is usually minimal, but occasionally the new connective tissue grows excessively for unknown reasons, to produce a **hypertrophic scar** or **keloid**.

Skin grafts can be used to cover areas from which skin has been lost. There are two kinds of graft, named from the thickness of the dermis that is included. In *split-skin grafts* the whole thickness of the epidermis but only the adjoining part of the dermis is included – the dermis has been split, with the lower part of it remaining at the donor site. In *whole thickness grafts*, the whole of the dermis as well as the epidermis is included. Special knives help the surgeon achieve the correct depth of graft. At the site to which the graft is applied, blood vessels grow into the graft and link up with the graft's own vessels, so restoring its circulation and keeping it alive; this enables the graft to 'take'. The grafts must be of the patient's own skin or from someone who, by tissue compatibility tests, has been shown to be suitable – if not, the graft will be rejected due to the immune response (p.69).

SKIN DISEASES

Any **skin disease** can be distressing due to unsightliness, and the visible surface can be affected in many ways. *Dermatitis* and *eczema* are names loosely applied to many conditions, with known or unknown causes, and skin specialists (dermatologists) recognize many different types. As illustrations of how skin structure and function may be altered in disease, two conditions may be mentioned: acne and psoriasis.

In *acne vulgaris*, cellular debris in the hair follicles and sebum from sebaceous glands accumulate and plug the tops of hair follicles; this causes swelling as the sebum cannot be discharged. Dust and dirt from the atmosphere adhere to the sticky surface of the plugs, forming blackheads (also called *comedos*). The hormonal changes associated with puberty increase the secretion of sebum, which is the reason why acne is so common in teenagers; this often causes distress out of all proportion to the severity of the disease at a time when personal appearances are becoming important. The condition eventually clears itself when hormonal stability is achieved, but since this may take some years it is no consolation to affected adolescents. Many helpful treatments can be prescribed.

In *psoriasis*, there are localized areas of excessive proliferation of epidermal cells and excessive production of keratin, with obvious 'flakes' of keratinized epidermis being shed from the affected areas.

To select just a few other conditions that illustrate the enormous range of skin diseases, the following may be mentioned: insect *bites* and *stings*, *urticaria* ('nettlerash') and other *allergic reactions*, *infections* such as impetigo (due to bacteria) and the *rashes* of the common childhood *fevers* such as measles and chickenpox (due to *viruses*), 'Athlete's foot' (due to a *fungus*), scabies (due to a *parasite*), and many kinds of *tumours*, both benign and malignant, including *melanoma* which can be one of the most rapidly spreading forms of cancer.

Smallpox is now of historic interest as an example of a dangerous viral disease (with a characteristic rash) that is now reported as having been eradicated from the world as a result of extensive immunization directed by the World Health Organization.

CHAPTER 4

SKELETON

The **skeleton** (**4.1**), which is formed by **bones** and **cartilages** that unite with one another at regions known as **joints** (p.31), is the supporting framework of the body, but it also has several other functions.

The skeleton provides protection for certain internal organs, such as the brain, which is inside the skull, and the heart and the lungs which are in the thorax (chest), although the main purpose of the thorax is not to protect but is to give a rigid frame within which the lungs can expand and contract during breathing (respiration).

Bones serve as a system of levers to which muscles are attached, enabling the control of body movements. They are also storehouses for minerals which are continually entering and leaving the store, and the cavities inside many bones (marrow cavities) are the sites for the formation of new blood cells (through the process of haemopoiesis).

BONES OF THE SKELETON

The bones of the adult skeleton number 200, or 206 if the three tiny bones of each ear (the auditory ossicles, p.169) are included in the total. They can be divided into the bones of the **axial skeleton** (the head and trunk of the body) and those of the **appendicular skeleton** or limbs.

Vertebrae, which form the central backbone of the body, are described below, but details of other bones are considered when dealing with the appropriate regions. Some parts of certain bones are relatively near the skin surface, and are liable to give rise to pressure sores, as described on p.60; the common possible sites are indicated in **4.1c**.

AXIAL SKELETON

The **axial skeleton** consists of the skull, the hyoid bone, the vertebrae forming the vertebral column, the ribs and costal cartilages, and the sternum.

SKULL

The **skull** is made up of 22 bones, one of which is mobile – the **mandible** or **lower jaw**, containing the lower teeth and making a joint (the temporomandibular or jaw joint) on each side of the skull. Of the remaining 21 skull bones, some are single and some paired. The two **maxillae** unite with one another to form the upper jaw, which bears the upper teeth. The **occipital bone** articulates with the first cervical vertebra (the atlas) at the two atlanto–occipital joints (one on each side), so joining the skull to the vertebral column. Further details of skull bones are given on pp.130–142.

HYOID BONE

The **hyoid bone** is a small, single U-shaped bone in the front of the neck. It is part of neither the skull nor the vertebral column, and is unique in being the only bone not joined to other bones by a joint; it is attached to the skull and to the cartilages of the larynx by ligaments and muscles (p.186).

VERTEBRAE

For most of its length, the **vertebral column** (also called the **spinal column**, **spine** or **backbone**) consists of individual **vertebrae** (**4.2–4.4**) connected, one above the other, by cartilaginous intervertebral discs and by ligaments and small joints (see below). There are 7 **cervical vertebrae** in the neck, 12 **thoracic vertebrae** in the thorax and 5 **lumbar vertebrae** in the lumbar region (the lower back), totalling 24 individual vertebrae. The rest of the vertebral column (the lower part) in the adult consists of two bones, the **sacrum** and the **coccyx** (**4.5**), representing the fusion of the 5 sacral and 4 coccygeal vertebrae of the fetus. Thus, the whole adult vertebral column consists of 26 bones, compared with 33 in the fetus.

The vertebrae of each region are numbered from above downwards, and each vertebra is frequently identified (as in this book) by a letter and a number, e.g. C6, T4, L3, to indicate its position in the cervical, thoracic or lumbar regions of the spine.

Parts of Vertebrae

A vertebra typically consists of a **body** – the thick front part – and a **vertebral arch** (also called a **neural arch**) at the back; the arch in turn consists of a pair of **pedicles** (which are attached to the vertebra's body) and a pair of **laminae**, which unite at the back (with a projecting **spine**) to complete the arch (**4.2**). **Transverse processes** project at each side, with

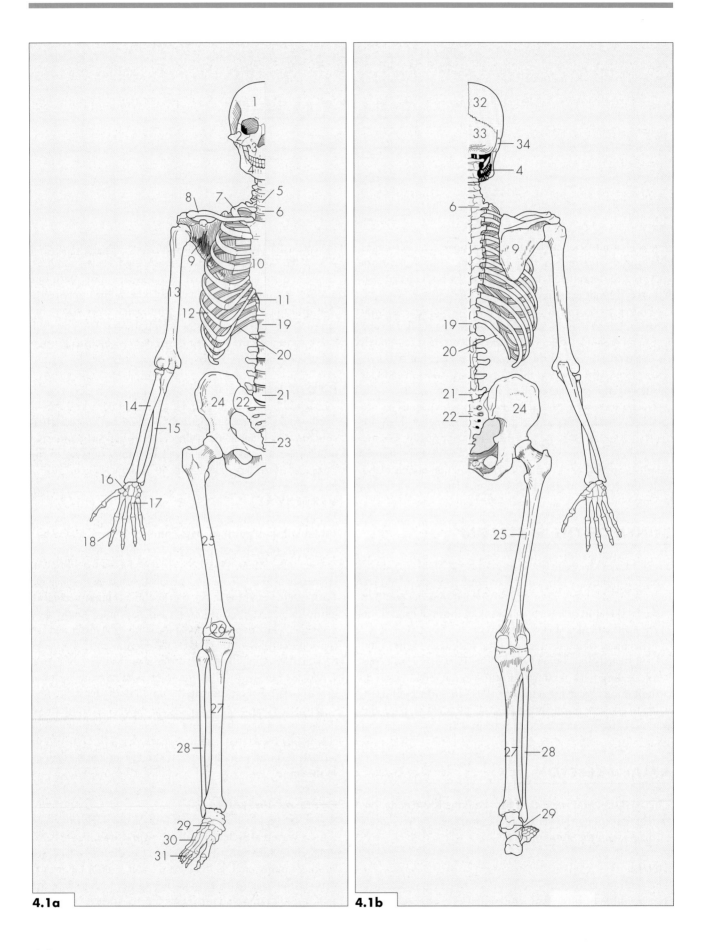

4.1a

4.1b

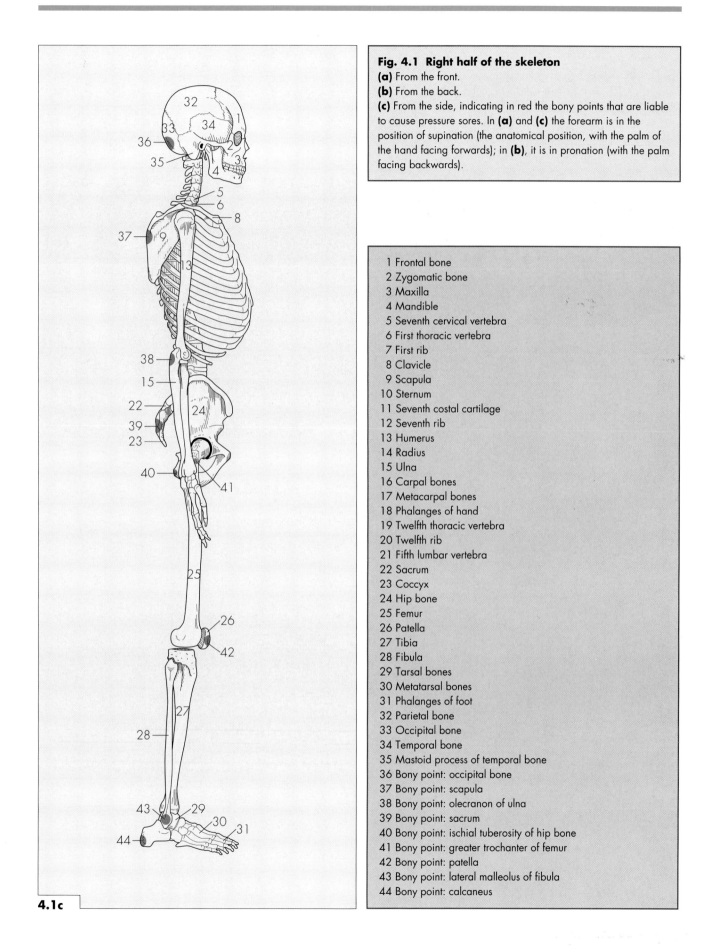

Fig. 4.1 Right half of the skeleton
(a) From the front.
(b) From the back.
(c) From the side, indicating in red the bony points that are liable to cause pressure sores. In **(a)** and **(c)** the forearm is in the position of supination (the anatomical position, with the palm of the hand facing forwards); in **(b)**, it is in pronation (with the palm facing backwards).

1 Frontal bone
2 Zygomatic bone
3 Maxilla
4 Mandible
5 Seventh cervical vertebra
6 First thoracic vertebra
7 First rib
8 Clavicle
9 Scapula
10 Sternum
11 Seventh costal cartilage
12 Seventh rib
13 Humerus
14 Radius
15 Ulna
16 Carpal bones
17 Metacarpal bones
18 Phalanges of hand
19 Twelfth thoracic vertebra
20 Twelfth rib
21 Fifth lumbar vertebra
22 Sacrum
23 Coccyx
24 Hip bone
25 Femur
26 Patella
27 Tibia
28 Fibula
29 Tarsal bones
30 Metatarsal bones
31 Phalanges of foot
32 Parietal bone
33 Occipital bone
34 Temporal bone
35 Mastoid process of temporal bone
36 Bony point: occipital bone
37 Bony point: scapula
38 Bony point: olecranon of ulna
39 Bony point: sacrum
40 Bony point: ischial tuberosity of hip bone
41 Bony point: greater trochanter of femur
42 Bony point: patella
43 Bony point: lateral malleolus of fibula
44 Bony point: calcaneus

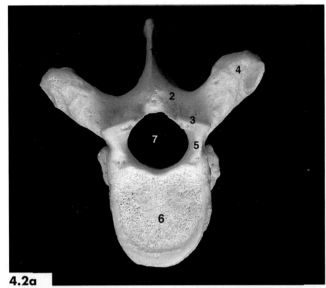

4.2a

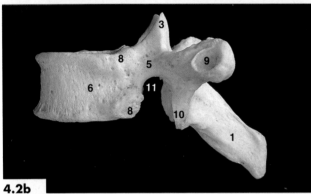

4.2b

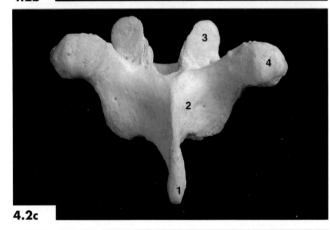

4.2c

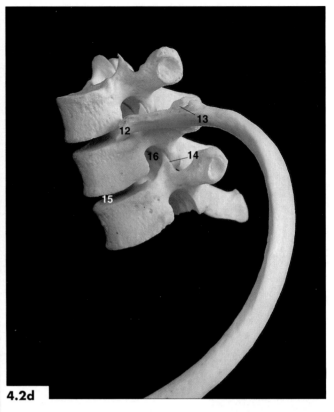

4.2d

Fig. 4.2 Typical thoracic vertebra (seventh).
(a) From above
(b) From the left side
(c) From the back
(d) From the front and the left, articulated with adjacent vertebrae and the seventh rib (for description of the parts of the ribs see p.97).

1 Spine, pointing downwards
2 Lamina
3 Superior articular process
4 Transverse process, with articular facet in side view (**b**9)
5 Pedicle The two pedicles and two laminae (2) form the vertebral arch
6 Body
7 Vertebral foramen, between the body and vertebral arch and rounded in shape
8 Costal facets of body, for articulation with part of the head of a rib (**d**12)
9 Costal facet of transverse process (**a**4), for articulation with tubercle of rib (**d**13) (for rib details see p.97)
10 Inferior articular process
11 Notch under pedicle, forming part of the intervertebral foramen (**d**16)
12 Head of rib, forming joint with costal facets (**b**8) of two vertebrae
13 Tubercle of rib, forming joint with transverse process (**b**9)
14 Facet joint, between superior and inferior articular processes (**a**3 and **b**10)
15 Position of intervertebral disc
16 Intervertebral foramen, between the pedicles (**a**5) of adjacent vertebrae, with the facet joint (14) behind and part of the vertebral body and intervertebral disc (15) in front

articular processes passing upwards and downwards to make small joints with their adjacent companions. Where the articular processes of adjacent vertebrae come into contact with one another, their surfaces are smooth, forming the **articular facets**.

The space between the body and the arch is the **vertebral foramen**; when the vertebrae are strung together to make the vertebral column, the individual vertebral foramina collective-ly form the **vertebral canal**. The vertebral foramina must not be confused with the highly important **intervertebral foramina**, which are the spaces between adjacent vertebrae at the sides, through which the spinal nerves emerge (p.40).

Regional Characteristics

The vertebrae in the cervical, thoracic and lumbar regions each have characteristic features.

In the **cervical** region (**4.3**), all seven have a foramen in the *transverse* process, and this alone distinguishes cervical vertebrae from all others. The first cervical vertebra (the

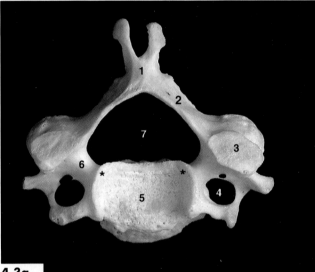

4.3a

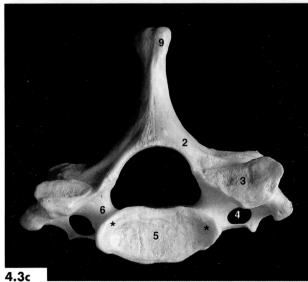

4.3b

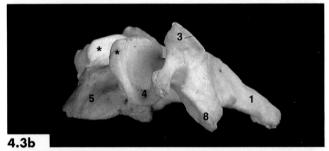

4.3c

Fig. 4.3 Cervical vertebrae.
(a) Typical (fifth), from above
(b) Slightly oblique left-side view
(c) Seventh, from above
(d) Two typical vertebrae articulated, from the front and left side

1 Spine, bifid unlike that of any other region
2 Lamina
3 Facet of superior articular process
4 Foramen in transverse process
5 Body, with posterolateral lip or uncus at asterisk
6 Pedicle. The two pedicles and two laminae (**a**2) form the vertebral arch
7 Vertebral foramen, between the body and vertebral arch and triangular in shape. Do not confuse with the foramen of the transverse process (**a**4) and the intervertebral foramen (**d**10)
8 Facet of inferior articular process, obliquely placed like that of the superior process (**a**3)
9 Spine with terminal tubercle, not bifid as in typical cervical vertebrae (**a**1) and usually the highest projecting spine when the neck is flexed
10 Intervertebral foramen, between adjacent pedicles as in thoracic and lumbar regions (**4.2d** 16, and **4.4d** 11)
11 Facet joint, between adjacent superior and inferior articular processes (**a**3 and **b**8), with obliquely placed joint line
12 Position of intervertebral disc

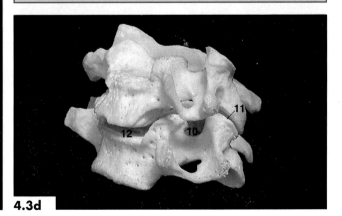

4.3d

atlas) has no body, and the second (the **axis**) has the **dens** (**odontoid process, 16.32c**) projecting upwards from the body. The other cervical vertebrae have a **posterolateral lip** or uncus on each side of the upper surface of the body, and they also have facets on the articular processes that are *obliquely* placed.

Thoracic vertebrae, in contrast (**4.2**), have *vertically* positioned articular facets. Another distinction of these vertebrae is that they have additional facets on the sides of the bodies and on the transverse processes, for joints with the ribs – these are called **costal facets** (**4.2d, 15.1b**).

Lumbar vertebrae (**4.4**) are the largest, with no costal facets but with large rectangular spines and articular processes that are *curved*.

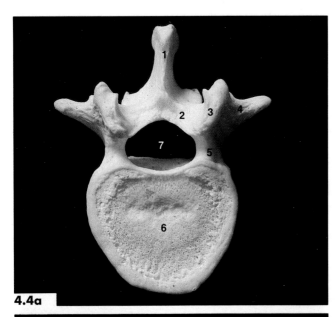

4.4a

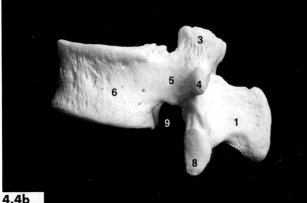

4.4b

Fig. 4.4 Lumbar vertebrae.
(**a**) First (typical) lumbar vertebra, from above
(**b**) From the left side
(**c**) Fifth lumbar vertebra, from above
(**d**) Two lumbar vertebrae, articulated, from the left side

---

1 Spine, rectangular on side view (**b**1)
2 Lamina
3 Superior articular process, vertical with a curved articular facet
4 Transverse process
5 Pedicle
6 Body
7 Vertebral foramen
8 Inferior articular facet, curved to fit a superior facet (**a**3)
9 Notch under pedicle
10 Transverse process, thick and merging with the side of the body – a feature unique to L5 vertebra
11 Intervertebral foramen, bounded above and below by pedicles (5), behind the facet joint (12), and in front by a vertebral body and intervertebral disc (13)
12 Facet joint, between superior and inferior articular processes (**a**3 and **b**8)
13 Position of intervertebral disc

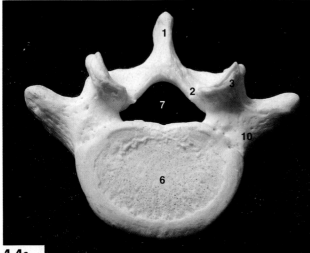

4.4c

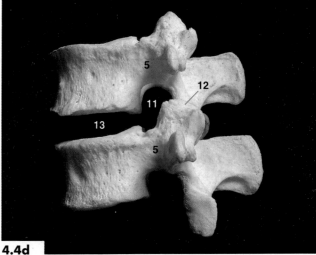

4.4d

Vertebral Column

The most important structure that unites vertebrae is the **intervertebral disc**. It consists of concentric rings of fibrocartilage that form the **annulus fibrosus**, and a central area of gelatinous material called the **nucleus pulposus** (**4.6a**). The discs are held in place by collagen fibres that extend from them and penetrate the adjacent vertebrae. Weakness of the cartilage sometimes allows the nucleus pulposus to project backwards (causing a *prolapsed disc*, commonly called 'slipped disc'); this is most common in the lowest disc (the disc between L5 vertebra and the sacrum –

the fifth lumbar or lumbosacral disc), and may cause irritation of the nerve roots that lie behind the disc, as explained in the legend to **17.5d**.

Other structures that hold vertebrae together are the **anterior** and **posterior longitudinal ligaments** (**4.6b**), which unite the bodies; the **ligamenta flava** (meaning 'yellow ligaments' because they contain elastic fibres) that unite adjacent laminae; **interspinous** and **supraspinous ligaments** that unite spines; and small synovial joints (usually called **facet joints**) between adjacent articular facets (**4.2d**, **4.3d**, and **4.4d**).

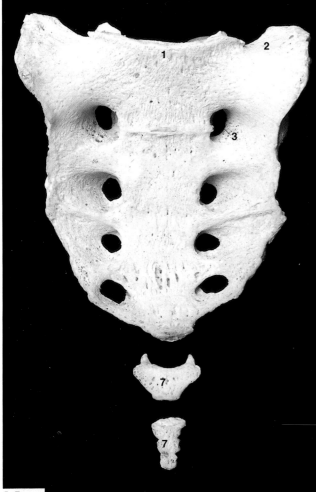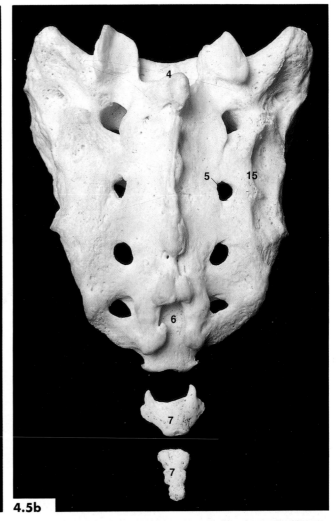

4.5a

4.5b

Fig. 4.5 Sacrum and coccyx.
(a) From the front
(b) From behind
The five sacral vertebrae that form the sacrum become fused together, leaving the sacral canal at the back, and four pairs of sacral foramina (front and back) which allow for the emergence of sacral nerves. The four coccygeal vertebrae forming the coccyx are small and degenerate, with no canal or foramina.

1 Sacral promontory, the upper margin of S1 vertebra, forming part of the pelvic brim (p.243)
2 Ala of sacrum, forming another part of the pelvic brim
3 Left first anterior sacral foramen
4 Sacral canal, upper end
5 Right second posterior sacral foramen
6 Sacral hiatus, the name given to the lower end of the sacral canal (4)
7 Coccyx, here in two pieces

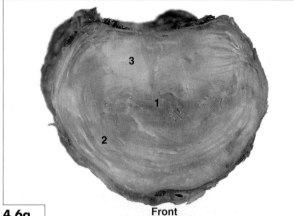

4.6a Front

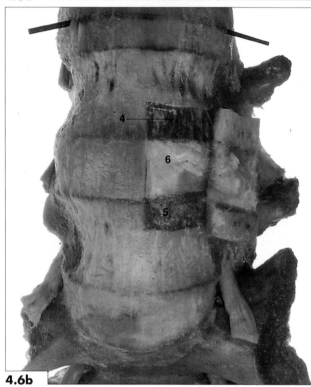

4.6b

Fig. 4.6 Intervertebral disc and anterior longitudinal ligament.

(a) Intervertebral disc, transverse section. Part of the disc has been shaved away at the back to show the cartilage plate on the top of the vertebral body.
(b) Lumbar vertebrae, viewed from the front, with discs and anterior longitudinal ligament. A window has been cut in the ligament and the flap turned back to show the underlying disc and vertebral bodies.

1 Nucleus pulposus	5 Vertebral body
2 Annulus fibrosus	6 Intervertebral disc
3 Hyaline cartilage	
4 Anterior longitudinal ligament	

important in helping to control the amount of flexion, i.e. when bending forwards from the upright position they act against gravity. The muscles have multiple attachments to the back of the sacrum, the arches of the vertebrae and the ribs. Strain that tears some of the fibres probably accounts for much of the 'low back pain', which is such a common complaint among those who, for example, try to lift heavy objects by bending the back instead of keeping the back straight and bending the knees.

Apart from some small muscles in the front of the neck, the main *flexors* of the trunk are the anterior abdominal muscles (the rectus abdominis and the external and internal obliques, **6.1a** and **6.1b**). They act mostly on the lumbar region by pulling the front of the thorax nearer to the pelvis. In the neck, sternocleidomastoid (**6.1a**) is a powerful *rotator*; the muscle on the *left*, for example, helps to turn the head to the *right*. Combinations of the oblique abdominal muscles produce rotation in the thoracic region because of their attachments to ribs.

THORACIC SKELETON

The thoracic vertebrae, costal cartilages, ribs and sternum together form the skeleton of the thorax (sometimes called the **thoracic cage**, p.97).

The 12 thoracic vertebrae articulate with the 12 pairs of ribs (**4.1a**, **4.2d** and **15.1b**). The upper 7 pairs of ribs are joined to the sternum by **costal cartilages**. The next three pairs have costal cartilages that join the cartilage above, while ribs 11 and 12 have very small cartilages at their ends which remain free.

The **sternum**, in the midline of the front of the chest (**4.1a** and **15.1e**), is made up of the **manubrium** and **body** (which are both made of bone) and the **xiphoid process** (which is cartilage, but which may become partly ossified in later life).

The ribs and sternum are further described with the thoracic walls (p.97).

Movements of the Vertebral Column

The amount of movement between individual vertebrae is small because of the above attachments, but collectively the movements add up to give a considerable range, especially for flexion and extension (p.5). Rotation to the left or right (as when turning the chest towards one side while keeping the pelvis fixed) is, perhaps surprisingly, greatest in the thoracic region and would be even greater if it were not for the splinting action of the ribs. In the cervical region, rotation is supplemented by head rotation at the atlantoaxial joints (p.174), while in the lumbar region it is negligible because of the curved shape of the articular facets.

The various parts of the erector spinae muscles (**6.2b**) act as *extensors* of the vertebral column, but they are also

APPENDICULAR SKELETON

The **appendicular skeleton** consists of the bones of the upper and lower limbs: 32 in each upper limb and 31 in each lower limb. They include the bones of the **limb girdles**, which are defined as the bones that connect the limb to the axial skeleton.

UPPER LIMB BONES

The **shoulder girdle** (also called the **pectoral girdle**) consists of the **clavicle** and the **scapula** (**4.1** and **18.1**). The clavicle is joined to the axial skeleton at the sternoclavicular joint – the only bony connection between the whole of the upper limb and the rest of the skeleton (p.216). The clavicle and scapula are united at the acromioclavicular joint (p.216), and the scapula is attached to the axial skeleton only by muscles (p.13).

The other bones of the upper limb (**4.1**) are the **humerus** (the bone of the arm or upper arm), the **radius** and the **ulna** (the bones of the forearm), the **carpal bones** (the wrist bones), the **metacarpal bones** and the **phalanges** (the bones of the hand).

The scapula and the humerus are joined at the shoulder joint (p.217).

The humerus, radius and ulna are joined at the elbow joint (p.227).

The upper ends of the radius and the ulna are joined at the proximal radioulnar joint (p.228), and their lower ends at the distal radioulnar joint (p.228).

The lower end of the radius (with the attached disc of the inferior radioulnar joint) and the proximal row of carpal bones) join at the wrist joint (p.230).

Carpal and metacarpal bones form various intercarpal and carpometacarpal joints with one another; the most important is the one at the base of the thumb (the first carpometacarpal joint, p.231), which helps to give the thumb its wide range of movement.

Metacarpal bones make metacarpophalangeal joints with the phalanges, and phalanges make interphalangeal joints with one another (p.238).

LOWER LIMB BONES

The **hip girdle** (also called the **pelvic girdle**) in the adult is the single **hip bone** (**4.1** and **20.1**), which consists of three bones (the **ilium**, the **ischium** and the **pubis**) that have become fused together during embryonic development.

The hip bone is joined to the axial skeleton at the sacroiliac joint (p.289), and to the opposite hip bone at the pubic symphysis in the front (p.289).

The other bones of the lower limb are the **femur** (the thigh bone), the **tibia** and **fibula** (the bones of the leg), the **tarsal** and **metatarsal** bones, and the **phalanges** (the bones of the foot).

The hip bone and the femur are joined at the hip joint (p.321).

The femur, the tibia and patella (i.e. the kneecap) are joined at the knee joint (p.324).

The upper ends of the tibia and fibula are joined at the superior tibiofibular joint (p.324); their lower ends joining at the inferior tibiofibular joint (p.333).

The tibia, fibula and talus join at the ankle joint (p.336).

Tarsal and metatarsal bones make various intertarsal and tarsometatarsal joints with one another; the most important are the joints beneath the talus, because inversion and eversion of the foot mainly take place here (p.338).

Metatarsal bones make metatarsophalangeal joints with phalanges, and phalanges make interphalangeal joints with one another; the most important are those of the great toe, because of its powerful push or 'toe-off' in walking and running (p.340).

CLASSIFICATION OF BONES

Bones are classified from their general shape as long, short, flat, irregular and sesamoid. *Long* and *short* bones are typically found in the limbs, and *flat* and *irregular* bones in the limb girdles, vertebral column and skull. *Sesamoid* bones (named after the shape, if not the size, of sesame seeds) are a kind that develop in certain tendons; the largest is the patella (**4.1a**), but they are usually much smaller, as in some hand and foot tendons (e.g. the pisiform bone at the wrist, see **18.12a**, in the tendon of the flexor carpi ulnaris muscle).

CHAPTER 5

JOINTS

The sites where bones and cartilages come together are called **joints** or **articulations** (from the Latin for 'joint'; *arthritis*, from the Greek, means 'inflammation of a joint'). The principal joints have been named in the previous chapter on the Skeleton (p.21).

Joints are classified into three main types: *fibrous*, *cartilaginous* and *synovial*. What most people understand by *joint* is the synovial kind; all of the limb joints are of this type, and display varying amounts of movement. The names of the three main types are derived from the type of tissue that lies between or around the bone ends.

FIBROUS JOINTS

In **fibrous joints** (**5.1**), the bones are connected together by **fibrous tissue**, and there is negligible or no movement. Examples are the joints between many skull bones (called **sutures**, see **16.8** and **16.18**) and the joint just above the ankle (the **inferior tibiofibular joint**, see **20.12**).

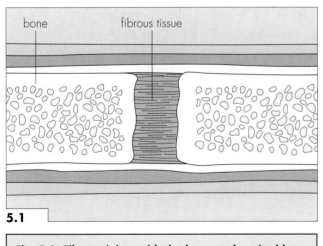

5.1

Fig. 5.1 Fibrous joint, with the bone ends united by fibrous tissue, as in sutures of the skull, allowing no movement.

bone   fibrous tissue

CARTILAGINOUS JOINTS

In **cartilaginous joints**, the bones are joined by **cartilage** – as between the bodies of vertebrae where the cartilage forms the intervertebral discs (p.27 and **4.6a**). This allows a small amount of movement between each vertebra, and also at the pubic symphysis at the front of the pelvis (p.289 and **5.2a**).

Such examples are often called **secondary cartilaginous joints**, to distinguish them from **primary cartilaginous joints**, of which the typical examples are the cartilage plates between the shafts and ends of growing bones (p.12, **5.2b**). Here there is no movement, and the cartilage is only temporary (during the growth period), being replaced eventually by bone. Alternative names for the two types of cartilaginous joints are **symphysis** (secondary cartilaginous joint) and **synchondrosis** (primary cartilaginous joint).

SYNOVIAL JOINTS

Synovial joints (**5.3**) have six characteristic features:
- The parts of the bone ends that make contact with one another are covered by cartilage that provides very smooth articulating surfaces; this enables the bones to move against one another with low friction. These 'caps' of cartilage are frequently called articular cartilage.
- The bone ends are enclosed by a sleeve-like connective tissue capsule that separates the joint from the surrounding tissues.
- The capsule encloses the **joint cavity**, which is the very small space around the bone ends inside the capsule.
- The inner surface of the capsule, and the surfaces of any parts of the bones within the joint cavity that are not covered by cartilage, are lined with **synovial membrane**, a tissue which secretes a small amount of **synovial fluid** for lubrication.
- The capsule is reinforced on the outside or inside, or both, by ligaments that help to unite the bones and/or assist in stabilizing the joint.
- The joint is capable of varying degrees of movement.

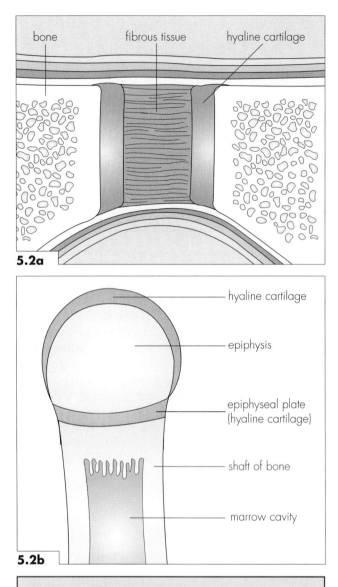

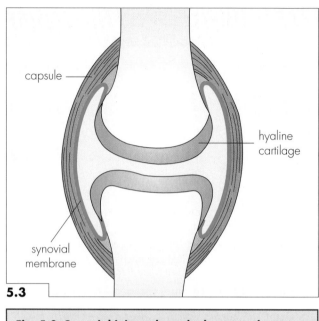

Fig. 5.2a — bone, fibrous tissue, hyaline cartilage

5.2b — hyaline cartilage, epiphysis, epiphyseal plate (hyaline cartilage), shaft of bone, marrow cavity

Fig. 5.2 Cartilaginous joints.
(a) Secondary cartilaginous joint, where bone ends are covered by hyaline cartilage and united by fibrous tissue, as at the pubic symphysis (illustrated) and the intervertebral discs, with limited movement.
(b) Primary cartilaginous joint, where bone and hyaline cartilage meet, allowing no movement. The figure shows the cartilage plate between the shafts and ends of growing bones. Other examples are the junctions between ribs and costal cartilages.

5.3 — capsule, hyaline cartilage, synovial membrane

Fig. 5.3 Synovial joint, where the bones ends are covered by hyaline cartilage and enclosed by a capsule lined by synovial membrane, allowing a range of movement.

VARIETIES OF SYNOVIAL JOINTS

Synovial joints can be subdivided into a number of varieties, depending upon the shapes of the bony surfaces and the kinds of movement that the surfaces make possible.

A **hinge joint**, such as the elbow, allows only bending and straightening. In **plane joints**, where the surfaces are more-or-less flat (as between individual carpal bones or the tarsal bones of the foot), only a small amount of gliding movement occurs. A **pivot joint** allows rotation, as where the atlas rotates round the dens of the axis, or the head of the radius against the side of the ulna at the proximal radioulnar joint during pronation and supination. In **ball-and-socket joints (spheroidal joints)**, the rounded end of one bone fits into a socket in the other, as in the hip and shoulder joints, where a wide range of movement in all directions is possible. **Condyloid joints** are similar to the ball-and-socket variety as far as bone shapes are concerned, but the articulating surfaces are elliptical rather than spherical, thus excluding the possibility of rotatory movement; the **metacarpophalangeal joints** are of this variety.

SYNOVIAL FLUID

Synovial fluid is a clear viscous liquid, rather like the white of an egg (from which it gets its name – the Latin for 'egg-like'). Surrounding tissues keep the capsule of a synovial joint closely applied to the structures inside the joint, with negligible empty space, so that the amount of synovial fluid in a joint is very small. The largest such joint is the knee joint, and the amount of fluid within the normal knee joint is less than 0.5 ml – which is merely a lubricating film – so synovial joints are not 'full of fluid', except after injury or disease, when the amount may increase considerably (as in 'water on the knee' following a knee joint injury).

SYNOVIAL SHEATHS AND BURSAE

Synovial membrane is not only found in joints; it is also present in **synovial sheaths**, which envelop certain tendons at the wrist and ankle (**18.13b** and **20.13a**) to provide smooth lubricated tubes within which tendons can glide freely across bones and joints.

Closely allied to synovial sheaths are small flattened sac-like structures known as **bursae**. They are like rounded, collapsed balloons, a few centimeters in diameter with a lubricated inner surface, and are found under parts of some muscles or skin. They act as protective cushions where skin or muscle passes over a bony prominence and are sometimes in direct communication with a synovial joint cavity. The best known is the **olecranon bursa** at the back of the elbow (p.225 and **18.11c**).

CHAPTER 6

MUSCULAR SYSTEM

The **muscular system** is made up of the individual skeletal muscles that are under voluntary nervous control, and that make up almost half of the body weight. Most are illustrated in **6.1** and **6.2**, and details of many that are particularly important are described with their related parts of the body. (See Appendix also.)

At first sight, the names of the individual muscles make strange reading for those who have not studied Latin or Greek. The names are usually derived from the muscle's shape, position or action, or a combination of these features. By modern custom in the English-speaking world, the anglicized versions of the Latin are sometimes used, e.g. external oblique (one of the abdominal muscles in **6.1a**) instead of *obliquus externus* (the name in the internationally recognized Anatomical Nomenclature), but the official Latin terms are used for most muscles.

MUSCLES

Each **muscle** is composed of bundles of **muscle fibres** (p.13) that are held together by **connective tissue** through which run the muscle's blood vessels, lymphatics and nerve fibres. It is the connective tissue, usually at the ends of a muscle, that forms the **tendons** by which it is attached to the skeleton. The collagen fibres of the tendon pass through the periosteum of the bone into the bone matrix, so anchoring the tendon firmly. The sites of a muscle's attachments are its *origin* and *insertion*; the attachment site that remains fixed during the usual movement of the muscle is the origin, and the attachment site that moves is the insertion.

Thus, the brachialis muscle which helps to bend (i.e. flex) the elbow by bringing the ulna nearer to the humerus is said to have its origin on the front of the humerus and its insertion on the front of the ulna. However, it is important to note that, functionally speaking, origins and insertions can become reversed; for example, if the forearm was fixed and the brachialis was helping to bring the humerus nearer to the forearm, the attachment to the humerus could be said to be the insertion and the ulnar attachment the origin (because the humerus is now moving and the ulna is the fixed bone).

It is simply a long-established convention to name the site most commmonly fixed as the origin and the opposite site as the insertion. Usually the origin is the upper (proximal) attachment and the insertion is the lower (distal) attachment.

While many limb muscles have rounded tendons of insertion, others have a rather extended flat or sheet-like attachment called an **aponeurosis** – the *neuro* part of the word suggests nerve, but the Greek *neuron* could mean either nerve or tendon.

MUSCLE SPINDLES

In most muscles, groups of very small, specialized muscle fibres are bound by connective tissue into microscopic cigar-shaped structures called **muscle spindles**. These are scattered among the ordinary muscle fibres; they act as sensors for the degree of tension in muscles, and are important in reflex activities and the control of posture (pp.50, 52 and 201).

MOVEMENTS

Movement at any particular joint depends upon the action of many muscles. The muscles producing a desired movement are the *prime movers,* and those capable of doing the exact opposite are the *antagonists*. Thus, if the desired movement at the elbow is flexion, the brachialis is acting as a prime mover and the triceps is an antagonist; if extension at the elbow is the desired movement, the triceps is now the prime mover and the brachialis is an antagonist. However, it must be remembered that gravity often assists movements; in the example just given (extending the elbow) brachialis may actually be contracting more powerfully than triceps in order to control the degree of movement.

To allow these movements at the elbow, the humerus and the shoulder must be kept in an appropriate position, and the muscles controlling the humerus and scapula are acting as *fixators*; they hold steady the origins of the prime-mover muscles. A muscle whose tendon crosses more than one joint can also act as a *synergist* – a special kind of fixator assisting prime movers by preventing unwanted movement. For example, muscles whose long tendons flex the fingers cross the wrist joint and can also flex that joint; if finger flexion

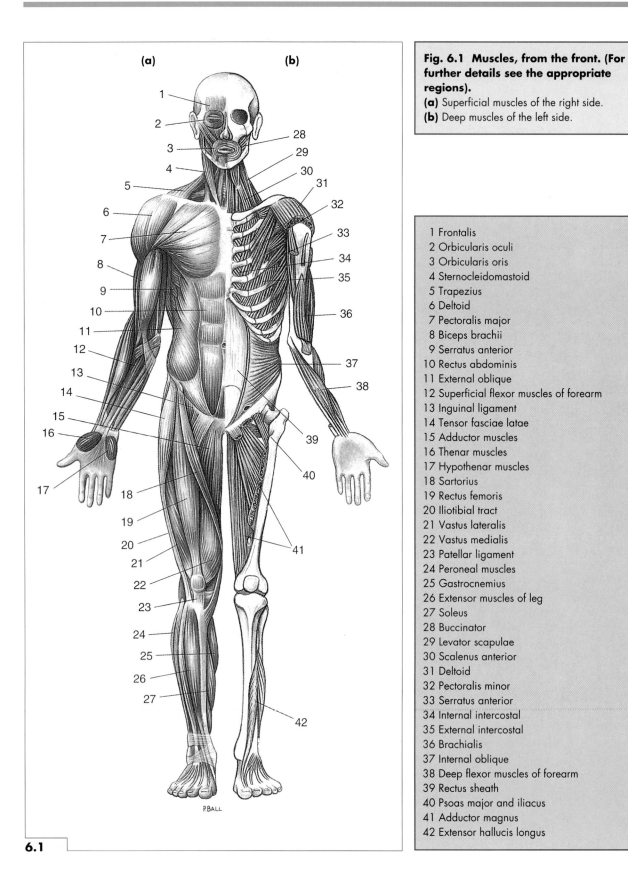

(a)   (b)

P.BALL

Fig. 6.1 Muscles, from the front. (For further details see the appropriate regions).
(a) Superficial muscles of the right side.
(b) Deep muscles of the left side.

1 Frontalis
2 Orbicularis oculi
3 Orbicularis oris
4 Sternocleidomastoid
5 Trapezius
6 Deltoid
7 Pectoralis major
8 Biceps brachii
9 Serratus anterior
10 Rectus abdominis
11 External oblique
12 Superficial flexor muscles of forearm
13 Inguinal ligament
14 Tensor fasciae latae
15 Adductor muscles
16 Thenar muscles
17 Hypothenar muscles
18 Sartorius
19 Rectus femoris
20 Iliotibial tract
21 Vastus lateralis
22 Vastus medialis
23 Patellar ligament
24 Peroneal muscles
25 Gastrocnemius
26 Extensor muscles of leg
27 Soleus
28 Buccinator
29 Levator scapulae
30 Scalenus anterior
31 Deltoid
32 Pectoralis minor
33 Serratus anterior
34 Internal intercostal
35 External intercostal
36 Brachialis
37 Internal oblique
38 Deep flexor muscles of forearm
39 Rectus sheath
40 Psoas major and iliacus
41 Adductor magnus
42 Extensor hallucis longus

6.1

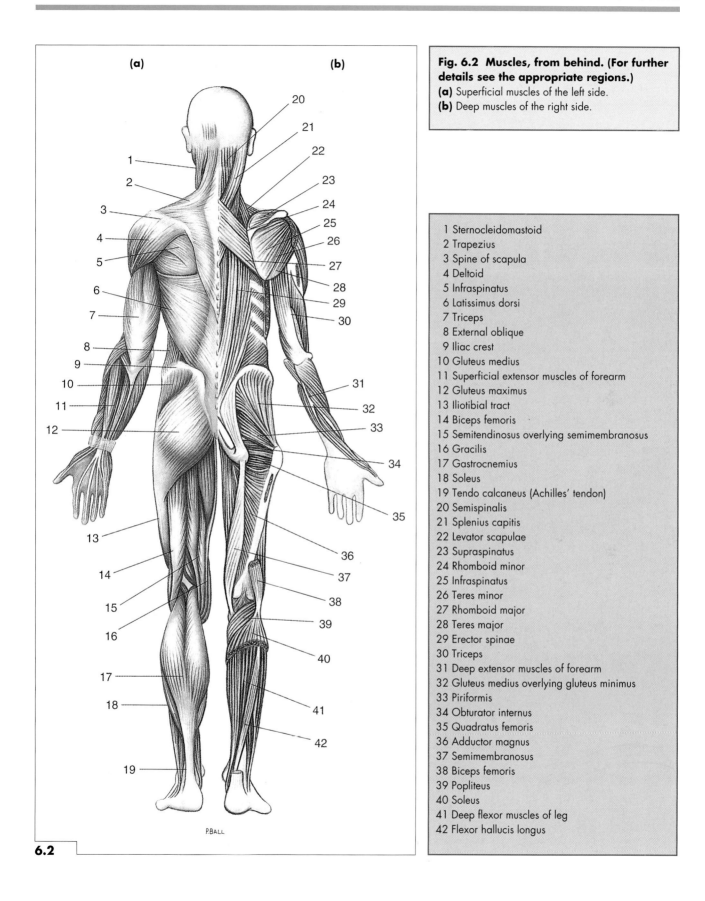

(a) (b)

P.BALL

6.2

Fig. 6.2 Muscles, from behind. (For further details see the appropriate regions.)
(a) Superficial muscles of the left side.
(b) Deep muscles of the right side.

1 Sternocleidomastoid
2 Trapezius
3 Spine of scapula
4 Deltoid
5 Infraspinatus
6 Latissimus dorsi
7 Triceps
8 External oblique
9 Iliac crest
10 Gluteus medius
11 Superficial extensor muscles of forearm
12 Gluteus maximus
13 Iliotibial tract
14 Biceps femoris
15 Semitendinosus overlying semimembranosus
16 Gracilis
17 Gastrocnemius
18 Soleus
19 Tendo calcaneus (Achilles' tendon)
20 Semispinalis
21 Splenius capitis
22 Levator scapulae
23 Supraspinatus
24 Rhomboid minor
25 Infraspinatus
26 Teres minor
27 Rhomboid major
28 Teres major
29 Erector spinae
30 Triceps
31 Deep extensor muscles of forearm
32 Gluteus medius overlying gluteus minimus
33 Piriformis
34 Obturator internus
35 Quadratus femoris
36 Adductor magnus
37 Semimembranosus
38 Biceps femoris
39 Popliteus
40 Soleus
41 Deep flexor muscles of leg
42 Flexor hallucis longus

only is the required movement, extensors of the wrist must act as synergists to hold the wrist steady while the flexors move the fingers by acting as prime movers.

MECHANISM OF CONTRACTION

The filaments of **myosin** and **actin** (p.13) – the **contractile proteins** – do not individually shorten to produce contraction. Instead, they are arranged in groups that overlap one another (interdigitate), and it is the increase in the amount of overlap that causes the change in length (**2.5d**). This is known as the *sliding filament mechanism* of muscular contraction.

The *chemical energy* required to produce contraction comes from the breakdown of glycogen, which is derived from the digestion of carbohydrate in food (p.84). The stimulus for contraction (p.49) causes the conversion of ATP to ADP (p.83), with the release of the energy that is required to cause the myofilaments to 'claw their way' along one another and so produce contraction.

During glycogen breakdown, which in chemical terms is an *oxidation process*, pyruvic acid is formed. When the muscles have sufficient oxygen from the bloodstream, the pyruvic acid undergoes further breakdown to the final products: carbon dioxide and water. However, if there is insufficient oxygen, as in violent exercise where even increased bloodflow cannot provide enough oxygen, the pyruvic acid becomes converted into lactic acid. This accumulates in the muscles and surrounding tissues and produces the feeling of fatigue or even cramp, which is a type of muscle spasm. The lactic acid that is absorbed into the bloodstream stimulates the respiratory centre in the brainstem to increase the rate of breathing (p.75) and, hence, the amount of oxygen in the blood. It may take some time to absorb enough oxygen to deal with the further breakdown of lactic acid (i.e. to repair the oxygen debt), which is why the increased respiratory rate continues for some time after the exercise itself has stopped.

CHAPTER 7

NERVOUS SYSTEM

The chief function of the **nervous system** is to enable the individual to detect what is going on round about, and to react to it. It also monitors changes within the body, in the various organs and tissues, and initiates responses to them. The principal part, the **brain**, coordinates most of the nervous system's activities (whether conscious or unconscious), which include such 'higher functions' as thinking, learning and memory, which have all played their part in enabling humans to become the most dominant creatures on earth.

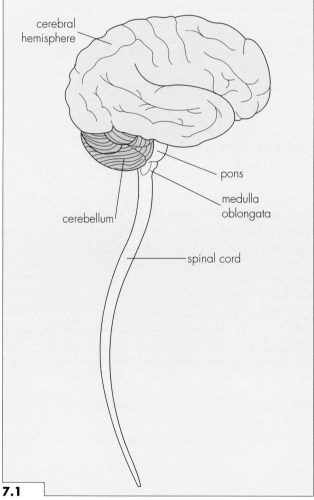

cerebral hemisphere

pons

medulla oblongata

cerebellum

spinal cord

7.1

CENTRAL AND PERIPHERAL NERVOUS SYSTEMS

For purposes of study, the **nervous system** can be considered in *two parts*, the central and peripheral nervous systems.

The **central nervous system** consists of the brain and the spinal cord, which are continuous with one another (**7.1**). The **brain** is inside the skull; part of it, the **brainstem**, passes downwards through the foramen magnum in the base of the skull to become the **spinal cord** which is inside the vertebral column (in the vertebral canal, p.25).

The **peripheral nervous system** consists of all of the other nervous tissue outside (or 'peripheral to') the brain and spinal cord. Its chief components are 12 pairs of **cranial nerves** which are attached to the brain (**17.4**), and 31 **pairs of spinal nerves** which are attached to the sides of the spinal cord (**17.5**). In addition, there are some other nerves and ganglia associated with the autonomic nervous system (see below), which, since they are not part of the brain or spinal cord, must be included in the peripheral nervous system.

While it may be convenient for descriptive purposes to divide the nervous system into central and peripheral parts, or somatic and autonomic parts (see below), there is really only one nervous system and the parts must not be considered as being separate from one another.

SOMATIC AND AUTONOMIC NERVOUS SYSTEMS

Just as the nervous system can be divided into central and peripheral parts, it can also be divided in a different way, according to the types of tissues with which it makes contact and over which it exerts control. According to this method of division, the **somatic nervous system** provides nerve

Fig. 7.1 Brain and spinal cord, from the right.
The pons and medulla oblongata constitute the major part of the brainstem (the upper part, the midbrain, is not visible in this view).

supply to skin, bones and skeletal muscle and controls movements, whereas the **autonomic nervous system** provides nerve supply chiefly to glands and internal organs, and controls automatic activities such as the heart rate, sweating, stomach contractions and the size of the pupil of the eye.

FIBRES, NERVES AND TRACTS

Bundles of **nerve fibres** within the brain and spinal cord are usually called **tracts**, whereas, outside the brain and spinal cord, the bundles constitute **nerves**; each cranial or spinal nerve is thus simply a bundle of nerve fibres. By forming tracts and nerves, nerve fibres form pathways of varying lengths that conduct impulses between different parts of the central nervous system, and between the central nervous system and other parts of the body.

A nerve fibre cannot function unless it remains connected to its own healthy cell body (**2.6**). If any part of a nerve fibre becomes cut off from its parent cell body (by injury or disease), the fibre distal to the injury will degenerate, and changes will also occur in the cell body. It is these degenerative changes (called *chromatolysis* in cell bodies and *Wallerian degeneration* in fibres) that have made it possible to map out microscopically the tracts and their cells of origin within the central nervous system. By correlating such changes found at autopsy with the patient's signs and symptoms during life, information about the function of the different cell groups and fibres has thus been gradually accumulated.

Fibres that conduct nerve impulses from various kinds of sensory receptors (see below) to the brain and spinal cord are *sensory* or *afferent* fibres (from the Latin for 'carrying towards'). Fibres that pass out from the central nervous system to cause a response in muscles or glands are *motor* or *efferent* fibres (from the Latin for 'carrying away'). Most nerves are a mixture of afferent and efferent fibres. The corresponding neurons of which these fibres are a part are sensory (afferent) neurons and motor (efferent) neurons. Within the central nervous system, and helping to form connections between the main afferent and efferent neurons, are many other neurons, often with very short processes; these neurons are collectively called **interneurons**. The sites where neurons communicate with one another (not by direct continuity but by means of chemical substances collectively called neurotransmitters) are known as **synapses**, and are described below (p.48).

Many of the ends of sensory neurons in peripheral nerves are specialized to form **sensory receptors**; they are essential for the nervous system's function of detecting changes both inside and outside the body. Several kinds of receptors can be distinguished histologically. Those in skin can detect the sensations of touch, pressure, pain, and heat and cold; those in muscles, tendons and joint tissues provide information on joint positions (kinaesthetic sense); others, for example in parts of the vascular system, detect changes in blood pressure and the amount of oxygen and carbon dioxide in blood. The special senses like vision and hearing each have their specific types of receptor (p.207).

CRANIAL NERVES

The twelve pairs of **cranial nerves** are numbered and named in order from front to back; by long tradition, Roman numerals are often used when numbering them. All but the first two pairs are attached to the brainstem. The cranial nerves are summarized in *Table* **7.1** with their principal functions, and with page references to further descriptions.

Note the following points:
* Nerves III, IV and VI are the ones responsible for eye movements.
* The trigeminal nerve (V) is the sensory nerve of the face, but the facial nerve (VII) is the motor nerve to the facial muscles and does not supply facial skin. Do not confuse facial muscles (supplied by the facial nerve) with mastication muscles (supplied by the trigeminal nerve).
* The vagus is the most widely distributed cranial nerve (the name means 'wandering'), supplying thoracic and abdominal viscera as well as head and neck structures, but its main importance is in supplying the larynx (for speaking), for stimulating gastric secretion and movement, and for slowing the heart.

SPINAL NERVES AND NERVE PLEXUSES

A **spinal nerve** is formed by the union of ventral (anterior) and dorsal (posterior) **nerve roots**, which emerge from the side of the cord (**7.2**). Any part of the cord that gives rise to a pair of roots on each side is called a **segment** of the cord. A spinal segment is named from the nerve to which it gives rise; thus the fifth cervical segment (C5 segment) gives origin to the fifth cervical nerve (C5 nerve). There are 8 cervical segments, 12 thoracic, 5 lumbar, 5 sacral and 1 coccygeal, with corresponding pairs of nerves. Usually, spinal nerves emerge *below* the pedicles of their respective vertebrae, e.g. the T1 nerve emerges below the pedicle of T1 vertebra, but in the cervical region there are 7 cervical vertebrae and 8 cervical nerves. The C1 nerve emerges above the C1 vertebra (the atlas), and C8 nerve below the pedicle of C7 vertebra.

The **ventral** roots contain motor (efferent) fibres and the dorsal roots contain *sensory* (afferent) fibres. The two roots of any one nerve pass laterally towards the appropriate intervertebral foramen. On the dorsal root is situated the **dorsal root ganglion** (**7.2**), within which are the cell bodies

			Table 7.1 Cranial nerves and their principal functions
I	Olfactory	Smell	Not a single nerve but about 20 small filaments passing through the roof of the nose to the olfactory bulb on the under surface of the brain (p.155).
II	Optic	Vision	Passing back from the retina of the eye to the optic chiasma on the under-surface of the brain (p.168).
III	Oculomotor	Motor/ parasympathetic	To four of the muscles which move the eye, and also containing parasympathetic fibres (p.46) which constrict the pupil and alter the curvature of the lens (pp.168–9).
IV	Trochlear	Motor	To one of the eye muscles (superior oblique) (p.167).
V	Trigeminal	Sensory/motor	Main sensory nerve of the head including the face and the surface of the eye, and the motor nerve to muscles of mastication (chewing), moving the lower jaw (pp.143, 147 and 168).
VI	Abducent	Motor	To one of the eye muscles (lateral rectus) (p.167).
VII	Facial	Motor/sensory/ parasympathetic	To the muscles of the face, and containing some taste fibres and parasympathetic fibres for lacrimal, salivary and nasal glands (pp.46 and 142).
VIII	Vestibulocochlear	Motor/sensory	Combined nerve for balance (vestibular part) and hearing (cochlear part) (p.169).
IX	Glossopharyngeal	Sensory/ parasympathetic	Some taste fibres, and other sensory fibres for the lining of the throat, and small but important parasympathetic fibres for reflex control of blood pressure (pp.54, 150 and 181).
X	Vagus	Motor/ parasympathetic	To larynx, pharynx and soft palate (for speech and swallowing), and parasympathetic fibres for gastric secretion and movement, and slowing heart rate. Afferent from many thoracic and abdominal viscera (pp.54, 115, 181, 185, 188 and 253).
XI	Accessory	Motor	The spinal part goes to the sternocleidomastoid and the trapezius, with other fibres (the cranial part) joining the vagus to supply the larynx, pharynx and soft palate (pp.181, 185 and 188).
XII	Hypoglossal	Motor	To tongue muscles (pp.150 and 181).

of the sensory (afferent) fibres of the nerve. The ganglion lies *in* the intervertebral foramen (**17.5**), and immediately beyond the ganglion the ventral root joins the dorsal root to form the spinal nerve. Note that there are no synapses in dorsal root ganglia; the structure is called a ganglion simply because it is the site of nerve cell bodies.

At an early period of embryonic life the cord and the vertebral column are the same length, but the vertebral column grows at a greater rate; at birth the lower end of the cord is at the level of L3 vertebra and in adult life at about the level of the lower border of L1 vertebra. Thus from above downwards the nerve roots have increasingly farther to go

before they reach their appropriate intervertebral foramina (**17.5c** and **17.5d**). This is particularly obvious for lumbar and sacral nerve roots (**17.5d**), which collectively form the *cauda equina* ('horse's tail') below the level at which the spinal cord ends. Note that the cauda is made up not by spinal nerves but by spinal nerve roots; the actual spinal nerves are not formed until the intervertebral foramina are reached.

As soon as the nerve roots have united within the intervertebral foramen to form the spinal nerve, the nerve divides into a ventral (anterior) and a dorsal (posterior) ramus (**7.2**). The smaller **dorsal rami** are the less important; they supply skin and muscles near the midline of the back. The

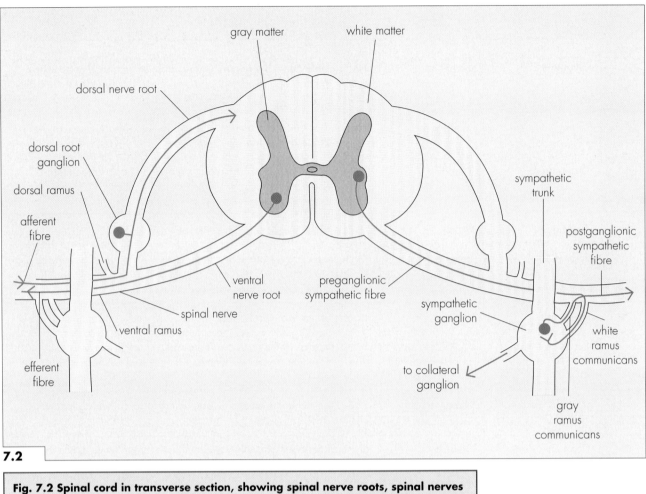

gray matter

white matter

dorsal nerve root

dorsal root ganglion

dorsal ramus

afferent fibre

ventral nerve root

preganglionic sympathetic fibre

spinal nerve

ventral ramus

efferent fibre

sympathetic trunk

postganglionic sympathetic fibre

sympathetic ganglion

white ramus communicans

to collateral ganglion

gray ramus communicans

7.2

Fig. 7.2 Spinal cord in transverse section, showing spinal nerve roots, spinal nerves and connections with the sympathetic trunks (for further details of the spinal cord and nerves see p.199).

larger **ventral rami** are highly important: they supply most of the body musculature and skin, and are the ones that unite to form the great **nerve plexuses** (**7.3**) that are largely responsible for innervating the limbs (*plexus* is the Latin for an 'entwinement' or 'plait'). The ventral rami of the nerves that form each plexus constitute the roots of the plexus (not to be confused with the roots of the spinal nerves themselves) and the way that the roots unite and divide is characteristic for each plexus.

The relatively small **cervical plexus** (p.182) supplies some neck muscles and skin, but also gives rise to one of the most important of all nerves – the **phrenic nerve** – that supplies the diaphragm which is the main muscle of respiration (p.101).

The **brachial plexus** (**7.4**) supplies the upper limb. Its largest branches are the **axillary**, **radial**, **ulnar**, **median** and **musculocutaneous nerves**. Their main supplies are summarized on p.214, and they are described in the appropriate regions.

The **lumbar** and **sacral plexuses** (**7.5** and **7.6**) supply the lower limb. The largest branches of the lumbar plexus are the **femoral** and **obturator nerves**. The sacral plexus, apart from supplying various pelvic structures (p.290), gives rise to the largest of all nerves – the **sciatic nerve** – which divides into the **tibial** and **common peroneal nerves**. The main supplies of the limb nerves are summarized on p.314, and they are described in the appropriate regions.

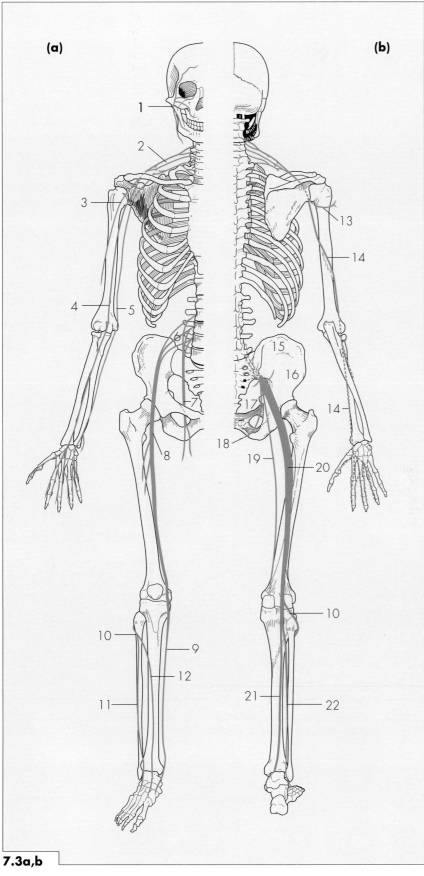

(a)

(b)

Fig. 7.3 Some major nerves, shown with the right half of the skeleton.
(a) From the front
(b) From the back

1 Facial n.
2 Brachial plexus
3 Musculocutaneous n.
4 Median n.
5 Ulnar n.
6 Lumbar plexus
7 Obturator n.
8 Femoral n.
9 Saphenous n.
10 Common peroneal n.
11 Superficial peroneal n.
12 Deep peroneal n.
13 Axillary n.
14 Radial n.
15 Sacral plexus
16 Superior gluteal n.
17 Inferior gluteal n.
18 Pudendal n.
19 Posterior femoral cutaneous n.
20 Sciatic n.
21 Tibial n.
22 Sural n.

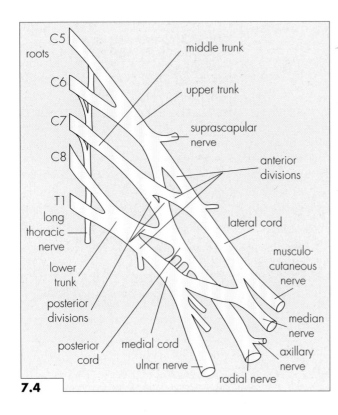

7.4

Fig. 7.4 Left brachial plexus and major branches, from the front.

The parts of the plexus are the roots, trunks, divisions and cords. The upper two roots unite to form the upper trunk; the middle (C7) root continues as the middle trunk; and the lower two roots form the lower trunk. Each trunk then divides into anterior and posterior divisions. The three posterior divisions unite to form the posterior cord, leaving two anterior divisions to form the lateral cord and one to continue as the medial cord. Only the largest branches of the plexus are named.

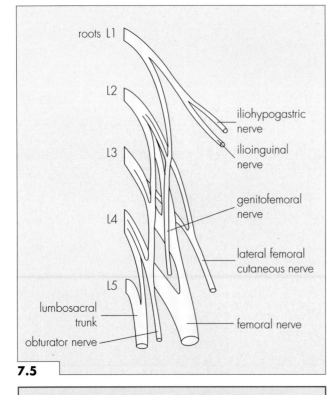

7.5

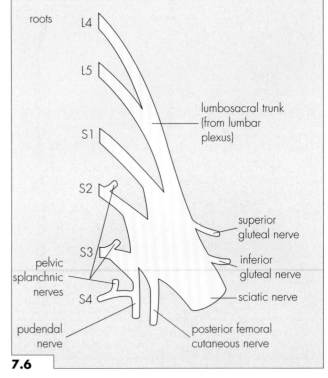

7.6

Fig. 7.5 Left lumbar plexus and major branches, from the front.

The lumbosacral trunk is the contribution that the lumbar plexus makes to the sacral plexus.

Fig. 7.6 Left sacral plexus and major branches, from the front.

THORACIC NERVES

The **ventral rami** of **thoracic nerves** (apart from T1) do not form plexuses but remain single, forming the **intercostal nerves** that supply the thoracic and most of the abdominal walls. They run round from the back to the front, just below their respective ribs, between the middle and innermost layers of thoracic muscles (p.100); the lower six pass into the anterior abdominal wall. All give off cutaneous and muscular branches, supplying the overlying skin and thoracic and abdominal muscles.

DERMATOMES

The area of skin supplied by the sensory fibres of any one spinal nerve (i.e. by fibres from the dorsal root ganglion of that nerve) is a **dermatome**; 7.7 illustrates the approximate distribution of the various dermatomes. The fifth cervical dermatome (C5 dermatome) lies over the outer aspect of the upper arm, and T10 dermatome includes the strip of skin containing the umbilicus.

Despite what may be suggested by diagrams such as these, there is no rigorous demarcation between one dermatome

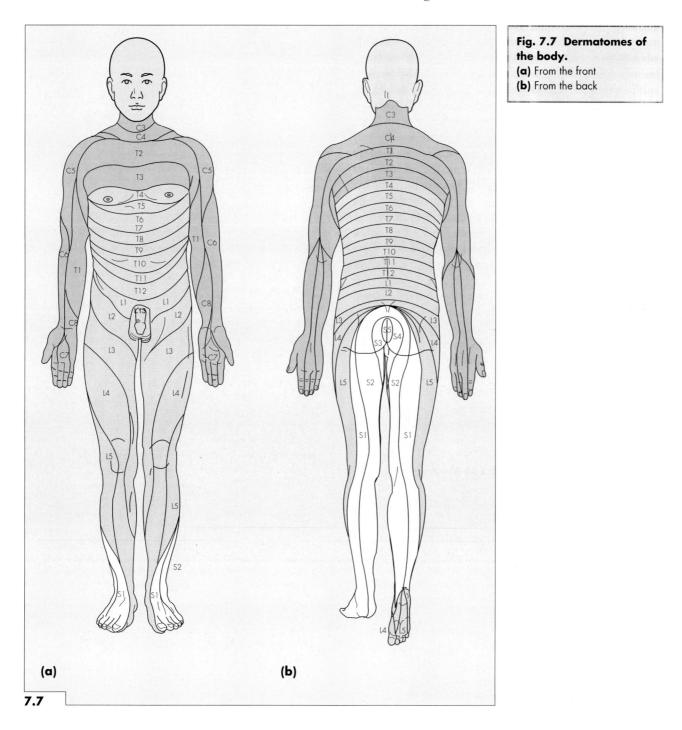

Fig. 7.7 Dermatomes of the body.
(a) From the front
(b) From the back

(a)   (b)

7.7

and another; there is always a certain amount of overlap, especially on the thoracic and abdominal walls where, in order to produce an area of local anaesthesia by injection, at least three adjacent nerves may have to be injected. Knowledge of the position of the dermatomes helps to establish, for example, the site of nerve and spinal cord injuries.

AUTONOMIC NERVOUS SYSTEM

The parts of the nervous system collectively called *autonomic* are functionally distinct because they are concerned not with supplying skeletal muscle but with supplying cardiac muscle, smooth muscle and glands; autonomic nerve fibres thus control activities such as heart rate, pupil size and gastric secretion. Autonomic nerves contain sensory (afferent) fibres as well as motor (efferent) fibres, and may take part not only in reflex activities (p.50), but are also concerned with the conduction of pain impulses from viscera to the central nervous system (p.210).

Somatic motor nerve fibres pass directly – within cranial or spinal nerves – from their cells of origin in the brainstem (p.195) or ventral horns of the spinal cord (p.201) to skeletal muscle fibres (**7.2**). The great difference between this (somatic) innervation and **autonomic innervation** is that autonomic pathways from the brainstem or spinal cord are always *interrupted* by synapses in ganglia before the target organ is reached. There are thus two groups of neurons on autonomic motor pathways, usually described as *preganglionic* and *postganglionic* (**7.8**).

The *preganglionic* cell bodies are those in certain parts of the brainstem and spinal cord (i.e. they are within the central nervous system), and the *postganglionic* cell bodies are in certain ganglia outside the brainstem and cord (i.e. outside the central nervous system). In considering the autonomic innervation of any structure, it is always necessary to define the sites of these two cell groups.

SYMPATHETIC AND PARASYMPATHETIC SYSTEMS

The autonomic nervous system is subdivided into two parts, the *sympathetic* and *parasympathetic*, which in general have opposing functions. Thus stimulation of the *parasympathetic* fibres to the heart acts to slow down the rate of the heart beat, and *sympathetic* stimulation increases it.

Apart from such functional differences, there are characteristic anatomical differences in the positions of the cell bodies.

In the parasympathetic system, the preganglionic cell bodies are in the brainstem (p.195) and in the sacral part of the spinal cord (p.201 and **7.8**), and from here their axons pass out of the central nervous system through cranial nerves III, VII, IX and X and certain sacral nerves (S2–S4) in order

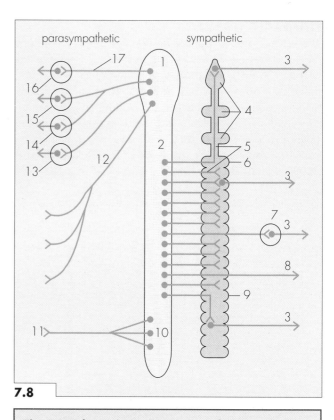

7.8

Fig. 7.8 Schematic representation of preganglionic and postganglionic neurons.
Parasympathetic neurons on the left, sympathetic neurons on the right. See text for further details.

1 Brainstem, with preganglionic parasympathetic cell bodies in cranial nerve nuclei
2 Spinal cord, with sympathetic cell bodies in T1–L2 segments
3 Postganglionic sympathetic fibres
4 Cervical sympathetic ganglia
5 Preganglionic sympathetic fibres
6 First thoracic sympathetic ganglion
7 Collateral sympathetic ganglion
8 Preganglionic sympathetic fibres to adrenal medulla
9 Second lumbar sympathetic ganglion
10 Preganglionic parasympathetic cell bodies in sacral segments 2–4
11 Pelvic splanchnic (parasympathetic) nerves to ganglia in pelvic viscera
12 Preganglionic vagal (parasympathetic) fibres to ganglia in viscera (e.g. heart, lung, stomach)
13 Otic ganglion, with postganglionic neurons for parotid gland
14 Submandibular ganglion, for submandibular and sublingual glands
15 Pterygopalatine ganglion, for lacrimal and nasal glands
16 Ciliary ganglion, for iris and ciliary body
17 Preganglionic parasympathetic fibres from cranial nerve nuclei

to reach their 'target organs'. In many cases, the preganglionic fibres do not terminate until they reach the target organ itself (e.g. the heart, lungs and gut); here they make synaptic connections with postganglionic cell bodies that form minute ganglia actually in the walls of the organs innervated. The postganglionic fibres are therefore microscopically short. In other cases, the preganglionic fibres end just before reaching the organ to be innervated, and the synapses occur in discrete ganglia close to, but not in, the organs concerned. There are four such discrete **parasympathetic ganglia** in the head, supplying the eye and the lacrimal gland, as well as the salivary glands and glands of the nasal lining.

Most of the preganglionic fibres of the parasympathetic system travel out towards their target organs in the four cranial nerves mentioned above. The few fibres that leave the central nervous system through sacral spinal nerves (S2–S4) leave the ventral rami of these nerves soon after they emerge from their anterior sacral foramina, and form a group called the **pelvic splanchnic nerves**. These nerves provide parasympathetic innervation to pelvic viscera and the lower part of the digestive tract.

In the sympathetic system, the preganglionic cell bodies are in the thoracic and upper lumbar parts of the spinal cord (p.201), and their axons pass out through spinal nerves and through connections called **white rami communicantes** (**7.12b**) enter the **sympathetic trunks**, which are a pair of structures, one on each side of the vertebral column (**7.8**, **15.26a** and **15.27a***)*. Each trunk is a chain of ganglia connected to one another like a string of beads, but with some distance – a centimeter or two – between the 'beads'. The preganglionic axons either make synaptic connections with postganglionic cell bodies in the ganglia or, in some cases, they pass through the trunk and its ganglia to certain other nearby ganglia – collectively called collateral ganglia – where they synapse with postganglionic cell bodies. In either case the postganglionic fibres have to travel some distance to get to the structures that they innervate, and run usually along blood vessels to the part concerned. (A third possibility, for a few lower thoracic preganglionic fibres, is that they innervate cells of the adrenal medulla directly – p.281.) Blood vessels themselves are among the principal structures receiving sympathetic fibres that control the degree of constriction and thus the amount of bloodflow through them. For the innervation of limb structures and the body surface (blood vessels, sweat glands and arrector pili muscles), the postganglionic fibres join spinal nerves by **gray rami communicantes** (**7.12b**) and are distributed with their branches, often via the great plexuses.

The *transmitter substance* at the synapses (p.48) between all autonomic preganglionic fibres and postganglionic cells, and between parasympathetic postganglionic fibres and their target organs, is **acetylcholine**, but at the ends of sympathetic postganglionic fibres the transmitter is nearly always **norepinephrine** (also called **noradrenaline**). All preganglionic neurons, and postganglionic neurons of the parasympathetic system, are therefore *cholinergic* neurons, whereas the majority of sympathetic postganglionic neurons are *adrenergic*. (There are some exceptions: a few sympathetic postganglionic neurons are cholinergic, notably those to most sweat glands).

The fact that some sympathetic ganglia are some distance from their target organs may allow sympathetic denervation to be achieved by the surgical removal of appropriate ganglia (*sympathectomy*). Thus, excessive axillary sweating, or excessive constriction of the blood vessels of the fingers, can be abolished by removing the appropriate part of the thoracic sympathetic trunk, an operation often called *cervical sympathectomy* when it is carried out through the neck (although it is part of the thoracic, not the cervical, trunk that is being removed; *cervix* is the Latin for 'neck').

NERVE IMPULSES

The conduction of **impulses** in neurons is an electrical phenomenon, and depends upon the movement of ions across the boundary membranes. In the resting state there are many more potassium ions (K^+) inside the cell than outside, while the reverse is true for sodium ions (Na^+) (**7.9a**). Owing to a small but continuous loss of potassium ions to the outside – through molecular channels in the membrane – the inside of the membrane is electrically negative with respect to the outside and the membrane is said to be *polarized*.

Upon adequate stimulation of the fibre, membrane channels that are specific for sodium open up; sodium ions diffuse into the fibre, thereby decreasing the negativity inside (because of their positive charge), and thus *depolarizing* the membrane. Very soon the influx of positively charged ions reverses the charge difference across the membrane, making the inside positive with respect to the outside. Subsequent closure of the sodium channels, and concomitant opening of specific potassium channels, stops the influx of sodium and promotes the efflux of potassium. The resultant reduction of positive charge inside the fibre returns the membrane to its original polarized state. This very brief change in electrical gradient across the cell membrane (which takes only a few milliseconds) is the action potential or nerve impulse, and it can be conducted along the whole length of the fibre. Under normal circumstances, it always travels in the same direction in any given fibre (for example, towards the central nervous system in afferent fibres or away from it in efferent fibres).

Many nerve fibres are covered by **myelin**, which is a fatty material formed by the cell membranes of certain non-neuronal cells – Schwann cells in peripheral nerves, and oligodendrocytes in the central nervous system (p.15 and **2.7**). In such *myelinated* fibres, the entry and exit of ions can

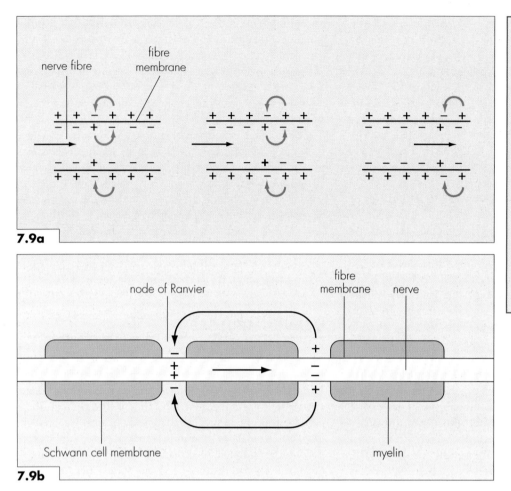

7.9a

7.9b

Fig. 7.9 Propagation of a nerve impulse.
(a) Unmyelinated fibre. The progressive change of the electrical charge between the inside and outside of the nerve fibre enables the impulse to move along the fibre.
(b) Myelinated fibre. Because of the insulating effect of myelin, the electrical changes can only occur at the nodes of Ranvier, the minute gaps between adjacent Schwann cells where the fibre is bare; the impulse 'jumps' from one node to the next.

occur only at regions where the nerve fibre is exposed through gaps in the myelin sheath – the **nodes of Ranvier**. Impulse transmission in myelinated nerves (**7.9b**) occurs by the action potential 'jumping' from one node to the next (called *saltatory conduction*, from a Latin word meaning 'to jump or dance', and nothing to do with salt). *Unmyelinated* fibres, though lacking myelin, are nonetheless enclosed in a single-layer wrapping of cell membrane and cytoplasm that is again derived from Schwann cells or oligodendrocytes.

The rate of conduction of nerve impulses is always the same for any given nerve fibre, and varies in different fibres from 1–100 meters per second (in contrast to electricity in a wire, which travels at 300 million meters per second). Conduction in myelinated fibres is faster than in unmyelinated fibres.

SYNAPSES

Despite the fact that nerve impulses are electrical and that it is common to talk about some nerve pathways as circuits, it would be wrong to consider the nervous system as being exactly similar to a series of electrical circuits, or like a telephone exchange. Electrical circuits rely for conduction

on complete physical contact, giving direct continuity between one element and another, but this is not the case with nerve cells. Nerve cells and fibres communicate with one another at junctional zones known as **synapses** (**7.10**). There is no actual continuity between one neuron and another; a minute gap exists between them – the **synaptic cleft** – across which a 'message' must be sent in the form of a chemical substance that is called a **neurotransmitter**.

At junctions between two neurons, the axon of the first neuron (the *presynaptic* neuron) branches, and the branch endings (the **axon terminals**) come to lie in close apposition to the cell membrane of the second neuron (the *postsynaptic* neuron). Each axon terminal is expanded into a small swelling, the **terminal bulb** or **bouton** (commonly called the **synaptic bag**), in which are stored vesicles containing the neurotransmitter.

When a nerve impulse travels down the axon and reaches the axon terminal, the neurotransmitter is released into the synaptic cleft and diffuses across to the cell membrane of the postsynaptic neuron where it binds to receptors. This action causes specific ion movements across the cell membrane of the postsynaptic neuron and consequent changes in the degree of polarization of the membrane; it may become depolarized or hyperpolarized depending upon the type of

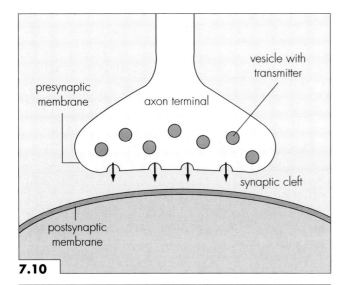

7.10

Fig. 7.10 Synapse.
The axon terminal or synaptic bag, the bulge at the end of the presynaptic nerve fibre, contains vesicles of neurotransmitter substance. The arrival of the nerve impulse causes the release of transmitter into the synaptic cleft. Binding of the transmitter to the postsynaptic membrane causes a change in the postsynaptic neuron (excitation or inhibition, depending upon the type of neurotransmitter involved). The small arrows indicate the release of neurotransmitter from the axon terminal: synaptic vesicles move to the presynaptic membrane and fuse with it, allowing the release of transmitter into the synaptic cleft.

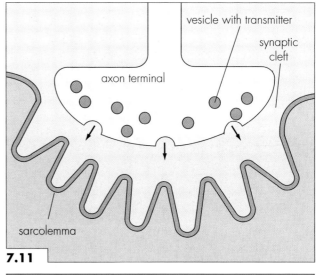

7.11

Fig. 7.11 Neuromuscular junction.
Neurotransmitter is released from nerve fibre terminations (as indicated by the small arrows) and binds to the membrane (sarcolemma) of the skeletal muscle cell, causing a response (action potential) in the muscle cell.

along nerve fibres; in nerve networks or circuits where there are many synapses, 'synaptic delay' accounts for much of the transmission time.

NEUROMUSCULAR JUNCTIONS

Skeletal muscles receive their innervation from cholinergic, somatic motor neurons. The site at which the end of the motor nerve fibre comes to lie adjacent to the membrane (i.e. the sarcolemma) of the muscle fibre is the **neuromuscular junction** (**7.11**), which is very like a synapse; there is no continuity of cytoplasm between the nerve fibre and muscle cell, but always a cleft between the two. When a nerve impulse arrives at the junction, about 1 million molecules of acetylcholine are released from synaptic vesicles and diffuse across the gap. Binding of the transmitter to receptors on the sarcolemma causes a depolarization of the sarcolemma that is of sufficient magnitude to initiate an action potential within it, with subsequent contraction of the muscle fibre. To prevent the continued action of the released acetylcholine, it is destroyed immediately by the enzyme **acetylcholinesterase** that is stored in the sarcolemma. The big difference between impulse transmission at synapses and at neuromuscular junctions is that at synapses a summation of impulses is required (see above), whereas at neuromuscular junctions a single impulse is sufficient to generate an action potential in the muscle cell membrane.

neurotransmitter. If it becomes depolarized, the postsynaptic cell becomes more likely to generate an action potential, but a single excitation is never sufficient to trigger off conduction through the postsynaptic cell; a number of impulses, quickly repeated from one synapse or from several different synapses (a *summation of impulses*), is required before there is sufficient depolarization to set up transmission.

There are usually thousands of synapses from many different neurons converging upon a single nerve cell. As pointed out above, not all are *excitatory*; some are *inhibitory*, helping to prevent impulse transmission. How a neuron finally responds is the result of a large number of often conflicting influences, and it is this that makes the unravelling of function in the nervous system so difficult and at the same time so fascinating.

For many years it was believed that there were only two transmitters, acetylcholine and norepinephrine (noradrenaline), but it is now known that there are several others. However, acetylcholine remains one of the commonest and most important, and neurons that release it from their axon terminals are therefore called *cholinergic* neurons. Those releasing norepinephrine (noradrenaline) are called *adrenergic*. Impulse transmission across synapses is much slower than

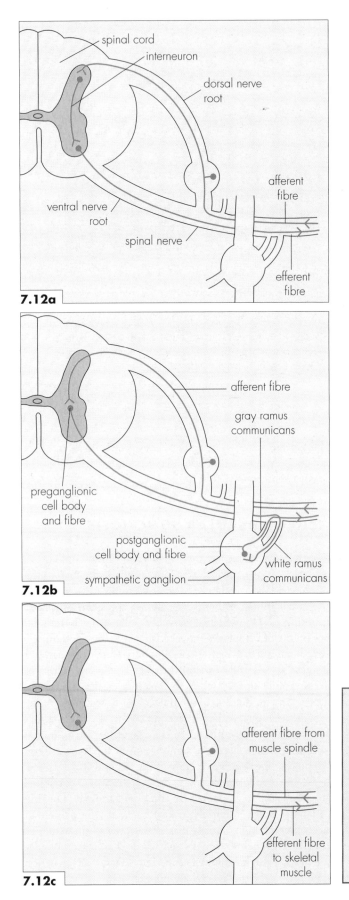

7.12a

spinal cord
interneuron
dorsal nerve root
afferent fibre
ventral nerve root
spinal nerve
efferent fibre

7.12b

afferent fibre
gray ramus communicans
preganglionic cell body and fibre
postganglionic cell body and fibre
sympathetic ganglion
white ramus communicans

7.12c

afferent fibre from muscle spindle
efferent fibre to skeletal muscle

REFLEXES

Reflexes are involuntary responses to a stimulus, and depend upon an arc or circuit of nervous tissue (**7.12**) consisting, in its simplest form, of an afferent neuron (which receives a stimulus) making synaptic connection with a motor neuron (that produces a response). Such an arc, with two neurons and one synapse, is referred to as a **monosynaptic reflex arc** (**7.12c**); other arcs may have one or more neurons intervening between the afferent and efferent (receptor and effector) neurons, and hence are called *multisynaptic* (**7.12a**). Most reflexes are multisynaptic, including sympathetic reflexes (e.g. for vasoconstriction, as in **7.12b**). The body's only examples of monosynaptic reflex arcs are the tendon reflexes, otherwise known as *stretch reflexes* or tendon 'jerks'.

TENDON REFLEXES

The *tendon reflex* is elicited by tapping the relaxed tendon with a rubber tendon-hammer (**7.13**). The tap on the tendon stretches the muscle spindles within the muscle, and the spindles' afferent fibres send impulses into the spinal cord, where the fibres synapse with the motor neurons supplying the ordinary muscle fibres (**7.12a**), thus causing the muscle to contract and produce the characteristic 'jerk'. Note that it is the muscle spindles within the muscle that are stimulated by stretching the tendon; the reflex has nothing to do with the tendon's own afferent nerves.

Testing tendon reflexes is an essential part of the neurological examination of a patient. Diminished (or absent) or exaggerated responses indicate some kind of abnormal function, and the physician must then localize the site where the arc has been damaged or interrupted, and establish the cause. A cut peripheral nerve would be an obvious cause for an absent reflex, since both the afferent and efferent sides of the arc would be interrupted. In the spinal cord itself, conditions such as tumour or multiple sclerosis (p.212) could interfere with any part of the arc, and give diminished or absent reflexes depending on the number of fibres involved. Exaggerated reflexes are characteristic of

Fig. 7.12 Reflex arcs. (For details of the internal structure of the spinal cord see p.201.)
(a) Typical pathway for a reflex arc. For simplicity, only one interneuron is shown between the afferent and efferent neurons but there are usually several, i.e. the pathway is multisynaptic (with more than one synapse).
(b) Pathway for a sympathetic reflex (multisynaptic), with the afferent fibre synapsing with the preganglionic cell body in the spinal cord, and the preganglionic fibre synapsing with the postganglionic cell body in a sympathetic ganglion.
(c) Pathway for a typical stretch reflex (tendon jerk, **7.13**), which is monosynaptic (with only one synapse, in the spinal cord).

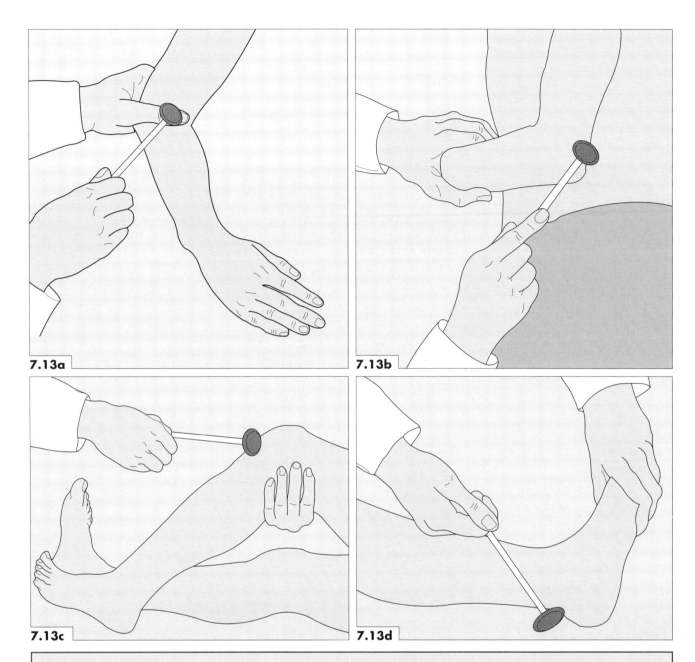

7.13a

7.13b

7.13c

7.13d

Fig. 7.13 Tendon reflexes.
(a) Biceps jerk, tapping the end of the thumb held against the biceps tendon (p.222). The pathway is mainly through C6 segment of the cord.
(b) Triceps jerk, tapping the triceps tendon (p.222). The pathway is mainly through C7 segment of the cord.

(c) Knee jerk, tapping the patellar ligament (p.315). The pathway is mainly through L3 segment of the cord.
(d) Ankle jerk, tapping the Achilles' tendon (p.336). The pathway is mainly through S1 segment of the cord.

upper motor neuron lesions (p.205), because the responsiveness of the cord's anterior horn cells (the motor neuron cell bodies) has been enhanced by interference with their normal control by corticospinal and extrapyramidal fibres (p.206).

POSTURE

Although it may not be apparent to the eye, when standing upright the body is swaying very slightly backwards and forwards. The maintenance of this upright posture depends on stimulation of the muscle spindles, acting in much the same way as in the tendon reflexes described above. The tendency to fall forwards stimulates the spindles in the muscles on the back of the lower limb; the muscles contract to pull the body backwards. This backward motion stretches the spindles in the muscles on the front of the limb, so that these muscles can now contract and pull the body forward. The constant alternation of slight contractions at the front and back maintains the upright position.

CHAPTER 8

CARDIOVASCULAR SYSTEM

The **cardiovascular system** consists of the **heart** and **blood vessels**, and contains **blood** that circulates through them. Some of the general features of the heart and circulation and of the blood are described here; details of the heart itself begin on p.107, and further information on the course and distribution of the major vessels is given with each region.

HEART, ARTERIES AND VEINS

The **heart** is a four-chambered muscular pump that causes blood to move through the vessels to all parts of the body, and then to return to the heart (**8.1**). The vessels are called **arteries** or **veins**, according to the direction of bloodflow within them: arteries conduct blood *away from* the heart and veins return blood *to* the heart. The vessels that connect the smallest arteries (which are called **arterioles**) to the smallest veins (called **venules**) are the **blood capillaries**. It is only through capillaries that substances can diffuse out of or into the blood; all the other vessels are simply conducting tubes leading to or from the networks of capillaries.

The **chambers** of the heart are the **left atrium** and **right atrium** and the **left ventricle** and **right ventricle** (**8.1**). The left atrium and left ventricle communicate with one another through the **mitral (bicuspid) valve**, and the right atrium and right ventricle through the **tricuspid** valve. (The two atria do not communicate with one another, nor do the two ventricles.)

In general, arteries contain blood with a high oxygen content (*oxygenated blood*), and the pumping action of the heart delivers it to all parts of the body. On the other hand, veins return blood to the heart; in most cases this blood has given up a significant proportion of its oxygen and is therefore called *deoxygenated blood* (although it has not, in fact, lost all of its oxygen), and it has also gained a good deal of carbon dioxide. There is *one important exception* to this description of the content of arteries and veins: the *pulmonary arteries* take deoxygenated blood to the lungs so that it can take up oxygen and give off carbon dioxide, while the *pulmonary veins* return the newly oxygenated blood to the heart (**8.5**). Thus, the circuit that carries blood to the lungs and back to the heart – the **pulmonary circuit** or

pulmonary circulation, from right ventricle to left atrium – is distinct from that which circulates blood to all other parts of the body – the **systemic circuit** or **systemic circulation**, from left ventricle to right atrium; not only is the content of the arteries and veins different in the two circuits, the circuits themselves are actually separate from one another.

The two atria thus receive blood from veins, and the two ventricles pump blood out into arteries. The **superior** and **inferior venae cavae** enter the top and bottom of the *right* atrium respectively, and the four **pulmonary veins** (two on each side) enter the *left* atrium. The **aorta** leaves the top of the *left* ventricle, and the **pulmonary trunk** (which divides into the **right** and **left pulmonary arteries**) leaves the top of the *right* ventricle. All the above-mentioned vessels are commonly called the 'great vessels' of the heart.

CARDIAC CYCLE

In the pumping action of the heart, both atria contract together to propel blood into the ventricles, and then the ventricles contract to force blood out. The sequence of atrial and ventricular contraction – the *cardiac cycle* – normally takes about 0.8 seconds, giving a heart rate of over 70 beats per minute. The term *systole* (Greek for 'contraction') is the medical word for the contraction of an atrium or ventricle, and *diastole* (Greek for 'dilatation') means the return of the chamber to its resting size. Atrial systole occupies the first 0.1 seconds of the cycle, and is accompanied by ventricular diastole; this is followed, over the next 0.3 seconds, by ventricular systole with atrial diastole; in the remaining 0.4 seconds, all of the chambers are in a diastolic phase.

On the *left* side of the heart (**8.1**), the mitral (bicuspid) valve opens during atrial systole but is closed at all other times of the cycle to prevent the oxygenated blood from returning to the left atrium. During ventricular systole, blood passes out of the left ventricle into the aorta through the aortic valve, whose cusps are so arranged that they prevent regurgitation into the ventricle when contraction ceases – the back pressure of the blood in the aorta forces them to close. The rhythmic contractions of the left ventricle cause waves of increased pressure within the arteries, and the pulsations so

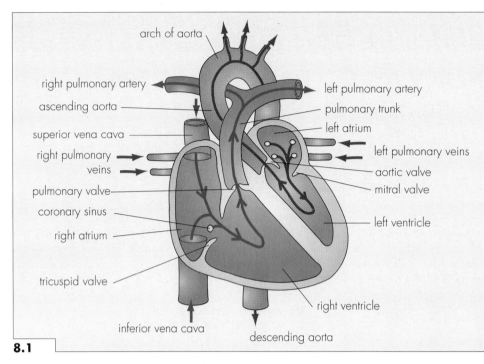

arch of aorta

right pulmonary artery

ascending aorta

superior vena cava

right pulmonary veins

pulmonary valve

coronary sinus

right atrium

tricuspid valve

inferior vena cava

descending aorta

left pulmonary artery

pulmonary trunk

left atrium

left pulmonary veins

aortic valve

mitral valve

left ventricle

right ventricle

Fig. 8.1 Diagrammatic representation of the heart and great vessels. The arrows indicate the direction of bloodflow. Red: oxygenated blood. Blue: deoxygenated blood

8.1

caused can be felt in some arteries that are sufficiently near to the skin's surface. The commonest site for 'feeling the pulse' is the radial artery at the front of the wrist (p.231).

On the *right* side of the heart (**8.1**), the tricuspid valve opens during atrial systole but is otherwise closed to prevent the deoxygenated blood from returning to the right atrium. During ventricular systole, blood passes out into the pulmonary trunk through the pulmonary valve, whose cusps, like those of the aortic valve, are closed by the back pressure of blood as ventricular contraction ceases. The pressure in the pulmonary system is much lower than in the systemic system (p.61), and, because the pulmonary vessels are deep in the thorax, there is no way of feeling a 'pulmonary pulse'.

Although in theory the words *systole* and *diastole* apply respectively to contraction and relaxation of either the atria or the ventricles, in practice these terms often refer to activity in the ventricles alone, since ventricular contraction is much more powerful than atrial contraction and tends to overshadow activity in the atria. Thus *systole*, if used alone, should be taken to mean the phase of ventricular contraction, and *diastole* to mean ventricular relaxation.

When the heart chambers contract, they do not completely empty. Each ventricle, for example, holds about 120–130 ml of blood when full, and ejects about 70 ml during ventricular systole, leaving about 50–60 ml in the ventricle. The volume ejected by each ventricle (about 70 ml) is the *stroke volume*; with a heart rate of over 70 beats per minute, over 5 litres of blood are pumped out of each ventricle every minute – this is the *cardiac output*. Since the right ventricle pumps blood into the pulmonary circuit, and

the left into the systemic circuit, cardiac output can be thought of as the volume of blood flowing through either the pulmonary or systemic circuit every minute. These two volumes may differ from one another slightly at any given moment but, over time, they should be equal. (Note that cardiac output refers to the volume pumped out by *either* the right *or* the left ventricle, not the total amount pumped by both ventricles.) The cardiac output will vary with changes in stroke volume or heart rate – an increase in either will increase the output, and a decrease in either will decrease output.

CONTROL OF HEART RATE

Specialized nerve receptors (p.40) – **baroreceptors** – in the walls of the internal carotid arteries (the carotid sinuses, see p.178) and in the arch of the aorta (p.116) constantly monitor the blood pressure. Other similar receptors – called **chemoreceptors** – in the carotid and aortic bodies are mainly concerned with monitoring the amount of oxygen in the blood. Through their nerve supplies by the vagus and glossopharyngeal nerves (p.181), information from all of these receptors reaches the **reticular formation** in the brainstem (p.195), so that any necessary changes in heart rate can be made. For example, with exercise when more oxygen is required than when at rest, the heart rate increases to increase the blood supply and therefore the oxygen supply; after a sudden haemorrhage which lowers blood pressure, the heart rate increases to compensate for the reduced pressure and keep up an adequate blood supply to the tissues.

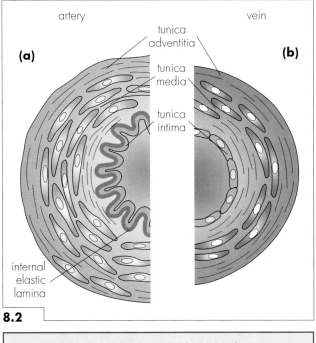

8.2

> **Fig. 8.2 Histological structure of a typical artery (a) and vein (b).**

STRUCTURE OF BLOOD VESSELS

While the heart is essentially composed of cardiac muscle (p.13), blood vessels (except for the capillaries) contain **smooth muscle** in their walls (**8.2**). The walls of **arteries** are described as having three coats (or layers). The inner coat (**tunica intima**), forming the layer in contact with the blood, consists of very flattened endothelial cells (the name given to the type of epithelium that lines vessels) which provide a smooth lining over which blood can flow easily, and a minimal amount of connective tissue. The middle layer (**tunica media**) is composed mainly of smooth muscle arranged in a circular fashion; when the muscle contracts the caliber of the vessel is made smaller – this process is called *vasoconstriction*. In the largest vessels, such as the aorta and its main branches, a large amount of elastic tissue is intermixed with the muscle fibres. The outer layer (**tunica adventitia**) has no muscle, being composed solely of connective tissue.

Veins have the same three layers as arteries but the tunica media is very much thinner.

Capillaries consist only of endothelial cells. Depending upon differences in pressure and in the concentration of substances in the blood and in the surrounding tissues, fluid and other substances can move through capillary walls (either inwards or outwards). Thus, capillaries (and the **capillary beds**) are the essential sites of exchange between the blood and the tissues.

SOME DEFINITIONS

The smaller branches of vessels often unite with one another – they are said to *anastomose*, to form an *anastomosis* (from the Greek meaning 'to make a mouth'). Arteries that do not unite with branches from adjacent areas (i.e. that do not anastomose with other vessels) are **end-arteries**.

Vessels that become obstructed by disease may cause the area supplied to become *ischaemic* (from the Greek meaning 'to keep back blood'), and the tissues involved may become *necrotic* – undergoing *necrosis* or dying (from the Greek for 'killing').

Any area supplied by vessels which anastomose is less likely to become necrotic than one supplied by an end-artery, because in the former there is a chance for the capillary bed to have several sources of supply, not just one as with an end-artery. The most important examples of end-arteries are those of the retina of the eye (p.165); complete blockage will cause a blind spot in the affected area.

PRINCIPAL ARTERIES

The **principal arteries** are illustrated in **8.3a**, and are summarized below. Those whose pulsations can be felt (see below) are indicated in **8.3b**. Further details are given with the appropriate regions or organs.

- From the left ventricle of the heart, the **ascending aorta** becomes the **arch of the aorta** and then the **descending** or **thoracic aorta**. It then continues into the abdomen as the **abdominal aorta** and ends by dividing into the two **common iliac arteries**.
- The **ascending aorta** gives off the **right** and **left coronary arteries**, which supply the heart.
- The **arch of the aorta** gives off the **brachiocephalic trunk** and the **left common carotid artery** and the **left subclavian artery**. The **brachiocephalic trunk** divides into the **right common carotid artery** and the **right subclavian artery**.
- The **common carotid artery** on each side divides, in the neck, into the **internal** and **external carotid arteries** which supply head and neck structures.
- Each **subclavian artery** gives off the **vertebral** and **internal thoracic arteries** and then continues as the **axillary artery** which in turn becomes the **brachial artery**, to supply the upper limb.
- The **brachial artery** divides at the elbow into the **radial** and **ulnar arteries** which continue into the hand.
- The **thoracic aorta** gives off **posterior intercostal arteries** on each side, supplying much of the chest wall. Additional blood supply to the chest wall comes from the **anterior intercostal arteries**, which are small branches from the **internal thoracic vessels** of each side.

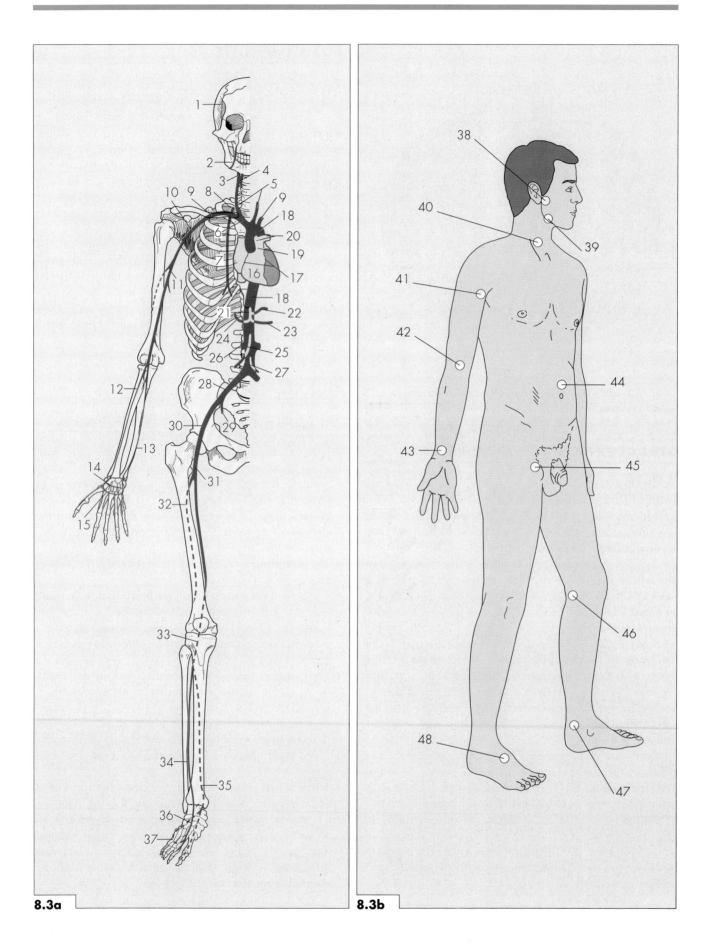

8.3a

8.3b

- The **abdominal aorta** gives off, from its anterior surface, the **coeliac trunk** and the **superior** and **inferior mesenteric arteries**, all of which supply the gastrointestinal tract. The largest branches from the side of the aorta are the **right** and **left renal arteries** (which supply blood to the kidneys), and there is a considerably smaller pair of **gonadal arteries** (**testicular** in the male or **ovarian** in the female) to each testis or ovary respectively.
- The **common iliac artery** divides into the **internal** and **external iliac arteries**. The **internal iliac artery** supplies pelvic structures. The **external iliac artery** continues into the lower limb as the **femoral artery**.
- The **femoral artery**, after giving off the **profunda femoris artery** which supplies the thigh, continues as the **popliteal artery** behind the knee, and then divides into the **anterior** and **posterior tibial arteries**. The anterior tibial artery continues on to the dorsum of the foot as the **dorsalis pedis artery**.

- The **posterior tibial artery** gives off the **peroneal artery** below the knee, and behind the ankle divides into the **medial** and **lateral plantar arteries** for the sole of the foot.

PRINCIPAL VEINS

The principal veins are illustrated in **8.4** and are summarized below. Further details are given with the appropriate regions or organs.

- The **superior vena cava**, which collects blood from the upper part of the body (except from the lungs) and enters the right atrium of the heart, is formed by the union of the **right** and **left brachiocephalic veins**.
- The **brachiocephalic vein** is formed by the union of the **internal jugular** and **subclavian veins**.
- The **internal jugular vein** is the main vein of the head and neck.
- The **subclavian vein** is the continuation of the **axillary vein** at the level of the first rib.
- The **axillary vein** is the continuation of the **brachial vein** of the arm, and receives the **cephalic vein**, which is the superficial vein of the lateral side of the limb.
- The **basilic vein** is the superficial vein of the medial side of the upper limb and joins the brachial vein.
- The **azygos vein** on the right side of the thorax drains into the **superior vena cava**. On the left side of the thorax, the **hemiazygos** and **accessory hemiazygos veins** (not shown in **8.4**) drain into the **azygos vein**.
- The **inferior vena cava**, which collects blood from the lower part of the body, is formed in the lower abdomen by the union of the **right** and **left common iliac veins**, and runs up to pass through the diaphragm into the right atrium of the heart. Its largest tributaries are the **right** and **left renal veins** (from the kidneys) and the **hepatic veins** from the liver.
- The **portal vein**, which takes blood to the liver from the gastrointestinal tract, is formed by the union of the **superior mesenteric vein** and the **splenic vein**. The **inferior mesenteric vein** joins the **splenic vein**.
- The **common iliac vein** is formed by the union of the **internal iliac vein** (which drains pelvic structures) with the **external iliac vein** which is the continuation of the **femoral vein** from the thigh into the abdomen.
- The **femoral vein** is the largest vein of the lower limb, with tributaries corresponding to the branches of the femoral artery.
- The largest superficial vein of the lower limb is the **great saphenous vein**, which drains into the **femoral vein** at the top of the front of the thigh.
- The **small saphenous vein** on the back of the leg drains into the **popliteal vein** behind the knee.

Fig. 8.3 Arteries and pulses.
(a) Principal arteries, shown with the heart and right half of the skeleton, from the front. The left ventricle is in red stipple.
(b) Pulses normally palpable, with page references for further details.

1 Superficial temporal a.	27 Inferior mesenteric a.
2 Facial a.	28 Common iliac a.
3 Internal carotid a.	29 Internal iliac a.
4 External carotid a.	30 External iliac a.
5 Common carotid a.	31 Femoral a.
6 Brachiocephalic trunk	32 Profunda femoris a.
7 Internal thoracic a.	33 Popliteal a.
8 Vertebral a.	34 Anterior tibial a.
9 Subclavian a.	35 Posterior tibial a.
10 Axillary a.	36 Dorsalis pedis a.
11 Brachial a.	37 Plantar arch
12 Radial a.	38 Superficial temporal
13 Ulnar a.	(p.130)
14 Deep palmar arch	39 Facial (p.142)
15 Superficial palmar arch	40 Common carotid (p.178)
16 Heart	41 Axillary (p.220)
17 Coronary a.	42 Brachial (p.226)
18 Aorta	43 Radial (p.231)
19 Pulmonary trunk	44 Aorta (p.253)
20 Pulmonary a.	45 Femoral (p.249)
21 Coeliac trunk	46 Popliteal (p.328)
22 Left gastric a.	47 Posterior tibial (p.339)
23 Splenic a.	48 Dorsalis pedis (p.339)
24 Common hepatic a.	
25 Superior mesenteric a.	
26 Renal a.	

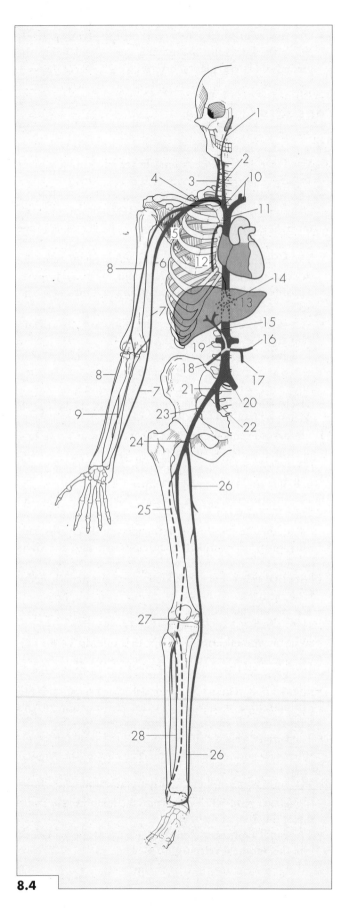

8.4

1 Facial v.	16 Splenic v.
2 Internal jugular v.	17 Inferior mesenteric v.
3 External jugular v.	18 Superior mesenteric v.
4 Subclavian v.	19 Renal v.
5 Axillary v.	20 Inferior vena cava
6 Brachial v.	21 Common iliac v.
7 Basilic v.	22 Internal iliac v.
8 Cephalic v.	23 External iliac v.
9 Median forearm v.	24 Femoral v.
10 Brachiocephalic v.	25 Profunda femoris v.
11 Superior vena cava	26 Great saphenous v.
12 Azygos v.	27 Popliteal v.
13 Liver	28 Small saphenous v.
14 Hepatic v.	
15 Portal v.	

BLOOD PRESSURE

Because of the constant tension in the walls of arteries (due to the muscle and elastic tissue) and the resistance offered to the passage of blood as it passes into smaller and smaller vessels (*peripheral resistance* – see below), the blood inside the arteries and their smaller branches is under pressure, even when the left ventricle is not contracting. With ventricular contraction, there is a surge of pressure that causes the larger arteries to distend momentarily and then recoil due to their own elasticity, so causing a pulsation (often palpable as the *pulse* – see below) which helps to keep the blood moving on into the smaller branches.

Three main factors help to maintain the blood pressure: cardiac output (p.54), blood volume (p.61), and peripheral resistance. Perpipheral resistance is the resistance offered to the flow of blood by the smaller arteries – especially the arterioles – whose caliber is controlled by the smooth muscle in their walls. The contractile activity of this smooth muscle is in turn affected by both the autonomic nerves supplying it (p.46) and the vasoconstrictor substances in the blood – in particular the angiotensin produced by the renin–angiotensin system of the kidney (p.286).

A fall in the blood volume, such as that which occurs after severe haemorrhage, leads to a fall in blood pressure, a rise in pulse rate, and vasoconstriction of peripheral vessels – especially in the limbs – which are all the signs of *shock*. The immediate need is to restore the blood volume to a normal level, hence the giving of intravenous fluid as an emergency measure by those who may be the 'first on the scene'. Even

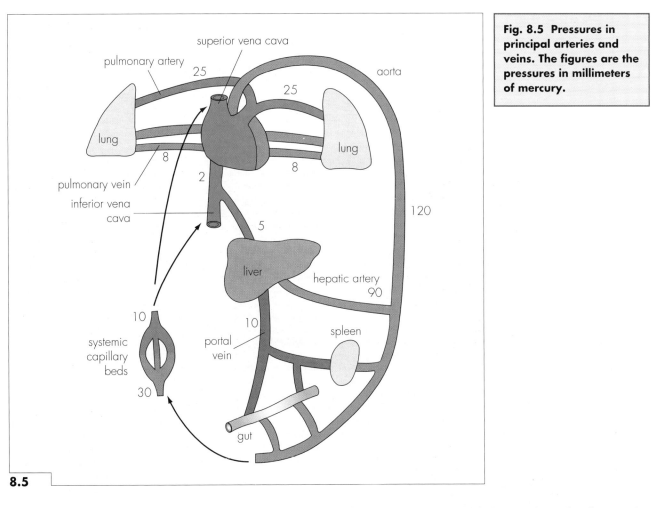

Fig. 8.5 Pressures in principal arteries and veins. The figures are the pressures in millimeters of mercury.

8.5

when the transfusion of blood itself is required, fluid such as 5% glucose solution or 0.9% sodium chloride (*physiological saline*) can be given to tide the patient over while being transported to a medical centre or while blood is being cross-matched (p.64).

As arteries divide and branch their diameters become smaller, and the blood pressure inside them becomes lower; by the time the arteries have branched sufficiently to be considered **arterioles**, the pressure is about 30 mmHg, which is the pressure at the arterial end of a capillary network (**8.5**). At the venous end, the pressure is about 10 mmHg, and becomes even lower in the larger veins until, in the inferior vena cava, it is negligible; the slight negative pressure in the thoracic cavity helps to propel blood into the right atrium.

TAKING THE BLOOD PRESSURE

The *arterial blood pressure* (commonly referred to as simply the *blood pressure*) is usually determined in the brachial artery by the use of a *sphygmomanometer*. A sphygmomanometer is an instrument with an inflatable cuff that is connected to a pressure gauge which is calibrated in millimeters of mercury (mmHg) or, if modern SI units are used, in kilopascals (kPa).

The cuff is wrapped round the arm above the elbow, and is inflated to compress the artery, thus preventing blood flowing through it (p.222). The air in the cuff is released slowly, while bloodflow (or the lack of it) is listened for with a stethoscope over the artery at the elbow (p.226). As blood begins to flow through the artery again it produces sounds (p.116) that correspond to the pressure waves of the pulse (see below); the pressure at which the sounds are first heard is noted – it is called the *systolic blood pressure*. With the further release of air from the cuff, there comes a time when the beats are no longer audible, and the pressure at which this happens is also noted – this is the *diastolic blood pressure*.

The systolic pressure represents the pressure when the left ventricle contracts, and is normally about 120 mmHg (16 kPa). The diastolic pressure is the pressure remaining when the ventricle is relaxed, and is normally about 75 mmHg (10 kPa). Using these examples, the blood pressure is recorded in writing as 120/75, which in words is spoken as 'one twenty over seventy-five' or 'one twenty seventy-five'. The difference between the systolic and diastolic pressures is the *pulse pressure*, which in the above example would be 45 mmHg (6 kPa).

TAKING THE PULSE

The pulsation produced by left ventricular contraction is 'the pulse', which can be felt in the larger arteries near the surface of the body when they are gently pressed against underlying firm structures. The artery used most commonly for 'taking the pulse' is the radial artery at the wrist – giving the radial pulse (p.231) – but several other pulses are normally palpable (**8.3b**). Because of the distance from the heart, the pulsation of, say, the posterior tibial artery at the ankle (p.339) will be felt a fraction of a second later than that of the radial artery at the wrist, but both, of course, depend upon the left ventricle contracting sufficiently strongly to distend the larger arteries.

HYPERTENSION

High blood pressure (*hypertension*) exists when the blood pressure is 140/90 or more. It is the commonest of all cardiovascular disorders, but in most cases the cause is unknown – this is *primary* or *essential hypertension*. In some cases, however, hypertension is known to be due to renal disease, and rarely to a tumour of the adrenal gland.

In the common type, many patients may have no symptoms, but the condition is potentially dangerous since it can lead to arterial disease (especially of the heart and brain) and to heart failure. The detection of hypertension is important because antihypertensive therapy can reduce the risk of these complications. Often, relatively simple measures are effective, such as attention to weight loss and reduction of the use of alcohol, tobacco and salt (all helping to reduce the load on the circulation), but drug treatment may be necessary. This includes the use of diuretics (to reduce the body's water and salt contents, p.284) and beta-blockers, which lower the heart rate and reduce the force of the heartbeat, so helping to lower blood pressure.

PRESSURE SORES

The very low pressure in **capillaries** means that they are easily compressed, with the effect of stopping blood from flowing through them. To see this effect, press on the back of a finger just below where the nail grows out from the skin, and, after releasing the pressure, note how the skin has become pale, taking a few seconds to regain its normal colour.

Prolonged pressure over bony prominences (**4.1c**) may interfere seriously with the blood supply of the skin and underlying tissues, and may lead eventually to tissue breakdown and ulceration – *pressure sores* or *decubitus ulcers* (**8.6**). Sites such as the heels and the back over the sacrum are particularly likely to be affected in those who are bed-ridden. Constant attention must be given to unconscious or otherwise immobile patients, moving them at regular intervals into different positions to prevent this kind of tissue damage, which is entirely preventable with sufficient care. It must be remembered that skin itself has a better blood supply than underlying tissues, so any pressure damage to skin indicates even more extensive damage at deeper levels.

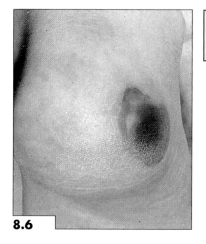

Fig. 8.6 Pressure sore on the heel.

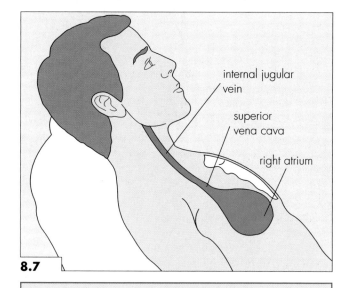

internal jugular vein

superior vena cava

right atrium

Fig. 8.7 Jugular venous pulse, due to contraction of the right atrium.
It is usually just observable (but not palpable) in the lower part of the neck when lying back at an angle of 45°, and is due to pulsation of the internal jugular vein (from contraction of the right atrium) transmitted through the overlying tissues of the neck.

JUGULAR VENOUS PULSE

The pressure in the right atrium (the *central venous pressure*) is normally about 5 mmHg, the equivalent of a column of blood 7 cm high. An indication of whether pressure in the right atrium is raised can be obtained simply by observing the jugular venous pulse. When sitting upright, the upper part of the internal jugular vein is collapsed but the lower part is distended for about 7 cm above the middle of the right atrium; this junction between the distended and collapsed parts is hidden behind the sternum and clavicle. When sitting back at an angle of 45° (**8.7**), the upper end of the distended part should be just visible above the clavicle and shows a slight pulsation – the *jugular venous pulse* (which is too weak to be palpable) – due to atrial contraction. Increased pressure in the vein (and therefore in the right atrium, as in right ventricular failure, p.119) will cause distension to a higher level.

PULMONARY CIRCULATION PRESSURE

In the pulmonary circulation, the blood pressure in the pulmonary artery is much lower than in the aorta – only 25/10 mmHg (8.5). It can be raised (giving rise to *pulmonary hypertension*) in such conditions as chronic lung diseases (chronic bronchitis or emphysema, p.125), where obstruction by lung tissues causes a greater and greater build-up of pressure in an attempt to maintain circulation, and with *pulmonary emboli* (blood clots in the pulmonary arteries, see p.332) which obstruct branches of the pulmonary arteries themselves.

PORTAL VENOUS PRESSURE

The pressure in the portal vein, which drains blood from the gastrointestinal tract and spleen to the liver, should be less than 10 mmHg (8.5); this is considerably more than the near-negligible pressure in the inferior vena cava into which the hepatic veins drain. Portal pressures higher than normal constitute *portal hypertension*. If due, for example, to 'strangulation' of veins in the liver (as in cirrhosis of the liver, where there is excessive fibrous tissue formation), it may result in the exudation of fluid from the surface of the liver and intestine into the peritoneal cavity (*ascites*), and to dilatation of veins at the sites of portal–systemic anastomosis (p.273).

BLOOD

The purpose of **blood** is to carry substances to and from the tissues of the body. It is a special type of connective tissue, consisting of a fluid part – **blood plasma** (comprising about 60% of the total amount of blood) – and a solid part – **blood cells** (making up the remaining 40%). Blood is contained within the cardiovascular system, but substances can be exchanged between blood and the surrounding tissues by passing through the walls of capillaries (p.51). The total amount of blood in the average body is about 5 litres; this is the *blood volume*, made up of 3 litres of plasma and 2 litres of cells.

BLOOD PLASMA

Blood plasma is 90% water. It contains a number of other constituents, among which are a variety of **mineral electrolytes**, with the most common being sodium and chloride ions.

Some of the most important constituents of plasma are the **plasma proteins**: albumin, globulin, fibrinogen and prothrombin. These proteins are responsible for the stickiness (viscosity) of blood, and their concentration in the plasma exerts an *osmotic pressure* that normally prevents too much fluid from passing out of the blood capillaries into the tissues, thus helping to control blood volume and blood pressure.

Plasma serves a very important function in *transport*. Most of the body's **carbon dioxide**, for example, is carried in plasma (p.77), in the form of **bicarbonate ions**. In addition, the products of digestion are absorbed into plasma and transported around the body, as are many other substances such as enzymes, hormones, waste products and antibodies.

BLOOD CELLS

Blood cells are of three main types: red blood cells (**erythrocytes**), white blood cells (**leucocytes**) and blood platelets (**thrombocytes**). All are developed from cells in bone marrow (p.11).

Erythrocytes

Red cells have the shape of discs that are concave on each side (8.8) and are about 7 μm in diameter. They have no nuclei, and are present in vast numbers – normally about 5 million per cubic millimeter of blood. They contain **haemoglobin**, a protein that contains iron and can combine with oxygen to form **oxyhaemoglobin** (p.76), so transporting this necessary element to all parts of the body. Oxyhaemoglobin is bright red in colour – hence the normal colour of arterial blood; haemoglobin that has given up its oxygen (**reduced haemoglobin**) is more purple – hence the more bluish colour of venous blood. Most of the carbon dioxide from the tissues is transported in the blood plasma; only a very small amount combines with the haemoglobin in the red cells (p.77). Red cells are not rigid structures; they can be made to change shape, so that they can easily be squeezed through the smallest capillaries.

The life span of erythrocytes is about 120 days; the constant production of new cells by bone marrow and their release into the bloodstream is matched by the destruction of old cells by the spleen and lymph nodes. The iron of the haemoglobin molecule is released in the liver, and can return in the bloodstream to bone marrow to be used again for new red cells. Some of the iron that is not reused in this way is converted in the liver to bile pigments which become excreted in the faeces (p.276).

Leucocytes

White cells are larger than red cells and all have nuclei; they are much less numerous, and there are three main types: **polymorphonuclear leucocytes**, **monocytes** and **lymphocytes**.

Polymorphonuclear leucocytes (from the Greek for 'many-shaped nuclei') have nuclei with a variable, lobed appearance, rather than the usual round shape (8.8a, b, c). They are also known as **granulocytes** because of the granules

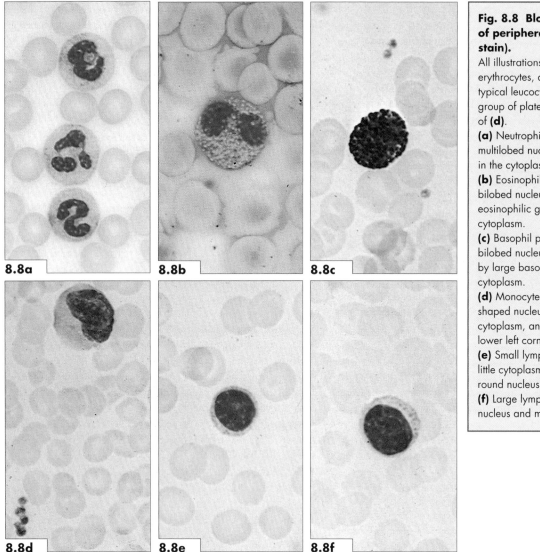

8.8a 8.8b 8.8c

8.8d 8.8e 8.8f

Fig. 8.8 Blood cells, in film of peripheral blood (Wright's stain).
All illustrations include many erythrocytes, and each shows typical leucocytes, with a small group of platelets in the lower part of **(d)**.
(a) Neutrophilic polymorphs, with multilobed nuclei and fine granules in the cytoplasm.
(b) Eosinophil polymorph, with bilobed nucleus and large eosinophilic granules in the cytoplasm.
(c) Basophil polymorph, with bilobed nucleus almost obscured by large basophilic granules in the cytoplasm.
(d) Monocyte, with a kidney-shaped nucleus and non-granular cytoplasm, and platelets in the lower left corner.
(e) Small lymphocyte, with very little cytoplasm surrounding the round nucleus.
(f) Large lymphocyte, with a larger nucleus and more cytoplasm.

that may be seen in their cytoplasm when they are stained for microscopic examination. There are three kinds of polymorphonuclear leucocytes, named after the staining reactions of their granules:

- **Neutrophilic polymorphonuclear leucocytes** (commonly called **neutrophils**, **PMNs** or simply '**polymorphs**'; 8.8a) account for 65% of all white cells, and are supremely important as the first line of defence against infection. *Leucocytosis*, which strictly means an increase in the total number of white cells, is usually taken to mean an increase in the number of neutrophils, and is a characteristic feature of infections. At infection sites, neutrophils pass through capillary walls into the tissues, where they ingest bacteria. Enzymes within the neutrophils digest and destroy what has been ingested, with the aim of bringing the infection under control. The process of cellular ingestion and destruction is *phagocytosis*, and any cell that carries out this function can be called a *phagocyte*. Neutrophils are the commonest phagocytes in the blood, and are attracted in large numbers to infection sites; in a septic finger or a boil, for example, the yellowish material called **pus** is a mass of phagocytes that have been helping to 'mop up' the infection. Neutrophils that circulate in the blood have a life span of only a few hours.

- **Eosinophilic polymorphonuclear leucocytes** (commonly called **eosinophils**, 8.8b) form about 4% of all white cells. Unlike neutrophils, they are *not* phagocytic; their numbers increase in some allergic and parasitic infections.

- **Basophilic polymorphonuclear leucocytes** (commonly called **basophils**, 8.8c) form about 1% of all white cells. They are not phagocytic, but instead secrete heparin and histamine which are concerned in the inflammatory response to disease and injury.

Monocytes (**8.8d**) are the largest of all white cells, and form about 5% of the total; they have usually rather horseshoe-shaped or kidney-shaped nuclei. Like polymorphs, they are phagocytic, migrating from capillaries to become **tissue macrophages** (the name given to phagocytic cells when they have left the bloodstream).

The remaining white cells (about 25% of the total) are the **lymphocytes** (**8.8e** and **f**). They have round nuclei and very little cytoplasm. Note that the standard laboratory stains for blood cells (such as that used for **8.8**) cannot distinguish between the B type and T type of lymphocyte, which are responsible for the body's immune responses (p.69); instead, special immunological methods are necessary.

Thrombocytes

Thrombocytes, more commonly known as **blood platelets**, are much smaller than red cells, and in fact are merely fragments of cytoplasm that have broken away from large cells in the bone marrow and entered the circulation. They are involved with the clotting of blood.

BLOOD CLOTTING

As part of the body's defence mechanisms, damage to blood vessels that causes the escape of blood sets up a series of reactions aimed at stopping further blood loss; the whole process is commonly called *haemostasis*. The ends of cut vessels constrict to narrow the escape route, and platelets adhere to the damaged endothelium to form a plug which, in capillaries, may alone be sufficient to stop bleeding – this is *primary haemostasis*, and occurs within 5 minutes of injury. The time until bleeding is stopped is called the *bleeding time*.

Further mechanisms are usually necessary to ensure the permanent elimination of blood loss, with *blood clotting* (*blood coagulation*) included in the list. Damaged vessels and platelets liberate an enzyme (**thromboplastin**) which, in the presence of calcium and other factors in the blood and local tissues, converts the plasma protein **prothrombin** into **thrombin**. Thrombin is another enzyme, and converts the plasma protein **fibrinogen** into **fibrin**, which is a thread-like substance that serves to trap red cells and platelets in its meshes, so forming a blood clot – this is *secondary haemostasis*, taking about 10 minutes. The time until clotting is completed is referred to as the *clotting time* – not to be confused with the bleeding time mentioned above. Later, the clot retracts, squeezing out some **serum** (plasma from which fibrinogen has been removed) and, if on the skin surface, a hardened scab eventually forms.

The above account has emphasized the principal steps in clotting, but various other substances (officially called **factors**) are involved at different stages of the process. One in particular, **factor VIII**, must be mentioned, since its deficiency results in *haemophilia* (the commonest congenital blood disorder). Haemophilia is associated with often-severe haemorrhages into various tissues such as skin, joints and internal organs. Treatment of factor VIII deficiency involves the injection of a stored form of factor VIII, which is prepared from frozen plasma (**cryofactor VIII**).

While after injury the process of blood coagulation is obviously beneficial, there are other circumstances when steps must be taken to prevent it or diminish it, e.g. after deep venous thrombosis (p.332), in haemodialysis machines (p.287), or in blood taken for laboratory examination or stored for transfusion (see below). There are several possible ways in which the sequence of clotting events can be interrupted. **Heparin** is an anticoagulant that is normally present in the blood in small quantities; it acts by interfering with the formation of thrombin, and it can be given therapeutically to increase the thrombin concentration. The fact that **calcium** is necessary for the conversion of prothrombin into thrombin is made use of in preserving blood for transfusion; if the calcium is removed, thrombin will not form. Sodium citrate is added to the donor's blood as it is withdrawn; the calcium reacts with the sodium citrate to become calcium citrate and so is no longer free to take part in the mechanism of coagulation.

BLOOD CELL FORMATION

The formation of erythrocytes (*erythropoiesis*) takes place in red bone marrow which, in normal adults, is found in the ends of long bones, the bodies of vertebrae, and flat bones such as the sternum and the ilium of the hip bone (the last two sites being used for obtaining specimens of bone marrow).

Primitive stem cells in the marrow give rise to **erythroblasts**, cells that are 'committed' to developing into erythrocytes. During the course of their development, there is repeated and rapid cell division, with each generation of cells accumulating more and more haemoglobin. The last generation of erythroblasts, called **normoblasts**, eventually discard their nuclei and are then known as erythrocytes. The newly formed erythrocytes, however, are distinguishable from the more mature forms (into which they develop) by special staining methods; these early erythrocytes are called **reticulocytes**. (With special stains, the residual RNA in their cytoplasm appears as a network, or 'reticulum'; as the cells mature, all of this RNA is gradually lost.)

In a film (microscope slide) of normal blood, 99% of red cells are mature erythrocytes, while 1% are reticulocytes. An increased number of reticulocytes in the peripheral blood indicates increased red cell production; most of them remain normally in bone marrow, as do all of the earlier nucleated forms of developing red cells.

Among the ingredients necessary for erythropoiesis are **iron, folic acid, vitamin B$_{12}$, intrinsic factor** and **erythropoietin. Iron** is required for the formation of the haemoglobin of red cells (p.61), and is obtained by absorption from the small intestine. **Folic acid** and **vitamin B$_{12}$ (cobalamin)** are necessary for normal erythropoiesis, and are also obtained from the diet. However, vitamin B_{12} can only be absorbed by the intestine in the presence of **intrinsic factor**, which is secreted by the parietal cells of the stomach (see below). **Erythropoietin (EPO)** is a hormone that is secreted primarily by the kidneys, and which is responsible for starting off the process of erythropoiesis from the primitive bone marrow cells, and regulating the rate of red cell production. There have been recent reports of the use of EPO to increase athletic performance by increasing the number of erythrocytes and, hence, the oxygen-carrying capacity of the blood (p.76).

The various **white blood cells** also develop from stem cells in red bone marrow. At a very early stage, the primitive cells become 'committed' to developing along one of a set of possible routes, with each route producing one or other of the different kinds of granular cells, monocytes or lymphocytes. Blood platelets are formed from exceptionally large marrow cells – the **megakaryocytes**.

Many factors influence blood cell production, and there are many kinds of blood disorders that affect the different types of cell. Red cell production is influenced particularly by oxygen requirements, as evidenced by those who live at high altitudes and exhibit *erythrocytosis (polycythaemia)* – an increased number of circulating red cells – in order to compensate for the lower pressure of oxygen. Air travellers who find themselves suddenly in a high altitude area may be unduly breathless for some days (the period of acclimatization, p.77). This lasts until the bone marrow has had time to respond to the relative oxygen lack (*hypoxia*) by releasing more red cells into the circulation to compensate for the smaller amount of oxygen carried by each cell.

Bone marrow, like any other organ or tissue, has an arterial blood supply and venous drainage, and its capillaries are usually dilated blood spaces (**sinusoids**). When red cells and white cells are ready to be released, they traverse the walls of the sinusoids to gain access to the vascular space. Normally only the fully developed cells (and a few reticulocytes) are released into the veins to join the general circulation, but in some blood diseases (see below) immature forms may leave the marrow as well.

BLOOD DISEASES

Anaemia is characterized by a reduction in the normal amount of haemoglobin; this may occur either because the haemoglobin content of the red cells is lowered, or because the number of red cells is lowered.

There are many types and causes of anaemia, with the commonest being *iron-deficiency anaemia*. This type of anaemia is usually due to some kind of chronic blood loss (e.g. from bleeding ulceration in the gastrointestinal tract or from heavy menstrual periods), or may occur when the amount of iron in the diet is not sufficient to compensate for the blood loss – dietary supplements of iron will be needed in this case, especially in menstruating females, who require twice as much dietary iron as males.

Pernicious anaemia (Addisonian anaemia, vitamin B_{12} deficiency anaemia) is much less common, and is usually due to malfunction of the parietal cells of the stomach lining (p.257). These cells fail to secrete intrinsic factor, the agent necessary for vitamin B_{12} absorption. Without vitamin B_{12}, cell division in the bone marrow is delayed, the erythroblasts grow larger than usual between divisions (and are called **megaloblasts**) and the red cells in the blood that are derived from them are also enlarged. (Coincidentally, malfunction of the parietal cells also leads to inadequate hydrochloric acid production in the stomachs of afflicted individuals.) Giving vitamin B_{12} by intramuscular injection (not by mouth, since it cannot be absorbed) rapidly restores the blood to normal.

Diseases of the white blood cells include the various kinds of *leukaemia*, in which there is uncontrolled (cancerous) production of leucocytes in bone marrow and lymphoid tissues. The lymphocytic cells are more commonly involved than the granulocytes, with the two types of the disease being called *lymphoid leukaemia* and *myeloid leukaemia* respectively. Modern treatment includes controlling the bone marrow through chemotherapy and irradiation, or destroying it and replacing it by bone marrow transplants from a suitably matched donor (or even from the patient during a period of remission). The marrow is obtained from the donor's iliac crest, and is transfused intravenously; marrow cells circulate and settle in the old marrow spaces, producing new cells in the bloodstream in about two to three weeks.

For haemophilia, see p.63.

BLOOD GROUPS AND TRANSFUSION

Blood cannot be taken from one person and given safely to another – *transfused* – without first checking to see whether the blood of the patient (the *recipient*) and the blood of the *donor* are compatible. Checking must be carried out because red blood cells carry **antigens** on their surfaces, and blood plasma contains the **antibodies** appropriate for them (p.69). Precisely which antigens and antibodies are carried is determined genetically by inheritance from parents, and is thus 'built in' to an individual's blood. (In contrast, the usual mode of antibody production requires the stimulus of the antigen and the participation of B lymphocytes, see p.69.)

ABO Blood Groups

Red blood cells contain protein molecules on their surfaces that act as antigens (p.69); they are known as **A** and **B agglutinogens**. When red cells carry the A agglutinogen, the blood in which they occur is said to belong to *group A*. If the B agglutinogen is present, the blood belongs to *group B*. If both A and B occur, the blood is *group AB*, while if neither is found the blood belongs to *group O*. These are the four ABO *blood groups*, or *blood types*.

Blood plasma contains antibodies known as **anti-A** and **anti-B agglutinins**; these are capable of reacting with A and

B agglutinogens (an antigen–antibody reaction) resulting in a clumping-together or *agglutination* of red cells, followed by their breakdown (*haemolysis*). Obviously, in any one person's blood the red cells do not react with the plasma. Thus, people with group A red cells have anti-B in their plasma (if they had anti-A they would destroy their own cells), those with group B cells have anti-A in plasma, those with AB cells have no plasma agglutinins, and those with group O cells have both anti-A and anti-B in plasma.

In blood transfusion, what matters is the effect that the patient's plasma will have on the donor's cells. Since patients with group AB cells have plasma with no agglutinins, such people are called *universal recipients* and can receive blood of any group. By contrast, patients with group O blood can receive blood only from other group O individuals; the anti-A and anti-B agglutinins in their plasma would attack the red cells donated by Type A, Type B or Type AB people. Type A individuals can receive group A and group O blood (the anti-A agglutinins in the group O plasma are diluted sufficiently during transfusion so that they do not damage the recipient's own red cells), and Type B people can receive group B and group O blood. From the foregoing it is perhaps clear why people with group O blood are called *universal donors*.

Rhesus Factor

The ABO antigens are not the only ones that may be present on red cells. Among many others of lesser importance, there is one that is of great significance in pregnancy, the *rhesus (Rh) factor*. About 75% of Caucasians have the Rh factor by inheritance, and are said to be *rhesus positive (Rh+)*; those without the antigen are *rhesus negative (Rh-)*.

There is no naturally occurring (inherited) rhesus antibody in blood plasma, but its formation may be stimulated by the transfusion of Rh+ blood or by pregnancy. If a Rh- female becomes pregnant by a Rh+ male, the fetus may be Rh+ and at birth some fetal red cells can cross the placenta into the mother's plasma and so stimulate an antibody response with the production of anti-Rh antibody – called *anti-D* – which will now persist in the mother's blood throughout her life. This has no immediate effect, but in the next pregnancy, the antibody may pass back to a Rh+ fetus through the placenta and destroy (haemolyse) the baby's red cells. This haemolytic disease of the newborn (*erythroblastosis fetalis*) may occur in varying degrees; in the severest cases the child dies or is born dead, sometimes there may be jaundice (due to the breakdown products of haemoglobin from the red cells, see p.276), and sometimes there may be no apparent effect at all. Babies jaundiced due to this condition can be given an exchange tranfusion of Rh- blood. It is thus important that Rh- females of child-bearing age are not given transfusions of Rh+ blood; this at least prevents one of the causes of antibody formation. It would also of course be prevented if Rh- females did not become pregnant by Rh+ males, but an enquiry into blood groups is not a normal preliminary to love-making!

BLOOD EXAMINATION

Specimens of blood for laboratory examination are usually obtained in a syringe, by introducing the needle into a vein (*venepuncture*) in the elbow region (p.225); the sample is then tranferred to a storage tube containing a suitable anticoagulant. If only a drop or two is required, as for making a *blood film* (blood smear) for microscopy, then pricking an ear lobe or the pulp of a finger (or the side of the heel in an infant) will provide a sufficient sample.

The commonest tests include the *complete blood count*, which involves a red blood cell count (RBC), white blood cell count (WBC, including the differential count to determine the proportion of each cell type), platelet count, estimations of the haemoglobin (Hb) and haematocrit (Hct), and the *erythrocyte sedimentation rate* (ESR).

The *haematocrit*, otherwise known as the *packed-cell volume* (PCV), is an estimation of the percentage of red cells in whole blood. It is either determined by centrifuging blood in a special tube, or is calculated using an electronic blood counting machine, and is useful for assessing the degree of anaemia.

The ESR is determined by placing blood that contains an anticoagulant into a narrow tube, and observing how far red cells fall towards the bottom of the tube in one hour. A normal result is less than 15 mm; a higher result suggests some kind of infection (without specifying which kind), but the test can be a useful indicator of the need to look for an inflammatory focus.

CHAPTER 9

LYMPHATIC SYSTEM

The **lymphatic system** (**9.1** and **9.2**) is concerned with the *production*, *storage* and *recirculation* of **lymphocytes** – the cells that are chiefly responsible for the immune response (see below) – the *storage* of **macrophages** (**phagocytes**), the *drainage* of **surplus tissue fluid** into the bloodstream, and the *transport* of **absorbed fat** from the intestine to the bloodstream. The principal organs of this system – often called the **lymphoid organs** – are the the **lymph nodes**, the **tonsils**, the **spleen** and the **thymus**. In addition, the system includes some aggregations of lymphoid tissue in non-lymphoid organs, such as the digestive tract. Finally, there is an extensive network of lymphatic channels (**lymphatics**) that resemble blood vessels but contain the fluid lymph instead of blood.

All tissues and organs, with the exception of the brain, spinal cord, eye and ear, drain lymph by way of lymphatics to adjacent lymph nodes; this *lymphatic drainage* assumes major importance, because it is a possible pathway for the spread of cancer cells. The successful treatment of the common cancers – skin, breast, lung, colon, stomach, uterus – depends to a large extent on whether the disease can be 'caught' early enough, before there has been lymphatic (or vascular) spread. It is unfortunate that in the anatomical dissecting room it is difficult to appreciate the importance of lymphatic channels because they are rarely identifiable; the autopsy room is the best place for seeing the effects of lymphatic spread.

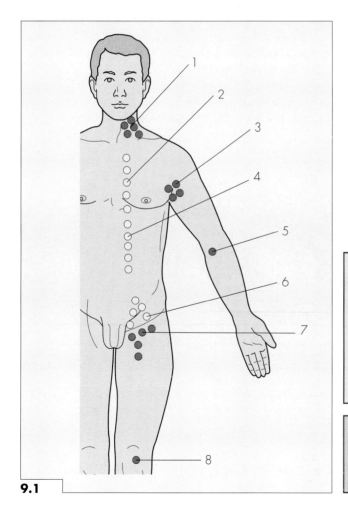

9.1

Fig. 9.1 Major sites of lymph nodes.
Those nodes that are (or may become) palpable are indicated by red dots, and those that are impalpable even when diseased are shown as yellow dots. The illustration is intended to convey the general positions of nodes and not their numbers, which are variable; e.g. there may be about 30 in the axillary group and 12 or so in the inguinal group, but only two in the popliteal group and there is only a single epitrochlear node behind the elbow.

1	Cervical	5	Epitrochlear
2	Parasternal	6	Iliac
3	Axillary	7	Inguinal
4	Aortic	8	Popliteal

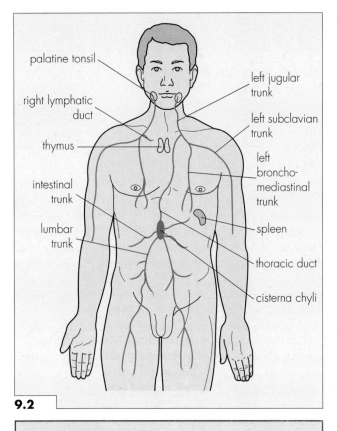

9.2

Fig. 9.2 Major lymphatic channels, and the tonsils, thymus and spleen.
The smaller lymphatic vessels that run with or near arteries and veins are not shown.

LYMPHOID ORGANS

Lymph nodes (**9.1** and **9.3a**), which are small bean-like structures, are found grouped together in certain areas such as the neck, axilla and inguinal region – where, when affected by disease, they are palpable – and in parts of the thorax, abdomen and pelvis – where they cannot be felt. They consist of a connective tissue framework, within which are embedded **lymphoid follicles**; these are rounded collections of lymphocytes with a central region (the **germinal centre**) of cells that are capable of undergoing division and of producing new lymphocytes. The nodes also contain many macrophages. There are lymphatic channels leading into and out of the nodes, which can thus filter the lymph passing through them. Infective agents such as bacteria, that may be present in the lymph, are filtered out and destroyed. Lymph nodes are described further in the appropriate regions.

The **tonsils** (properly called the **palatine tonsils**, **9.2** and **9.3b**) are in the oral part of the pharynx and are visible through the open mouth. The **pharyngeal tonsil** (which when enlarged is commonly called the **adenoids**) is on the posterior wall of the nasopharynx – too high to be seen through the open mouth unless an inspection mirror is used. Tonsils have a similar structure to lymph nodes, but are partly covered by stratified squamous epithelium. They are further described with the pharynx (p.182). Groups of lymphoid follicles in the back of the tongue (p.149) are often called the **lingual tonsil**.

The **spleen** (**9.2** and **9.3c**) lies in the upper left part of the abdomen beside the left kidney, well under cover of the costal margin, and is not palpable unless grossly enlarged. It also

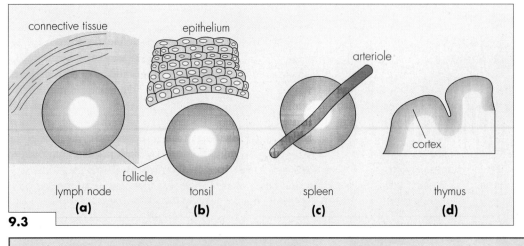

9.3

Fig. 9.3 Diagrammatic representation of the essential histological features of lymphoid organs.
(a) Lymph nodes: lymphoid follicles with connective tissue on the surface.
(b) Tonsil: lymphoid follicles with overlying stratified squamous epithelium.
(c) Spleen: lymphoid follicles with arterioles passing through them.
(d) Thymus: no follicles but a continuous cortex of lymphoid tissue.

contains many lymphoid follicles, but here they have characteristically small arterioles running through them. The spleen is further described on p.279.

The **thymus** (**9.2** and **9.3d**) lies in the front of the upper part of the thorax, in front of the heart and the great vessels, and extending into the lower part of the neck. It is a prominent organ up to the age of puberty, after which it slowly regresses and is mostly replaced by fatty tissue. It is responsible for forming the T lymphocytes that migrate from it to colonize other lymphoid tissues (see below). It is described further on p.103.

Apart from being present in lymph nodes, tonsils and spleen, lymphoid follicles are found scattered singly in mucous membranes – especially those of the alimentary tract (including the appendix). In the terminal part of the small intestine, a number become aggregated together to form **Peyer's patches**. As in the lymph nodes and other lymphoid organs, all of these follicles are the site of lymphocyte production and house macrophages.

LYMPHATIC VESSELS AND LYMPH

Lymphatic vessels (**9.2**) resemble very thin-walled veins, and contain many valves to ensure one-way flow. They form communications between adjacent lymph nodes and drain fluid (lymph) from most body tissues as well as transporting lymph and lymphocytes from nodes and other lymphoid organs.

Lymph is essentially surplus tissue fluid that has become collected into the lymphatic channels by passing through the walls of the smallest of them (the **lymphatic capillaries**), and contains lymphocytes that have escaped from the nodes. Lymph flow depends largely upon the pressure from surrounding structures, since there is very little smooth muscle in the walls of even the largest lymphatics. Eventually, lymph from most of the body reaches the venous bloodstream via the **thoracic duct** – the body's largest lymphatic channel.

The duct begins in the upper abdomen (p.103) and runs up, in front of the vertebral column, to the left side of the root of the neck, where it drains into the junction of the internal jugular and subclavian veins (p.179). Lymph from the right upper limb, the right side of the thorax and the right side of the head and neck follows a much shorter channel – the **right lymphatic duct** – which joins at the junction between the right internal jugular vein and the subclavian vein.

Lymph from the gastrointestinal tract contains most of the absorbed fat, which thus does not reach the liver by the portal venous blood like other absorbed substances, but via the thoracic duct and the systemic blood circulation (p.85).

IMMUNE RESPONSE

In the section on blood (p.61) it has been mentioned that polymorphs and monocytes are phagocytic cells. Phagocytosis is one of the body's two great defence mechanisms. The other is the *immune response*, for which lymphocytes are responsible but in which phagocytosis also plays a part. There are two types of immune response – *humoral* and *cellular* – that differ in whether molecules or cells are the essential agents.

HUMORAL IMMUNE RESPONSE

When substances such as bacteria and other micro-organisms enter the body, they are not only engulfed by macrophages in an attempt to destroy them, but are also recognized as 'foreign' substances (i.e. not part of the body's own 'self') and another reaction occurs in an attempt to destroy them. The material that induces this defensive reaction is known as an **antigen**, and the substance produced to react to it is an **antibody**.

Antibodies are *protein molecules* that are manufactured in large quantities by **plasma cells**. (Plasma cells are cells that are derived by proliferation from the type of lymphocytes called **B cells**, but which are under the influence of other lymphocytes – a type of **T cell**.) The antibody molecules enter the bloodstream and circulate with the blood plasma as **immunoglobulins**. They leave the blood eventually, and become attached to the antigens that have become exposed on the surface of the ingesting macrophage; the combination (in the presence of certain other complex plasma components, known as **complement**) can be destroyed by phagocytosis. Macrophages and certain other cells, including the Langerhans cells of skin (p.18), are necessary for preparing the antigen in such a way that the antibody can combine with it. The production of antibody *molecules* constitutes the *humoral immune response* (from the old use of the word 'humour' meaning 'fluid' – the molecules are released from cells into tissue fluid and blood plasma). Each antigen induces the formation of its own particular antibody, which is effective only against its own antigen, and no others.

The body is continually subjected to hundreds of thousands of antigenic insults (through the respiratory and alimentary tracts, skin wounds, etc.), resulting in hundreds of thousands of different antibodies being produced, especially in early life. The amount of lymphoid tissue in a child of about 10 years is twice as great as that in adult life, reflecting this immune activity. Many lymphocytes are short-lived, but some remain in the lymphoid tissues and, when an antigen invades again, those cells with a 'memory' for it will recognize it and rapidly begin the production of new antibody. This is the basis of *immunization* against certain diseases such as measles, whooping cough and diphtheria. Preparations of the causal organisms that have been rendered harmless, but which remain antigenic, are injected into the body – as *vaccines* – so that some B lymphocytes can be programmed to produce the appropriate antibodies; if and when the real (harmful) infection enters the body, it will at once be recognized and more antibodies can be formed without delay, so suppressing the infection before it has time to develop.

The antigen–antibody reaction is also the basis of *allergic reactions*, which may be local or general in their effects. In these reactions, the antigens are substances such as certain pollens, dust, animal fur or even foods, each stimulating their own antibody production. The ensuing reaction varies greatly, but with pollen for example the result is hay fever (see p.161).

CELLULAR IMMUNE RESPONSE

The second type of immune reaction, the *cellular immune response*, depends not upon the production of antibody molecules, but on *cells* – in this case a type of T lymphocyte. These cells circulate in the blood and lymph, and either destroy the antigen (e.g. the 'foreign' bacteria) themselves, or stimulate macrophages to destroy it by phagocytosis.

It is this type of reaction that is responsible for the rejection of grafted tissue that occurs when the grafts are between individuals who are not identical twins. The grafted tissue is antigenic, since it is recognized as 'non-self' by the recipient. Where possible, grafts such as skin grafts are taken from the patient's own skin so that there will be no immune reaction. However, for transplanting an organ such as a kidney – when no identical twin is available – *tissue typing* (see below) must be carried out to choose a donor whose tissue, immunologically speaking, is as close as possible to that of the patient. In such a case, the graft rejection process is minimal and can be suppressed by an 'immunosuppressive' drug such as cyclosporin, which prevents the multiplication of T cells and so reduces the number in circulation.

ORIGIN OF LYMPHOCYTES

All lymphocytes are initially produced in bone marrow, but they may mature in different sites. **B cells** complete their maturation in bone marrow itself, and then leave, via the bloodstream, to take up residence in the lymphoid tissues. **T cells,** by contrast, leave the bone marrow as immature cells, and then mature in the thymus. From here, mature T cells migrate to the lymphoid tissues, which thus come to house a mixture of B and T cells. Both B and T cells are capable of *recirculation*, and leave the lymphoid tissues periodically via the lymphatics, entering the bloodstream along with the lymph (p.69) and reaching the lymphoid tissues once again via the blood.

The T cells are so named because they depend on the **T**hymus for their development and, since T cells are responsible for cellular immunity, this kind of immunity is dependent upon the thymus. There are several subgroups of T cells, and the whole subject has given rise to the science of *immunology* which is one of the most active areas of current research in the whole of medicine.

AUTOIMMUNITY

Occasionally, instead of just reacting to 'foreign' material, the body's own lymphocytes appear to attack their own body tissues – giving rise to *autoimmune diseases*; the reason why they do this is not yet clear. Conditions that are likely to be the result of autoimmunity include rheumatoid arthritis, multiple sclerosis, thyroid diseases (such as myxoedema and thyrotoxicosis), pernicious anaemia (plus some other blood diseases), and various skin diseases. Corticosteroids may be helpful in rheumatoid arthritis because they suppress the action of B and T lymphocytes (as well as being anti-inflammatory).

AIDS

The human immunodeficiency virus (HIV) prevents the proliferation of certain T cells; this is the fundamental defect in AIDS – the *Acquired Immune Deficiency Syndrome*. The body's immune system gradually fails, so the usual resistance to infections is lost, and even infective organisms that would normally have no adverse effect (because the immune system destroys them) are allowed to develop unchecked.

TISSUE TYPING

Apart from having a compatible ABO (red cell) blood group, those who are prospective donors for graft or transplant tissues or organs must also be tested for lymphocyte compatibility. Each individual has a specific set of genes (the **Major Histocompatibility Complex – MHC**) that carries the code for a particular family of glycoproteins which, when inserted into cell membranes, play an important role in the recognition of 'self versus nonself'. These cell-surface glycoproteins were called the HLA antigens (**Human Leucocyte-Associated antigens**) because they were first demonstrated on leucocytes, but it is now known that at least three of them are present on all nucleated cells, and not only on leucocytes.

In any given individual, the major HLA antigens are identical on each cell, but in another individual a different set will be found. Because of the enormous diversity of HLA antigens in the human population, the chances of finding a perfectly matched pair of individuals is rare indeed – unless, of course, they are identical twins. Therefore, finding a donor for a transplant patient is a difficult task that involves *tissue typing* – a set of tests that are designed to determine the degree to which the HLA antigens differ between the potential donor and the recipient.

LYMPHOID DISEASES

Apart from involvement in diseases of other systems by lymphatic spread, the organs of the lymphatic system are affected by their own diseases. Among the commonest are *lymphoid leukaemia*, where there is excessive production of lymphocytes (p.64), and *Hodgkin's disease* (*lymphadenoma*), which is of unknown cause, where there is generalized enlargement of lymph nodes and organs – usually first recognized by painless enlargement of the cervical nodes, and in which there may be chest symptoms due to enlargement of thoracic nodes. Combinations of radiotherapy and chemotherapy can now offer good chances of cure when the condition is recognized early.

The virus infection causing AIDS has been mentioned above, together with some other examples of conditions involving the immune response.

CHAPTER 10
RESPIRATORY SYSTEM

The purpose of the **respiratory system** is to transfer *oxygen* (O_2) from the air into the bloodstream, and to transfer *carbon dioxide* (CO_2) from the blood into the air. This exchange of gases takes place in the **alveoli** (air sacs) of the two **lungs**, which occupy each side of the thorax (thoracic cavity or chest). The thorax provides a firm but slightly mobile container within which the lungs can expand and contract during breathing (*respiration*).

A lubricated membrane – the **pleura** – lines the interior of the thoracic cavity on each side, and also covers the outer surface of each lung. The parts of the pleura in these two locations are referred to as the **parietal pleura** (lining the cavity, from the Greek 'parietes' meaning 'wall'), and the **visceral pleura** (covering the lungs, which are included among the body's internal organs or viscera).

Breathing is brought about mainly by the **diaphragm** – the sheet of skeletal muscle that separates the thorax from the abdomen. Air is conducted to and from the lungs by the rest of the respiratory system (the **respiratory tract**), which is essentially a conducting pathway without any gaseous exchange. The tract modifies the incoming air in a protective manner, by adjusting its temperature, making it moist and trapping dust particles. Part of the tract (the **larynx**) has the important function of producing speech.

RESPIRATORY ORGANS

The **respiratory organs** (10.1) consist of the **nose** and **paranasal air sinuses**, the **pharynx, larynx, trachea, bronchi** and **lungs**.

The **nose** consists of the **external nose** – the projection on the face with two openings (**nostrils** or **anterior nares**) – and the **nasal cavity**, which is the internal part which is divided into right and left halves by the **nasal septum**. Each half of the nasal cavity communicates with the **paranasal air sinuses** (air-filled spaces in the skull within the maxillae and the frontal, ethmoid and sphenoid bones) via small openings, and by a large opening at the back (the **posterior naris** or **choana**) with the pharynx. Further details of the nose and sinuses begin on p.153.

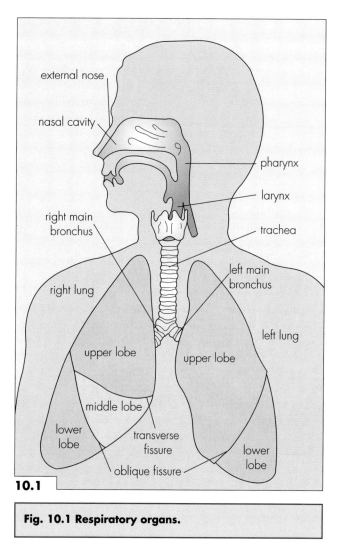

10.1

Fig. 10.1 Respiratory organs.

The **pharynx** is a muscular tube (of skeletal muscle) about 12 cm (5 inches) long, which extends down from the base of the skull, consisting of nasal, oral and laryngeal parts. The nasal part (the **nasopharynx**), into which the nasal cavities open, belongs exclusively to the respiratory tract, but the oral and laryngeal parts (the **oropharynx** and the **laryngo-**

pharynx), commonly called the **throat**, belong to both the respiratory and alimentary tracts. During swallowing, the soft palate closes the nasopharynx off from the oropharynx. Further details of the pharynx begin on p.182.

At its lower end, the **laryngopharynx** opens into two structures: the larynx anteriorly, and the oesophagus directly below. (The oesophagus belongs to the digestive system and is described on p.103.) The **larynx**, which is the organ of speech, opens off from the front of the laryngopharynx and contains the **vocal folds** (or **vocal cords**) whose movements produce sounds. The larynx has a framework consisting of various cartilages; the largest is the **thyroid cartilage** which produces the bulge at the front of the neck commonly called the **Adam's apple** (**laryngeal prominence**). Further details of the larynx begin on p.186.

At the level of C6 vertebra, the lower end of the larynx continues into the **trachea** (**windpipe**), which passes from the lower neck into the upper thorax. It is a muscular tube about 10 cm (4.5 in) long, whose wall contains U-shaped strips of cartilage (called 'rings' – but they are never complete circles) which keep the lumen continuously open.

Just below the level of T4 vertebra, the trachea divides into the right and left main or **principal bronchi**, which enter the lungs.

The **left lung** is divided into *two* lobes (upper and lower) by an oblique fissure, and is somewhat smaller than the right lung because the heart bulges towards the left.

The **right lung** is divided into *three* lobes (upper, middle and lower) by oblique and transverse fissures.

The region of each lung where the main bronchus enters is called the **hilum**. Other important structures that pass through this region are the two pulmonary veins (leaving the lung) and the single pulmonary artery (entering the lung) (see **15.26** and **15.27**).

Within the lungs, the main bronchi divide to form **lobar bronchi**, one for each lobe, and each in turn divides into **segmental bronchi** (see **15.25**). Further subdivision results in a profusion of smaller tubes (**bronchioles**) that eventually open into the microscopically small air sacs (**alveoli**) through whose thin walls gaseous exchange can occur with the plasma and red cells of the blood in adjacent capillaries (**10.2**). Due to its extensive branching pattern, the system of bronchi and bronchioles within each lung is often referred to as the **bronchial tree**.

Further details of the trachea and lungs begin on p.120.

RESPIRATION

Breathing in and out (*inspiration* and *expiration*, together called *respiration* or *external respiration*) is essential for taking in O_2 and getting rid of CO_2. The diaphragm and intercostal muscles (p.100) are normally used for this purpose.

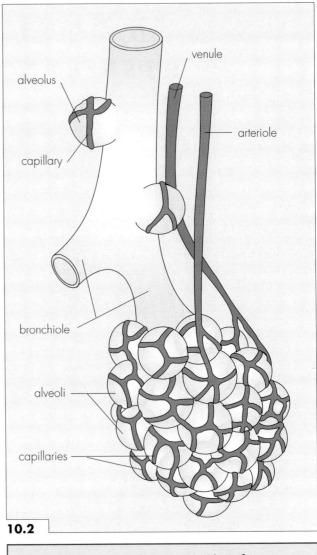

10.2

Fig. 10.2 Diagrammatic representation of bronchioles, alveoli (air sacs) and blood capillaries. Two single alveoli with overlying capillaries are seen opening off a bronchiole, with a cluster of alveoli and vessels at the end of the bronchiole.

In quiet *inspiration* at rest, the domes of the diaphragm move down about 1.5 cm, and some of the intercostal muscles elevate the ribs; both of these movements increase the internal capacity of the thorax. The visceral and parietal layers of the pleura are kept in contact with one another by a film of fluid so that, as the thoracic walls expand, the lungs also expand and draw in air. The **pleural cavity** is thus not a completely empty space, but is a closed space with a slightly negative pressure; it contains a very small amount of tissue fluid which, by its surface tension, maintains contact between the two layers of the pleura. In *expiration*, the thoracic capacity decreases as the inspiratory muscles relax – the lungs then shrink by their own elasticity. The two layers of pleura remain in contact at all times.

In deep or forced respiration, as in vigorous exercise or disease, other muscles can act as 'accessory muscles of respiration' to assist the diaphragm and intercostals. The range of downward movement of the diaphragm can increase to as much as 9 cm: sternocleidomastoid and the scalene muscles (pp.175–176) help to elevate the sternum and upper ribs; the quadratus lumborum (p.253) stabilizes the twelfth rib and (with the arms abducted) the pectoralis major and latissimus dorsi (p.213) help to lift the ribs outwards.

In certain injuries or diseases (such as a stab wound of the chest wall or the bursting of an emphysematous bulla, p.125) the negative pressure within the pleural cavity is lost – resulting in a condition called *pneumothorax*. As the pressure in the pleural cavity becomes the same as atmospheric pressure, the surface tension of the fluid film between the two layers of pleura is no longer sufficient to keep them in contact. The natural elasticity of lung tissue will then cause the lung to collapse, 'breaking away' from the parietal pleura. This is why, with pleural drainage via a tube inserted into the pleural cavity, the tube must be led into a bottle of fluid so that the cavity does not communicate with the outside atmosphere (**15.27**).

RESPIRATORY RATE

The normal rhythm of breathing is controlled by groups of nerve cells in the brainstem (p.195), called the **respiratory centres**; these nerve cells send impulses down the spinal cord to act on the spinal nerve fibres that supply the diaphragm and intercostal muscles. The movement of air into and out of the lungs (*pulmonary ventilation*) enables the necessary exchange of gases to occur by *diffusion* (see below). The repeated cycles of inspiration followed by expiration (*respiratory cycles*) occur in adults at rest about 12 –16 times per minute (the *respiratory rate*), with inspiration lasting approximately 2 seconds and expiration 3 seconds.

If disease or injury cuts off the nervous control of respiration, it must be restored by artificial means, or death will ensue. In anaesthesia, the respiratory muscles are often deliberately paralyzed and an artificial respirator (a *ventilator*) is used to keep pulmonary ventilation going. As an emergency measure in cardiac arrest, artificial respiration by mouth-to-mouth breathing is part of the process of *Cardiopulmonary Resuscitation* (CPR) – see p.126.

EXCHANGE OF GASES

The **alveoli** (p.124) are the only parts of the lung where gaseous exchange can occur (**10.2**); the rest of the bronchial tree is simply a system of delivery tubes leading to them. There are perhaps 300 million alveoli in the lungs, with a total surface area of about 80 square metres (the size of a tennis court, say). Since lung capillaries come into contact

with about half of this, the area available for the passage of oxygen and carbon dioxide is also about half of this – it is still enormous considering the relatively modest size of the lungs.

Air is a mixture of gases: it is mostly nitrogen (N_2) which is of no importance as far as normal respiration is concerned, but has a content of O_2 which is essential for life, and a very small amount of CO_2 (see below). The purpose of breathing is to enable the O_2 that is breathed in to be transferred from air to blood so that it can then be transported all over the body by the arterial (oxygenated) blood. At the same time, venous (deoxygenated) blood with a low O_2 content but a high content of CO_2 (the ultimate breakdown product of the chemical activities within body cells) is brought to the lungs so that the CO_2 can be discharged into the air when breathing out. The whole process of transferring O_2 and CO_2 between air and tissue cells thus depends on two systems: the respiratory system, which acts between air and blood, and the cardiovascular system, which acts between blood and tissues. Thus, disease that affects either of these two systems, respiratory or cardiovascular, may interfere with the essential delivery of O_2.

In ordinary quiet breathing, the volume of air inspired is about 500 ml, and the same volume is expired; this amount is called the *tidal volume* (**10.3**). Multiplying this by the number of respirations per minute gives the *minute volume* – the amount of air inspired in one minute (e.g. 500 ml × 12 = 6 litres). In *forced inspiration*, i.e. breathing in (inhaling) as much air as possible, an additional 3000 ml may enter; this is the *inspiratory reserve volume* or *complemental air*. In *forced expiration*, i.e. breathing out (exhaling) as much air as

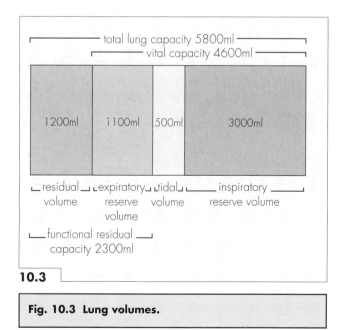

10.3

Fig. 10.3 Lung volumes.

possible, about 1100 ml can be expelled in addition to the tidal volume; this additional amount is the *expiratory reserve volume* or *supplemental air*. These three amounts added together: tidal volume (500 ml), inspiratory reserve volume (3000 ml) and expiratory reserve volume (1100 ml) give the *vital capacity* – the maximum amount of air that can be expired (about 4600 ml) after taking in the deepest possible breath. However, the lungs can never be completely exhausted of air; some always remains, and the so-called *residual volume* can amount to as much as 1200 ml. Adding this 1200 ml to the vital capacity of 4600 ml gives 5800 ml (nearly 6 litres) – the *total lung capacity*. This obviously varies with body size.

As there is always some residual air in the lungs, any newly inspired air must become mixed with what is already there, i.e. with the residual volume of 1200 ml and with the expiratory reserve volume of 1100 ml – totalling 2300 ml – which is the *functional residual capacity*; the purpose of this residual air is to prevent extreme and sudden changes in the concentrations of O_2 and CO_2. About 150 ml of the air in the whole respiratory tract never reaches the alveoli, where diffusion actually takes place; it remains in the nose, pharynx, larynx and bronchial tree, all collectively known (as far as respiration is concerned) as the *respiratory dead space*. Thus, of the 500 ml of air inspired in a single breath, 350 ml is available for mixing with the 2300 ml already in the functional (alveolar) part of the lung.

Atmospheric air is normally (i.e. at sea level) at a pressure of 760 mmHg (100 kPa, using the S.I. system of units) and contains approximately 79% N_2, 21% O_2 and 0.05% CO_2. There is always a small amount of water vapour (up to 3%). The amount of each gas present can be expressed in terms of *pressure* rather than percentage, because it is the differing pressures between the air, blood and tissues that determine in which direction the molecules of gas diffuse. Pressure and percentage are directly related according to *Dalton's law*: in a mixture of gases, each gas exerts a pressure proportional to its concentration in the mixture. What matters most are the O_2 and CO_2 pressures. For atmospheric O_2 (which makes up 21% of air), 21% of 760 mmHg is 160 mmHg, and this is called the *partial pressure of O_2*, usually written as PO_2. Similarly the PCO_2 in atmospheric air is 0.3 mmHg (0.05% of 760 mmHg).

In alveolar air within the lungs (**10.4**) the PO_2 is 100 mmHg, but in the blood entering lung capillaries it is only 37 mmHg. Therefore, because of this pressure difference, O_2 diffuses from the alveoli into the blood, meaning that in the blood leaving the lung capillaries the PO_2 is virtually the same as in alveolar air (100 mmHg). In contrast, the PCO_2 of venous blood is 46 mmHg and in alveolar air it is 40 mmHg, so CO_2 diffuses out of the blood into the alveolar air. It is for these two fundamental processes of diffusion of O_2 and CO_2 that the lungs exist; they convert **deoxygenated**

venous blood with *low O_2* and **high CO_2** content into **oxygenated arterial blood** with **high O_2** and **low CO_2** content.

Because of the exchange of gases within the lung, expired air contains 16% O_2 (compared with 21% in inspired air) and about 5% CO_2 (compared with 0.05%).

The tissue that allows molecules of gas to pass between alveolar air and blood in the lung capillaries must obviously be extremely thin. It consists essentially of the very flattened **alveolar epithelial cells** and the equally flattened **endothelial cells** of the blood **capillaries**; it is about 0.5 μm in total thickness. The time taken for the diffusion of gases as described above is 0.2 seconds and, as blood takes about 1 second to pass through the capillaries, there is plenty of time for the exchange to occur. The size of the lung capillaries is such that red blood cells (i.e. erythrocytes – those that carry O_2) have to go through one after the other, and not side by side, so that they pass as close as possible to the alveoli.

Erythrocytes (p.61) are able to 'carry' O_2 because it combines chemically with the iron in the *haem* part of the haemoglobin molecules of the cells by forming *oxyhaemoglobin*. About 97% of all the O_2 that passes into blood from the alveoli of the lungs is combined in this way; the remaining 3% dissolves in the blood plasma. The total amount of O_2 that can be taken up by haemoglobin is limited, and depends on the PO_2 in the blood. With the maximum possible amount of O_2 being carried – when the PO_2 is high, as in lung capillaries – the haemoglobin is said to be *fully saturated* and remains bound to the O_2; with less O_2 and a lower PO_2 – as in tissue capillaries in the rest of the body – it is *partially saturated reduced haemoglobin* and gives up oxygen for diffusion into the tissues – this process

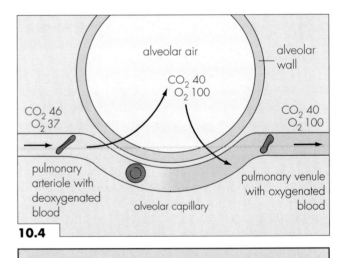

10.4

Fig. 10.4 Gaseous exchange between alveolus and blood capillary (pressures in millimeters of mercury). Due to the pressure differences, CO_2 diffuses out of the blood into the alveolar air (46 to 40 mmHg), and O_2 from air to blood (100 to 37 mmHg).

is called *oxygen–haemoglobin dissociation*. Despite giving up O_2 to the tissues, the haemoglobin in venous blood at rest remains about 75% saturated; it is by no means entirely depleted of O_2. Exercise results in more oxygen being released from the haemoglobin, as factors such as temperature and blood pH (acidity) (both of which rise with exercise) also affect oxygen dissociation.

In contrast to O_2, most of the CO_2 in blood (about 70% of it) is carried in blood plasma in the form of bicarbonate ions. Of the rest, 7% is dissolved in the plasma and 23% combines with the globin part of haemoglobin as *carbaminohaemoglobin*. In lung capillaries, where the PCO_2 becomes low, CO_2 diffuses out of the blood plasma, it is released from carbaminohaemoglobin, and is produced from the bicarbonate ions by a reversal of the chemical reactions which formed the bicarbonate. All of this CO_2 diffuses into the alveoli and so into the air that is expired.

CYANOSIS

If capillary blood contains more reduced haemoglobin (p.76) than normal, the reddish colour that is usually observed in certain skin areas (such as the fingertips and toes in the case of those with fair skin) and mucous membranes (i.e. mouth and tongue) is replaced by a purplish shade – this is called *cyanosis*. There are two types of cyanosis, central and peripheral.

Central cyanosis indicates either a poor uptake of oxygen due to lung disease or a right-to-left cardiac shunt (p.119) with deoxygenated blood passing into the systemic circulation instead of going to the lungs; it affects mucous membranes as well as the extremities.

Peripheral cyanosis, which is seen in the extremities but not in mucous membranes, indicates poor circulation, as in heart failure or as the 'blue hands and feet' of a cold day. It should be noted that those who are severely anaemic cannot display cyanosis, because the amount of reduced haemoglobin is not sufficient to give the bluish colour.

HIGH ALTITUDE AND AVIATION

As the altitude above sea level increases, air pressure decreases, but its composition remains the same. At 5500 m (18000 feet), pressures are halved, with an air PO_2 of 80 mmHg; at 11000 m (36000 feet), about the height at which jet aircraft fly, they are halved again. Those who live at high altitudes (such as the Andes or the Himalayas) develop *polycythaemia* (increased numbers of erythrocytes) to increase the O_2-carrying capacity. Those who arrive at high altitudes after low-level living experience varying degrees of mountain sickness due to hypoxia (relative O_2 shortage) – with such symptoms as headache, lassitude, and increases in heart and respiratory rates – until they become acclimatized; the hypoxia stimulates the release of erythropoietin (p.64), which increases red cell production. Aircraft cabins are pressurized but not quite to ground level, resulting in the ascent and descent being recognized by 'popping' in the ears (p.169).

DIVING

In shallow swimming with a 'snorkel' (a breathing tube that extends from the mouth to above the surface), respiration must be deeper than usual (i.e. the tidal volume must be increased) because the capacity of the tube adds to the respiratory dead space (p.76).

Below water, the pressure doubles every 10 m (33 feet), and even a few feet below the surface the inspiration of air would become impossible because of pressure on the chest wall. Scuba-diving (SCUBA – self-contained underwater breathing apparatus) with apparatus such as an aqualung allows breathing to be maintained because the gases are under pressure. Since gases are compressed upon descent and expand upon ascent, it is necessary to **exhale** when ascending to avoid overinflating the lungs; overinflation can have serious consequences, such as pneumothorax (p.75) or *air embolism* (in which gas enters the pulmonary veins and the arterial blood, and gas bubbles enter the cerebral arteries and block the blood flow, with often fatal consequences).

Although the N_2 in air is normally inert and of no interest, it becomes highly important for those breathing air under pressure, such as in diving bells or caissons; it dissolves in body tissues and unless the return to normal atmospheric pressures is very slow, the N_2 (which does not escape back into the lungs) forms bubbles within the tissues, causing varying degrees of pain commonly known as 'the bends' (properly called *decompression sickness* or *caisson disease*). Involvement of any part of the nervous system, such as the spinal cord, is particularly serious. Immediate *recompression* in a pressure chamber is essential, so that the return to normal can take place very slowly. For naval and other professional divers, there are strict regulations for the duration and depth of dives, and for the rates and times of ascent.

CHAPTER 11

DIGESTIVE SYSTEM

The **digestive system** is concerned with the *breakdown of food and its absorption*. A constant intake of food is necessary for the body's *metabolism* – a term that includes the processes whereby physical and chemical reactions produce the energy and heat necessary for the many kinds of cellular activity required to keep the body alive (see below).

The essential foodstuffs are proteins, fats, carbohydrates, mineral salts, vitamins and water. The first three are complex substances that cannot be absorbed unless they are reduced to smaller and simpler molecules, but the others can be directly absorbed. It is the function of *digestion* to convert the larger molecules into smaller ones that are suitable for absorption.

The main component of the digestive system is a tube, the **digestive tract** (the **alimentary canal**, **11.1**), within which digestion and absorption take place. The tract begins at the mouth, where food is taken in, and ends at the anus, from which unwanted material is discharged. Associated with the tract are a number of separate **glands** that assist the digestive process – the salivary glands, the liver and the pancreas. Digestion depends upon the secretion of various *enzymes* by the tract and its glands; these have the effect of breaking down the larger molecules (*Table* **11.1**). The control of enzyme secretion is carried out both by nerves and hormones (the latter being produced by endocrine cells, *Table* **11.2**).

DIGESTIVE TRACT

The main parts of the digestive tract (**11.1**) are the **mouth, pharynx, oesophagus, stomach, small intestine,** and the **large intestine**, which includes, at its lower end, the **rectum** and **anal canal**, ending at the **anus**. 'Gut' is a rather vague general term, often taken to mean the small and large intestines together ('the guts'). The term **gastrointestinal tract** (**GI tract**) is often used synonymously with digestive tract, although strictly speaking it should refer to the part of the tract from the stomach to the end of the large intestine.

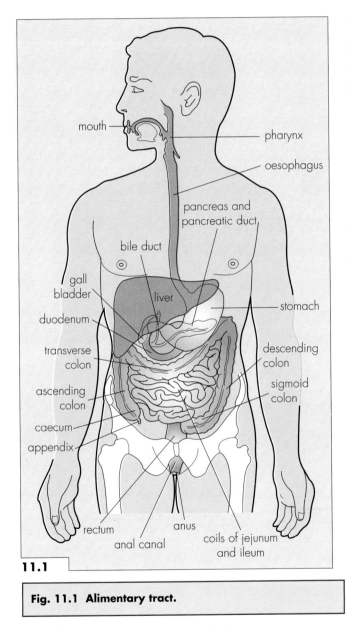

mouth
pharynx
oesophagus
pancreas and pancreatic duct
bile duct
gall bladder
liver
duodenum
stomach
transverse colon
descending colon
ascending colon
sigmoid colon
caecum
appendix
rectum
anus
anal canal
coils of jejunum and ileum

11.1

Fig. 11.1 Alimentary tract.

Table 11.1 Principal intestinal enzymes		
Source	Enzyme	Action
Salivary glands	Amylase	Breakdown of starch to maltose
Stomach (body)	Pepsin	Converted from pepsinogen by HCl; breakdown of proteins to peptides
Pancreas (exocrine part)	Trypsin	Converted from trypsinogen by enterokinase of intestinal mucosa; breakdown of proteins to peptides
	Amylase	Breakdown of starch to glucose
	Lipase	Breakdown of fats to fatty acids
Intestinal mucosa	Peptidases	Breakdown of peptides to amino acids
	Disaccharidases	Breakdown of carbohydrates to glucose and other monosaccharides
	Enterokinase	Conversion of trypsinogen to trypsin

Table 11.2 Principal intestinal hormones			
Hormone	Source	Stimulus	Action
Gastrin	G cells of pyloric antrum and duodenum	Vagus nerves	Release of HCl
CCK	Duodenum and jejunum	Proteins and fats	Release of pancreatic enzymes
Secretin	Duodenum and jejunum	Acid duodenal contents	Release of pancreatic bicarbonate
GIP (gastric inhibitory peptide)	Duodenum and jejunum	Glucose and fat in duodenum	Inhibition of gastric secretion
Somatostatin	Islets of pancreas and GI tract epithelium	Gastric acid	Inhibition of islet and GI hormones

The **mouth** (p.147) contains the **tongue** and the **teeth** which manipulate food and prepare it for swallowing. The secretions of the three pairs of main salivary glands – the **parotid**, **submandibular** and **sublingual** glands (pp.144 and 147) – assist by moistening the food.

The act of *swallowing (deglutition*, p.185) passes food out of the mouth into the **pharynx** (which also serves as part of the respiratory system, p.182), and then into the **oesophagus** (p.103). The oesophagus is a channel about 25 cm (10 inches) long, running from the neck through the thorax and passing food on to the stomach which, like most of the digestive system, is situated in the abdomen.

The **stomach** (p.253) is the widest part of the digestive tract, and acts as a receptacle and mixer; it is where digestion really begins. The contents of the stomach are passed on by degrees into the small intestine.

The part of the **small intestine** that is continuous with the stomach is the **duodenum** (p.257). Here, bile from the liver and secretions from the pancreas enter by the bile and pancreatic ducts respectively. The rest of the small intestine, the **jejunum** and **ileum** (p.260), is a hosepipe-like tube whose length in life is about 2.4 m (8 ft). Most of the

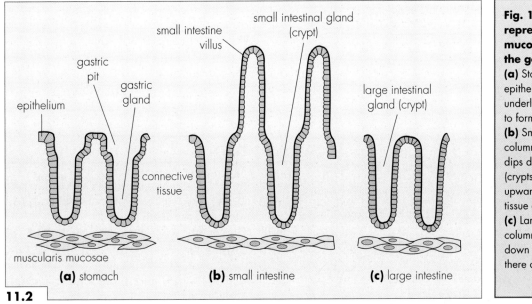

epithelium

gastric pit

gastric gland

small intestine villus

small intestinal gland (crypt)

large intestinal gland (crypt)

connective tissue

muscularis mucosae

(a) stomach

(b) small intestine

(c) large intestine

11.2

Fig. 11.2 Diagrammatic representation of the mucous membrane of the gastrointestinal tract.
(a) Stomach. The columnar epithelium dips down into the underlying connective tissue to form pits and glands.
(b) Small intestine. The columnar epithelium not only dips down to form glands (crypts) but also projects upwards with connective tissue cores, forming villi.
(c) Large intestine. The columnar epithelium dips down to form glands (crypts); there are no villi.

processes of digestion take place in the small intestine, and this is also where absorption of the modified chemical substances into the blood and lymphatic systems occurs.

Unabsorbed material passes from the ileum into the **large intestine** (p.263), which is about four feet (1.2 m) long, and consists of the **caecum** (with its small outgrowth, the **appendix**), the ascending, transverse, descending and sigmoid parts of the **colon**, the **rectum** and the **anal canal**. The main functions of the large intestine are the absorption of water and the storage of the semi-solid end-products of digestion – the **faeces** – that are eventually discharged from the body through the **anus** (the opening at the lower end of the anal canal) in the act of *defaecation*.

STRUCTURE OF THE DIGESTIVE TRACT

Apart from the mouth and pharynx, which have their own special features, the general structure of the digestive tract is similar in all parts; there is an internal lining or **mucous membrane** (mucosa), an underlying **submucous layer** (submucosa) of connective tissue, two layers of smooth muscle (inner circular and outer longitudinal, collectively forming the **muscular layer**), and finally an outer connective tissue layer. If there is no covering epithelium, then this connective tissue is the final layer and is called the **adventitia**. If there *is* a thin covering layer of epithelium, then the connective tissue and epithelium together are called the **serosa**, or **peritoneum**. (Peritoneum is the tissue which lines the entire abdominal cavity and covers the organs suspended in it, and is described further on p.243.)

It is the character of the mucous membrane that principally distinguishes one part of the gut from another, and also which part is responsible for each of the different functions. The gut mucosa consists of **epithelium**, followed by a layer of connective tissue (the **lamina propria**, meaning 'the layer nearest the epithelium'), and then a thin layer of smooth muscle (the **muscularis mucosae**, which is not to be confused with the main muscular part of the wall, which is properly called the **muscularis externa**).

In the **oesophagus**, the mucosa has a lining of **stratified squamous epithelium** that is many layers thick (**2.2c**); it is a food conduit only, with no digestive function – moreover, it must protect the underlying tissues from abrasive or extremely hot (or cold) items of food or drink that may be swallowed.

From the **stomach** down to the upper part of the **anal canal**, the epithelium is single-layered, and forms innumerable test-tube-like glands (**11.2a**). There are **mucus-secreting epithelial cells** in all parts; other cells in the stomach secrete *hydrochloric acid* and *digestive enzymes*. In the **small intestine**, the enzymes from its own epithelial cells are supplemented by those from the **pancreas**, and by *bile* from the **liver**. Apart from glands, which are downgrowths of epithelium, the small intestine also has projections – the **villi** (**11.2b**) – which increase the surface area for absorption. The **duodenum** has one particularly distinctive feature: there are collections of **mucus-secreting glands (Brunner's glands)** within the submucosa. The large intestine has the largest concentration of mucus-secreting cells, whose secretions assist the passage of material that will be stored there before being discharged from the body.

In all parts of the gut, the epithelium is constantly migrating upwards and being shed from the surface, to be renewed by constant mitotic activity in the glands. The rate of renewal varies in different parts; it is greatest in the small intestine, where the epithelium on the villi is replaced about every two days.

DIET AND DIGESTION

Any intake of food substances is a *diet*, although the word is often misused, as though it should only be applied to food intake that is restricted or special in some way. A *balanced diet* is one that is sufficient for the body's needs without a wasteful excess to be stored or eliminated. From the point of view of body metabolism, it does not matter whether particular molecules have been derived from a piece of meat or a bowl of rice; diets vary enormously, but the fundamental chemical processes are the same for everyone.

The dietary *proteins* become reduced to small peptides and amino acids, *fats* to fatty acids and glycerol, and *carbohydrates* to monosaccharides – principally glucose, fructose and galactose. The minerals and vitamins are absorbed unchanged, and *water* is a universal accompaniment of everything absorbed.

The role played by the various parts of the alimentary tract in the digestion and absorption of foodstuffs is described with each organ, but an overall summary is given here. (*Tables* **11.1**, **11.2** and **11.4** list the principal digestive enzymes and hormones, and the vitamins.)

The digestion of protein begins in the stomach and continues in the small intestine. The digestion of fat and carbohydrate takes place in the small intestine, and the products of protein, fat and carbohydrate digestion are absorbed through the small intestine. The large intestine is mainly concerned with water absorption and the discharge of waste products. The following paragraphs bring together the principal features, with page references to fuller descriptions.

The very small amount of *salivary amylase* that is present in the mouth has an insignificant effect on carbohydrate digestion, which occurs essentially in the small intestine under the influence of *pancreatic amylase* and various enzymes in the *epithelial cells* (pp.262 and 278).

Protein digestion begins in the stomach (p.255), where *hydrochloric acid* (from the parietal cells) converts *pepsinogen* (from chief cells) into *pepsin*, which is an active *proteolytic enzyme*. Digestion continues in the small intestine where pancreatic *trypsinogen* is converted to *trypsin* (another proteolytic enzyme) by the *enterokinase* that is produced by small intestinal epithelium, p.262).

Fat digestion takes place in the small intestine by pancreatic and intestinal *lipases* (p.262), assisted by *bile* from the liver which acts as an emulsifying agent (it lowers surface tension and makes fat droplets smaller – p.276).

The large intestine acts as a site of bacterial activity, breaking down some substances that are not affected by enzyme activity in the small intestine. This applies particularly to the cellulose of vegetables, which provides important bulk or roughage and assists peristalsis. It is the products of this bacterial digestion (such as ammonia, methane and indole) that give the odour to faeces and flatus.

ABSORPTION

Most of the breakdown products of digestion, together with other ingested substances such as minerals, vitamins and water, are **absorbed** by the **small intestine** – mainly by the jejunum. It is important to note that the small intestine of the newborn child is able to absorb whole proteins for the first few days after birth, so allowing antibodies (which are very large protein molecules) to be taken in to the infant's body from the mother's milk, and thus provide passive immunity against infection (p.69).

Most absorbed digestive products enter the **portal bloodstream** (p.269) for direct transport to the liver. However, most of the absorbed fat enters **intestinal lymphatics,** and so reaches the systemic circulation via the **thoracic duct,** which enters the junction of the internal jugular and subclavian veins in the root of the neck (p.179). Thus the fat, entering the right side of the heart, must pass through the lungs before returning to the left side of the heart and into the arterial blood, from which some will reach the liver by the hepatic artery – a long way round to the liver compared with most absorbed substances.

The **large intestine** absorbs water and electrolytes and perhaps some amino acids, but not fat or carbohydrate. Most of the water absorption takes place in the ascending and transverse colon; the contents of the caecum are fluid, but by the time the splenic flexure is reached they are becoming semisolid, so the rest of the large intestine is a storage organ.

NUTRITION AND METABOLISM

The essential features of *metabolism* are that carbon and hydrogen from food, and oxygen from air, combine to form carbon dioxide and water; during the process, energy – including heat, which is a form of energy – is released.

The formation of new molecules (*synthesis*) requires *energy*, and synthetic activities can be collectively called *anabolic reactions*; the manufacture of proteins from amino acids is an example of *anabolism*. Drugs that stimulate such reactions are likewise called anabolic; those such as anabolic steroids, which can assist in the build-up of muscle and other tissues and have many legitimate medical uses, have gained notoriety from their (illegal) use to enhance athletic performance. The breakdown of molecules (*decomposition*) releases energy, and such activities are *catabolic*; the digestion of foodstuffs is an example of *catabolism*.

The breakdown of food to its ultimate end-products (carbon dioxide and water) does not occur, as it were, in one fell swoop, but via a whole series of intermediate products, each a little smaller than its predecessor (in molecular terms), and each an essential part of the chain of reactions. As the organic molecules are broken down, some of the energy released is transferred to a small but highly important molecule, *ATP* (*adenosine triphosphate*). ATP is the universal 'energy transfer' molecule in cells: it transfers the chemical energy of the fuel molecules to the energy-requiring processes of the cell (e.g. contraction by a muscle cell). When ATP is hydrolyzed, the terminal phosphate group is removed (thus converting ATP to *adenosine diphosphate*, *ADP*), and energy is made available for a cellular function.

Since each ATP molecule carries a rather small amount of energy, and the total amount of ATP in a cell at any one time is also small – ATP must be continually resynthesized by the body to supply the energy needs of the cells. Synthesis is closely coupled to the breakdown of fuel molecules, as the energy in the latter's chemical bonds can be transferred to ATP for use in cellular activities. Cells can use all three of the major types of fuel molecules – carbohydrates, lipids and proteins – for ATP synthesis, but the most important 'storage forms' of fuel are carbohydrate and fat. A small amount of glucose can be stored – particularly in the liver and in muscles – as the polysaccharide *glycogen* but the greatest reserve of fuel is in the form of fat in adipose tissue (see below).

ENERGY AND CALORIES

The scientific unit that is now used for measuring energy is the joule, or often the kilojoule, which is 1000 joules; for the human body, however, it is still common to use the calorie, which is a unit of heat. One small **calorie** (spelt with a 'small c') is equivalent to 4.2 joules, and one large **Calorie** (with a capital 'C') corresponds to 1000 calories or 4.2 kilojoules. When considering the body and its nutritional requirements, it is always the large Calorie that is used, even though in this context it is often spelt with a small c, as it will be in the rest of this section.

Food must contain adequate *nutrients* (from the Latin meaning 'to nourish') – substances that the body can use to provide the calories necessary for all its chemical and physical activities. The calories are provided by the fat, carbohydrate and protein in the diet, and the number of calories is directly related to the food intake: one gram of fat produces 9 calories, and one gram of carbohydrate and protein each produces 4 calories. Alcohol has a high calorie value, producing 7 calories per gram. In the western world, over half the daily requirement of calories comes from carbohydrate, about 35% from fat and the rest from protein; in less developed countries, 90% may come from carbohydrate (such as rice and maize).

Table **11.3** gives selected examples of the calorie value of various foods, to show how greatly the values vary.

The daily energy requirements obviously vary with age and

Table 11.3 Calorie values of some common foods 25 g (1 oz) or 30 ml (1 fl. oz)	
Butter	200
Margarine	200
Roasted peanuts	170
Milk chocolate	140
Bacon	130
Sugar	110
Cheese	110
Boiled rice	100
Grilled steak	100
Fruit cake	100
Cornflakes	100
Honey	80
Boiled ham	80
Jam	80
Fried potatoes	70
Whisky, gin	70
Bread	65
Liver	60
Roast chicken	45
Boiled egg	45
Sweet wine	30
Boiled potatoes	25
Milk	20
Apple	15
Orange	12
Beer	12
Tomato	10
Cabbage	5
Carrot	5
Lettuce	2
Diet cola	0
Water	0

activity and many other factors, but a food intake that produces something like 2800 calories per day is needed for an adult. A growing child of 12 years requires as many calories as an adult. A manual labourer might need 6000 calories or more, and a patient lying in bed only 1000. Female requirements are a few hundred calories less than for males of equivalent age, because of their generally smaller body size, although an increase will be needed in pregnancy and lactation.

For an adult at rest but awake and 12 hours after taking food (when digestion and absorption have ceased) about 1700 calories are required to keep the body 'ticking over'. This is the *basal metabolic rate* (*BMR*). The everyday activities of moving about account for the additional daily requirements. A diet containing 375 grams of carbohydrate (375 × 4 calories = 1500 calories), 100 grams of fat (100 × 9 grams = 900 calories) and 100 grams of protein (100 × 4 grams = 400) would provide the 2800 calories mentioned in the paragraph above.

Ideally, the food intake should balance the energy requirement; an excessive intake will lead to the storage of excess calories as fat. The extensive records of hospitals and insurance companies show that, in people who are considerably overweight for their age and height, there are increased risks of cardiovascular and respiratory diseases. In those with hypertension or diabetes, even small increases above average weight carry serious risks. While it is true that for many people every gram of excess weight is due to overeating, there are others whose weight increase cannot be adequately explained.

Since most calories are derived from carbohydrates, cutting down on these elements in the diet is a common way of reducing the calorie intake; this encourages the removal of fat from body stores to make up any deficit in the calorie requirement. Since fat produces more than twice as many calories as the other main nutrients, reduced fat consumption can make an important contribution to reducing body weight, but a completely fat-free diet is unattractive because of the lack of taste, and because another source for the fat-soluble vitamins must be found. Excessive reduction of protein intake is not advisable, because its nitrogen content is essential. The 'calorie-controlled diet' has become a well-worn phrase, but its practical success depends on much self-discipline!

CARBOHYDRATE METABOLISM

Carbohydrates are complex molecules containing carbon, hydrogen and oxygen, and include such substances as *starch* (found in bread, potatoes and rice) and various *sugars* (in sugar cane, sweet fruits, milk and honey). Only certain sugars – glucose, galactose and fructose – can be absorbed from the digestive tract; more complex carbohydrates must therefore be broken down into these simple monosaccharides, or they will be left behind in the lumen of the gut (see below).

After absorption, it is the fate of *glucose* that is of primary interest, since the other sugars are either converted into glucose or enter the same metabolic pathways.

The level of glucose in the blood (*blood sugar* means 'blood glucose') is maintained within fairly constant limits (60–100 mg glucose per 100 ml blood, or 3.3–5.5 mmol per litre). The level is important, because the nerve cells of the brain have glucose as their sole food source; with blood glucose levels below 40 mg, the patient lapses into *hypoglycaemic coma*. If the blood glucose rises above normal, as after a meal, the excess is converted into glycogen and stored in the liver. For this process to occur, *insulin* from the islets of Langerhans of the pancreas is necessary. A rise of blood glucose stimulates the release of insulin, so stimulating glycogen formation. If there is insufficient insulin, as occurs in diabetes mellitus (p.279), the blood glucose remains high (*hyperglycaemia*) and exceeds the threshold for reabsorption by the kidney tubules (180 mg per 100 ml of blood); hence, glucose appears in the urine (p.286). Liver glycogen can be formed not only from carbohydrate but from fat by *gluconeogenesis* – meaning 'new glycogen formation'.

When the liver's store of glycogen is full, the excess glucose is converted into fat; this is what usually happens in anyone who is overweight (excess protein can also be converted into fat). The usual fat stores, like the buttocks and anterior abdominal wall, have to store this fat.

If the blood glucose falls below normal, liver glycogen is converted to glucose and enters the blood to restore normality. For this conversion, another pancreatic islet hormone is necessary – *glucagon* – whose release is stimulated by the low blood sugar.

The glycogen of muscle (p.38) is also formed from blood glucose, and requires the presence of insulin. In contrast to liver glycogen, muscle glycogen cannot be used to maintain blood glucose levels.

Certain indigestible carbohydrates form what is now called *dietary fibre*. This provides the roughage that seems to be necessary for the progress of material through the colon. In those who habitually have constipation, an increase in dietary fibre is often beneficial.

PROTEIN METABOLISM

Proteins consist of *amino acids*, which contain atoms of carbon, hydrogen, oxygen, nitrogen, and often sulphur and phosphorus. *Nitrogen*, which is an essential element of living cells, is found only in proteins, and not in carbohydrates or fats. The amino acids are linked together to make molecules of very widely varied sizes, the smaller ones being called *peptides*. One of the smallest proteins is the hormone *TSH* which is produced by the pituitary gland (p.138); it consists of just three amino acids. Other proteins may contain hundreds or thousands; the haemoglobin molecule of red blood cells contains over 500, and collagen contains many thousands.

There are about 20 different amino acids and, of course, in large protein molecules, any particular amino acid may occur many times; the precise numbers of each, and the precise order in which they are linked together, determines why one protein differs from another. Nine of the 20 are called *essential amino acids*, because they are essential to human life; they cannot be synthesized in the body (as the others can), and must be present in the diet. Protein foodstuffs that contain good quantities of all the essential amino acids are known as *high-quality* or *first-class proteins*; they are the animal proteins such as meat, eggs and dairy products (cheese and milk). Those that contain very little or only some of the essential amino acids are *low-quality* or *second-class proteins*; they are the plant proteins such as wheat and the pulses (peas and beans).

The diet recommended for normal bodily growth and maintenance usually contains some first-class animal protein, although by choice (as in vegetarians) or due to geographical circumstance, only the second-class variety may be available. The precise origin of the necessary molecules does not matter as long as they are obtained somehow. Deficiencies lead to malnutrition and eventually death.

Proteins that are broken down by the digestive tract (p.82) are reduced to their constituent amino acids, which are then transferred to the liver by the portal bloodstream. Some remain there for the liver's own use (such as for the manufacture of plasma proteins), and others pass into the systemic circulation for distribution to all parts of the body, where they can be built up into whatever proteins are required for cell growth and maintenance.

Any excess of protein that is not required for cell use is reduced to carbon dioxide, water, heat and energy. The nitrogen of the excess amino acid molecules is removed by *deamination*: it is converted by all of the body's cells into ammonia, which in turn is converted into *urea* by the liver and is then excreted by the kidneys (p.287).

FAT METABOLISM

Fat is composed of *triacylglycerols* (*triglycerides*), which are one of the major subclasses of lipids in the body. A triacylglycerol molecule consists of three *fatty acids* that are linked to a *glycerol* molecule; it thus contains predominantly carbon and hydrogen. Fat in the diet comes from both animal and plant sources – in fatty meat and dairy products, and in oils such as olive oil and nut oils. The animal fats contain the fat-soluble vitamins A, D, E and K.

Fats are not soluble in water, so absorption from the digestive tract depends not only upon their breakdown by pancreatic and intestinal *lipase*, but also on the detergent action of *bile*; bile makes possible a mixture of water and fat (an emulsion) that is absorbable into the lymphatics of the gut and thence via the thoracic duct into the bloodstream.

Transport in the bloodstream relies upon fats combining with certain proteins (*lipoproteins*). The liver further processes the absorbed material so that it can either be broken down into the usual end-products – carbon dioxide and water, with the release of energy – or be used in the build-up of tissues such as cell membranes, bone marrow and fat depots.

Like some amino acids, some fatty acids cannot be synthesized in the body and are termed *essential*, because they are needed for the formation of *prostaglandins*. These substances, which are themselves varieties of fatty acids, are widely distributed in the body, and have local hormone-like actions (however, they do not circulate in the blood like true hormones). Their main effects seem to be on smooth muscle – e.g. some cause uterine muscle to contract and bronchial muscle to relax. They are the subject of much current research, some of which has revealed that one of the commonest of all drugs, aspirin, appears to act by inhibiting prostaglandin synthesis in the brain.

It is important to note that the breakdown of fat to carbon dioxide and water can **only** take place if some glucose breakdown is going on at the same time. If it is not, the fat breakdown is incomplete and results in the accumulation in the blood of ketone bodies (*ketosis*). Ketones are toxic substances that affect brain function. The impaired carbohydrate metabolism in diabetes (p.286) may lead to severe ketosis and hence to diabetic coma; the coma is due to the accompanying alteration in fat metabolism.

Cholesterol is a particular type of lipid that has achieved prominence because of its possible association with arterial disease. Although some is present in food (such as in eggs and meat), most is synthesized by the liver. It is a component of cell membranes, and both bile salts and steroid hormones are derived from it. It is also present in the walls of diseased arteries; there appears to be a correlation between blood cholesterol levels and coronary artery disease, although some physicians still consider this to be a controversial matter.

VITAMINS

Vitamins are a group of substances that are essential for life but are not sources of body fuel. Rather, they are the sources of *coenzymes*, which are compounds that are essential participants in certain enzyme-mediated reactions in all cells. They are all required in very small quantities, and most average diets contain more than enough; however, in those who are chronically underfed there may obviously be deficiencies. The common names of the vitamins and their functions are summarized in *Table* **11.4**.

There may be specific circumstances in which dietary supplements of vitamins may be justified, such as in pregnancy and prolonged illnesses, but it is wrong for most people to consider they can do themselves a good turn by adding them to a normal diet. There are usually limits to storage, and excess will simply be excreted. Large amounts of some vitamins, especially A and D, can be positively harmful, especially in children.

Table 11.4 Vitamins		
Name	**Main sources**	**Importance**
Vitamin A (retinol)	Liver, milk products, fruit, leafy vegetables. Added to margarine.	Necessary for light receptors of retina and night vision. Deficiency damages retina and cornea.
Vitamin B1 (thiamin)	Cereals, meat	Assists carbohydrate metabolism. Deficiency causes beri-beri.
Vitamin B2 (riboflavin)	Milk, cheese	Cell growth
Niacin (nicotinamide)	Meat, liver, cereals	Assists cell metabolism. Deficiency causes pellagra.
Pantothenic acid	Eggs, liver	Assists cell metabolism
Vitamin B6 (pyroxidine)	Meat, liver, cereals	Assists protein metabolism
Vitamin B12 (cyanocobalamin)	Liver, meat, milk	Essential for red blood cell development and myelin formation. Gastric intrinsic factor required for absorption. Deficiency causes anaemia.
Folate (folic acid)	Vegetables, wholemeal bread, meat	Necessary for red blood cell formation. Deficiency causes anaemia.
Vitamin C (ascorbic acid)	Fruits, vegetables	Necessary for integrity of blood vessels and connective tissues. Easily destroyed by cooking. Deficiency causes scurvy.
Vitamin D (calciferol)	Fish liver oils. Added to margarine.	Formed by action of ultraviolet light on skin. Deficiency causes rickets.
Vitamin E	Vegetable oils, cereals	Necessary for red blood cell formation
Vitamin K (phytomenadione)	Vegetables	Necessary for the liver's production of blood-clotting factors. Deficiency causes haemorrhagic diseases.

MINERALS

Minerals are absorbed by the gut with water and the other food substances. Many minerals are essential to life and the functions of most of them are well defined. Of the major minerals required, *sodium* (Na) and *potassium* (K) are needed because they are the principal ones concerned in maintaining a proper electrolyte balance, which is controlled by the kidney (p.284), and in the conduction of nerve impulses (p.47). They are widely distributed in foodstuffs, and common salt (sodium chloride, NaCl) is frequently added during cooking. *Calcium* (Ca) is necessary as a constituent of bone (p.12), for proper nerve function (p.192) and for blood clotting (p.63). It is present in dairy products such as eggs, milk and cheese, and in green vegetables. Vitamin D (p.18) is necessary for its absorption; the level of calcium in the blood is controlled by

parathyroid hormone (p.192) and by calcitonin from the thyroid gland (p.191).

Some substances are necessary but only in small amounts, and so are called *trace elements*. *Iron* (Fe) is needed for the formation of haemoglobin in red blood cells (p.61), and is found in green vegetables, red meat and egg yolk. *Cobalt* (Co) is a component of vitamin B_{12} and is found in liver, meat and milk, and is essential for red cell development and the formation of myelin (p.47). *Iodine* (I) is essential for the synthesis of thyroxine by the thyroid gland (p.191), and is present in seafoods and some green vegetables; it is often added to commercial preparations of common salt. The role of copper, manganese, nickel, silicon and some others has yet to be defined.

WATER

The all-important control of body *water* by the kidney is described on p.284; the daily movement of water in the gastrointestinal tract is summarized in *Table* **11.5**. Apart from food and drink, a surprisingly large amount of water enters the gut every day from its own glands. Almost all is absorbed, so that the overall loss in the faeces is only about 200 ml.

ENTERAL AND PARENTERAL FEEDING

When patients are unable to take food by mouth (e.g. due to unconsciousness or GI tract operations), periods of keeping up the body's nutritional requirements other than by normal mouth feeding may be necessary.

Enteral feeding (*enteral replacement therapy*) refers to feeding via a tube inserted into the stomach or the intestine (usually through the nose). Suitably macerated foods can thus be introduced into the gut, which must itself be functioning normally.

When digestion and absorption are not normal, *parenteral feeding* (*parenteral replacement therapy*, *total parenteral nutrition*, *TPN*) may be required; *parenteral* is from the Greek for 'outside the gut', and means *intravenous feeding*. The solutions that are used usually consist of dextrose with certain fats and amino acids, and are administered via a peripheral vein; the sublcavian vein is often used if prolonged therapy for some days is anticipated.

Table 11.5 Daily water and the gastrointestinal tract	
Ingested in food and drink	2500 ml
GI tract secretions	
Salivary secretion	1500 ml
Gastric secretion	2500 ml
Intestinal secretion	1000 ml
Pancreatic secretion	1500 ml
Bile	500 ml
Daily total in GI tract	9500 ml
Absorption from GI tract	
Jejunal absorption	5500 ml
Ileal absorption	2500 ml
Colonic absorption	1300 ml
Daily absorption from GI tract	9300 ml
Balance excreted in faeces	200 ml

CHAPTER 12

URINARY SYSTEM

The essential purpose of the **urinary system** is to control the *composition* and the *volume* of the *blood* so that the environment of the body tissues can be preserved within the required narrow limits of normality. The end result is that water and dissolved substances, including waste products, are eliminated from the body as *urine* in the act of *micturition* (*urination*). Ancillary to the control of body fluid and blood volume, the kidneys play an important part in the control of *blood pressure* (p.58) by secreting an enzyme, *renin*, which acts on a plasma protein in what is now usually called the *renin–angiotensin system* (described on p.286). They also have a role in the formation of red blood cells by secreting the hormone *erythropoietin* (*EPO*) (p.64).

URINARY ORGANS

The **urinary organs** (**12.1**) are the pairs of kidneys and ureters, and the single urinary bladder and urethra. The noun 'kidney' is of Anglo-Saxon origin, but the Latin and Greek for kidney, *'ren'* and *'nephros'*, give rise to the adjective *'renal'* and words such as *'nephritis'*, meaning inflammation of the kidney.

Each **kidney** (p.282) lies in the upper posterior part of the abdomen. The region where the blood vessels and ureter enter or leave is the **hilum**.

The functional units of the kidney are the **nephrons** (2 million in each kidney), which are delicate coiling tubules (**12.2**) that form the urine and pass it on to the **collecting tubules**, from which it eventually reaches the ureters. Each nephron is intimately associated with a **glomerulus**, a tuft of blood capillaries which, during development, indents the blind end of the nephron. As blood courses through the glomerulus, fluid and many dissolved materials filter out of the capillaries and into the lumen of the nephron. The filtrate is further modified by selective absorption and secretion as it passes through the rest of the nephron and then finally into the collecting tubule. The formation of urine thus depends essentially on *glomerular filtration* and *tubular reabsorption*, and is described on p.284.

Each **ureter** (p.288) is a muscular tube (of smooth muscle), about 25cm (10 inches) long, that passes down on the posterior abdominal wall into the pelvis to enter the urinary bladder.

The **bladder** (p.294) is a muscular storage bag (again of smooth muscle) that lies in the pelvis behind the pubic symphysis – in front of the upper part of the vagina in the female or in front of the rectum in the male.

The bladder empties, via the **urethra**, which is 4 cm (1.5 inches) long in the *female* (p.294). The urethra runs in the front wall of the vagina and is surrounded by the **external urethral sphincter** (of skeletal muscle) to open at the **external urethral meatus** at the front of the vagina 2.5 cm (1 in) behind the clitoris.

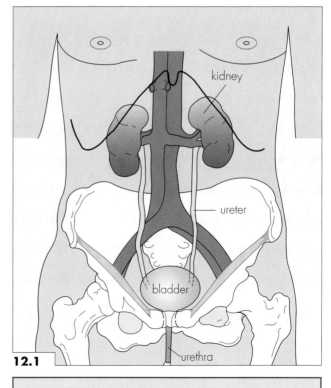

12.1

Fig. 12.1 Urinary tract.

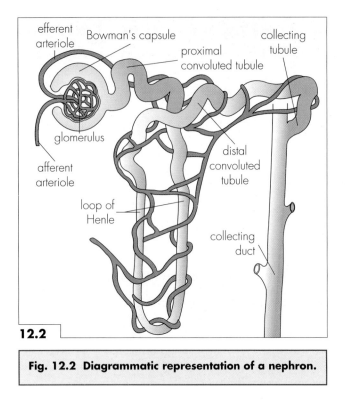

efferent arteriole

Bowman's capsule

collecting tubule

proximal convoluted tubule

glomerulus

afferent arteriole

distal convoluted tubule

loop of Henle

collecting duct

12.2

Fig. 12.2 Diagrammatic representation of a nephron.

The **urethra** in the *male* (p.295) is about 20 cm (8 inches) long. The first 3 cm is the **prostatic part**; it runs through the prostate (a large gland that lies below the bladder, see p.308), where it is joined by the ejaculatory ducts (p.309) – from here onwards the urethra is a common pathway for urine and seminal fluid. At the beginning of the prostatic part, the male urethra is surrounded by the **internal urethral sphincter** (of smooth muscle), which prevents regurgitation of semen into the bladder during ejaculation (p.310). The short **membranous part**, about 2 cm long and surrounded by the **external urethral sphincter** (of skeletal muscle), continues into the **penile part** within the corpus spongiosum of the penis (p.309), to open on the glans penis at the **external urethral meatus**.

CHAPTER 13

REPRODUCTIVE SYSTEM

The male and female **gonads**, the **testes** and **ovaries**, produce the sex hormones and the **gametes, spermatozoa** and **ova** that are necessary for reproduction. The remainder of the male and female reproductive systems serve to transport the gametes and, if an ovum is fertilized, to support its development into a new individual within the female.

FEMALE ORGANS

The **female reproductive organs** (**13.1**) consist of the **ovaries, uterus** and **vagina** which form the internal reproductive organs (the **internal genitalia**, within the pelvis), and a number of structures which make up the external organs (**external genitalia**) including the **mons pubis, labia majora, labia minora, clitoris, bulbs of the vestibule, greater vestibular glands** and the **vestibule** of the **vagina**. These are situated in the **perineum** (p.290), and the part of the perineum containing the external genitalia is the **vulva** (p.301).

Each **ovary** (p.296) lies near the side wall of the pelvis and is suspended from the back of the peritoneal fold that supports the uterus. Its function during reproductive life is to discharge **ova** that are capable of being fertilized by spermatozoa, and also to secrete the *female sex hormones, oestrogen* and *progesterone*.

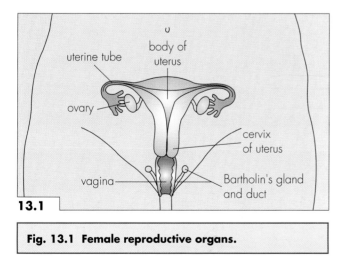

uterine tube

body of uterus

ovary

cervix of uterus

vagina

Bartholin's gland and duct

13.1

Fig. 13.1 Female reproductive organs.

The **uterus** (p.299) lies above the urinary bladder, with its narrow end, the **cervix**, opening into the top of the vagina. From each upper corner of the uterus a **uterine tube** (**Fallopian tube**) extends towards the ovary, to receive liberated ova. The mucous membrane of the uterus, the **endometrium**, undergoes cyclic changes during every month of reproductive life (the *menstrual cycle*) to prepare for the possible reception of a fertilized ovum. In the absence of a fertilized ovum, the endometrium breaks down to form a discharge of blood and tissue (during *menstruation*) before regenerating itself in preparation for the next cycle.

The **vagina** (p.301) is the female organ of copulation, and receives the erect penis of the male during sexual intercourse; this allows the spermatozoa that are discharged in the seminal fluid during ejaculation to migrate into the uterus and the uterine tube to fertilize an ovum. It also receives the products of menstruation and forms the birth canal during childbirth (*parturition*, p.306).

The lower end of the vagina that opens onto the vulva is the **vestibule of the vagina**, and is guarded on either side by two pairs of skin folds, the **labia minora** and **labia majora** (p.302); the latter continue forwards to become the fatty skin (**mons pubis**) over the pubic symphysis. The urethra (p.294) opens into the front of the vestibule, and on either side of the vestibule are the **bulbs of the vestibule** (p.302), which are elongated masses of erectile tissue. Under cover of the back of each bulb is the **greater vestibular gland** (**Bartholin's gland**, p.302), which has a short duct opening into the side of the vestibule. The **clitoris** (p.302) is the female counterpart of the penis (but is not associated with the urethra); it is at the front ends of the labia minora.

MALE ORGANS

The **male reproductive organs** (**13.2**) consist of the **testis** (plural – **testes**), **epididymis, ductus deferens (vas deferens), seminal vesicle, ejaculatory duct, prostate gland, bulbourethral gland** and **penis**. All are paired except for the prostate and penis.

The **testes** (p.307) are suspended within the **scrotum**, a wrinkled sac of skin and smooth muscle below the pubic symphysis (p.252) and, together with the penis (p.309), they form the external reproductive organs (**external genitalia**). The other structures of the male reproductive system constitute the **internal genitalia**, which are within the pelvis – with the **ductus deferens** (p.307) passing from the testis, through the inguinal canal in the lower abdominal wall, to get into the pelvis. The testes produce spermatozoa and the *male sex hormone*, *testosterone* (p.308).

Spermatozoa migrate from the testis to the **epididymis** (p.307), which acts as a storage organ and site of maturation for sperm.

The epididymis continues as the **ductus deferens** (p.307) which is still commonly called by its old name – the **vas deferens**. This is a muscular tube (of smooth muscle) that passes, with other structures that form the **spermatic cord** (p.248), through the inguinal canal into the pelvis. Here it joins the duct of the **seminal vesicle** (the main source of **seminal fluid**, p.309) at the back of the **prostate** (a glandular organ that also produces some seminal fluid, p.308) to form the **ejaculatory duct** (p.309).

Both ejaculatory ducts run through the back of the prostate to open into the prostatic part of the urethra. From this point on, the **urethra** (p.295) is the common channel for urine and seminal fluid.

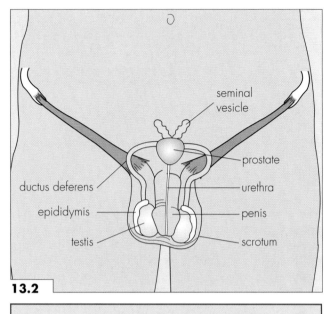

13.2

Fig. 13.2 Male reproductive organs.

CHAPTER 14

ENDOCRINE SYSTEM

Like the nervous system, the **endocrine system** is a control and communication system, but one that operates at a much slower pace than the nervous system. Endocrine tissues secrete a variety of **hormones** into the bloodstream; these are chemical substances ('chemical messengers') that exert their effect on other tissues (the 'target' tissues) by either stimulating or inhibiting their activity.

The endocrine tissues exist either as discrete glands, as groups of cells in other organs, or as single cells scattered in other organs. The main discrete **endocrine organs** (**14.1**) are the pituitary, adrenal (suprarenal), thyroid, parathyroid and pineal glands. Other endocrine tissues exist as groups of cells in other organs – e.g. the islets (of Langerhans) in the pancreas, the interstitial (Leydig) cells of the testis, follicular and luteal cells of the ovary, the placenta of the pregnant female, and endocrine cells of the kidney and thymus. Yet more **endocrine cells** are scattered singly in some organs – e.g. the endocrine cells of the stomach and intestine. Finally, some neurons (nerve cells) are capable of secreting hormones into the bloodstream, notably the **neuroendocrine cells** (**neurosecretory cells**) of the hypothalamus of the brain.

Although the endocrine cells of the gastrointestinal tract are seen on microscopic examination to be scattered singly among the other mucosal cells, it is likely that if they were all collected together they would form the largest of all endocrine organs.

All endocrine tissues are concerned in some way or other with *modifying metabolism*. The hormones that they produce belong to three main groups: amines, steroids and peptides. The *amine hormones*, which are derived from the amino acid *tyrosine*, are produced by the **thyroid gland** and by the **adrenal medulla**. The *steroid hormones*, derived from *cholesterol* (a lipid substance), are produced by the **kidneys**, the **adrenal cortex** and the **gonads**. The remainder are chiefly *peptides* (short chains of amino acids), although a few are small proteins (long-chain polypeptides).

The nervous and endocrine systems have two particularly important connections with one another: part of the brain (the **hypothalamus**, p.196) is connected, both directly and via a special system of blood vessels, with the **pituitary gland**, and the cells of the **medulla** (the central area) of the **adrenal gland** are modified **sympathetic nerve cells** that are supplied by preganglionic nerve fibres (p.47).

ENDOCRINE GLANDS

The **pituitary gland** is connected to the under-surface of the brain by the **pituitary stalk**, and lies in a small bony depression in the base of the skull, the **pituitary fossa** (p.134). The anterior and posterior parts of the gland (**anterior** and **posterior lobes** – often simply called the anterior and posterior pituitary) each have their distinct functions. For many years the pituitary was often called the 'leader of the endocrine orchestra' or the 'master gland' because it controls some (but by no means all) of the other major endocrine organs. For example, the anterior pituitary regulates the function of the thyroid gland, part of the cortex of the adrenal gland and the gonads. More recently, it has been demoted from 'master gland' status by the discovery that the pituitary, in its turn, is controlled to a large degree by the hypothalamus of the brain (p.196).

The pair of **adrenal glands** lie adjacent to the upper and medial parts of each kidney (p.280). Each has a peripheral part, the **adrenal cortex**, and a central part, the **adrenal medulla**, and each part has its distinct functions.

The **thyroid gland** lies in the front of the neck, with a narrow central part, the **isthmus**, overlying the upper part of the trachea, and two **lateral lobes**, one on each side of the larynx (p.189).

The four very small **parathyroid glands** (two on each side) are immediately behind the lateral lobes of the thyroid gland (p.192).

Each **ovary** (p.296) lies near the side wall of the pelvis, suspended from the back of the broad ligament of the uterus (p.299)

Each **testis** (p.307) is suspended from the end of the spermatic cord and lies in the scrotum.

HORMONES

The principal **hormones** of the main glands and other endocrine tissues, with their common abbreviations and alternative names, and their target tissues, are summarized in *Table* **14.1**, with page references to fuller descriptions. (Other hormones whose human functions are still being elucidated will be found in specialist texts.)

Table 14.1 Principal hormones of the main glands and other endocrine tissues

Posterior lobe of pituitary gland	*Vasopressin* (antidiuretic hormone, ADH, arginine vasopressin, AVP), reducing urine production by controlling water reabsorption by kidney tubules (p.286) *Oxytocin*, controlling uterine muscle contraction (p.306) and stimulating milk ejection from the breasts (p.107)
Anterior lobe of pituitary gland	*Growth hormone* (GH, somatotropin, STH), causing a general increase in the size and number of body cells (p.140) *Prolactin* (PRL, luteotropin, LTH), controlling breast development and milk production in the female (p.107) and assisting LH in the male (p.140) *Adrenocorticotropic hormone* (ACTH, corticotropin), controlling secretion of cortisol from the adrenal cortex (p.281) *Thyroid-stimulating hormone* (TSH, thyrotropin), controlling secretion of T3 and T4 from the thyroid gland (p.191) *Luteinizing hormone* (LH, interstitial-cell stimulating hormone, ICSH), controlling the corpus luteum of the ovary (p.296) or the interstitial cells of the testis (308) *Follicle-stimulating hormone* (FSH), controlling the development of ovarian follicles in the female (p.296) and spermatozoa in the male (308)
Hypothalamus	Neurosecretory cells producing the hormones of the posterior pituitary (p.135) Neurosecretory cells producing releasing (and inhibiting) hormones that control the release of hormones from the anterior pituitary (p.139)
Adrenal gland – cortex	*Aldosterone*, conserving water and sodium excretion by the kidneys (p.285) *Cortisol* (hydrocortisone), stimulating gluconeogenesis (p.84); anti-inflammatory and immunosuppressive (p.281) *Testosterone* and *oestrogen*, insignificant effects compared with production of these hormones by testis and ovary (see below)
Adrenal gland – medulla	*Adrenaline* (epinephrine), and *Noradrenaline* (norepinephrine), controlled by sympathetic nerves, stimulating sympathetic nervous activity (p.47)
Thyroid gland	*Thyroxine* (T4), the main thyroid hormone, and *Triiodothyronine* (T3), increasing metabolic rate (p.191) *Calcitonin*, lowering blood calcium (p.191)
Parathyroid gland	*Parathyroid hormone* (parathormone, PTH), raising blood calcium (p.192)
Islets of the pancreas) (islets of Langerhans	*Insulin*, lowering blood glucose and stimulating glucose storage (p.84) *Glucagon*, raising blood glucose and stimulating glucose production (p.84) *Somatostatin*, inhibiting release of insulin, glucagon and some intestinal hormones, and inhibiting gastro-intestinal motility (*Table **11.2*** and p.80)
Kidney	*Erythropoietin* (EPO), from glomerular epithelial cells, increasing erythropoiesis (p.64)
Thymus	*Thymin*, probably concerned with the maturation of T lymphocytes (p.70)
Testis	*Testosterone*, from interstitial (Leydig) cells, stimulating male sex organs and sexual characteristics (p.307) *Inhibin*, from Sertoli cells, inhibiting secretion of pituitary FSH and ICSH (p.308)
Ovary	*Oestrogen* (mainly oestradiol), from follicular and stromal cells, and corpus luteum (and placenta), stimulating female sex organs and sexual characteristics (p.298) *Progesterone*, from corpus luteum (and placenta), stimulating female sex organs (p.296) *Relaxin*, from corpus luteum (and placenta), loosening pelvic ligaments and relaxing uterine cervix at the end of pregnancy (p.289) *Inhibin*, from follicular fluid (and placenta), inhibiting secretion of pituitary FSH and LH (p.299)
Digestive tract	*Gastrin*, from G cells in the pyloric part of the stomach, stimulating secretion of hydrochloric acid (p.255) *Cholecystokinin* (CCK), from endocrine cells in the upper small intestine, stimulating pancreatic secretion (p.263, p.278) *Secretin.* from endocrine cells of the upper small intestine, assisting CCK in stimulating pancreatic secretion (p.263 p.278) *Gastric inhibitory peptide* (GIP), from endocrine cells of the duodenum and jejunum, inhibiting gastric secretion and motility (p.263)

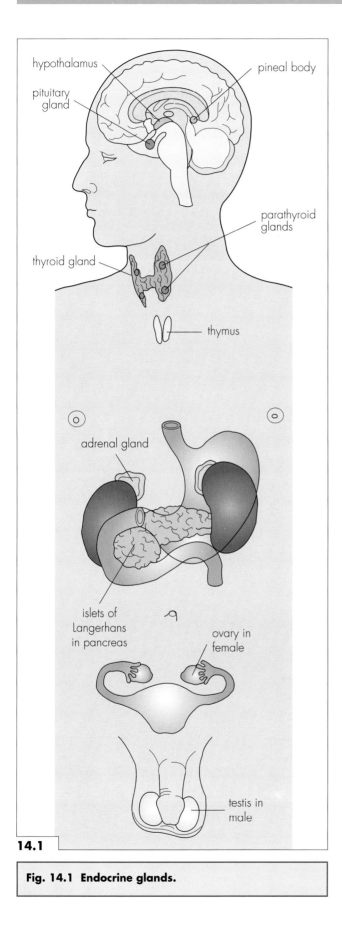

hypothalamus

pineal body

pituitary gland

parathyroid glands

thyroid gland

thymus

adrenal gland

islets of Langerhans in pancreas

ovary in female

testis in male

14.1

Fig. 14.1 Endocrine glands.

CHAPTER 15

THORAX

THORACIC WALLS AND THORACIC CAVITY

Consult the introduction to the Respiratory System (p.73).

The **thorax** (chest) is the section of the trunk between the neck and the abdomen. Some muscles of the upper limb and abdomen have attachments to the thoracic skeleton and lie under the skin on the front and side of the thorax; they include pectoralis major, serratus anterior, external oblique and rectus abdominis (**6.1**); such muscles are described with the upper limb (p.213) and anterior andominal wall (p.246). The breasts (mammary glands) are in the connective tissue under the skin of the front of the chest, and are described on p.106.

BONES AND JOINTS OF THE THORAX

The **skeleton** of the thorax (see **4.1a**) consists of the thoracic part of the **vertebral column** (the twelve thoracic vertebrae with their intervertebral discs and other ligaments), the twelve pairs of **ribs** with costal cartilages at their front ends, and the **sternum** which consists of three parts: the manubrium, body and xiphoid process. Although the ribs and sternum help to form a bony cage that protects the heart and lungs – the principal thoracic contents – the main reason for the existence of ribs is to assist respiration by providing a 'box' with firm but slightly mobile walls within which the lungs can expand and contract.

RIBS AND THEIR JOINTS

The main part of a typical **rib** (**15.1a**) is the body or **shaft**. The **head** at the vertebral end is joined to the body by the **neck**, and at the back of the junction of the neck and body is the **tubercle**. The bodies of most ribs have lateral and medial surfaces and have a groove at their lower borders – the *costal groove*. The first rib, however, has upper and lower surfaces (**15.1c**); it appears to be 'twisted' at right angles to the rest to form the top of the thoracic cage. The two first ribs with their costal cartilages, the first thoracic vertebra and the upper margin of the manubrium of the sternum are the boundaries of the **thoracic inlet** (**15.2**); this is an important aperture for the passage of several structures (e.g. the trachea and oesophagus) between the neck and the interior of the thorax. The thoracic inlet is about the same size and shape as a kidney – 12 cm broad and 5 cm deep (10 inches × 2 inches).

The heads of the ribs make small synovial joints with the sides of the bodies of the vertebrae (**joints of the heads** of the ribs), and the tubercles of the ribs articulate with the transverse processes of the vertebrae (**costotransverse joints** – **4.2d** and **15.1b**). At the front, the ends of the upper seven ribs are joined to the sternum by their **costal cartilages** (**15.2**). The eighth, ninth and tenth ribs have cartilages that do not reach the sternum, but each joins the cartilage above it, forming with the seventh cartilage the costal margin (see **4.1a**). The last two ribs have only very small cartilages at their tips and do not join any others ('floating ribs'); the twelfth rib is rather short and straight.

Injury to the chest wall that causes bruising of a rib (perhaps with haemorrhage and therefore tension under the periosteum) is painful; the pain may persist for a surprisingly long time (perhaps several weeks), which is presumably because the subperiosteal blood clot takes a long time to become resorbed. The danger in fracturing ribs lies in the fact that the jagged ends may puncture the lung, causing pneumothorax or haemothorax (p.125).

STERNUM AND ITS JOINTS

The central part of the body of the **sternum** (**15.1e**) is a narrow cavity filled with bone marrow; being in a convenient subcutaneous position, the body of the sternum is one of the common sites (like the iliac crest) from which specimens of bone marrow can be obtained (by *sternal puncture*). In this process, a special wide-bored needle is pushed through the outer layer of bone into the marrow cavity, a syringe is then connected and some marrow is sucked out. Care must be taken not to penetrate the back of the sternum with the aspirating needle, as this may introduce infection into the mediastinum (p.101).

The **manubrium** and the body of the sternum are held at a slight angle to one another (the **sternal angle** or **angle of Louis**) at a cartilaginous joint (the **manubriosternal joint** – **15.2**). The **xiphoid process**, which is normally cartilage, not bone, unites with the lower end of the body at the **xiphisternal joint**. The sternum presents two important

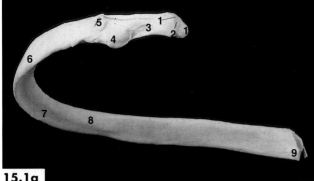

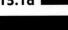

15.1a

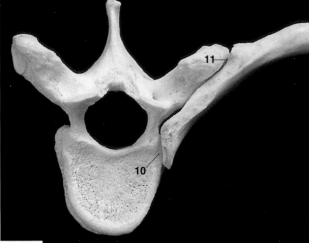

15.1b

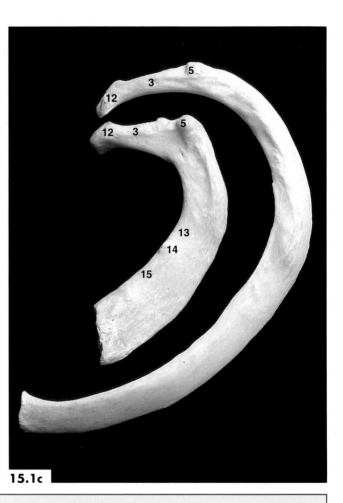

15.1c

Fig. 15.1 Ribs and sternum.
(a) A typical left rib, from behind.
(b) A typical left rib and thoracic vertebra articulated, from above.

(c) Left first and second ribs, from above.
(d) Left twelfth rib, from the front (above) and back (below)
(e) Sternum, from the front.

1 Articular facets of head, for joints with vertebral body facets
2 Crest of head, for articular ligament joining intervertebral disc
3 Neck
4 Articular facet of tubercle, for joint with transverse process (11)
5 Non–articular part of tubercle
6 Angle
7 Costal grove
8 Shaft
9 Anterior end, joining costal cartilage
10 Upper costal facet of vertebral body, joining lower facet of head of rib
11 Articular facet of transverse process, joining articular part of tubercle of rib (4)
12 Head

13 Groove for subclavian artery and first thoracic nerve
14 Scalene tubercle, for attachment of scalenus anterior and a landmark between the arterial and venous grooves (13 and 15)
15 Groove for subclavian vein
16 Manubrium of sternum
17 Jugular notch, an easily palpable landmark
18 Clavicular notch, for the sternoclavicular joint
19 Notch for first costal cartilage
20 Manubriosternal joint (sternal angle, angle of Louis)
21 Notches for second costal cartilage
22 Body of sternum
23 Notches for seventh costal cartilage
24 Xiphisternal joint
25 Xiphoid process

landmarks on the surface of the chest: the **jugular notch**, a shallow depression at the top of the manubrium, easily observed and palpated, and the sternal angle (described above) that makes a palpable ridge 5 cm below the notch.

The *second* costal cartilages join the sides of the manubrium and the body at the sternal angle, and ribs and costal cartilages can be counted downwards from the second. The first rib and cartilage cannot be clearly identified by palpation

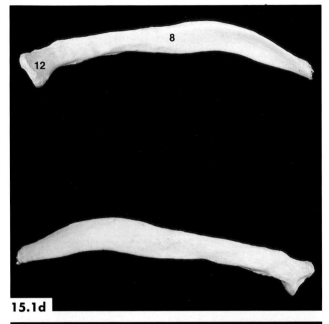

15.1d

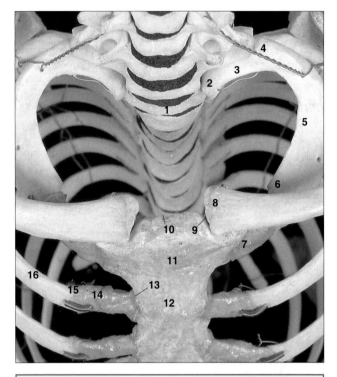

Fig. 15.2 Inlet of the thorax in an articulated skeleton, looking down from above and in front.

1 Body of T1 vertebra
2 Head
3 Neck
4 Tubercle ⎫ of first rib
5 Shaft ⎬
6 Anterior end ⎭
7 First costal cartilage
8 Sternal end of clavicle
9 Sternoclavicular joint
10 Jugular notch
11 Manubrium of sternum
12 Manubriosternal joint (sternal angle, angle of Louis), the most important palpable landmark on the front of the thorax (**15.7**)
13 Second sternocostal joint
14 Second costal cartilage
15 Costochondral joint
16 Second rib

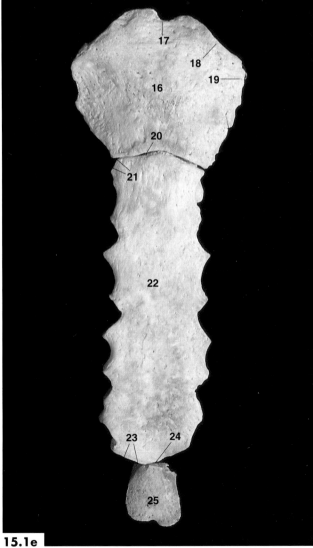

15.1e

because they are under cover of the clavicle, so, in order to identify any particular rib on the front of the chest, the second one is always chosen as the landmark for the others. The ability to 'count ribs' on a patient's chest is extremely useful, since they are landmarks for locating the positions of important viscera underneath (p.104). Other landmarks, also used frequently for this purpose, are the **midclavicular** and **midaxillary lines** (**15.3**); these are imaginary lines that are drawn vertically downwards from the midpoints of the clavicle and axilla.

All of the above costal (rib) and sternal joints allow the ribs to rise and fall with inspiration and expiration. In middle or old age, the sternal joints become less mobile and (like the xiphoid process) may even ossify, so slightly restricting rib movement.

INTERCOSTAL MUSCLES, VESSELS AND NERVES

The gaps between the ribs (the **intercostal spaces**) are filled in by the three layers of **intercostal muscles** (the external, internal and innermost layers) that run largely between one rib and another (**15.4a** and **b**). The innermost layer is broken up into three groups of muscles: subcostal muscles at the back, innermost intercostals at the side, and transversus thoracis at the front. It is usually considered that the external intercostals assist with inspiration and the internal intercostals with expiration, but apart from this, all of the intercostals help to prevent the non-bony parts of the chest wall from 'flapping in and out' when breathing.

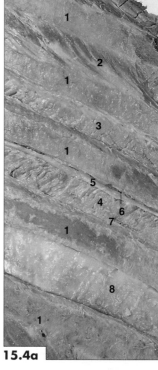

15.4a

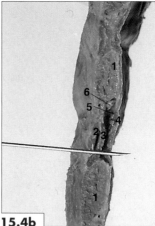

15.4b

Fig. 15.4 Intercostal spaces.
(a) Some spaces of the right side, dissected to show the three successive layers of muscles and the pleura.
(b) Cross section of two ribs and an intercostal space, showing the correct position for a needle entering the pleural cavity – immediately above the upper border of a rib, and avoiding the vessels and nerve (5 and 6) which are at a higher level.

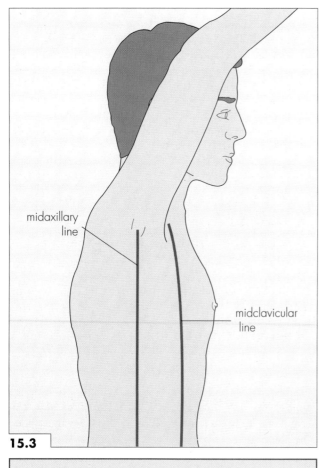

15.3

Fig. 15.3 Midclavicular and midaxillary lines, on the right side with the arm fully abducted.

1 Rib
2 Exernal intercostal muscle, the outer layer
3 Internal intercostal muscle, the middle layer, shown after removing the external intercostal (2) in **(a)**
4 Innermost intercostal muscle, the innermost layer, shown after removal of the external and internal intercostals (2 and 3) in **(a)**
5 Intercostal nerve, immediately below the rib
6 Posterior intercostal artery, partly covered by the rib. The accompanying vein is above the artery, completely covered by the rib
7 Position for insertion of needle into the pleural cavity (as in **b**), immediately above a rib and so well away from the major vessels and nerve (5 and 6)
8 Pleura, covering the ribs on their deep surfaces and seen after all three layers of muscles (2, 3 and 4) have been removed

The intercostal spaces are numbered, just as the ribs are: the gap between the first and second ribs is the first intercostal space, and so on.

The **intercostal vessels** and **nerves** pass round the chest wall largely under cover of their own rib – in the costal groove – and between the internal and innermost intercostal muscles. They lie in the order: vein, artery, nerve, from above downwards (**15.4b**).

The **intercostal nerves** are derived from the thoracic spinal nerves; they supply the intercostal muscles and pass right round to the front of the chest, supplying strips of skin segmentally. However, there is much overlap in the amount of skin supplied by any one nerve, and, to produce local anaesthesia of any one segment, at least three adjacent nerves must be anaesthetized.

The main **arteries** of the intercostal spaces are the **posterior intercostals**, which come mostly from the aorta. At the front there are smaller anterior intercostal arteries from the internal thoracic (p.55) which are important mainly because the upper ones give branches to the breast (p.106).

DIAPHRAGM

The **diaphragm**, the main muscle of the thorax, is a dome-shaped, muscular partition separating the thorax from the abdomen (**15.5** and **15.6**). Its muscle fibres originate from various peripheral structures and converge to a single central tendon. Points of origin are the left and right crus (plural *crura* – muscular bundles attached to the front of the upper lumbar vertebrae, **15.5b**), fibrous bands bridging the psoas and quadratus lumborum muscles (**15.5b**), the inner surfaces of the lower six ribs, and the back of the xiphoid process. The fibres then converge on the **central tendon** which lies below the heart, fused with the pericardium (p.111 and **15.5**). Due to the pressure of the liver and other abdominal contents, each half of the diaphragm bulges upwards into its own half of the thoracic cavity. The upper part of the diaphragm, and thus the upper part of the abdomen, extends *well above* the level of the costal margin, reaching as high as the fifth rib at the front on the right and the fifth intercostal space on the left; this is much higher than might be expected from the extent of the thoracic cage (see **19.2**).

The muscle of each half of the diaphragm is supplied from the cervical plexus by the **phrenic nerve** of its own side – one of the most important nerve supplies in the body (see below). That a structure located between the thorax and abdomen should be supplied by cervical nerves is perhaps unexpected. The explanation lies in the fact that the muscle fibres of the diaphragm are originally derived from the cervical region, from which they migrate down to their normal adult position, carrying their nerves with them.

The diaphragm acts as the main muscle of *respiration*. In quiet breathing, the domes of the diaphragm descend about 1.5 cm at each inspiration, so increasing the thoracic capacity and drawing air into the lungs (because of the negative pressure within the pleural cavities). Expiration occurs largely because of the elastic recoil of the lung tissues themselves, and the diaphragm rises to its original position due to relaxation of its muscle fibres. In the deep respiration that accompanies exercise, the extent of diaphragmatic movement (the respiratory excursion) may be as much as 9 cm.

MEDIASTINUM

The thoracic cavity is filled at both sides by the lungs, with each covered by their enclosing membrane, the visceral pleura (pp.73 and 120). The principal structures in the central region of the cavity are the heart and its great vessels (pp.107 and 115), the phrenic and vagus nerves (see below), the trachea (dividing into the bronchi, which enter the lungs – p.120), the oesophagus and thoracic duct at the back (in front of the vertebral column – see below), and the thymus at the front (see below), together with intervening connective tissue with numerous lymph nodes. This whole central region is the **mediastinum**, and is of great importance because infection within it can spread rapidly and is difficult to control.

An imaginary line drawn backwards from the manubriosternal joint to the lower border of T4 vertebra divides the area into an upper part, the **superior mediastinum**, and a lower part consisting of the **anterior**, **middle** and **posterior mediastinum** (**15.6**). The superior part contains the arch of the aorta, other great vessels, the trachea and the oesophagus, while the posterior part contains the continuation of the trachea and oesophagus. The middle mediastinum (a term which is not often used) consists of the pericardium and heart, while the anterior mediastinum is the very narrow space in front of the pericardium and behind the sternum, containing the thymus. The oesophagus, thoracic duct and thymus are described below, the vascular and respiratory organs on pp.107 and 120).

Phrenic and Vagus Nerves

To reach the diaphragm, the **phrenic nerves** must pass down through the whole length of the thorax, beneath the parietal pleura on each side of the mediastinum. From the cervical plexus in the neck (p.182), the **right phrenic** (**15.27a**) runs down on the right side of the superior vena cava and the right side of the heart (the right atrium – separated from it by the pericardium), and goes through the vena caval opening in the diaphragm. The **left phrenic** (**15.26a**) crosses the arch of the aorta and runs down on the pericardium (overlying the left ventricle), to pierce the muscle of the diaphragm. Both nerves enter the diaphragmatic muscle from below (**19.10**), and are the *only source of motor nerve fibres to the whole of the diaphragm*, including the crura. Although the peripheral part may receive fibres from intercostal nerves, these are purely sensory (afferent). The phrenics themselves have afferent fibres, not only from the diaphragm itself and the adjacent pericardium and pleura, but also from peritoneum on its

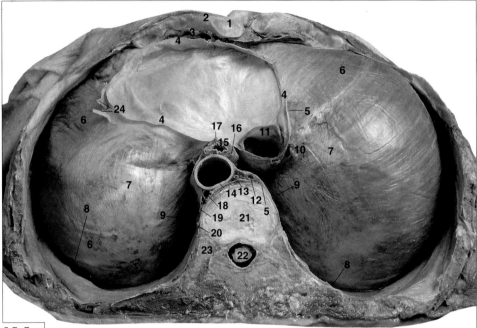

15.5a

Fig. 15.5 Diaphragm.
(a) Left and central regions seen from above after transecting the thorax at the level of the intervertebral disc between T9 and T10 vertebrae, and after removal of the lungs, heart and most of the pericardium.
(b) Central region, from below, showing origins from the crura and adjacent structures.

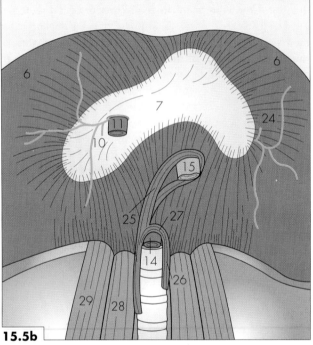

15.5b

9 Costomediastinal recess
10 Right phrenic nerve, passing through the vena caval foramen in the tendon of the diaphragm (not through the muscle)
11 Inferior vena cava, passing through its foramen just to the right of the midline in the tendon of the diaphragm, and therefore not subject to compression when the muscle contracts
12 Azygos vein, passing up from the abdomen into the thorax through the aortic opening of the diaphragm, approximately in the midline
13 Thoracic duct, also passing up through the aortic opening
14 Aorta, passing down through the thorax into the abdomen
15 Oesophagus, almost in the midline in **(a)** and passing down to its opening in the diaphragm which is often to the left of the midline, as in **(b)**
16 Posterior vagal trunk, behind the right edge of the oesophagus (15)
17 Anterior vagal trunk, adhering to the anterior wall of the oesophagus
18 Hemiazygos vein, the left–sided equivalent of the azygos vein (12)
19 Greater splanchnic nerve, derived from ganglia 5 to 9 of the sympathetic trunk (20)
20 Sympathetic trunk
21 Intervertebral disc
22 Spinal cord, within the vertebral canal
23 Head of ninth rib
24 Left phrenic nerve, piercing the muscle of the diaphragm (unlike the right phrenic, 10, which goes through the tendon)
25 Right crus, with fibres encircling the oesophageal opening
26 Left crus, smaller than the right
27 Median arcuate ligament, the union of the two crura (25 and 26) in front of the aorta (14)
28 Psoas major
29 Quadratus lumborum

1 Seventh costal cartilage
2 Internal thoracic artery. After giving off the musculophrenic artery (3) it continues into the abdominal wall as the superior epigastric artery
3 Musculophrenic artery
4 Cut edge of fibrous pericardium
5 Cut edge of pleura, overlying pericardium
6 Muscle of diaphragm
7 Tendon of diaphragm
8 Costodiaphragmatic recess of pleural cavity, which does not become occupied by the lung

lower surface and around the liver and gall bladder. This accounts for 'referred pain' to the tip of the shoulder (p.211) from disease in this area.

From the neck (p.181), the **left vagus nerve** runs down over the aortic arch, where it gives off the recurrent laryngeal nerve (p.188), and the **right** along the side of the trachea. Both nerves reach the back of the lung roots (giving branches to the cardiac plexus), and then join to form a plexus, mostly behing the lower oesophagus, before separating into the vagal trunks (**19.11**). These enter the abdomen and are mainly concerned with supplying the stomach (p.253).

Oesophagus

The **oesophagus** is the tubular connection between the pharynx in the neck and the stomach in the abdomen; it has a length of about 10 inches (25 cm). Its mucous membrane is lined by stratified squamous epithelium, and its outer muscular wall consists of skeletal muscle in the upper third and smooth muscle in the lower two-thirds. Some fibres are attached to the back of the cricoid cartilage (**16.37c**).

Beginning at the level of C6 vertebra, it runs down in front of the vertebral column (**15.26a** and **15.27a**) to the lower thorax (through the superior and then the posterior mediastinum on the way); here, it deviates slightly to the left usually, to pass through the diaphragm at the level of T10 vertebra; the lower 2 cm lie below the diaphragm. The oesophagus joins the stomach at the **cardia** (cardio-oesophageal junction, **19.14**). The trachea is in front of the upper part of the oesophagus, while the base of the heart (the left atrium) is in front of its lower part; an enlarged left atrium (from stenosis of the mitral valve) can press backwards, through the pericardium, and cause a radiologically detectable narrowing of the oesophagus.

The normal oesophagus is narrowest at its commencement (i.e. at the junction with the pharynx, p.184), which is 15 cm (6 inches) from the incisor teeth. Other regions in which some narrowing may be present are where the oesophagus crosses the right side of the arch of the aorta (22 cm, 9 inches from the teeth), where it is crossed by the left bronchus (27 cm, 11 inches from the teeth), and where it passes through the diaphragm (38 cm, 15 inches from the teeth). After a further 2 cm, the stomach is reached. These measurements are important when examining the interior of the oesophagus with the oesophagoscope or when passing instruments or tubes into the stomach; a stomach tube, for example, must be passed for at least 40 cm (16 in) from the front teeth before it reaches the gastric lumen.

Blood Supply and Lymph Drainage

The blood supply of the oesophagus comes from any adjacent arteries, together with their corresponding veins. One of these veins, the **left gastric**, is unusual in belonging to the portal system rather than the systemic circulation (as do the other veins); hence the lower oesophagus is a site of *portal–systemic anastomosis* (p.273). In fact, this is the most important of all the sites, because of the possible danger to life from rupture of enlarged veins (*oesophageal varices*).

Lymph drains from the oesophagus to adjacent nodes, such as the deep cervical, mediastinal and aortic nodes. There are both sympathetic and parasympathetic (vagal) nerve fibres present; oesophageal pain appears to be transmitted by both types, which is unusual, since pain fibres from viscera normally run only with sympathetic fibres (p.210).

Diseases

The normal process of swallowing is described on p.185. Difficulty in swallowing (*dysphagia*) of oesophageal origin may be due to various strictures or muscular disorders. *Strictures* may be benign, as following peptic ulceration or the after effects of swallowing corrosive liquids (whether accidental or in attempted suicide), or due to *carcinoma* which can occur in any part of the tube. Surgical removal may involve replacement by a length of intestine, but cure is complicated by the involvement of mediastinal lymph nodes.

Heartburn is a painful feeling behind the sternum which is due to the reflux of gastric contents into the oesophagus. It is usually of no significance but, as in the duodenum, the acid may cause peptic ulceration (p.257).

Achalasia (cardiospasm) is a neuromuscular condition of unknown cause, in which there is failure of muscular relaxation at the junction with the stomach. Instruments can be used to dilate the orifice.

Thoracic Duct

The **thoracic duct**, which is the largest lymphatic channel (**9.1**), begins as a slightly dilated *cul-de-sac* – the **cisterna chyli** – which lies in the abdomen under cover of the right crus of the diaphragm. The cisterna receives various lymph trunks both from the GI tract and from the rest of the abdomen. The duct enters the thorax through the aortic opening in the diaphragm; it then runs up in front of the vertebral column and behind the oesophagus to reach the left side of the neck. Here it curls round behind the common carotid artery and the internal jugular vein to enter the junction of that vein with the left subclavian vein (**16.35b**).

The duct contains many valves that direct the flow of lymph upwards, and so into the venous system. The last valve is not at the very end of the duct where it joins the venous junction, but a centimeter or two away from the junction; in the dissecting room, the end of the duct is filled with venous blood, and so may be confused with a vein.

Thymus

The **thymus** is a key element of the immune system; it is responsible for the maturation of **T-lymphocytes** (p.69), and is possibly under the influence of its hormone – thymin. It consists of two lobes lying closely side by side in the anterior mediastinum (**15.22**), in front of the upper part of the

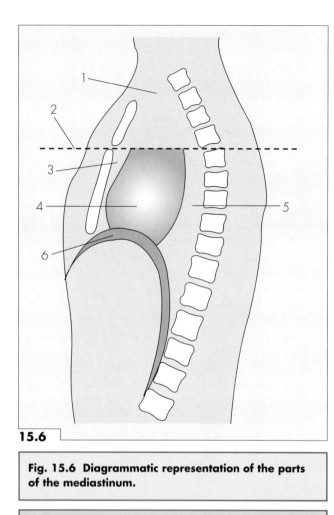

15.6

Fig. 15.6 Diagrammatic representation of the parts of the mediastinum.

1 Superior mediastinum
2 Manubriosternal joint line
3 Anterior ⎫
4 Middle ⎬ mediastinum
5 Posterior ⎭
6 Diaphragm

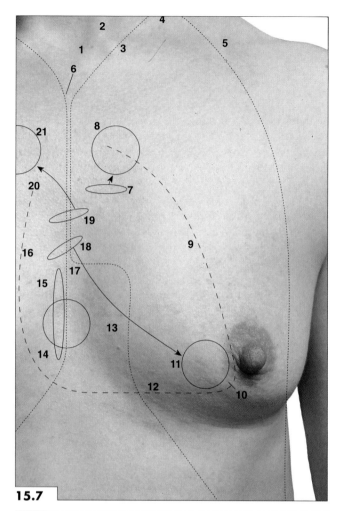

15.7

Fig. 15.7 Surface markings of the central and left part of the thorax.
The heart is outlined by the interrupted line and the pleurae by the dotted line. The heart valves are indicated by the ellipses and the positions where the valve sounds are best heard are indicated by the circles; the arrows indicate the direction of transmitted sounds.

pericardium and the great vessels. In children up to the age of puberty, it extends from the level of the fourth costal cartilage towards the neck, and may reach the lower border of the thyroid gland. In the adult, it usually becomes much reduced in size and is usually replaced by fatty tissue – it is often difficult to distinguish from adjacent mediastinal fat. It receives blood vessels from the inferior thyroid and internal thoracic arteries, and venous blood (containing thymic lymphocytes) drains into the corresponding arteries and into the left brachiocephalic vein.

Removal of the thymus (*thymectomy*) is often effective (for reasons not yet known) in controlling symptoms in *myasthenia gravis*, which is probably an autoimmune disease causing muscular weakness due to an acetylcholine defect at neuromuscular junctions (p.49).

SURFACE MARKINGS ON THE THORAX

The *surface markings* of the heart, great vessels and lungs are described with those structures, but it is *so* important to be able to visualize the positions of the principal thoracic contents in relation to the surface of the chest wall that they are summarized here (**15.7** and *Table* **15.1**), with page references to further descriptions. At first reading, the list should perhaps be regarded as an indication of 'things to come', rather than something to be fully memorized at this stage, though it can later be used for revision of essential facts.

1 Jugular notch of manubrium of sternum
2 Sternal head of sternocleidomastoid
3 Sternoclavicular joint, behind which the internal jugular and subclavian veins unite to form the brachiocephalic vein
4 Apex of pleura (and lung) extending into the neck for about 3 cm above the medial third of the clavicle (5)
5 Clavicle
6 Manubriosternal joint, a palpable landmark level with the second costal cartilages about 5 cm below the jugular notch (1) and where the two pleurae come to lie adjacent to one another
7 Pulmonary valve
8 Position where pulmonary valve sounds are best heard
9 Left border of heart, mostly left ventricle but with a small part of the left auricle at the upper end
10 Apex of the heart, in the fifth intercostal space about 9 cm from the midline

11 Position where sounds of the mitral valve (18) are best heard
12 Inferior border of the heart, mostly right ventricle
13 Area of pericardium not covered by pleura and lung
14 Level of sixth costal cartilage, where the inferior vena cava enters the right atrium
15 Tricuspid valve, lying vertically and the largest of the valve orifices. The valve sounds are best heard overlying it
16 Right border of the heart, formed by the right atrium
17 Level of fourth costal cartilages, where the left pleura deviates to the left
18 Mitral valve
19 Aortic valve
20 Third costal cartilage level, where the superior vena cava enters the right atrium
21 Position where sounds of the aortic valve (19) are best heard

Table 15.1 Surface markings on the thorax

Right border of the heart	at the right margin of the sternum from the third to the sixth costal cartilage (p.109).
Left border of the heart	from the second left costal cartilage at the left margin of the sternum to the left fifth intercostal space about 9 cm (3 1/2 in) from the midline (p.109).
Apex of the heart	left fifth intercostal space about 9 cm (3 1/2 in) from the midline, i.e. medial to the midclavicular line (p.110).
Lower border of the heart	from the lower border of the right sixth costal cartilage to the apex in the left fifth intercostal space (p.110).
Highest point of the arch of the aorta	midpoint of the manubrium (p.115).
Superior vena cava	at the right margin of the sternum from the first to the third costal cartilage (where it enters the right atrium of the heart) (p.115).
Inferior vena cava	enters the right atrium at the level of the right sixth costal cartilage (p.116).
Left brachiocephalic vein	from behind the left sternoclavicular joint to the right first costal cartilage (p.116).
Right brachiocephalic vein	from behind the right sternoclavicular joint to the right first costal cartilage (where it unites with its fellow to form the superior vena cava) (p.116).
Lung root	behind the third and fourth costal cartilages, level with the fifth to seventh thoracic vertebrae (p.123).
Oblique fissure of the lung	from the spine of the third thoracic vertebra and round the side of the chest to the sixth costal cartilage at the margin of the sternum. This line corresponds approximately to the position of the vertebral border of the scapula when the arm is raised above the head (p.122).
Transverse fissure of the right lung	transversely from the fourth costal cartilage at the right margin of the sternum to the point where it meets the line of the oblique fissure (p.122).
Left pleura	from the dome 3 cm above the inner third of the clavicle to the midline at the sternal angle (second costal cartilage), then straight down to the fourth cartilage level where the line deviates 2.5 cm to the left before running down to the sixth cartilage, then outwards to the eighth rib in the midclavicular line, tenth rib in the midaxillary line and twelfth rib at the lateral border of erector spinae (remembered by the even numbers from 2 to 12) (p.121).
Right pleura	similar to the left, except that there is no cardiac notch and the line runs straight down in the midline from the second to the sixth cartilage (p.121).
Lung	mostly follows the lines of pleural reflexion on each side, except that beyond the sixth costal cartilage the lower border of the lung is at a higher level than the pleura, reaching the eighth rib in the midaxillary line and tenth rib at the lateral border of erector spinae (remembered by the even numbers 2 to 10) (p.121).

SURGICAL APPROACHES THROUGH THE CHEST

As the intercostal vessels and nerves are situated at the lower border of a rib (see above), needles or tubes that are introduced through the chest wall (as in intubation of the chest, to remove fluid or air from the pleural cavity) are always inserted into the intercostal space immediately *above* a rib, so keeping as far away as possible from the vessels and nerve (**15.4**). For the removal of fluid, the site chosen is usually the eighth intercostal space in the midaxillary line, and for the removal of air (in pneumothorax, p.125), the second intercostal space just lateral to the midclavicular line. For local anaesthesia of an intercostal nerve, the anaesthetic solution must be introduced near the lower border of the rib (after aspiration to ensure that the needle is not in a vessel).

The surgical approach to organs within the chest involves either splitting the sternum longitudinally in the midline (*median sternotomy*) or entering through the 'bed' of a rib (*thoracotomy*). For the latter, the periosteum of the chosen rib is incised along its length and stripped back to expose the rib itself, which is then 'shelled out' of its periosteal sleeve and part of it removed. Subsequent incision through the periosteum in the 'bed' of the rib allows access to the pleural cavity. Afterwards, the incision is closed by suturing the two strips of periosteum together. (Owing to its osteogenic capacity (p.12) the periosteum will gradually regenerate a bony structure that bears some resemblance to a rib.) The intercostal muscles above and below are undisturbed, since their attachments to the periosteum have not been cut. This kind of incision, deep to a rib, heals better than one that incises the intercostal muscles.

BREAST

The **breasts** (mammary glands) exist in the female to provide milk for the newborn child, and are usually considered to be modified sweat glands. They are present in the male, but remain in a rudimentary state throughout life (though there may be some enlargement in endocrine disorders or with hormone treatment, e.g. for carcinoma of the prostate).

The adult *female* breast consists largely of an irregular framework of fibrous tissue (**15.8**) that contains a variable amount of fat and a number of blind-ending duct systems which, under the influence of the hormonal changes in pregnancy, develop into secretory acini. The breast lies in the subcutaneous tissue (superficial fascia) of the anterior thoracic wall, overlying pectoralis major and overlapping on to serratus anterior and with a small part over the rectus sheath and external oblique (**6.1a**). Strands of fibrous tissue attach the breast to overlying skin and the underlying fascia and help to maintain its normal form; cancerous involvement of these connections (sometimes called the **suspensory ligaments** of the breast) causes contraction and puckering of the

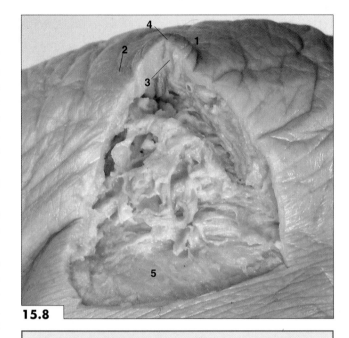

15.8

Fig. 15.8 Dissection of female breast to show the connective tissue framework (after removal of fat), and lactiferous ducts converging on the nipple.

1 Areola	4 Nipple
2 Areolar gland	5 Fascia over pectoralis
3 Lactiferous duct	major

skin. Although the size of the non-lactating breast is very variable (depending entirely on the fat content, not on glandular tissue), the extent of the **base** of the breast is constant: from near the midline to near the midaxillary line, and from the second to the sixth rib. A small part of the upper outer quadrant of breast tissue penetrates the fascia of the floor of the axilla, forming the **axillary tail** of the breast which comes to lie adjacent to some of the axillary lymph nodes.

About 15 **lactiferous ducts** (**15.8**) converge in a radial direction to open on the **nipple**, which is a projection just below the middle of the breast, and is surrounded by an area of pigmented skin – the **areola**. (Although some breast structure develops very early in embryonic life, it is only a small nipple and areola that are apparent in the young female.) A few large sebaceous glands (**areolar glands**) may form small elevations (tubercles) of the areola.

At **puberty**, under the influence of oestrogen and progesterone (p.296), the gland enlarges due to the deposition of fat and some increase in the size of the ducts and the primitive glandular acini. During menstruation there is some vascular engorgement and acinar dilatation in the first half of the cycle; this is followed by regression in the second half.

BLOOD SUPPLY AND LYMPH DRAINAGE

Perforating branches of the internal thoracic and intercostal arteries enter the breast through the second, third and fourth intercostal spaces – there are also corresponding veins.

Most of the lymph (75%) drains to axillary nodes, but some passes through the pectoralis major muscle (along the paths of the perforating blood vessels) to nodes within the thorax, especially those alongside the internal thoracic vessels near the sternum. It might have been expected that the lateral part drained to axillary nodes and the medial part to these parasternal nodes, but this is not so; lymph from any part of the breast can drain to any of these sites, because there is plenty of communication of lymphatic channels within the breast. Lymph from the overlying skin can pass across the midline from one breast to the other.

NERVE SUPPLY

The skin of the breast is supplied by intercostal nerves – usually T4 to T6. Sympathetic fibres supply the blood vessels of the glands, but the control of secretion is hormonal.

LACTATION

With pregnancy, there is a large increase in the acini and ducts (due to progesterone, oestrogen and prolactin), and the areola acquires a deeper pigmentation which remains throughout life. After birth, *lactation* (milk secretion and ejection) is induced by the sudden fall in circulating oestrogen, allowing prolactin to exert its secretory effect; for mothers who cannot or will not breast-feed, oestrogen can be given to stop lactation.

The stimulus of *suckling* by the baby is necessary to maintain the secretion and ejection of milk; suckling induces the production of prolactin by the anterior pituitary (causing milk secretion), and of oxytocin by the posterior pituitary, which causes milk ejection.

The first milk that is secreted for a day or two after birth is thin and watery (*colostrum*), but thereafter *true milk* is produced. Apart from proteins (mainly lactalbumin), carbohydrate (lactose), fats and minerals, milk also contains some maternal antibodies that may be important in preventing infection in the infant – an advantage that bottle (artificial) feeding cannot give. In comparison with human milk, cow's milk contains, in particular, less sugar but more sodium and potassium, so if given to a human infant the cow's milk must be diluted but have sugar added.

Lactation appears to inhibit ovulation, which does not recur until weaning; thus, in many nursing mothers, lactation has a contraceptive effect. However, it is also possible for ovulation to recur earlier than this. If lactation is suppressed after birth, menstruation usually returns after six weeks.

EXAMINATION

Clinical examination of the breasts includes *inspection* and *palpation*, with the patient sitting up, bending forward and lying down, and sitting up with the hands above the head. Any asymmetry and 'tethering' of swellings to skin or underlying tissues must be particularly noted. Palpation must include examination of the axillary and supraclavicular lymph nodes. Regular self-examination should be encouraged in all females, especially during reproductive life and in those with a family history of breast cancer, since a hereditary factor is undoubtedly present in this disease.

Specialized examinations include soft-tissue radiography (*mammography* and *xerography*), *ultrasound* and *thermography* (the viewing of 'hot spots' by infra-red photography).

DISEASES

The breast has for long been the site of the **commonest female cancer**, though that of the lung may now be overtaking it. A painless, irregular lump that eventually becomes fixed to the surrounding tissues, perhaps with discharge from the nipple, is a characteristic feature. As in most sites, the danger lies in *lymphatic spread*, especially to within the mediastinum, and early recognition is now aided by the publicity of screening programmes and less reticence on the part of modern females in seeking advice. Localized removal coupled with radiotherapy or chemotherapy is often considered as effective in controlling the condition as the complete removal (*mastectomy*) often carried out in the past. Plastic surgery, including the use of implants, does not appear to have any adverse effect on rates of cure and has obvious advantages in restoring not only physical form but self-respect.

Benign tumours are commoner than cancerous growths, and the commonest of all breast conditions is *fibrocystic disease* (*chronic cystic mastitis*). Although solitary cysts do occur, in most cases there are multiple, rounded nodules of varying size but often painful and tender to the touch. There is no specific treatment, but patients must be examined regularly since the incidence of carcinoma is greater in those who have fibrocystic disease. A *fibroadenoma* is another frequent but benign breast lump; it feels rather mobile in the surrounding tissue, and should be treated by excision. Sometimes, biopsy for microscopic examination is necessary to confirm the diagnosis of any breast tumour.

Infections of the ducts and acini (*acute mastitis*) are commonest during lactation, and should respond to antibiotics, but a large abscess may require surgical incision to drain away the pus.

HEART AND GREAT VESSELS

Consult the introduction to the Cardiovascular System on p.53, which includes a description of the pumping action of the heart (the cardiac cycle).

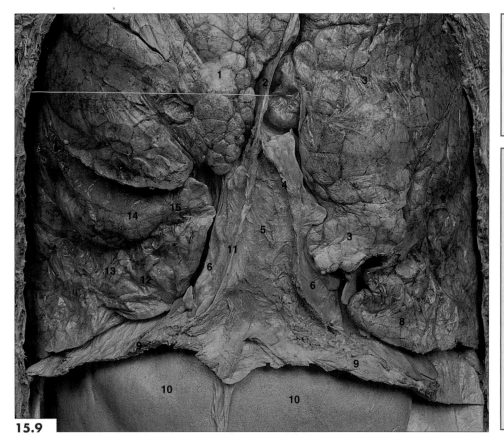

Fig. 15.9 Central part of the thorax, from the front.
The anterior chest wall has been removed, leaving the cut edges of the pleura and diaphragm.

1 Upper lobe of right lung
2 Cut edges of right and left pleurae in contact
3 Upper lobe of left lung
4 Cut edge of left pleura
5 Area of pericardium in contact with sternum
6 Pleura overlying pericardium
7 Oblique fissure
8 Inferior lobe of left lung
9 Cut edge of diaphragm
10 Liver
11 Cut edge of right pleura
12 Inferior lobe of right lung
13 Oblique fissure
14 Middle lobe of right lung
15 Transverse fissure

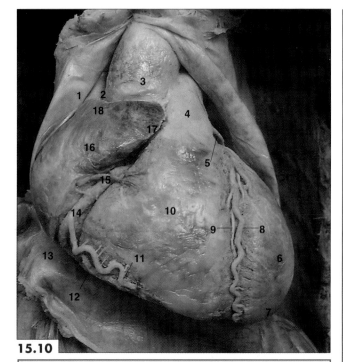

Fig. 15.10 Anterior surface of the heart.
The pericardium has been incised and turned back but remains attached to the great vessels at the top.

1 Pericardium
2 Superior vena cava, entering right atrium (16)
3 Ascending aorta, which has emerged from the left ventricle (6) behind the pulmonary trunk (4)
4 Pulmonary trunk, emerging from the upper part (infundibulum, outflow part) of the right ventricle (10)
5 Tip of auricle of left atrium, which is at the back (base) of the heart
6 Left ventricle, forming most of the left border
7 Apex, whose forward thrust when the ventricles contract produces the apex beat felt in the fifth intercostal space
8 Anterior interventricular artery in interventricular groove
9 Great cardiac vein
10 Right ventricle, forming most of the anterior surface
11 Marginal branch of right coronary artery
12 Small cardiac vein
13 Upper surface of diaphragm, here obscuring the entry of the inferior vena cava into the right atrium (16)
14 Right coronary artery in atrioventricular groove
15 Anterior cardiac vein, opening into right atrium (16)
16 Right atrium, forming the right border
17 Auricle of right atrium, covering the beginning of the right coronary artery (14)
18 Position of SA node in atrial wall

HEART

The **heart** is enclosed in a fibrous sac – the **pericardium** – and lies in the central part of the thoracic cavity (the middle mediastinum, p.101), more to the left than the right, behind the body of the sternum, in front of the oesophagus and vertebral column, and level with the fifth to eighth thoracic vertebrae (**15.6**, **15.7**, **15.9**, and **15.10**).

CHAMBERS OF THE HEART

Of the four chambers of the heart – the left and right atria, and the left and right ventricles (see **8.1**) – the two atria are separated from one another by the **interatrial septum**, and the two ventricles by the **interventricular septum**; there is normally no communication between the two sides. How-ever, during fetal development there is a stage during which the two sides *do* communicate (before the septa are complete) and sometimes the communication persists, most commonly between the two atria (the common type of 'hole in the heart', p.119).

The heart does not hang down from the great vessels with the ventricles directly below the atria; instead it is tilted *forwards* and twisted to the *left*, so that the atria are towards the back and right side of the heart, with the ventricles towards the front and left (**15.11** and **15.12**). The **right atrium** forms the right border of the heart, and when viewed from the front it lies just beside the right margin of the sternum, from the third to the sixth costal cartilage. The uppermost part of the right atrium at the front is the **right**

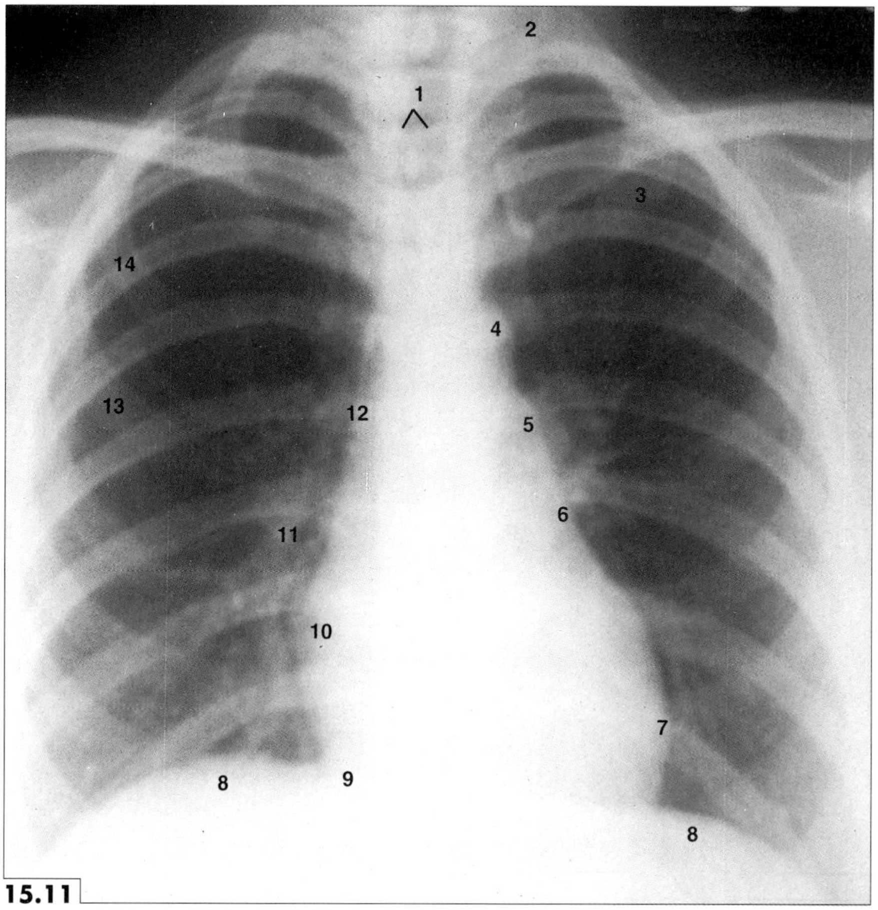

15.11

Fig. 15.11 Radiograph of the thorax.

This is the standard postero-anterior (PA) view, the 'straight X-ray' or 'plain film' of the chest, taken from behind with the X-ray plate at the front of the chest but viewed from the front, to show the outline of the heart and the lung fields.

1 Margin of trachea, translucent because of its contained air
2 Tubercle of first rib
3 Anterior end of first rib
4 Arch of aorta, passing backwards and producing the characteristic bulge known radiologically as the aortic knuckle
5 Pulmonary trunk
6 Tip of left auricle, whose outline is a slight concavity
7 Left ventricle
8 Dome of diaphragm
9 Inferior vena cava, entering right atrium (10)
10 Right atrium
11 Hilar shadows, due to vessels and bronchi of the lung root
12 Superior vena cava, passing down to enter the right atrium (10)
13 Anterior end of third rib
14 Posterior part of third rib. Note the overlapping of the shadows of the ribs as they pass obliquely forwards and downwards.

auricle. The **left ventricle** forms most of the left border, with a small prolongation of the left atrium (called the **left auricle**) at its upper end. The left border extends from the left margin of the sternum at the level of the second costal cartilage to the **apex** of the heart. This is the lower left corner, formed by the left ventricle, and is in the fifth intercostal space about 9 cm (3½ in) from the midline, where the *apex beat* is felt through the chest wall. Much of the front surface is the right ventricle, and this also forms most of the lower border, which extends from the right sixth costal cartilage to the apex.

The **base** of the heart is the *posterior* surface, made up chiefly of the left atrium. The top of the heart, where most of the great vessels enter and leave, has erroneously been called the base of the heart or even its apex, but it has no special name.

The left atrium and left ventricle communicate through the **left atrioventricular opening**, which is guarded by the **mitral valve** (a **bicuspid valve** – having two cusps, **15.12**); similarly there is a **right atrioventricular opening** with the **tricuspid valve** (with three cusps) between the right atrium and right ventricle (**15.13**). At the upper part of the heart, the left ventricle opens into the aorta with the aortic valve at the junction (**15.12**), and the right ventricle opens through

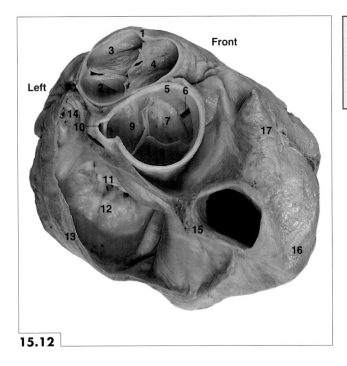

15.12

Fig. 15.12 Pulmonary, aortic and mitral valves, from above.
The pulmonary trunk, ascending aorta and superior vena cava have been cut off, and so has much of the left atrium. This view looking down from above shows the cusps of the three valves.

1 Pulmonary trunk	11 Anterior ⎱ cusp of
2 Left ⎱ cusp of pulmonary valve	12 Posterior ⎰ mitral valve
3 Anterior ⎰	13 Posterior wall of left atrium, forming the base of the heart
4 Right	
5 Ascending aorta	14 Auricle of left atrium
6 Marker in ostium of right coronary artery	15 Superior vena cava
7 Right ⎱ cusp of aortic valve	16 Right atrium, forming right border
8 Posterior ⎰	17 Auricle of right atrium
9 Left	
10 Ostium of left coronary artery	

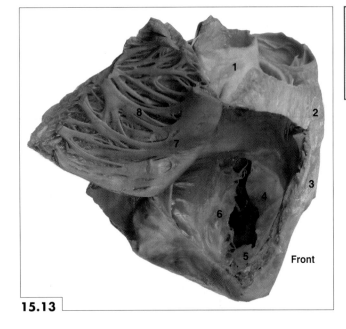

15.13

Fig. 15.13 Tricuspid valve and the right atrium.
A flap has been cut in the anterior wall of the atrium (as shown in **15.15**) and turned backwards. The view is looking towards the left, on to the cusps of the vertically placed tricuspid valve, separating the atrium from the right ventricle.

1 Superior vena cava	7 Crista terminalis*
2 Auricle of right atrium	8 Pectinate muscles*
3 Anterior wall of right atrium	
4 Anterior ⎱ cusp of tricuspid valve	*of anterior wall of right atrium
5 Posterior ⎰	
6 Septal	

the pulmonary valve into the pulmonary trunk (**15.12**). The aortic and pulmonary valves, which each have three cusps, are sometimes collectively called the **semilunar valves** (from the shape of the valve cusps).

Interior of the Chambers

Each chamber can be recognized by the features in its interior.

In the **right atrium** (**15.14**), most of the walls are smooth but the auricle and the anterior wall show muscular ridges (the **pectinate muscles** and the **crista terminalis**). In the middle of the interatrial septum is a circular depression, the **fossa ovalis**, representing the site of the foramen ovale of the embryo (p.119). The openings of the superior vena cava and the inferior vena cava are at the top and bottom corners, and just to the left of the inferior vena caval opening is the opening of the **coronary sinus**, the main vein of the heart itself (p.114). Farther still to the left is the large vertically placed **tricuspid opening** (**15.13**).

In the **right ventricle** (**15.15**), much of the wall shows muscular ridges (**trabeculae**), with some forming the **papillary muscles** which are connected to the tricuspid valve cusps by **chordae tendineae** (see below). At the front at the top is the **pulmonary valve**.

In the **left ventricle** (**15.16**), **trabeculae** are again prominent, with **papillary muscles** joined to the **mitral valve** cusps by **chordae tendineae**, and the aortic valve at the top of the chamber.

In the **left atrium** (**15.12**), the walls are smooth except in the auricle, with the **pulmonary veins** entering at each side and the **mitral opening** towards the bottom.

STRUCTURE

The **pericardium**(15.9), the sac containing the heart and the roots of the great vessels, consists of fibrous and serous parts. The fibrous outer part (**fibrous pericardium**) fuses underneath the heart with the central tendon of the diaphragm (**15.5**), and also fuses with the ends of the great vessels as they enter or leave, so helping to anchor the heart in its central position. The inner **serous pericardium** has two layers: the **parietal layer** is the part that adheres to the inner surface of the fibrous pericardium; over the great vessels it becomes reflected on to the outer surface of the heart as the **visceral layer**. This visceral layer of serous pericardium is sometimes called the **epicardium**. The adjacent surfaces of the serous pericardium are kept moist by a very small amount of **pericardial fluid** so that as the heart beats, the surfaces can glide over one another easily (like the layers of the pleura when the lungs move, p.120).

The walls of the chambers of the heart – collectively called the **myocardium** – are composed of **cardiac muscle**, which varies in thickness in the different chambers; it is thinnest in the two atria, thicker in the right ventricle, and thickest in the left ventricle. The wall of the left ventricle is three times as thick as that of the right because the blood pressure in the left ventricle is much higher than in the right (**15.15** and **15.16**; p.61). The inner surfaces of all the chambers are lined by endothelial cells similar to those of the blood vessels (p.55); in the heart these cells and the small amount of underlying connective tissue constitute the **endocardium**. Similar flattened cells and connective tissue on the outer surface of the heart form the **epicardium**, which was described above.

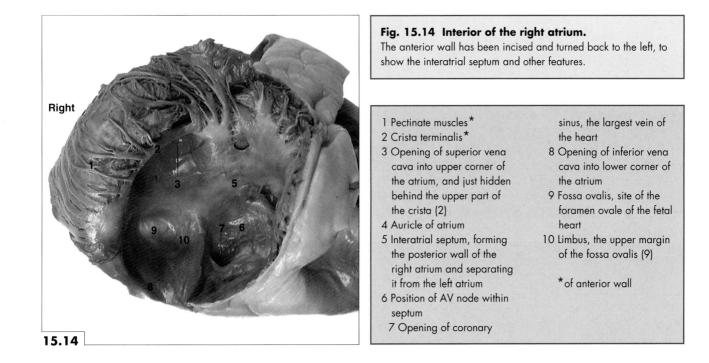

Right

15.14

Fig. 15.14 Interior of the right atrium.
The anterior wall has been incised and turned back to the left, to show the interatrial septum and other features.

1 Pectinate muscles*
2 Crista terminalis*
3 Opening of superior vena cava into upper corner of the atrium, and just hidden behind the upper part of the crista (2)
4 Auricle of atrium
5 Interatrial septum, forming the posterior wall of the right atrium and separating it from the left atrium
6 Position of AV node within septum
7 Opening of coronary

sinus, the largest vein of the heart
8 Opening of inferior vena cava into lower corner of the atrium
9 Fossa ovalis, site of the foramen ovale of the fetal heart
10 Limbus, the upper margin of the fossa ovalis (9)

*of anterior wall

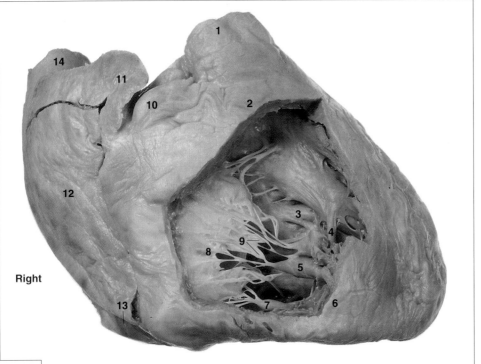

Right

Fig. 15.15 Right ventricle, opened from the front by removing most of the anterior wall. The specimen also shows the incision in the right atrium used for **15.13** and similar to that used for **15.14** (from a different specimen).

15.15

1 Pulmonary trunk	8 Anterior cusp of tricuspid valve, obscuring the posterior and
2 Infundibulum (outflow part) of right ventricle	septal cusps seen in **15.13**
3 Trabeculae on interventricular septum	9 Chordae tendineae
4 Septomarginal trabecula (moderator band), extending from	10 Cut edge of ascending aorta
the septum to the anterior papillary muscle (5)	11 Auricle of right atrium
5 Anterior papillary muscle, arising from the anterior wall	12 Right atrium, with incision lines for the flap seen in **15.13**
6 Anterior ventricular wall	13 Inferior vena cava
7 Posterior papillary muscle, arising from the floor	14 Superior vena cava

The muscle of the atria is rather surprisingly not in direct continuity with the muscle of the ventricles; at the junctions between the atria and ventricles, indicated on the surface of the heart by the **atrioventricular groove**, there is a figure-of-eight of dense connective tissue (the **fibrous framework** of the heart), forming rings round the atrioventricular openings, and giving attachment not only to the muscle fibres of the atria (above the rings) and ventricles (below the rings) but also to the margins of the mitral and tricuspid valves. A smaller, connective-tissue figure-of-eight lies at the beginning of the aorta and pulmonary trunk, and gives attachment to the cusps of the aortic and pulmonary valves.

Valve cusps consist of a connective tissue core which is covered on each side by endocardium. The shape of the cusps of the aortic and pulmonary valves (**15.12**) is such that, after blood has been squeezed past them by the contraction of the ventricles, the back pressure of blood in the aorta and pulmonary trunk brings the valve cusps together, so closing the gap and preventing regurgitation of blood into the

ventricles. The margins of the mitral and tricuspid valves are attached by fibrous tissue strands (**chordae tendineae**) to small muscular projections from the ventricular walls (**papillary muscles, 15.15** and **15.16**); when the ventricles contract, these muscles and chordae prevent the cusps from being turned 'inside out' and so prevent blood from returning to the atria. Thus, the only way blood can leave the contracting ventricles is through the aortic and pulmonary valves.

Conduction System

The rate at which the heart beats is controlled by a small area of specialized cardiac muscle – the **sinuatrial node** – which is commonly called the **SA node** or 'pacemaker of the heart'. This node is situated within the front wall of the right atrium, just below the opening of the superior vena cava (**15.17**). It receives nerve fibres from the vagus (parasympathetic) and sympathetic nerves.

Specialized muscle fibres in the SA node demonstrate the

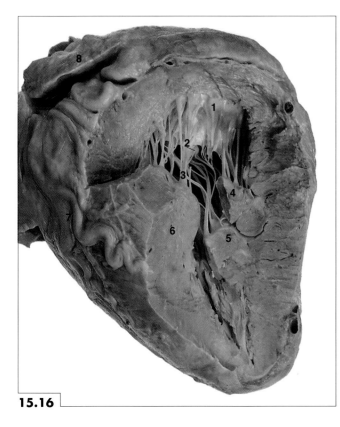

15.16

Fig. 15.16 Left ventricle, opened from the front and the left, looking upwards to the under surface of the mitral valve cusps.

1 Anterior ⎫
2 Posterior ⎬ cusps of mitral valve
3 Chordae tendineae
4 Anterior ⎫
5 Posterior ⎬ papillary muscle
6 Anterior ventricular wall, three times as thick as the right ventricular wall in **15.15**
7 Anterior interventricular branch of left coronary artery
8 Auricle of left atrium

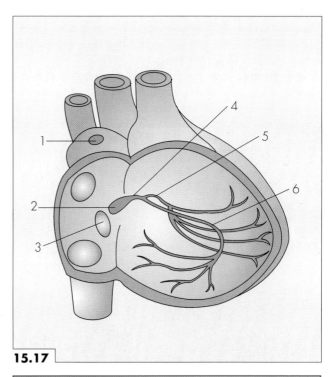

15.17

Fig. 15.17 Diagrammatic representation of the main components of the conducting system of the heart.
To avoid complicating the diagram, only a few short branches of the main limbs of the AV bundle are shown; in reality they spread throughout the walls of the respective ventricles.

1 SA node
2 AV node
3 Opening of coronary sinus
4 AV bundle
5 Left branch of AV bundle
6 Right branch of AV bundle

unusual property of *spontaneous depolarization* which leads to action potentials (p.47). These fibres are connected to the nearby, ordinary, atrial muscle fibres by gap junctions (p.14); the action potential generated in the SA node cells can be conducted to neighbouring fibres via this route, and can cause contractions in them. Since the ordinary atrial fibres are, in turn, connected to one another by gap junctions, waves of excitation – followed by contraction – spread all over the atria.

Impulses soon reach another area of specialized muscle – the **atrioventricular node** or **AV node** – which is situated in the lower part of the interatrial septum (**15.17**). From this point, specialized fibres continue into the interventricular septum as the **AV bundle** (**bundle of His**, named after the German anatomist who described it). Right and left bundle branches course down the two sides of the septum and give off many branches that spread through the walls of the ventricles. Therefore, when the wave of excitation reaches the AV node, it moves swiftly along this pathway to reach the ventricular muscle fibres, causing them to contract. Note that there is no muscle continuity between atria and ventricles; the only way impulses can pass from atria to ventricles is via the AV bundle. The SA and AV nodes, together with the AV bundle and its branches, collectively form the **conduction** or **conducting system** of the heart.

If any parts of the conducting system become diseased, the regularity of the heart beat will be disturbed; there are different kinds of *heart block*, each depending upon which parts of the system are affected. When deprived of the normal impulse for contraction, the atria and ventricles may still continue to beat but at their own inherent rhythms (about 70 beats/minute for the atria and 30 beats/minute for the ventricles). It is also possible for *fibrillation* of atria or ventricles to occur – exceptionally rapid beating at 200–300 beats/minute or more. Ventricular fibrillation is a common cause of cardiac arrest; the rapid 'quivering' of the ventricles does not allow proper contraction, so blood circulation ceases. The use of a *defibrillator* – a machine that delivers an electrical shock to the heart through the chest wall – may stimulate the return of normal rhythm and contraction.

BLOOD SUPPLY AND LYMPH DRAINAGE

The heart gets its own blood supply from the **right** and **left coronary arteries** (**15.10** and **15.18**); these are the first vessels to arise from the aorta, and do so just above the aortic valve. The main branches of the right coronary are the **right marginal artery** and the **posterior interventricular artery**; from the left coronary arise the **anterior interventricular artery** and the **circumflex artery**.

In the normal heart, their various branches do not make significant anastomotic connections with one another, so that any sudden blockage by thrombosis or other vascular disease damages the part of the heart wall supplied by that vessel.

However, *slow* occlusion of vessels may give time for functional anastomoses to open up, and so perhaps reduce the seriousness of a later blockage. It may be possible to bypass a blocked vessel – in a **coronary artery bypass** (**CAB**) operation (**15.19**) – by using a vein graft (i.e. part of the great saphenous vein, turned inside out or orientated such that any valves in it do not block the desired direction of bloodflow), or by anastomosing the internal thoracic artery from the anterior thoracic wall to the vessel beyond the point of blockage. It is perhaps fortunate that the coronary vessel most commonly affected by disease is the anterior interventricular branch of the left coronary artery; since it is on the front of the heart it is easy to expose surgically.

Most of the venous blood from the heart wall drains (via veins that often accompany the arteries but do not have the same names) into a vein at the back of the heart, the **coronary sinus** (**15.20**); this opens into the right atrium just to the left of the opening of the inferior vena cava. Although the arteries of the heart are so frequently affected by pathological changes, the cardiac veins remain singularly free from disease.

Lymph from the heart drains to mediastinal lymph nodes, but, as far as function and disease are concerned, the lymphatics of the heart are of little importance.

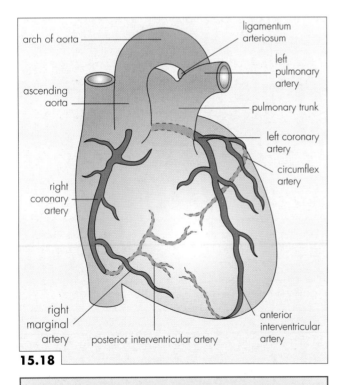

15.18

Fig. 15.18 Diagram of the arteries of the heart, as seen from the front (those not on the anterior surface are shown in interrupted line).

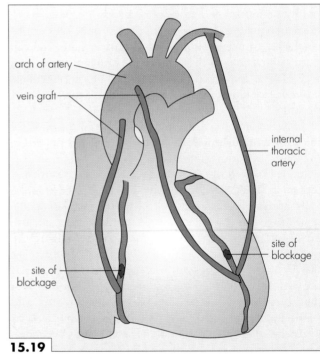

15.19

Fig. 15.19 Diagram of coronary artery bypasses. Obstructed vessels can be bypassed by vein grafts or by anastomosis with the internal thoracic artery from the chest wall.

NERVE SUPPLY

The heart receives parasympathetic and sympathetic nerve fibres from the **cardiac plexus**. This is a mass of nerve fibres derived from branches of the vagus nerves and the sympathetic trunks in the neck and upper thorax; they collect together under the arch of the aorta and the bifurcation of the trachea, and send branches mainly to the SA node and the coronary arteries. The vagus slows the heart and the sympathetic increases the heart rate (p.46).

GREAT VESSELS

At the upper end of the heart, the **superior vena cava** (see below) enters the upper corner of the right atrium (**15.10**), level with the right third costal cartilage. To the left of the vena cava the **ascending aorta** runs upwards to become the **arch of the aorta** (**15.21**). This rises as high as the middle of the manubrium of the sternum, and then passes backwards and slightly to the left, to run down as the **descending (thoracic) aorta**. To the left of the ascending aorta, the **pulmonary trunk** passes upwards from the top of the right ventricle and divides beneath the aortic arch into the **right** and **left pulmonary arteries** (**15.21**). Note that of these three great vessels, the aorta is in the middle, with the vena cava on the right and the pulmonary trunk on the left; although

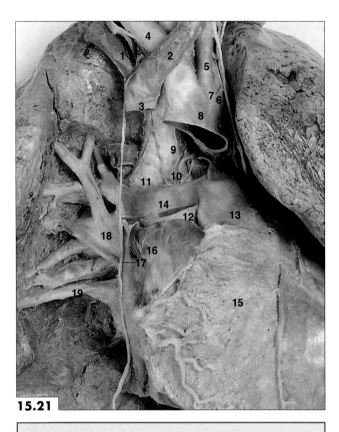

15.21

Fig. 15.21 Heart, lungs and great vessels, from the front.
Part of the aorta and most of the superior vena cava have been removed to show the bifurcation of the trachea and structures in the right lung root, displayed by dissecting away some lung tissue.

1 Right brachiocephalic vein
2 Left brachiocephalic vein, joining the right (1) to form the superior vena cava (3)
3 Superior vena cava
4 Brachiocephalic trunk
5 Left common carotid artery
6 Left subclavian artery
7 Left phrenic nerve
8 Arch of aorta, from which the three large arteries arise (4, 5 and 6)
9 Trachea
10 Left main bronchus, with an overlying bronchial artery
11 Right main bronchus
12 Ascending aorta (cut edge)
13 Pulmonary trunk, dividing into the two pulmonary arteries (right: 14; the left is hidden by the overlying lung)
14 Right pulmonary artery
15 Right ventricle
16 Right atrium
17 Right phrenic nerve
18 Superior pulmonary vein, lying in front of the branches of the pulmonary artery (14)
19 Inferior pulmonary vein

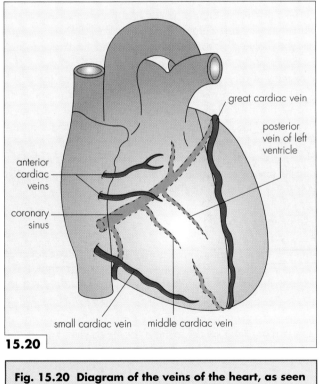

15.20

anterior cardiac veins

coronary sinus

great cardiac vein

posterior vein of left ventricle

small cardiac vein   middle cardiac vein

Fig. 15.20 Diagram of the veins of the heart, as seen from the front (those not on the anterior surface are in interrupted line).

the left ventricle forms the left border of the heart, the ascending aorta which arises from it spirals behind the pulmonary trunk and comes to lie on the right of the trunk.

From the top of the aortic arch arise the **brachiocephalic trunk**, the **left common carotid artery** and the **left subclavian artery**, in that order from right to left (**15.21**). The **left brachiocephalic vein** (formed behind the left sternoclavicular joint, p.216) runs in front of these arteries to unite with the **right brachiocephalic vein** (formed behind the right sternoclavicular joint) and so forms the **superior vena cava**, level with the right first costal cartilage. At the level of the right second costal cartilage, the superior vena cava is joined from behind by the arch of the **azygos vein**, curling over the top of the lung root (**15.27a**). This vein begins in the upper abdomen by the union of lumbar and subcostal veins, and runs up through the aortic opening in the diaphragm and on the right side of the thoracic vertebral bodies, collecting posterior intercostal veins on the way. On the left side in a similar position, the **hemiazygos vein** in the lower thorax and the **accessory hemiazygos vein** in the upper thorax (**15.26a**) cross over the vertebral column, usually about the levels of T7 and T8 vertebrae, to join the azygos vein.

In and around the wall of the aortic arch, there are specialized nerve receptors concerned with the control of the heart rate (p.54). Beneath the arch, the left pulmonary artery is joined to the arch by a band of tissue, the **ligamentum arteriosum** (**15.26a**). This represents the obliterated remains of the *fetal* ductus arteriosus. Because the lungs are not functional in fetal life, there is no need for a large pulmonary circulation, and the blood from the right ventricle is 'short-circuited' from the pulmonary trunk into the aorta, through the ductus arteriosus. Within a few hours of birth, the ductus should have become greatly constricted, so directing blood into the lungs, and within a few weeks it should have become a fibrous cord (the ligamentum arteriosum). Failure to close results in a **patent ductus arteriosus**, the commonest congenital anomaly of the heart and great vessels (p.119). A large patent ductus requires surgical closure to prevent the complications of mixing the pulmonary and systemic circulations.

As it crosses the arch of the aorta, the **left vagus nerve** (**15.26a**) gives off the highly important **left recurrent laryngeal nerve** (supplying the muscles of the left side of the larynx, p.188), which hooks round the ligamentum (or ductus) to pass up into the neck; it must be carefully preserved in operations in this region. (The **right recurrent laryngeal nerve** hooks under the right subclavian artery in the lowest part of the neck – **15.27a**.)

The **inferior vena cava** (p.253) comes up from the abdomen (**19.10**) to pass through the tendon of the diaphragm (so that it is not squeezed when the muscle contracts – **15.5a** and **15.5b**) and enters the lower corner of the right atrium on a level with the right sixth costal cartilage.

EXAMINATION OF THE HEART

The *examination* of cardiac function includes the clinical examination of the chest, with *inspection, palpation, percussion* and *auscultation* (as described on p.124 and in **15.5**), feeling the pulses (p.60) and taking the blood pressure (p.59). The commonest chest radiograph (**15.11**), which is taken from behind with the X-ray film at the front (*posteroanterior* or *PA view*), shows a 'cardiac shadow' that indicates the position and size of the heart, and any alterations from the normal shadow pattern can be noted – such as a bulging right atrium or left ventricle that indicates enlargement of these chambers. *Electrocardiography* (see below) is a common supplement to clinical examination, and for the specialist many other methods are available, including those involving *cardiac catheterization* (see below), *ultrasound* (echocardiography) and circulatory studies using radioactive isotopes.

Heart Sounds

The *sounds* of a beating heart as heard with a stethoscope are due to reverberations in the blood caused by the closures of the heart valves. There are normally *two* sounds in rapid succession, followed by a pause (which is twice as long as the time between the two sounds) before the sounds are repeated. The sequence is usually described in writing as 'lubb-dupp, pause, lubb-dupp, pause'. The *first* sound – the louder of the two – is due to the closure of the atrioventricular (mitral and tricuspid) valves immediately after the beginning of ventricular systole. The *second* and shorter sound is due to closure of the semilunar (aortic and pulmonary) valves as ventricular systole comes to an end. When valves become diseased, they fail to close properly and lead to unusual patterns of bloodflow and therefore to changes in the character of the sounds. These abnormal sounds are called *heart murmurs*; physicians can diagnose particular valvular diseases from the kind of sounds murmurs cause (although some murmurs can be innocent and do not always indicate heart disease). Very loud murmurs become palpable as *thrills*. Common valvular diseases include *mitral stenosis* (narrowing of the mitral valve) and *aortic incompetence* (incomplete closure of the aortic valve).

Electrocardiography

One of the commonest methods used by the physician for investigating cardiac function and its disorders is *electrocardiography*. The contraction of heart muscle is accompanied by electrical changes that can be detected by electrodes placed on the skin surface; they can be recorded as an electrocardiogram (ECG or EKG). There are various standard positions on the front of the chest, wrist and ankles on which the electrodes (suitably smeared with a jelly to ensure good electrical contact) are placed; **15.23** illustrates a typical normal ECG, which can be recorded on ECG paper or examined on a monitor. The main features of an ECG are the *P wave* (produced by atrial depolarization), the *QRS*

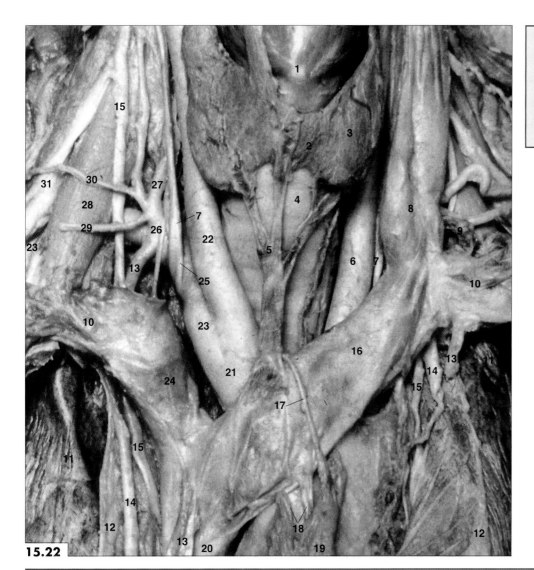

15.22

1 Arch of cricoid cartilage, at the level of C6 vertebra
2 Isthmus of thyroid gland
3 Lateral lobe of thyroid gland
4 Trachea
5 Inferior thyroid veins
6 Left common carotid artery
7 Vagus nerve
8 Internal jugular vein
9 Thoracic duct, joining the junction of the internal jugular and subclavian veins (8 and 10)
10 Subclavian vein
11 Lung, covered by visceral pleura
12 Cut edge of parietal pleura, stripped off thoracic wall
13 Internal thoracic vein
14 Internal thoracic artery
15 Phrenic nerve. On the right side (left of the picture) it is seen running down over the scalenous anterior (28), a landmark for its position in the neck
16 Left brachiocephalic vein, formed by the union of the left internal jugular and subclavian veins (8 and 10)
17 A thymic artery

18 Thymic veins
19 Thymus, lying in front of the upper part of the pericardium
20 Superior vena cava, formed by the union of the two brachiocephalic veins (16 and 24)
21 Brachiocephalic trunk, dividing into the right common carotid and right subclavian arteries (22 and 23)
22 Right common carotid artery
23 Right subclavian artery
24 Right brachiocephalic vein
25 Right recurrent laryngeal nerve, branching off the vagus nerve (7) and hooking round the subclavian artery (23). (The left recurrent laryngeal nerve from the left vagus hooks under the ligamentum arteriosum and the arch of the aorta, 8 in **15.26a**.)
26 Thyrocervical trunk
27 Inferior thyroid artery
28 Scalenus anterior
29 Suprascapular artery
30 Superficial cervical artery
31 Upper trunk of brachial plexus

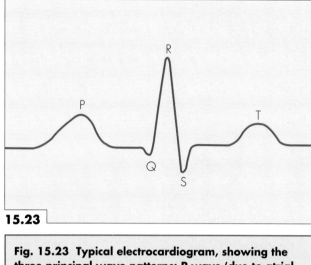

15.23

Fig. 15.23 Typical electrocardiogram, showing the three principal wave patterns: P wave (due to atrial depolarization and signifying atrial contraction), QRS complex (ventricular depolarization with ventricular contraction), and T wave (ventricular repolarization with ventricular relaxation).

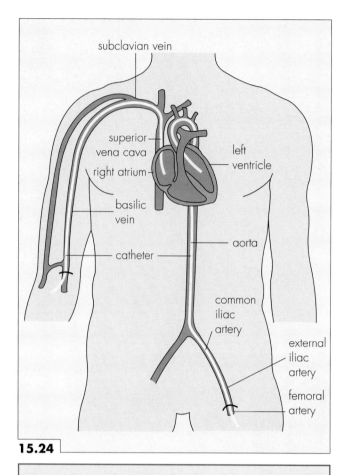

15.24

Fig. 15.24 Cardiac catheterization.
On the right side a venous catheter has been passed through the basilic vein into the right atrium, and on the left an arterial catheter enters the left ventricle via the femoral artery.

complex (produced by ventricular depolarization) and the *T wave* (produced by ventricular repolarizaton). Different heart diseases cause characteristic changes in the ECG pattern which are of great use to the cardiologist, especially for diagnosing myocardial infarction, disorders of rhythm, and alterations in the function of the chambers.

Cardiac Catheterization

For various specialized diagnostic procedures (such as the measurement of blood gas concentrations in the different chambers, or injection of contrast media for radiography of vessels), it may be necessary to pass *catheters* into the heart via veins or arteries (**15.24**). In all cases, the progress of the catheter is checked radiologically. The right atrium can be entered via the arm veins (p.225), and the catheter can also be pushed through the tricuspid valve into the right ventricle and on through the pulmonary valve into the pulmonary trunk and a pulmonary artery. A special type of catheter can also be made to pierce the interatrial septum to pass from the right atrium into the left atrium. The left ventricle can be entered via a catheter introduced through the femoral artery, pushing it into the external and then the common iliac artery into the abdominal aorta, and then right on through the thoracic aorta, aortic arch and aortic valve. For *coronary angiography*, the right brachial artery is often used, by directing the tip of the catheter into the orifice of the required coronary artery just above the aortic valve.

Angioplasty is a technique developed from catheterization, and is sometimes used for treating constricted coronary arteries. A special type of catheter with a minute balloon at its tip is introduced via the femoral artery and aorta into the affected vessel; when in position, the balloon is inflated to try to dilate the area. The full name for the procedure is *percutaneous transluminal coronary angioplasty (PTCA)*, meaning 'approach through the skin (*percutaneous*) to push the catheter into the lumen of the required vessel (*transluminal*) and alter the shape of the vessel (*angioplasty*)'.

HEART DISEASES

Of the many kinds of *cardiovascular disorders*, disease of the coronary arteries is the commonest cause of death in the West. Other common types of heart disease are congestive cardiac failure, disease of the heart valves, cardiac arrythmias, and congenital diseases.

Among the more important signs and symptoms of heart disease are breathlessness (*dyspnoea*), *pain* and *oedema*. Breathlessness may of course be due to respiratory as well as cardiovascular diseases, but the history of the condition coupled with clinical examination will usually enable the physician to reach a diagnosis which may then be confirmed by other tests.

Coronary Artery Disease

Inadequate arterial oxygen supply to the myocardium (*ischaemia of the myocardium*) causes discomfort or pain, typically aggravated by exertion (*angina pectoris*) and relieved by rest. The ischaemia may be sufficient to cause necrosis of an area of the myocardium (*myocardial infarction*, often called *coronary thrombosis* because of the formation of a thrombus – clot of blood – in the vessels of the affected area), and the pain is usually more severe and persistent than with ischaemia alone. These types of cardiac pain may be felt not only in the chest behind the sternum but often radiating down the arms or up into the neck (i.e. referred pain, due to the fact that the sympathetic nerves responsible for supplying the heart also have branches which run with the nerves of these parts, p.210).

Various vasodilator drugs, such as glyceryl trinitrate (sucked under the tongue for sufficient absorption through the mucous membrane or swallowed for intestinal absorption) can dilate the coronary vessels and so help to relieve ischaemic pain. Coronary artery bypass is described on p.114.

Heart Failure

Heart failure occurs when the power of the ventricles becomes inadequate to pump the blood that is received from the atria into the arteries. In left-sided failure (*left ventricular failure*), which may be due to hypertension or disease of the coronary arteries or aortic valve, pressure builds up in the left atrium and so in the pulmonary veins that open into it; the pressure in the pulmonary capillaries rises because of this. Eventually, the driving force for filtration (the movement of fluid out of the capillaries which is due to a hydrostatic pressure gradient) will exceed that for reabsorption (movement inward, due to an osmotic gradient), and fluid will accumulate in the lung tissues (*pulmonary oedema*). This interferes with gaseous exchange and makes breathing difficult (*dyspnoea*). It is easier to breathe when sitting up (*orthopnoea*) than when lying down, because, in the upright position, the fluid (and blood) tend to gravitate towards the bottom of the lungs, leaving the upper parts clearer for more normal exchange.

In right-sided failure (*right ventricular failure*), due, for example, to mitral stenosis or pulmonary hypertension, pressure builds up in the right atrium and so back into the systemic veins. Distension in the neck veins becomes obvious (p.61) and, because of the increased pressure in the systemic capillaries, fluid accumulates in the general body tissues (*generalized oedema* – in contrast to the pulmonary oedema described above). The oedema is typically seen first as a *swelling of the ankles* in patients who are still up and about, since the fluid gravitates to the lowest part of the body; in those confined to bed, the oedema accumulates in the sacral region. The subcutaneous tissues distend with fluid, and a few seconds pressure on the skin by the examiner's finger or thumb leaves an impression or indentation that may take several minutes to disappear – this is *pitting oedema*.

The poor tissue oxygenation that ensues from any kind of heart failure leads to disturbed kidney function with sodium and water retention (p.284); this further adds to the accumulation of body fluid. Thus treatment with diuretics is necessary to reduce the fluid volume, and can be supplemented by cardiac drugs such as digitalis to improve ventricular contraction.

Arrhythmias and Heart Block

Disorders of the **conducting system** (usually due to ischaemic disease) may prevent the impulse for contraction from reaching the ventricles; in this situation, they can only beat at their own inherent rate of about 30 beats per minute, which is not sufficient for even modest bodily activity such as walking. The ventricles then require stimulation by an *artificial pacemaker*. This electrical device is implanted in the chest wall underneath the pectoralis major muscle, and is connected to a wire electrode which has been passed into a neck vein and so into the right ventricle (via the superior vena cava and right atrium and through the tricuspid valve). The pacemaker gives regular electric shocks to the ventricular wall at about the normal rate of 70 or so per minute, thus simulating the normal stimulus to contraction.

Congenital Heart Disease

This includes abnormalities of the great vessels as well as of the heart itself. There are numerous kinds and degrees of defects in the interatrial and interventricular septa, and in the heart valves. Some are not compatible with life after birth, while others may not make their presence felt until well into adult life. One of the commonest and simplest defects is a *patent ductus arteriosus* (p.116), i.e. one that fails to constrict and close off during the first few hours of life, resulting in a useless *shunting* of newly oxygenated arterial blood from the arch of the aorta back to the lungs through the pulmonary arteries (left to right shunt). Surgical ligation of the duct restores the normal circulation.

Other left to right shunts occur with septal defects; the commonly called 'hole in the heart' is an *atrial septal defect* (ASD), where arterial blood in the left atrium passes into the right atrium and so back to the lungs through the right ventricle and pulmonary trunk. (In the fetus, where there is no aeration of blood in the lungs, blood passes from the right atrium to the left atrium through an opening in the septum – the foramen ovale – thus bypassing the lungs. At birth, the foramen ovale should close; the common septal defect is caused by failure to do so.)

Ventricular septal defects (VSD) will obviously allow communication between the two ventricles, and there may be accompanying abnormalities of valves. The commonest congenital heart disease associated with cyanosis (p.77) is *Fallot's tetralogy*, which is a combination of four structural features: VSD, stenosis (narrowing) of the pulmonary trunk, an overriding aorta (straddling the upper ends of both ventricles) and right ventricular hypertrophy (enlargement, due to the increased pressure required to force blood through the narrow pulmonary trunk). These and other defects can often be repaired by modern cardiac surgery.

Transplantation of the Heart

In certain patients with cardiac diseases – especially those involving the heart muscle (*cardiomyopathies*) – *transplantation* may now offer a realistic method of treatment. The procedure involves removing most of the diseased heart by cutting through the ascending aorta and the pulmonary trunk but leaving the posterior parts of both atria intact, so that the superior and inferior venae cavae and the four pulmonary veins are undisturbed; the part of the right atrium containing the SA node is also retained. The atria of the donor heart are trimmed to fit the remains of the patient's atria and appropriately sutured together. Finally the patient's aorta and pulmonary trunk must be sutured to those of the donor heart.

TRACHEA, BRONCHI AND LUNGS

Consult the introduction to the Respiratory System on p.73. The uppermost parts of the respiratory tract (nose, pharynx and larynx) are described on p.153.

TRACHEA

The **trachea** (windpipe) is the part of the respiratory tract that runs from the larynx in the neck (p.186) to the bronchi and lungs in the thorax. It is about 10 cm long and just under 2 cm in diameter, beginning at the level of the sixth cervical vertebra as the direct continuation of the larynx. It runs down into the thorax approximately in the midline (**10.1** and **16.35c**) and immediately in front of the oesophagus. At the level of the manubriosternal joint (opposite the lower border of the fourth thoracic vertebra) it divides into the **right** and **left main** or **principal bronchi** which enter their respective lungs (**15.21** and **15.25**). The upper end of the trachea is easily felt in the neck above the jugular notch of the sternum (**16.34a**); this is where it can be incised for tracheotomy – the making of an artificial opening for the insertion of a breathing tube when there is laryngeal obstruction.

In cross section the trachea resembles a capital 'D', being curved at the front and sides but flat at the back where it lies against the oesophagus. This shape is maintained by rings of hyaline cartilage. (Although called 'rings' they are never complete but rather U-shaped, and there is never any cartilage at the back of the trachea, where the wall includes smooth muscle.) The cartilage is necessary to keep the tube open as an airway. There is smooth muscle as well as connective tissue between the rings, and the epithelial lining, like that of most of the nasal cavity, is ciliated to assist the expulsion of mucus

and debris from the lungs. Infections that cause sore throats can spread down to affect the trachea (*tracheitis*), and are among the causes of irritable and painful coughs.

MAIN BRONCHI

The bifurcation of the trachea into the **main bronchi** (**15.21** and **15.25**) is like an inverted 'Y', but the two limbs of the 'Y' are not quite symmetrical. The **right bronchus** is more vertical than the left, so that foreign bodies (such as peanuts or extracted teeth) falling down the trachea are more likely to enter it than the **left bronchus** (which leaves the trachea at more of an angle). There is also a slight difference in length, the right bronchus being the shorter of the two (3 cm compared with 5 cm). Each bronchus enters its own lung at the **hilum**, the site where the vessels also enter or leave. Cancer of the lung (see below) is usually cancer of a bronchus (bronchial carcinoma).

LUNGS AND PLEURA

The **lungs** (**10.1**) are the respiratory organs in which the exchange of gases occurs: oxygen from the air delivered to them via the trachea and bronchi diffuses into the blood, and carbon dioxide leaves the blood to enter the air (p.75).

Each lung is enveloped by **pleura** (called **visceral pleura** where it adheres to the lung); this is a lubricating membrane that becomes reflected off the hilum of the lung to line the space within which the lung lies (where it is called **parietal pleura**, from the Greek for 'wall' – **15.22**). The lung is said to 'lie' in the **pleural cavity**, but is not quite as big as the whole cavity, leaving a part of the cavity between the periphery of the diaphragm and the chest wall – the **costodiaphragmatic recess** – unfilled by lung, even during the deepest respiration. For this reason, the surface markings of the pleura and lung (see below) are not identical in the lower thorax.

The **surfaces** of each lung are the **mediastinal** (**medial**) **surface** which contains the hilum (**15.26b** and **15.27b**), **costal surface** which is curved to fit the front, side and back of its own half of the thorax, and the **diaphragmatic** (**inferior**) **surface** which is curved to fit the upward bulge of its own half of the diaphragm. The **apex** of the lung is the upper part of the upper lobe and it extends into the neck about 3 cm above the inner third of the clavicle; stab wounds of the neck may injure this part.

Lobes and Fissures

The **left lung** is divided into *two* lobes (upper and lower), which are separated by the **oblique fissure**, and the **right lung** into *three* lobes (upper, middle and lower) separated by **oblique** and **transverse fissures** (see **10.1**). The left lung is smaller than the right because the heart bulges more towards the left. The main bronchi divide into **lobar bronchi**, and these in turn give rise to **segmental bronchi** (**15.25**), so named because they lead to the **bronchopulmonary segments** – wedge-shaped areas of lung tissue that are essentially independent of one another in terms of their air and blood supply. The patterns of division and segmentation are remarkably constant, and each lung has ten segments, each with its own number and name.

The arrangement of lobes and fissures is such that when listening with a stethoscope (see below) at the *back*, it is mainly the *lower* lobe that is being examined, while at the *front* the *upper* lobes (and middle lobe on the right) are the ones from which the breath sounds are most clearly heard. The lobular and segmental nature of the lung makes possible the surgical removal of a single lobe (*lobectomy*) or one or more segments (*partial lobectomy*), apart from total removal (*pneumonectomy*).

Surface Markings

The surface markings of the **pleura** (**15.7**) are usually remembered by the even numbers 2, 4, 6, 8, 10, 12. On each side, beginning at the dome of the pleura which extends into the neck *3 cm above* the inner third of the **clavicle**, the line of the pleura passes down to the level of the *second costal cartilage* in the midline of the sternum, then to the *fourth cartilage* level, where, on the left, it passes laterally for 2.5 cm (1 in) and then down to the *sixth cartilage* level, while on the right it continues straight down to the sixth cartilage. From here on, the two sides are the same: to the *eighth rib* in the midclavicular line, *tenth rib* in the midaxillary line, and *twelfth rib* at the lateral border of the erector spinae muscle.

For the surface markings of the **lungs**, the figures to remember are 2, 4, 6, 8 and 10. The marking are the same

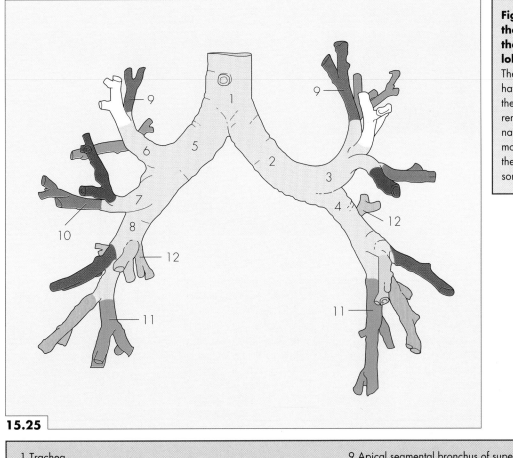

15.25

Fig. 15.25 Diagram of the bronchial tree, with the main bronchi and lobar bronchi identified. The various segmental bronchi have been coloured (and all their smaller branches removed); each has an official name and number, but for most students knowledge of them is not necessary and only some examples are given.

1 Trachea
2 Main bronchus ⎫
3 Superior lobar bronchus ⎬ of left lung
4 Inferior lobar bronchus ⎭
5 Main bronchus ⎫
6 Superior lobar bronchus ⎪
7 Middle lobar bronchus ⎬ of right lung
8 Inferior lobar bronchus ⎭

9 Apical segmental bronchus of superior lobe
10 Lateral segmental bronchus of middle lobe
11 Posterior basal segmental bronchus of inferior lobe
12 Superior segmental bronchus of lower lobe, important because it is the highest bronchus to arise from the posterior surface of any lobar bronchus; in a patient lying in bed, infected bronchial secretions may gravitate into it and so into the superior bronchopulmonary segment of the inferior lobe

as those for the pleura down to the sixth costal cartilage, and then the lung margin reaches the *eighth rib* in the midaxillary line and the *tenth rib* at the lateral border of erector spinae.

The surface marking for the **oblique fissure** of each lung is from the **spine** of *T3 vertebra* round the side of the chest to the *sixth costal cartilage*; this approximates to the line of the vertebral border of the scapula when the arm is raised above the head. For the **transverse fissure** of the right lung, the marking is from the *fourth costal cartilage* transversely backwards until it meets the line of the oblique fissure.

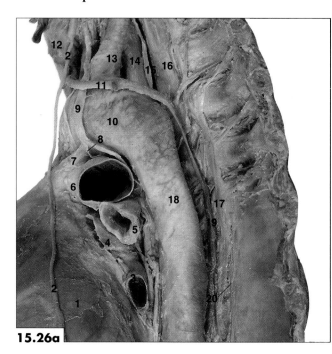

15.26a

Fig. 15.26 Left side of the mediastinum and the lung root.
(a) After removal of the pleura and lung.
(b) Diagram of the mediastinal surface of the left lung, showing the lung root and impressions made by adjacent structures.

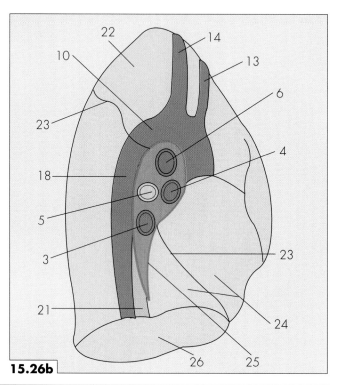

15.26b

1 Pericardium overlying left ventricle
2 Phrenic nerve
3 Inferior pulmonary vein, the lowest structure in the lung root
4 Superior pulmonary vein, the most anterior structure in the lung root
5 Main bronchus, the most posterior structure in the lung root
6 Pulmonary artery, the highest structure in the lung root
7 Ligamentum arteriosum connecting the arch of the aorta (10) to the left pulmonary artery
8 Recurrent laryngeal branch of vagus nerve (9) hooking round the ligamentum arteriosum (7) and under the arch of the aorta (10)
9 Vagus nerve, crossing the arch of the aorta (10) behind the phrenic nerve (2)
10 Arch of aorta
11 Superior intercostal vein, crossing the arch of the aorta (10) transversely and running superficial to the vagus nerve (9) but deep to the phrenic nerve to drain into the left brachiocephalic vein (12)

12 Left brachiocephalic vein
13 Subclavian artery, obscuring the trachea in (a)
14 Oesophagus
15 Thoracic duct, passing up in front of the vertebral column (16) behind the left margin of the oesophagus (14)
16 Vertebral column
17 Sympathetic trunk
18 Thoracic (descending) aorta
19 Accessory hemiazygos vein, in this specimen communicating with the superior intercostal vein (11)
20 Cut edge of pleura
21 Oesophagus, lying between the heart (24) and aorta (18)
22 Upper lobe
23 Oblique fissure
24 Cardiac impression
25 Cut edge of pleura
26 Diaphragmatic surface of lower lobe

Lung Roots

The **lung root** is the region where the structures that enter or leaving the hilum (see above) are attached to the mediastinum (p.101 and **15.26** and **15.27**). It is surrounded by pleura, and lies behind the third and fourth costal cartilages (at the level of T5–T7 vertebrae). The largest structures in the root are the **main bronchus**, the **pulmonary artery** and the **two pulmonary veins**. The veins carry freshly

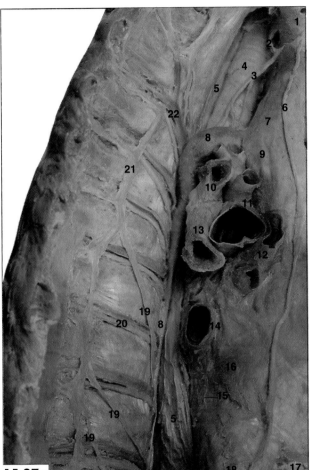

15.27a

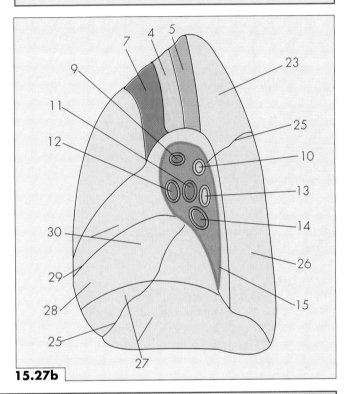

Fig. 15.27 Right side of the mediastinum and the lung root.
(a) After removal of pleura and lung.
(b) Diagram of the mediastinal surface of the right lung, showing the lung root and impressions made by adjacent structures.

15.27b

1 Subclavian artery, with the recurrent laryngeal branch (2) of the vagus nerve (3) hooking underneath it
2 Recurrent laryngeal nerve
3 Vagus nerve, running obliquely downwards and backwards across the trachea (4)
4 Trachea
5 Oesophagus
6 Phrenic nerve, running down the side of the superior vena cava (7) and, lower down, on the pericardium overlying the right atrium (16)
7 Superior vena cava
8 Azygos vein, arching forwards above the lung root to join the superior vena cava (7)
9 Branch of pulmonary artery (11) to upper lobe
10 Upper lobe bronchus, branching off the main bronchus (13)
11 Pulmonary artery, the most central structure in the lung root
12 Superior pulmonary vein, the most anterior structure in the lung root
13 Main bronchus, the most posterior structure in the lung root

14 Inferior pulmonary vein, the lowest structure in the lung root
15 Cut edge of pleura
16 Pleura and pericardium overlying right atrium
17 Diaphragm
18 Inferior vena cava, passing through its foramen in the tendinous part of the diaphragm to enter the right atrium
19 Splanchnic branches of sympathetic trunk (21)
20 A posterior intercostal artery and vein
21 Sympathetic trunk
22 Superior intercostal vein
23 Upper lobe
24 Trachea and oesophagus
25 Oblique fissure
26 Lower lobe
27 Diaphragmatic surface
28 Middle lobe
29 Transverse fissure
30 Cardiac impression

oxygenated blood to the left atrium of the heart (p.53), while the artery conveys deoxygenated blood from the right ventricle to the lungs (via the pulmonary trunk). The artery and veins divide within the lung, following the divisions of the bronchi and bronchioles, to end in the pulmonary capillaries. This *pulmonary circulation* is concerned purely with the oxygenation of blood, and is obviously of major importance. There is, however, a second circulation in the lungs which is much smaller. It is the *bronchial circulation* which provides blood supply to the lung tissue itself (especially the bronchial tree and lung connective tissue). Small *bronchial arteries* arise from the aorta and one of the posterior intercostal arteries, while corresponding *bronchial veins* drain mostly into the azygos veins (p.116). There is normally little communication between the bronchial and pulmonary circulations, but such connections may become important in some forms of congenital heart disease in getting as much blood as possible into the pulmonary capillaries.

The lung root contains not only *lymphatic vessels* which collect lymph from all over the lung, but *lymph nodes* as well. From them, lymph passes to other mediastinal nodes (around the trachea and beside the vertebral column), and it is their involvement by spread from bronchial carcinoma which makes eradication of this disease so difficult. Autonomic nerves that assist in respiratory reflexes (p.75) also pass through the lung root.

Structure

Lung tissue is like an extremely fine sponge; the main bronchi divide into smaller and smaller tubes (the 'bronchial tree') which eventually open into the **alveoli** (air sacs, the 'spaces' of the sponge); it is through their walls that gases diffuse into or out of the blood capillaries which lie on the surface of the alveoli in the intervening (interstitial) tissue of the lung (**10.2**). The main bronchi are structurally just like the trachea, but as other bronchi become smaller with repeated divisions, the amount of cartilage in their walls becomes lower and eventually disappears; bronchi then change their name to **bronchioles**.

The smallest bronchioles are called **respiratory bronchioles** because they lead not only into the alveoli (the truly respiratory structures of the lung), but a few alveoli actually branch off from their walls. The alveoli themselves have extremely thin walls; by this stage the epithelial cells have lost their cilia and have become as flattened as the endothelial lining cells of blood capillaries – as little tissue as possible intervenes between the air in the alveoli and the blood in the capillaries. Bronchi and bronchioles (right down to respiratory bronchioles, but not alveoli) have smooth muscle fibres in their walls and, in the interstitial tissue filling in the gaps between the various parts of the bronchial tree, there are elastic fibres which assist in expiration. For further details of respiration, see p.74.

EXAMINATION OF THE CHEST

The time-honoured sequence of personal investigations by the physician – inspection, palpation, percussion and auscultation – is the cornerstone of any chest examination (whether for cardiac or respiratory disease).

Inspection involves observing the movements of both sides of the thorax and its muscles, and the rate of respiration.

Palpation of the chest wall includes detection of the apex beat of the heart (in the left fifth intercostal space), and of the trachea (at the jugular notch, **15.7**); both may be displaced by lung conditions.

In *percussion*, one (warm) hand is laid flat against the chest wall and the middle phalanx of the middle finger is tapped with the tip of the opposite middle finger. This technique gives different audible degrees of resonance; the resonance over normal air-filled lung tissue becomes duller over areas that are airless (consolidated, as by pneumonia or collapse) or overlaid by fluid (pleural effusion).

Auscultation (listening) with the stethoscope enables the examiner to hear the breath sounds, which are the vibrations transmitted from the vocal cords through the trachea, bronchi, lungs and chest wall, and which vary according to the state of the tissues.

The *straight X-ray* of the chest (**15.11**) is the principal supplement to any personal thoracic examination, but it must be remembered that the radiograph itself does not make a diagnosis. The X-ray plate shows only certain shadows produced by the tissues that the beam has traversed, but experience has shown that certain types of shadow indicate certain diseases. Varying shapes and varying degrees of opacity all have their meaning, but modern scanning methods are adding greatly to the precision of thoracic examination.

Bronchoscopy using fibreoptic illumination allows direct examination of the larger bronchi and can be used for the removal of foreign bodies, and for biopsy of bronchial tissue (*transbronchial biopsy*), especially for diagnosing carcinoma. Biopsy by a needle inserted into the lung through the chest wall (*percutaneous biopsy*) enables microscopic examination to be made of the lung tissue.

LUNG DISEASES

Many different lung conditions can interfere with normal function and lead to respiratory and/or circulatory disturbances. About 5% of the epithelial cells of the alveoli are not of the very flat lining variety but are a special secretory type producing *surfactant* – a substance that reduces surface tension and is particularly important in the newborn child taking the first breaths. Fetal lungs are full of fluid (partly tissue fluid and partly amniotic fluid which has been swallowed); surfactant allows the alveoli to expand and so become capable of gaseous exchange. If there is insufficient surfactant (as in premature infants) and therefore poor alveolar expansion, there will be respiratory difficulty (*infantile respiratory distress syndrome* (RDS)) – sometimes called *hyaline membrane disease* because the unexpanded alveoli have the appearance of opaque glass), leading possibly to death from a lack of oxygen getting through to the bloodstream.

Bronchitis (inflammation of the bronchi) is usually part of an *upper respiratory infection* (URI, p.153), leading to excessive production of mucus and hence to coughing in an attempt to get rid of it. It may be acute (of short duration) as when it follows a cold or sore throat, or chronic as in cigarette smokers in whom the smoke is a constant irritant to the bronchial tree.

Bronchial carcinoma, commonly called *lung cancer*, is the commonest male cancer, with an incidence 20 times as great in cigarette smokers when compared with non-smokers; it also appears to be overtaking breast cancer as the commonest female cancer. It usually begins in the epithelium of one of the main or other large bronchi, and it may take several years for a tumour to reach a size of 1 cm in diameter, by which time it may have already spread by lymphatics or the bloodstream to the mediastinum and organs such as the liver or brain (hepatic or cerebral metastases). The local effects on the lung itself are those of obstruction, leading to infection or collapse. If detected early, surgical removal may be successful – either of a whole lung (*pneumonectomy*) or a single lobe (*lobectomy*) – but metastatic spread is one of the hazards of this and other types of cancer. The lung itself may be a site for metastases from a primary growth elsewhere, especially from bone or the prostate.

Pneumonia is the name given to infection involving the alveoli, where they and the adjacent small bronchioles and bronchi become like a mass of miniature test-tubes containing pus; in the affected parts, gaseous exchange is obviously impossible. In *lobar pneumonia*, the infection is limited to the alveoli of a lobe, but in *bronchopneumonia* it is more extensive; in *double pneumonia* both lungs are involved. Treatment with antibiotics is usually successful, but in the old and debilitated it is frequently a terminal illness.

Tuberculosis of the lung (pulmonary TB) is a specific infection, with the tubercle bacillus (*Mycobacterium tuberculosis*) leading to the breakdown of lung tissue and the formation of cavities, especially in the apical part of the lung. The cavities give a characteristic radiographic appearance. The condition is dangerous because the infection is airborne; coughing and sneezing spread the bacilli in droplets which can be inhaled, and people living in overcrowded conditions are therefore particularly susceptible to being infected by those who (perhaps unknowingly) are harbouring the bacilli. In recent years, the treatment of TB has been transformed by the discovery of drugs such as Rifampicin and Isoniazid which specifically kill the bacilli. Two or three of such drugs are often given in combination in case resistance to one of them develops. Those who are infectious (with tubercle bacilli detectable in sputum) are required to be isolated until sputum tests for the bacilli become negative.

Bronchial asthma (often simply called asthma) is usually an allergic condition causing spasm of the smooth muscle of the smaller bronchi; this leads to wheezing and difficulty with **expiration** (not inspiration) for periods ranging from minutes to hours. In other cases, both in children and adults, no allergic basis can be discovered and a psychological background may be present; emotional stress, even in those with a demonstrable allergy, is often a complicating factor. Its severest form, *status asthmaticus*, lasting for many hours, requires emergency treatment with bronchodilator drugs (such as isoproterenol or salbutamol); these are given by a pressurized ventilator so that they reach the constricted bronchi as quickly as possible. In less severe attacks and for maintenance therapy for some weeks after an attack, drugs can be given via a nebulizer – a miniature aerosol spray which can be squirted into the mouth so that the spray can be inhaled.

Bronchiectasis is a complication of lung infections in which the elastic and muscular tissue in the walls of parts of the bronchial tree become lost, leading to dilatation of bronchi and bronchioles; these become reservoirs for infected mucus. The destruction of tissue which leads to enlargement of alveoli (as opposed to bronchi and bronchioles) results in *emphysema*, in which alveoli become ballooned out into pea-like or grape-like vesicles (*emphysematous bullae*). Obstruction of any part of the bronchial tree may give rise to collapse of segments, lobes or a whole lung (*atelectasis*).

The inhalation of different kinds of dust particles (from coal, asbestos, silica, etc.), over periods of years in those who work in industries such as mining and sandblasting, can cause various types of *pneumoconiosis* such as silicosis and asbestosis; these are among the most dangerous of occupational diseases. The particles are ingested by the lung macrophages and, because they cannot be broken down by the usual enzyme activity, the particles accumulate to cause obstruction and interference with gaseous exchange. The pathological changes in the lungs are irreversible, so that treatment must be essentially preventive; many countries now have legislation for 'safety at work' which is designed to eliminate industrial hazards.

In *cystic fibrosis*, one of the commonest genetic diseases, there are alterations in many glandular secretions, especially those of the mucous glands of the respiratory tract, leading to obstruction and chronic infection in the lungs.

If air enters the pleural cavity (in what is called *pneumothorax*), the lung collapses because there is no longer a negative pressure within the cavity (p.74). Possible causes of this include injuries of the chest wall such as stab wounds, and the rupture of emphysematous bullae, which are dilatations of air spaces with thinning and destruction of their walls. *Haemothorax* indicates the escape of blood into the pleural cavity. The lung will obviously collapse in thoracic surgery involving the pleural cavity, but here the ventilating

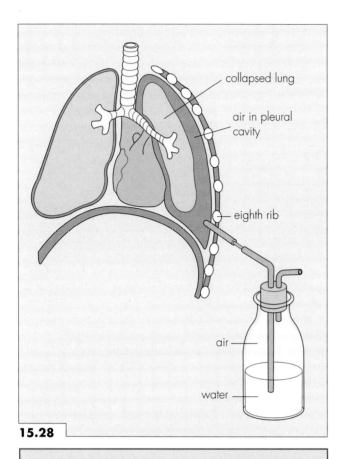

collapsed lung

air in pleural cavity

eighth rib

air

water

15.28

Fig. 15.28 Diagram of drainage of the left pleural cavity.
The tube must enter the water in the collecting bottle below the fluid level in order to prevent air from entering the pleural cavity.

machine that is used for anaesthesia can control gaseous exchange mechanically and can be used to inflate the lung at the end of the operation when the chest wall is closed.

Lung disease that affects the pleura on the surface of the lung and the adjacent chest wall (*pleurisy*) may cause extreme pain because the pleural surfaces can no longer glide over one another smoothly. Fluid may collect in the pleural cavity (*pleural effusion*) and may have to be removed by aspiration with a needle and syringe or by more prolonged drainage through a tube inserted into the cavity (*intubation* – **15.28**).

Pulmonary emboli are referred to on p.331.

CARDIOPULMONARY RESUSCITATION

When the heart suddenly ceases to beat (*cardiac arrest*) and breathing stops (*cardiopulmonary arrest*), usually as a result of injury or myocardial infarction, immediate measures are required to help keep the patient alive and to prevent irreversible brain damage which must be considered to occur within four minutes of the loss of blood circulation through the brain. The steps to be taken constitute **cardiopulmonary resuscitation**, commonly called CPR. It can be divided into *basic life support* (BLS), which can be taught to lay people as well as to all those in the health care professions, and *advanced cardiac life support* (ACLS) which, in addition to the elementary measures of BLS, also requires the use of drugs and hospital equipment.

Everyone should have a clear understanding of the background to the immediate steps required for CPR, and they are conveniently summarized by 'the ABC of CPR' – 'A' for Airway, 'B' for Breathing, and 'C' for Circulation.

AIRWAY

Breathing is not possible if the airway is obstructed, and in unconscious patients, especially those lying on the back, the commonest cause for airway obstruction is the tongue falling backwards to close off the pharynx (**15.29a** and **15.29b**). Tilting the head backwards and lifting the lower jaw forwards helps the tongue to come forwards and so restores a free passage for air. Of course, there may be other causes of airway obstruction such as foreign bodies or vomit, and methods of dealing with these taught in CPR courses, but '*A for Airway*' is the first thing to think of in CPR.

BREATHING

If the patient is not breathing, as judged by looking for chest movements, listening for breath sounds and feeling for expired air using the back of the hand, mouth-to-mouth breathing (*ventilation*) must be begun as soon as the airway is clear – '*B for Breathing*'. Two slow breaths (mouth-to-mouth, while holding the patient's nose shut, **15.29c**) are recommended to inflate the lungs (watch to see that the chest moves), and a breath every five seconds should be given until spontaneous breathing occurs.

CIRCULATION

If the patient is pulseless, as judged by feeling for the carotid pulse (p.178) for five seconds, blood circulation must be restored – '*C for Circulation*'. A blow to the lower part of the sternum with the side of a clenched fist (*precordial thump*) may restore normal beating if the arrest was due to some abnormality of rhythm, but usually *external cardiac compression* is required. The palms of both hands, one on top of the other, are placed over the lower part of the body of the sternum which is then compressed backwards for 4–5 cm (2 in) at a rate of 15 times per minute. The compression not only presses the ventricles between the sternum and the vertebral column (**15.30**), helping to press blood out into the great vessels and to stimulate the chambers to beat on their own again, but also increases the intrathoracic pressure, helping blood to pass from the lungs to and through the heart.

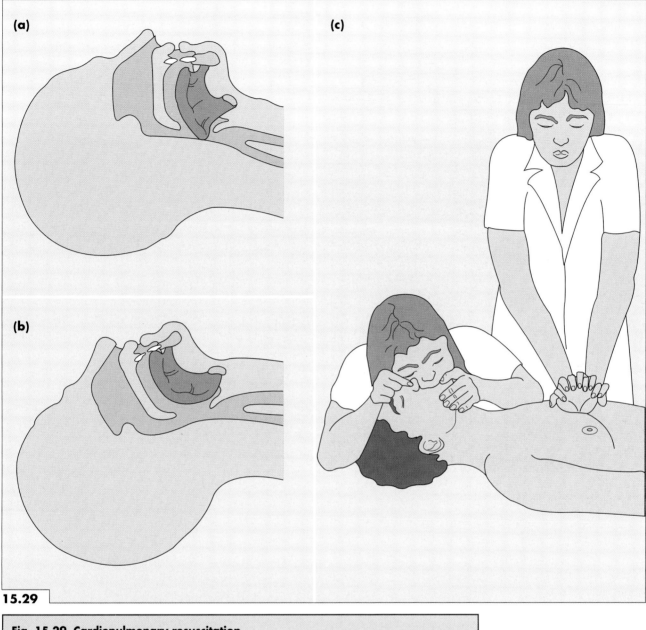

15.29

Fig. 15.29 Cardiopulmonary resuscitation.
(a) Obstruction of the airway by the tongue falling back to the posterior pharyngeal wall.
(b) Tilting the head back and the mandible upwards brings the tongue forwards and opens up the airway.
(c) Ventilation (mouth-to-mouth breathing) and compression over the lower sternum to restore circulation.

Ideally two people should be involved in CPR, one dealing with breathing and one with circulation but, if only one is available, compression and lung ventilation should be carried out as 15 compressions followed by two ventilations, then another 15 compressions and two ventilations and so on.

In hospital or with an emergency ambulance team, the basic life support initiated above can be supplemented by giving oxygen to restore respiration, and defibrillation (p.114) to restore cardiac activity.

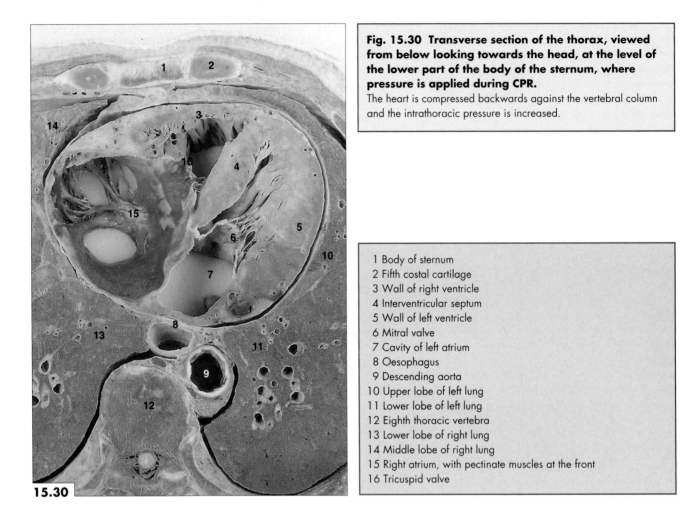

Fig. 15.30 Transverse section of the thorax, viewed from below looking towards the head, at the level of the lower part of the body of the sternum, where pressure is applied during CPR.
The heart is compressed backwards against the vertebral column and the intrathoracic pressure is increased.

1 Body of sternum
2 Fifth costal cartilage
3 Wall of right ventricle
4 Interventricular septum
5 Wall of left ventricle
6 Mitral valve
7 Cavity of left atrium
8 Oesophagus
9 Descending aorta
10 Upper lobe of left lung
11 Lower lobe of left lung
12 Eighth thoracic vertebra
13 Lower lobe of right lung
14 Middle lobe of right lung
15 Right atrium, with pectinate muscles at the front
16 Tricuspid valve

15.30

CHAPTER 16

HEAD AND NECK

SCALP

The **scalp** is the soft tissue covering the vault of the skull and is usually the hairiest part of the body. It extends from the eyebrows to the back of the head; the forehead, from eyebrows to hairline (or where the hairline ought to be), belongs both to the scalp and the face (p.142), but unlike the rest of the scalp it appears hairless.

LAYERS

The *five layers* that make up the scalp (**16.1**) are conveniently remembered by the five letters of its name: **S**kin, **C**onnective tissue, **A**poneurosis, **L**oose connective tissue, **P**ericranium.

Skin forms the outer layer, most of which contains many hair follicles, sweat glands and sebaceous glands (p.18). While the skin over most of the body is 1–2 mm thick, it is

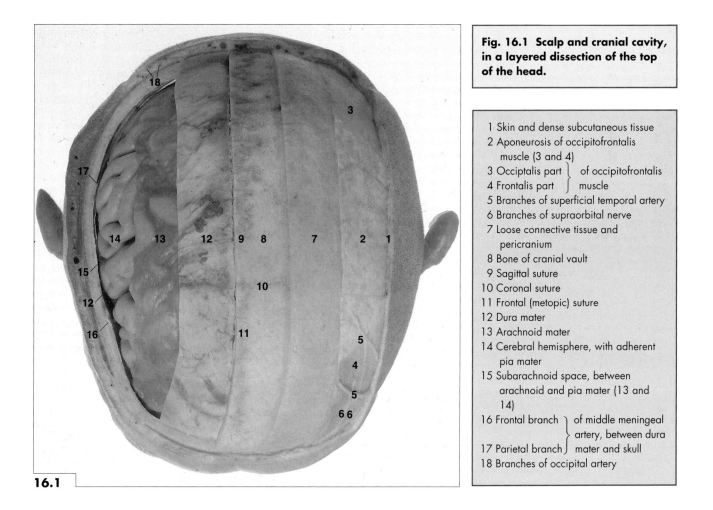

Fig. 16.1 Scalp and cranial cavity, in a layered dissection of the top of the head.

1 Skin and dense subcutaneous tissue
2 Aponeurosis of occipitofrontalis muscle (3 and 4)
3 Occiptalis part ⎫ of occipitofrontalis
4 Frontalis part ⎬ muscle
5 Branches of superficial temporal artery
6 Branches of supraorbital nerve
7 Loose connective tissue and pericranium
8 Bone of cranial vault
9 Sagittal suture
10 Coronal suture
11 Frontal (metopic) suture
12 Dura mater
13 Arachnoid mater
14 Cerebral hemisphere, with adherent pia mater
15 Subarachnoid space, between arachnoid and pia mater (13 and 14)
16 Frontal branch ⎫ of middle meningeal
  ⎬ artery, between dura
17 Parietal branch ⎭ mater and skull
18 Branches of occipital artery

16.1

3–7 mm thick on the scalp, and thickest at the back (occipital region).

Beneath the skin is **dense connective tissue** that binds it firmly to the third layer, which consists of a fibrous **aponeurosis** with muscle both at the back (occipitalis) and at the front (frontalis). The **occipitalis muscle** has a bony attachment to the skull but **frontalis** does not; the latter is the muscle responsible for the transverse wrinkles of the forehead.

Beneath the muscles and aponeurosis is a thin layer of **loose connective tissue** that allows the rest of the scalp to move on the deepest layer, the **pericranium** – the name given to the periosteum on the vault of the skull. The loose tissue layer forms the plane of cleavage for 'scalping', which may occur as an industrial accident when hair gets caught in machinery.

BLOOD SUPPLY AND LYMPH DRAINAGE

The arteries of the scalp enter round its edges; these have accompanying veins. In addition, there are a few small veins that penetrate the vault of the skull through **emissary foramina** (such as the parietal foramen) and so provide communication between venous sinuses *inside* the skull and the scalp on the *outside* – and hence a possible route for infection to reach the inside of the skull. The main vessels run in the dense tissue between the skin and the aponeurosis–muscle layer; when severed, the cut ends of the vessels are prevented from constricting because of their adherence to this connective tissue, and so wounds of the scalp bleed profusely. Scalp vessels make good anastomoses with one another and, because of its good blood supply, wounds of the scalp heal well.

The principal arteries on each side are: the **supraorbital** (from the ophthalmic branch of the internal carotid) which enters at the supraorbital margin (**16.8**), two fingerbreadths from the midline; the **superficial temporal** (from the external carotid) at the side, and palpable just in front of the tragus of the ear (**16.11**); and the **occipital** (from the external carotid) at the back.

There are no lymph nodes within the scalp, but there is good lymphatic drainage by channels which reach occipital, retroauricular, parotid, submandibular and deep cervical nodes. Infections and infestations of the scalp are therefore among the common causes of enlargement of any of these nodes.

NERVE SUPPLY

There are several **sensory nerves** (from the **trigeminal nerves** at the front and **cervical nerves** at the back) which, like the arteries, all enter the scalp at its periphery. The **muscles** are supplied by the **facial nerve**; its temporal branch passes out from the parotid gland (**16.11**) to reach the frontalis, and another small branch passes backwards to the occipitalis.

HAIR

Hair follicles (p.19) on the scalp may have a growing phase of two to three years, followed by a resting phase of a few months during which time the old hair falls out before the matrix begins to make a new hair. Adjacent follicles are out of phase with one another so that the pattern of renewal and replacement is not obvious; some hair loss is thus a normal phenomenon, and finding hairs on the brush and comb every day does not mean they are all going to fall out.

There may be many reasons for hair loss (i.e. baldness or *alopecia*), but the common male pattern of increasing baldness is familial (genetically determined) and depends on the presence of the male sex hormone testosterone. There is as yet no means of stopping or reversing its progress (apart from castration – eunuchs do not grow bald). Baldness is also part of the aging process.

DISEASES

The commonest skin diseases affecting the scalp are seborrhoea and psoriasis (p.20); neither of these causes baldness. *Seborrhoea* is an itchy scaling condition whose mildest form is commonly called dandruff. Because of the numbers of hair follicles and sebaceous glands in the scalp, *sebaceous cysts* (rounded swellings due to obstruction of the ducts damming back the secretion) are commoner on the scalp than on any other part of the body.

CRANIAL VAULT AND CRANIAL CAVITY

For protection, the brain is enclosed in the skull. The domed upper part above the eyes and ears is the **cranial vault** (**16.1**, **16.2** and **16.8**) – the frontal, parietal, occipital, temporal and sphenoid bones take part in its formation. The cranial vault covers the upper part of the brain; the lower part of the brain lies over the inside of the base of the skull. Most of the bone of the vault consists of inner and outer layers (tables) of compact bone with an intervening layer of spongy or cancellous bone (the **diplöe** – **16.9**) containing bone marrow. At the side of the skull, above the zygomatic arch, the bone is thinner and single-layered with no diplöe.

MENINGES

The brain is kept in its normal position by partial partitions of fibrous tissue, the **falx cerebri** and **tentorium cerebelli** (**16.2a** and **16.3**). These structures are formed by folds of **dura mater**, itself a tough fibrous membrane. The dura mater lines the inside of the skull and extends down through the foramen magnum in the base of the skull to surround the spinal cord within the vertebral canal (p.199). It is one of three tissue layers collectively forming the **meninges**; in contact with the inside of the dura is the **arachnoid mater**, a much thinner fibrous layer; adhering to the surface of the

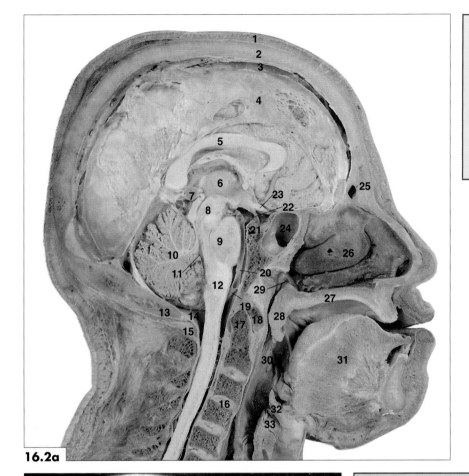

16.2a

Fig. 16.2 Sagittal section of the head.
(a) Midline section, looking at the left half of the head, with the nasal septum removed.
(b) Magnetic resonance image of a living head. Compare with **(a)** and with **17.2a** and note how well this modern imaging technique can display internal features.

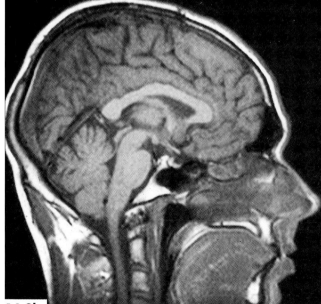

16.2b

1 Scalp
2 Cranial vault
3 Superior sagittal sinus
4 Falx cerebri, the fold of dura mater separating the two cerebral hemispheres
5 Corpus callosum
6 Thalamus, in the lateral wall of the third ventricle
7 Pineal body
8 Midbrain, with the aqueduct of the midbrain leading from the third ventricle to the fourth ventricle
9 Pons
10 Cerebellum
11 Fourth ventricle
12 Medulla oblongata
13 Margin of foramen magnum
14 Cerebellomedullary cistern (cisterna magna), part of the subarachnoid space

15 Posterior arch of atlas
16 Intervertebral disc
17 Dens of axis
18 Anterior arch of atlas
19 Vertebral artery
20 Basilar artery, sectioned throughout its length
21 Pituitary gland
22 Pituitary stalk
23 Optic chiasma
24 Sphenoidal sinus
25 Frontal sinus
26 Middle nasal concha
27 Hard palate
28 Soft palate
29 Opening of auditory tube, in nasal part of pharynx
30 Oral part of pharynx
31 Tongue
32 Epiglottis
33 Inlet of larynx

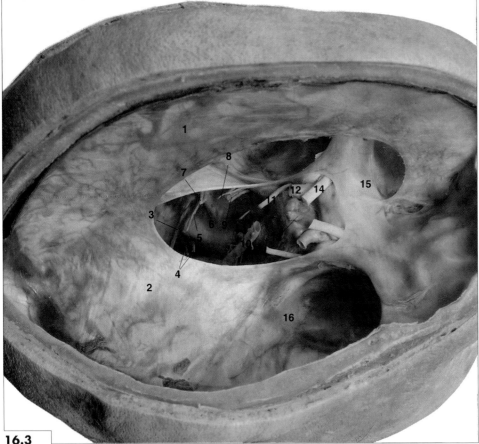

Fig. 16.3 Cranial cavity and dura mater.
The cerebral hemispheres and brainstem have been removed, leaving in place the folds of dura mater and the cut ends of some cranial nerves and vessels, viewed from the right and above and looking slightly forwards.

16.3

1 Falx cerebri, the fold of dura separating the two cerebral hemispheres
2 Tentorium cerebelli, the fold of dura forming the roof of the posterior cranial fossa and separating the cerebral hemispheres from the cerebellar hemispheres (which lie below the tentorium). The brainstem passes down through the gap between the free (medial) margins of the tentorium
3 Spinal part of accessory nerve (XI)
4 Hypoglossal nerve (XII)
5 Glossopharyngeal, vagus and cranial part of accessory nerves (IX, X and XI)
6 Vestibulocochlear nerve (VIII)

7 Facial nerve (VII)
8 Trochlear nerve (IV)
9 Trigeminal nerve (V)
10 Abducent nerve (VI)
11 Oculomotor nerve (III)
12 Internal carotid artery
13 Pituitary stalk, piercing the diaphragma sellae, the fold of dura forming the roof of the pituitary fossa, in the central part of the middle cranial fossa
14 Optic nerve (II)
15 Anterior cranial fossa
16 Lateral part of middle cranial fossa

brain and spinal cord and intimately following all their surface undulations is an even finer layer, the **pia mater**. The space between the arachnoid and pia is the **subarachnoid space** which is filled with **cerebrospinal fluid**, so forming a 'waterbath' which helps to cushion the brain within its bony box.

One of the most important arteries inside the skull is the **middle meningeal artery**. It enters through the foramen spinosum in the floor of the middle cranial fossa (**16.6**), and runs between the dura mater and the bone (**16.1** and **16.4**), dividing into two main branches which pass backwards at the side of the skull where they are liable to be damaged by

fractures (see below). It supplies bone and meninges, but not the brain.

CEREBROSPINAL FLUID

Cerebrospinal fluid (CSF) is a clear, watery fluid that is secreted by special groups of blood capillaries (**choroid plexuses**) within parts of the ventricular system of the brain (p.196). CSF escapes from the brain through openings in the roof of the fourth ventricle into the subarachnoid space.

Out of a total of approximately 130 ml of CSF, about 30 ml is within the ventricles of the brain and 100 ml in the subarachnoid space – 25 ml in the cranial part of the space

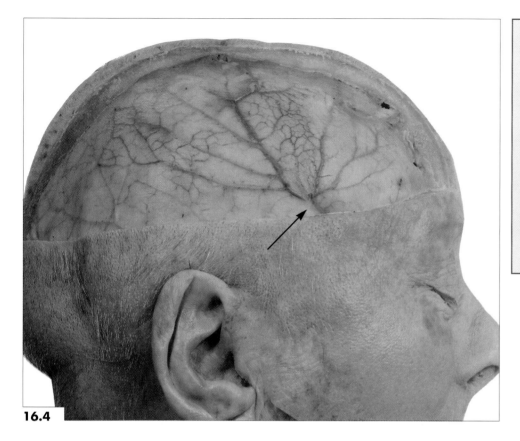

Fig. 16.4 Branches of the right middle meningeal vessels, shown after removal of part of the vault of the skull, leaving the dura mater intact. The arteries and accompanying veins are closely applied to one another, and may be ruptured (as at the arrow) by injuries to the side of the head, causing extradural haemorrhage (p.134) and pressure on the brain.

16.4

surrounding the brain, and 75 ml in the spinal part around the spinal cord. Because CSF is constantly being produced it must be constantly reabsorbed, and this occurs mostly into the venous blood of the superior sagittal sinus (see below) through projections of arachnoid (**arachnoid villi** or **granulations** – **16.2** and see **17.2a**) that penetrate the dura mater forming the wall of the sinus. Some CSF also seeps away through the sheaths of spinal nerves. If CSF is prevented from leaving the brain, e.g. by congenital malformation, tumour or infection of the meninges (*meningitis*), the ventricular system or parts of it may become grossly enlarged (*internal hydrocephalus*). If its circulation outside the brain is obstructed, the subarachnoid space may expand and so compress brain tissue (*external hydrocephalus*).

VENOUS SINUSES

In certain areas, the dura mater splits to enclose venous channels – the **intracranial venous sinuses** – which drain much of the venous blood from the brain (p.199). Like any other vessels, they have an internal lining of endothelium. The most extensive is the **superior sagittal sinus**, which runs in the midline below the bony vault (at the top of the falx cerebri, **16.2**) from front to back. It ends where the upper margin of the falx cerebri joins the tentorium cerebelli, a region at which several sinuses come together to form the **confluence of the sinuses**.

At this point, most of the blood in the superior sagittal sinus enters the **right transverse sinus**, which courses transversely until, in the region of the mastoid process, it turns downwards to become the **sigmoid sinus (16.6)**. This vessel leaves the skull through the jugular foramen to become the **right internal jugular vein**. The much smaller **inferior sagittal sinus** is in the lower margin of the falx, and is joined by the **great cerebral vein** to form the **straight sinus** which runs in the junction between the falx and the tentorium cerebelli. At the confluence of the sinuses the straight sinus turns to the left as the **left transverse sinus**, in turn becoming the sigmoid sinus and internal jugular vein of the left side. Apart from small cranial veins from the skull itself, the sagittal and sigmoid sinuses receive numerous **cerebral veins** from the brain (p.199).

Among the other sinuses, the most important are the **cavernous sinuses (16.7)**, lying one on each side of the pituitary gland and the adjacent part of the sphenoid bone. The internal carotid artery , the three nerves that supply the eye muscles, and the ophthalmic and mandibular branches of the trigeminal nerve all pass through the sinus, which only contains about 1.5 ml of blood. The cavernous sinuses are important because among their tributaries are veins from the orbit and the face, which act as possible pathways for infection from the *outside* to the *inside* of the skull (p.42). Before the days of antibiotics, septic *cavernous sinus thrombosis* was invariably fatal; it is still a serious condition, like any pathological process within the closed space of the skull.

INTRACRANIAL HAEMORRHAGE

Blood vessels within the skull and brain are subject to injury or disease giving rise to four kinds of haemorrhage: *extradural*, *subdural*, *subarachnoid* and *cerebral*.

Extradural Haemorrhage

Extradural haemorrhage is due to rupture of the middle meningeal vessels (**16.4**) by blows on the side of the head that fracture the relatively thin bone of this part of the skull – usually at the **pterion** (**16.18**), an area of the skull with an 'H'-shaped pattern of suture lines formed by parts of the frontal, parietal, temporal and sphenoid bones and which overlies the anterior branch of the middle meningeal artery. *Arterial* blood escapes **rapidly** between the bone of the skull and the dura, causing a swelling that increases intracranial pressure and may, for example, press on the motor area of the cerebral cortex (p.193), so causing a spastic type of paralysis of arm or leg depending on the area affected (p.206). Operation to remove the mass of clotted blood and relieve the intracranial pressure involves making a *burr hole* (see below) at the pterion to expose the ruptured vessels and control further bleeding.

Subdural Haemorrhage

Subdural haemorrhage is usually due to rupture of cerebral veins as they enter the superior sagittal sinus, leading to bleeding into the subdural space between the dura and arachnoid. The result is a swelling, which causes pressure on the underlying brain. However, since the bleeding is **slow venous** rather than rapid arterial, the effects are usually less severe and take longer to develop. A *trephine* or *bone flap* (see below) may be required to deal with the condition.

Subarachnoid Haemorrhage

Subarachnoid haemorrhage is usually due to rupture of a small *aneurysm* (pea-like dilatation) of some part of the arterial circle at the base of the brain (**17.4b**). The blood bursts out into the subarachnoid space, causing the cerebrospinal fluid to become blood-stained, and there is increased intracranial pressure with decreased vascularity of the brain. The condition may be acute, leading to death in a few hours, or chronic lasting for weeks or months.

Cerebral Haemorrhage

Cerebral haemorrhage or *thrombosis*, commonly called a *stroke*, is the commonest of all types of intracranial haemorrhage, and is due to rupture or blockage of one or more of the small arteries that supply the part of the cerebral hemisphere (internal capsule, p.195) through which pass the principal nerve fibres controlling body movements (p.199).

FRACTURES AND BRAIN DAMAGE

Fractures of the cranial vault range from hairline fractures (so called because they are barely distinguishable on radiographs) to obvious depressed fractures with splintering of bone and damage to the underlying brain. Head injuries without skull fracture can still cause severe brain damage because of the way the brain may be jolted within its bony box, and include 'contre-coup' injuries – damage to one side from a blow on the opposite side.

SURGICAL APPROACH

Surgical access to the inside of the skull is usually gained through some part of the vault. After appropriate incisions in the overlying scalp, avoiding the major nerves and blood vessels, the cranial cavity can be reached through burr holes, trephines or bone flaps. *Burr holes* (up to 15 mm in diameter) are made by drilling (which destroys the bone), but *trephining* removes a circular disc of bone (up to 5 cm in diameter) which can be replaced. For wider access, approximately rectangular *bone flaps* can be removed (*craniotomy*) by drilling several burr holes and then cutting the bone between adjacent holes (**16.5**). These flaps can also be replaced by stitching their pericranium to that of the surrounding skull. Which method of approach is used will obviously vary with the site and nature of the condition being treated. Dealing with a ruptured blood vessel (as in the example given above) may require only a burr hole, but removal of a cerebral tumour will require a more extensive bone flap.

PITUITARY GLAND

The **pituitary gland** (**hypophysis cerebri**) lies in the **pituitary fossa** in the base of the skull (**16.2** and **16.6**). It is a more or less rounded structure, less than 1 cm in diameter, and is connected to the under surface of the brain by the **pituitary stalk**, which is about 1 cm long (**16.3** and **17.2a**). Removing the brain in the dissecting room or mortuary invariably tears the pituitary stalk and leaves the gland behind in its fossa. A cavernous sinus (p.133) lies on either side of the fossa, and the fossa usually projects downwards into one or both sphenoidal air sinuses. The optic chiasma (p.195) is just above and behind the gland; pituitary tumours growing upwards may press upon the chiasma and cause visual defects (p.195).

LOBES

Developmentally and functionally, the pituitary is really two glands stuck together. The **posterior part** (**posterior lobe, posterior pituitary**), which develops from the brain, is the part that is directly connected with the hypothalamus of the brain by nerve fibres that run in the pituitary stalk. The **anterior part** (**anterior lobe, anterior pituitary**), which

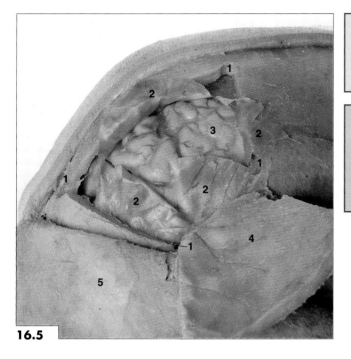

Fig. 16.5 Craniotomy – surgical exposure of the brain – at the front of the left side of the head.
After cutting away a bone flap, the dura mater has been incised to expose the arachnoid overlying the cerebral hemisphere.

1 Burr hole
2 Flap of dura mater
3 Arachnoid mater, overlying cerebral hemisphere. Cerebral veins are visible on the deep surface of the arachnoid
4 Bone flap, turned down and back
5 Scalp flap, turned down

16.5

develops from the pharynx, adheres to the front of the posterior lobe without any direct connection with the brain; the brain 'communicates' with it by hypothalamic hormones which are secreted into a system of blood vessels (the **hypophysial portal vessels**) that run down the stalk to join the capillaries of the anterior lobe.

POSTERIOR PITUITARY

The **posterior lobe** does not synthesize its own hormones; rather, it stores and releases hormones that have been manufactured in the **hypothalamus**. Here, the synthesis occurs in the cell bodies of certain *neurosecretory cells* (p.93) whose axons run down the pituitary stalk to end in the posterior pituitary. Newly synthesized hormones are transported down the axons and stored in their terminals, from which they are released when certain stimuli impinge on the cell bodies and on dendrites in the hypothalamus (as described below). The two hormones are *antidiuretic hormone* (ADH, also known as *vasopressin, arginine vasopressin* or *AVP*) and *oxytocin*.

Antidiuretic Hormone

The main function of *ADH* is to regulate the amount of water that is *reabsorbed* by kidney tubules (p.286) and so *prevent diuresis* (excessive production of urine). Its other action, constricting small blood vessels, is much less important in the amounts normally secreted, but accounts for its more common alternative name, vasopressin (meaning 'increasing pressure within vessels').

There are special sensory receptors (**osmoreceptors** – detecting changes in osmotic pressure) in blood vessels of the hypothalamic region which respond to changes in the amount of water in the blood. If the body is short of water, the receptors send nerve impulses to the neurosecretory cells and ADH secretion is stimulated so that the kidney tubules reabsorb more water and less urine is produced. If there is too much water, ADH release is suppressed so the kidneys reabsorb less water and more urine is produced.

A failure of ADH secretion (which is very uncommon – possibly due to head injuries or tumours in the hypothalamic region) leads to large quantities of body fluid being lost as urine, and this is accompanied by excessive thirst and the drinking of large amounts of fluid in an attempt to compensate for the loss. The urine is very pale and dilute, and the condition is named *diabetes insipidus* (not to be confused with the very common type of diabetes whose proper name is diabetes *mellitus*, p.279). Giving ADH by injections or even as a nasal spray (which is absorbed into the blood through the mucous membrane) enables the condition to be controlled effectively.

Oxytocin

Oxytocin causes contraction of the pregnant uterus (p.203), and its normal secretion is the stimulus for labour to begin (although what causes the stimulus for secretion is not known; it can be given by injection to accelerate delayed labour). It also causes the breasts to release milk (p.107).

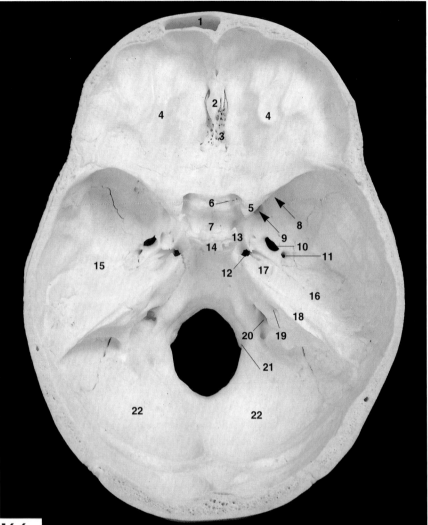

Fig. 16.6 Interior of the base of the skull.

16.6

1 Frontal sinus
2 Crista galli, to which the front of the falx cerebri is attached
3 Cribriform plate of ethmoid bone, pierced by filaments of the olfactory nerve
4 Anterior cranial fossa
5 Anterior clinoid process, for the attachment of part of the tentorium cerebelli. The internal carotid artery passes up to the brain on the medial side of this process
6 Optic canal, for optic nerve and ophthalmic artery
7 Pituitary fossa, lodging the pituitary gland
8 Superior orbital fissure, for the ophthalmic branch of the trigeminal nerve, the nerves for the extra-ocular muscles that move the eye (oculomotor, trochlear and abducent), and ophthalmic veins
9 Foramen rotundum, for the maxillary branch of the trigeminal nerve
10 Foramen ovale, for the mandibular branch of the trigeminal nerve
11 Foramen spinosum, for the middle meningeal vessels

12 Foramen lacerum, through the upper part of which the internal carotid artery enters the middle cranial fossa
13 Posterior clinoid process, for attachment of part of the tentorium cerebelli
14 Dorsum sellae, forming the posterior wall of the pituitary fossa
15 Middle cranial fossa (lateral part)
16 Roof of middle ear cavity (tegmen tympani)
17 Trigeminal impression, for the trigeminal ganglion
18 Petrous part of temporal bone
19 Internal acoustic meatus, for the facial and vestibulocochlear nerves
20 Jugular foramen, for glossopharyngeal, vagus and accessory nerves and sigmoid sinus (becoming the internal jugular vein as it leaves the skull)
21 Hypoglossal canal, for the hypoglossal nerve
22 Posterior cranial fossa
23 Foramen magnum, for the medulla oblongata, spinal part of the accessory nerves and the vertebral arteries

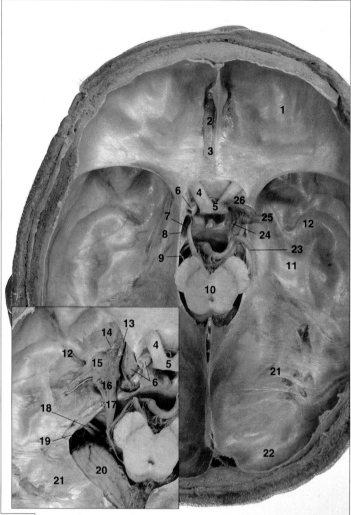

16.7

Fig. 16.7 Cranial fossae.
The brainstem is sectioned through the upper part of the midbrain. Inset, an area of dura mater, including the roof and lateral wall of the cavernous sinus, has been removed to show the trigeminal ganglion and its three branches.

1 Anterior cranial fossa
2 Olfactory bulb
3 Olfactory tract
4 Optic nerve
5 Optic chiasma, formed by the union of the two optic nerves
6 Internal carotid artery
7 Oculomotor nerve, entering the roof of the cavernous sinus
8 Lateral wall of cavernous sinus
9 Trochlear nerve
10 Midbrain
11 Middle cranial fossa
12 Middle meningeal vessels, seen deep to the dura mater after emerging through the foramen spinosum
13 Ophthalmic nerve, passing forwards to enter the superior orbital fissure
14 Maxillary nerve, passing forwards to enter the superior orbital fissure

15 Mandibular nerve, passing downwards to enter the foramen ovale
16 Trigeminal ganglion
17 Trigeminal nerve, passing forwards to the ganglion over the apex of the petrous part of the temporal bone
18 Facial nerve ⎫ passing laterally to enter
19 Vestibulocochlear nerve ⎬ the internal acoustic meatus
20 Cerebellum
21 Tentorium cerebelli
22 Transverse sinus
23 Posterior cerebral artery ⎫ for the pattern of these
24 Posterior communicating artery ⎬ vessels when dissected
25 Middle cerebral artery ⎬ away from the brain
26 Anterior cerebral artery ⎭ and skull, see **17.4b**

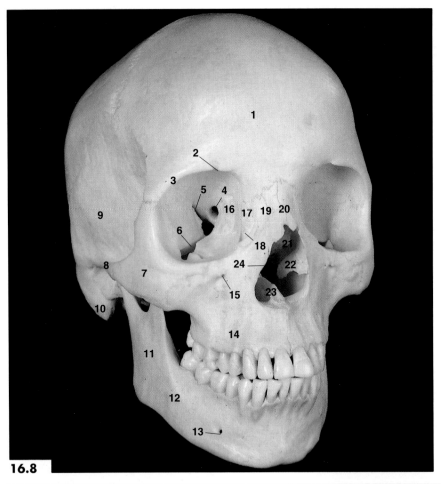

Fig. 16.8 Skull, from the front and the right, looking into the right orbit.

16.8

1 Frontal bone	13 Mental foramen, for the mental nerve
2 Supraorbital notch, sometimes a foramen, for the supraorbital vessels and nerve	14 Maxilla, bearing the upper teeth
3 Supraorbital margin	15 Infraorbital foramen, for the infraorbital nerve
4 Optic canal	16 Lateral wall of ethmoidal sinus, with air cells visible through the paper-thin bone (lamina papyracea)
5 Superior orbital fissure	17 Lacrimal bone
6 Inferior orbital fissure	18 Lacrimal groove, for the lacrimal sac
7 Zygomatic bone	19 Orbital process of maxilla
8 Zygomatic arch	20 Nasal bones
9 Squamous part of temporal bone	21 Middle nasal concha
10 Mastoid process of petrous part of temporal bone	22 Inferior nasal concha
11 Ramus of mandible	23 Lower part of bony nasal septum
12 Body of mandible, bearing the lower teeth	24 Margin of anterior nasal aperture (piriform aperture)

ANTERIOR PITUITARY

The **anterior pituitary** produces six main hormones, commonly named as follows (with alternatives in brackets):
- Growth hormone (GH, somatotropin, STH)
- Prolactin (PRL, mammotropic hormone, luteotropin, LTH)
- Adrenocorticotropic hormone (ACTH, corticotropin)
- Thyroid-stimulating hormone (TSH, thyrotropic hormone, thyrotropin)
- Luteinizing hormone (LH, sometimes known in the male as interstitial-cell stimulating hormone – ICSH)
- Follicle-stimulating hormone (FSH)

Growth hormone affects body tissues in general, and prolactin is concerned with breast function; all of the others act on specific endocrine glands and are collectively called *trophic hormones*. Those acting on gonads are *gonadotrophins* or *gonadotrophic hormones*.

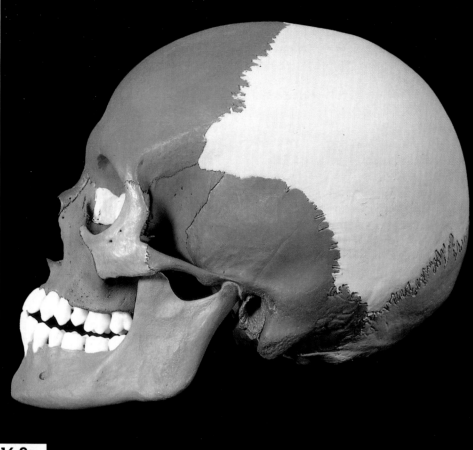

16.9a

Fig. 16.9 Skull bones.
(a) From the left side, with individual bones coloured.
(b) Parietal bone, dissected to show the diplöe, the cancellous bone between the inner and outer tables of compact bone.

Red – frontal
Gray – parietal
Orange – occipital
Red brown – temporal
Blue – sphenoid
Pink – mandible
Green – maxilla
Light brown – zygomatic
Dark brown – nasal
Dark gray – Lacrimal
Yellow – ethmoid

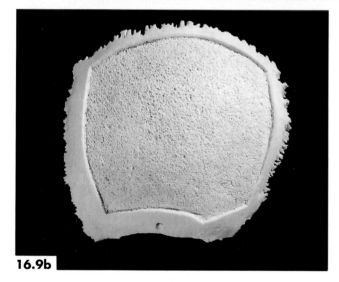

16.9b

cells by a special system of blood vessels (the *pituitary* or *hypophysial portal system*). It might be expected that one particular type of cell under the influence of its own controlling substance would always produce one particular hormone, but it is not yet certain whether this is true. So far, the controlling substances have been named after the type of hormone produced by the cells upon which they act; thus TRH, meaning thyrotropin releasing hormone, is the hypothalamic hormone that acts on the pituitary cells which secrete TSH (thyroid-stimulating hormone, or thyrotropin). GnRH, meaning gonadotrophin releasing hormone, acts on the cells producing the gonadotrophins, FSH and LH.

It appears that GH and PRL are unusual in that their release is under dual control: as well as ***releasing*** hormones (GH-RH and PRH), there are ***inhibiting*** ones (GH-IH and PIH). GH-IH, originally discovered in the hypothalamus, is now known as *somatostatin*, and has been found in pancreatic islets and also various endocrine cells of the gastrointestinal tract, from which it is released not only into the bloodstream but also into the lumen of the gut – a hitherto unsuspected site for a hormone. A further unusual feature is that GH appears to exert at least some of its effects not directly on the target tissues, but by causing the liver to secrete proteins called *somatomedins* which are the effective agents.

The secretion of all the anterior pituitary hormones is controlled by substances produced by neurosecretory cells in the hypothalamus (p.196). Unlike the similar cells associated with the posterior lobe, their axons are very short and extend only a short distance into the pituitary stalk. The controlling substances (usually called *hypothalamic releasing hormones*) are transported from the neurosecretory cells to the anterior lobe

A seventh hormone (MSH, *melanocyte stimulating hormone*), coming from a small intermediate part of the pituitary between the anterior and posterior lobes, is concerned with changes in skin pigmentation in animals but its function in man is uncertain, but it has nothing to do with suntanning.

Growth Hormone

Growth hormone is responsible for the general growth of body tissues during childhood and adolescence. ***Too much*** GH in a ***child*** (as caused by certain pituitary tumours) produces an excessively tall person (*gigantism*, like the biblical Goliath), but such giants are very rare. Most unusually tall people are simply expressing a hereditary tendency to tallness which is nothing to do with pituitary disease. ***Too little*** GH in a ***child*** leads to *pituitary dwarfism*, another rare condition (typically seen in the dwarfs of the circus); there is no tumour and the rest of the pituitary functions normally. There are many causes of lack of growth in the young, and most children who are apparently small for their age have no pituitary disorder; if blood tests ***do*** prove a GH deficiency, the repeated injection of GH throughout the normal growth period will stimulate growth.

In ***adults***, an ***excess*** of GH (from a pituitary tumour) leads to *acromegaly*. Because the epiphyses of long bones have fused, there can be no increase in height, but the limbs and face become enlarged with coarse-looking features. If surgical removal of the tumour is not possible, treatment may be by radiotherapy, e.g. by implanting radon capsules within the gland.

Although growth hormone is chiefly known for its effects on growth, it also has effects on the metabolism of foodstuffs (p.82), assisting in fat breakdown and elevating blood sugar.

Prolactin

Prolactin stimulates the synthesis and secretion of milk in the breasts, provided that the breast tissue is at a stage of development suitable for milk production. Like GH, it appears to be controlled by both a releasing hormone and an inhibiting one. Under normal conditions, the inhibitory hormone (PIH) is the dominant one, and prolactin secretion is thus kept quite low. Its secretion increases if the pituitary cells producing it are released from inhibition, as happens, for example, after childbirth. Pituitary tumours (even in males as well as females) and some drugs including the contraceptive pill can cause excessive prolactin secretion.

ACTH

The *ACTH* (adrenocorticotropic hormone) that is secreted by the anterior pituitary controls the secretion of cortisol by the adrenal cortex (p.281), but ***not*** the aldosterone of the cortex which is controlled by angiotensin (p.286).

TSH

TSH (thyroid-stimulating hormone) controls the secretion of thyroid hormone by the thyroid gland (p.191).

Gonadotrophins

The ***gonadotrophins***, as their name implies, exert their effects on the gonads – the testes and ovaries. In general, they regulate the development of spermatozoa and ova, and control the secretion by the gonads of the sex hormones: testosterone, oestrogen and progesterone. FSH (*follicle-stimulating hormone*) derives its name from its essential role in the growth of ovarian follicles (p.296), while LH (*luteinizing hormone*) was named because it is needed for the development and maintenance of the corpus luteum (an ovarian structure, p.296); both FSH and LH, however, have other roles as well. LH in the male is sometimes called ICSH (*interstitial-cell-stimulating hormone*) because it stimulates testosterone secretion by the interstitial (Leydig) cells of the testis (p.308).

---

1 Root ⎫	14 Zygomatic arch
2 Dorsum ⎪	15 Head of mandible
3 Apex ⎪	16 Auriculotemporal nerve and superficial temporal vessels, with the artery giving a palpable pulse
4 Septum ⎬ of external nose	17 Tragus of ear, landmark for the superficial temporal pulse (16)
5 Ala ⎪	18 Parotid duct emerging from gland
6 Nostril (aperture) ⎪	19 Parotid duct turning medially at anterior border of masseter
7 Alar groove ⎭	20 Philtrum
8 Frontal notch (or foramen) and supratrochlear nerve and vessels	21 Mental foramen, nerve and vessels
9 Supraorbital notch (or foramen), nerve and vessels	22 Lower border of body of mandible
10 Lateral part of supraorbital margin	23 Anterior border of masseter, and facial artery and vein, with the artery giving a palpable pulse
11 Medial palpebral ligament in front of lacrimal sac	24 Lower border of ramus of mandible
12 Infraorbital margin	25 Angle of mandible
13 Infraorbital foramen, nerve and vessels	

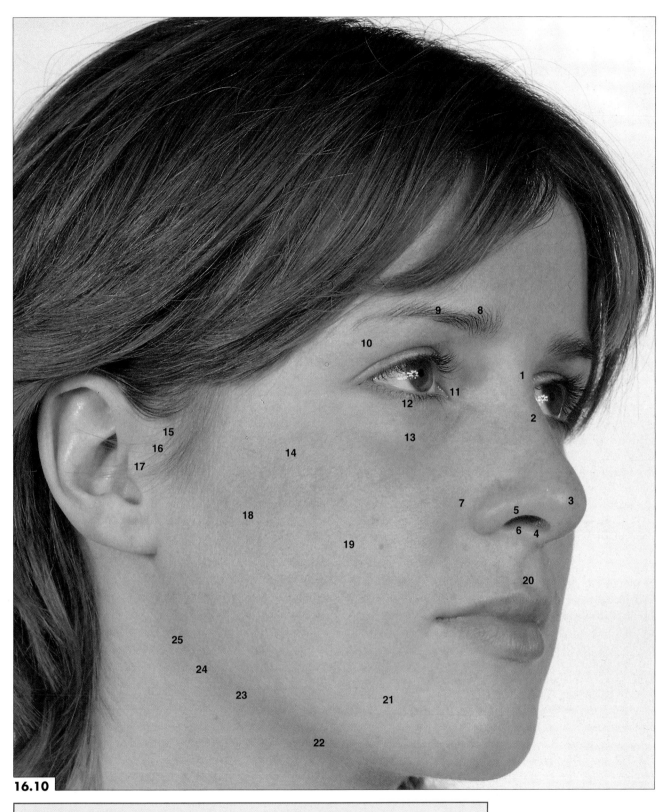

16.10

Fig. 16.10 Face, from the right and front, showing the surface markings of underlying structures.
Compare with the dissection in **16.11** and the skull in **16.9**. For details of the eye see **16.25a**.

FACE

FACIAL SKELETON

The **face** (**16.10**) extends from the hairline (or where the hairline ought to be) to the chin, and from ear to ear. Its bony framework is the front part of the skull (**16.8**) including the **mandible**, which is the only movable bone of the skull. The upper part of the nose is formed by the two small **nasal bones**, but the lower part is *cartilaginous* and so is relatively mobile (and missing from the dried skull). The facial skeleton shows, in its centre, the **nasal aperture** with a **maxilla** on each side, and above this are the **orbits** (orbital cavities) in which are lodged the eyes. At the upper margin of each orbit is the **frontal bone** which forms the bony part of the forehead, and the rest of each orbital margin is completed by the maxilla and (on the outer side) by the **zygomatic bone** (commonly called the cheek bone). The two maxillae bear the upper teeth and form the **upper jaw**, and the mandible with the lower teeth forms the **lower jaw**. The lower part of the mandible in the front forms the **chin**, while at the sides the head of the mandible articulates with part of the temporal bone at the **temporomandibular joint** (jaw joint, p.144).

FACIAL SKIN AND MUSCLES

Although everyone looks different (unless they have an identical twin!), **facial muscles** are the same in everyone; the differences are due to the underlying bone structure and the overlying connective tissues and skin, and depend largely on genetic factors. **Skin** and **connective tissues** adhere closely to the underlying muscles, but the amount of **subcutaneous fat** is variable. The chubby cheek of the infant is due to a particularly large fat pad (the **buccal pad**) which probably aids sucking by giving support to the cheek. All parts of the facial skin except the lips and eyelids have hair follicles, even the forehead, although here the hair produced is very fine and does not rise above the skin surface. All areas except the lips have sebaceous glands and sweat glands; the sweat glands of the forehead, like those of the axillae and palms of the hands, respond to emotional stimuli.

The appearance of the **facial skin**, more than that of any other part of the body, often has an important bearing on human behaviour. The commonest disease is *acne*, which may affect the neck, shoulders and back as well as the face, and is described on p.20.

Among the more important superficial muscles of the face (**16.11**) are **orbicularis oculi** (surrounding the eye, and responsible for closing and 'screwing up' the eye), **orbicularis oris** (surrounding the mouth and which, with other muscles, assists with lip movements), and **buccinator** ('the trumpeter', the muscle of the cheek which is important in blowing and in keeping food between the teeth so that it can be chewed). Note that the terms 'facial muscles' and 'muscles of facial expression' refer to the superficial muscles attached to the skin, and does not include the 'muscles of mastication' which move the lower jaw (p.145).

BLOOD SUPPLY AND LYMPH DRAINAGE

The main vessels (**16.11**) are the **facial artery** and the **superficial temporal artery**, with the **supraorbital** and **supratrochlear** vessels above the orbits.

The **facial artery** (from the external carotid) should be palpable as it comes on to the face (**16.10**), crossing the lower border of the mandible 2.5 cm in front of the angle of the mandible. It runs beneath the facial muscles towards the side of the nose and the inner angle of the eye, with the facial vein behind it. It is characteristic that the *artery is tortuous* while the *vein is straight*. The vessels make good anastomoses with their fellows on the opposite side, especially by the **superior** and **inferior labial branches** which make a vascular ring within the tissues of the lips.

The **superficial temporal artery** (from the maxillary branch of the external carotid) runs upwards, immediately in front of the tragus of the ear, where it is easily palpable (**16.10**).

The main veins drain to the internal jugular in the neck (p.179), but it is *highly important* to note that veins in the region of the nose and orbit (the 'danger area' of the face) communicate with those within the orbit and hence with veins *inside the cranial cavity*. There is thus a possible pathway for infection to spread, say, from a septic spot on the face beside the nose, to the cavernous venous sinus within the skull, causing a dangerous thrombosis (p.134).

Facial lymph drains to deep cervical nodes, either directly or (at the front) via submandibular and submental nodes (p.181).

NERVE SUPPLY

All of the facial **muscles** are supplied by the **facial nerve** (i.e. the seventh cranial nerve). The nerve passes through the parotid gland below the ear and fans out from the front border of the gland (**16.11**) in five groups of branches that run to the various muscles. The facial nerve has nothing to do with the sensory supply of facial skin, which is largely from the trigeminal nerve (the fifth cranial nerve – see below). In *facial paralysis* the main features are drooping of the corner of the mouth on the affected side with uncontrolled dribbling of saliva, and the inability to close the eye (p.162) and to clear food out of the vestibule of the mouth (p.147). *Bell's palsy*, the commonest of all cranial nerve paralyses, is a type of facial nerve paralysis of unknown cause; it is associated with varying degrees of recovery. Facial paralysis may also result from a stroke (p.199) if the fibres that control the facial nerve within the brain are affected. Note that drooping of the upper eyelid (*ptosis*) is **not** part of a facial nerve paralysis; the muscle responsible for elevating the upper lid (the levator palpebrae superioris) belongs to the muscles of the orbit (p.162) and is supplied by the oculomotor nerve (the third cranial nerve).

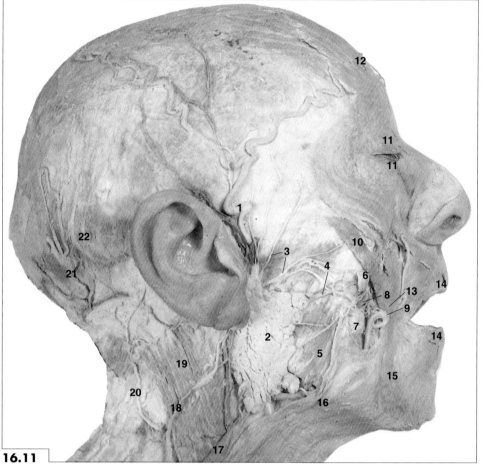

Fig. 16.11 Dissection of the right side of the face. Only the more important facial muscles have been named.

1 Superficial temporal artery and auriculotemporal nerve. The artery is the main supply to the side of the scalp
2 Parotid gland
3 Branches of facial nerve emerging from parotid gland to supply facial muscles (but not the overlying skin)
4 Parotid duct, emerging from the gland to turn medially at the anterior border of masseter (5) and pierce buccinator (7)
5 Masseter
6 An accessory parotid gland, a common feature just above the duct
7 Buccal fat pad overlying buccinator
8 Facial vein, behind the artery (9)
9 Facial artery
10 Zygomaticus major
11 Orbicularis oculi
12 Occipitalis part of occipitofrontalis
13 Levator anguli oris
14 Orbicularis oris
15 Depressor anguli oris
16 Platysma, labelled where it overlies the facial artery (9)
17 External jugular vein
18 Great auricular nerve, from the cervical plexus, supplying much of the skin of the ear and the skin over the angle of the mandible – the only part of the facial skin not supplied by branches of the trigeminal nerve
19 Sternocleidomastoid
20 Lesser occipital nerve, from the cervical plexus
21 Occipital artery, the main supply to the back of the scalp
22 Occipitalis part of occipitofrontalis

The *sensory* supply of most of the facial skin comes from the three main branches of the **trigeminal nerve**. The **ophthalmic branch** supplies the part above eye level (and also a strip down the centre of the nose), the **maxillary branch** the part between eye and mouth, and the **mandibular branch** the area below the mouth and upwards in front of the ear. Disease that affects the trigeminal nerve may illustrate very clearly the distribution of its branches; thus the rash of *herpes zoster* (*shingles*) is often found in the area supplied by the ophthalmic and maxillary nerves.

COSMETIC SURGERY

The good healing properties of the face and scalp (due to their profuse blood supply) contribute to the excellent results of operations carried out for injury or disease, or for cosmetic reasons. A common procedure is *facelift* (*facialplasty*), which is carried out to disguise the creases in face and neck that inevitably appear as part of the aging process. Incisions are made just behind the hairline and ears so that the skin, together with the underlying platysma muscle, can be undermined and pulled back to 'take up the slack'; the excess tissue at the incision line is removed before suturing the cut edges. Great care must be taken to avoid damage to the branches of the facial nerve that fan out from the front of the gland and supply the facial muscles (see above) when elevating the skin in front of the parotid gland.

PAROTID GLAND AND TEMPOROMANDIBULAR JOINT

There are three major pairs of **salivary glands** – **parotid**, **submandibular** and **sublingual** – and many minor glands embedded in the mucous membrane of the mouth and tongue. All help to keep the inside of the mouth moist to assist in chewing, and, although some of their secretions contain enzymes as well as mucus, the contribution that saliva makes to digestion of food is negligible. The moisture is also important in those who wear dentures since the mucus helps to keep them in place.

PAROTID GLAND

The **parotid glands** are the largest salivary glands, lying one on either side of the face (**16.11**), tucked in behind the ramus of the mandible below the ear and in front of the mastoid process. Underneath the skin, each gland overlaps part of the masseter muscle which covers the ramus of the mandible. The **facial nerve** and its main branches are *embedded* within the gland, as are the end of the **external carotid artery** (dividing into the superficial temporal and maxillary branches), and the **retromandibular vein**; branches of these vessels supply the gland. Some lymph nodes may also lie within the gland as well as on its surface. Unless affected by disease, the gland is not obvious on palpation.

The gland discharges its secretion into the mouth via the **parotid duct**. This is 5 cm long and, from the front of the gland, it runs forwards over the masseter and then turns inwards in front of the ramus of the mandible to pierce the buccinator muscle obliquely and open into the mouth opposite the crown of the second upper molar tooth. The pinpoint opening can be seen when examining the inside of the mouth. The *surface marking* of the duct (**16.10**) is along the middle third of a line drawn from the tragus of the ear to the midpoint of the philtrum.

The nervous stimulus to secretion is parasympathetic (p.47), and is effected by impulses that run in the glossopharyngeal nerve (the ninth cranial nerve) and eventually 'hitch-hike' to the gland via the mandibular branch of the trigeminal nerve (the fifth cranial nerve). Note that secretion has nothing to do with the facial nerve, which is so obviously associated with the gland.

Diseases

The commonest disease of the gland is *mumps*, a virus infection causing painful swelling of the gland – it is painful because the gland is enclosed in a dense connective tissue capsule; it is the increased tension within this tissue that causes the pain. Although commonest in children, it can affect any age group and spreads by contact with the infected saliva.

Parotid tumours require surgical removal, which is a delicate exercise in dissection because as far as possible the facial nerve and its branches within the gland should be preserved to prevent a disfiguring facial paralysis. The gland may also have to be removed when lymph nodes of the neck are involved in cancer metastases, because some nodes are embedded within the gland and they cannot be dissected out from it.

MANDIBLE

The main parts of each half of the **mandible** (lower jaw, **16.12**) are the **body**, which is the horizontal part bearing the teeth, and the **ramus**, the rectangular part at the back. The lower corner at the back is the **angle** of the mandible, and the central part at the front forms what is commonly called the chin. The ramus divides at its upper end into the **coronoid process** at the front and the **condyle** at the back; the condyle consists of the head and the neck. The **head** is the smooth curved surface taking part in the temporo-mandibular joint, and the **neck** is the narrower part joining the head to the rest of the ramus. At birth the two halves of the mandible are bony but separated from each other by a disc of cartilage; within two years, this cartilage has become completely replaced by bone.

TEMPOROMANDIBULAR JOINT

The **temporomandibular joint** (jaw joint, **16.13** and **16.9a**) is formed by the articulation between the **head** of the mandible and the **mandibular fossa** and **articular tubercle** on the base of the skull. The deeply spoon-shaped fossa does not lie completely transversely, but is on a line that is tilted slightly backwards at its inner end; this helps to stabilize side-to-side movements of the mandible. The mandible does not make direct contact with the fossa because there is an intervening **disc** of fibrocartilage (**16.13b**); this creates two separate joint cavities – one between fossa and disc, and one between disc and mandible. The disc is attached to the connective tissue capsule surrounding the joint. Opening the mouth a small amount, as in talking, involves a hinge

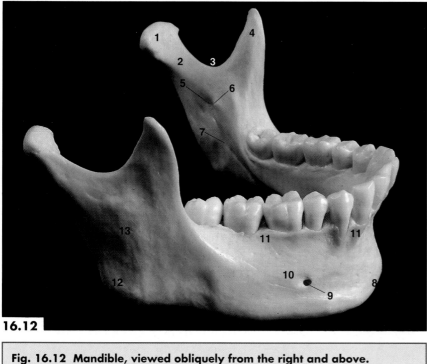

1 Head ⎱ together forming
2 Neck ⎰ the condyle
3 Mandibular notch
4 Coronoid process
5 Mandibular foramen, for the inferior alveolar nerve and vessels supplying all the lower teeth
6 Lingula, at the entrance to the foramen (5)
7 Mylohyoid groove, for the nerve to mylohyoid
8 Mental protuberance, forming the tip of the chin
9 Mental foramen, for the mental nerve and vessels
10 Body, forming with the ramus (13) the main part of the bone
11 Alveolar process, the upper part of the body bearing the teeth
12 Angle, at the lower posterior part of the ramus
13 Ramus, bearing at the top the condyle (1 and 2) and coronoid process (4)

16.12

Fig. 16.12 Mandible, viewed obliquely from the right and above. For the names of the teeth see **16.17**.

movement between the head of the mandible and the disc, but when the mouth is opened wide the head of the mandible is pulled forwards so that the head comes to lie on the part of the disc that is in front of the fossa, on the articular tubercle. Closing the mouth restores the normal position. In dislocation of the jaw from injury (or sometimes an unusually wide yawn!), the head of the mandible gets stuck in the forward position outside the fossa, and the whole mandible must be pressed downwards and backwards to get it back into the normal position.

MUSCLES OF MASTICATION

The muscles that are mainly responsible for moving the jaw are the group of four (on each side) collectively known as the **muscles of mastication: temporalis, masseter** and the **medial** and **lateral pterygoid muscles**. Of these, only the lateral pterygoid is involved in *opening* the mouth. (This action also involves other small muscles of the neck, the digastric and mylohyoid, sometimes called *accessory* muscles of mastication.)

The **lateral pterygoid (16.13b)** can assist in opening the mouth because its fibres run backwards (from the lateral pterygoid plate and the adjacent part of the base of the skull) to be inserted into the joint capsule, the disc and the neck of the mandible. Its contraction can thus pull the head of the mandible *forwards*, and at the same time the tip of the chin tilts downwards and backwards, which is what happens in opening the mouth wide.

The other three muscles help to *close* the mouth because they all pull the mandible upwards. The large, fan-shaped **temporalis (16.13a)** comes from the side of the skull and passes under the zygomatic arch to be attached to the coronoid process of the mandible and the front of the ramus. The *lowest* fibres of origin of this muscle first run *horizontally* and then take a 90° turn downwards round the root of the zygomatic arch; these are the fibres responsible for pulling the head of the mandible *back* into the fossa after wide opening of the mouth.

Masseter (16.13a) is a rectangular muscle running from the zygomatic arch to the ramus of the mandible and so is obviously well placed for closing the mouth.

The **medial pterygoid (16.13b)** passes downwards and backwards from the lateral pterygoid plate to be inserted into the inner side of the angle of the mandible, and so helps to close the mouth.

The two pterygoid muscles of each side are also important in being able to move the jaw from side to side, producing the grinding movements between the teeth which complement the crushing part of the chewing mechanism. Parts of the temporalis and masseter can often be seen and felt in action under the skin, but the pterygoids are too deep.

The pterygoid muscles occupy the region below the base of the skull behind the maxilla known as the **infratemporal fossa**. When most of the ramus of the mandible is removed to allow dissection of this area (**16.13b**), two large and important branches of the mandibular nerve are seen

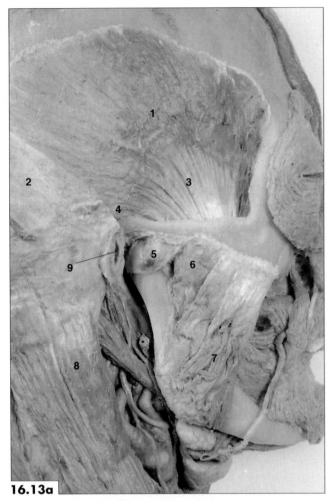

16.13a

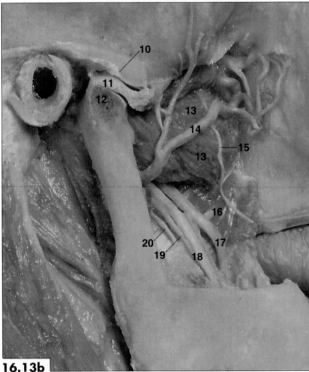

16.13b

Fig. 16.13 Muscles of mastication of the right side.
(a) Temporalis, masseter and the temporomandibular joint, after removal of the parotid gland.
(b) Deep dissection after removal of the parotid gland, temporalis and masseter and much of the ramus of the mandible, to show the two pterygoid muscles, occupying the region below the base of the skull known as the infratemporal fossa.

1 Temporalis, arising from the temporal fossa
2 Temporalis fascia
3 Temporalis tendon, passing down deep to the zygomatic arch (7) to the coronoid process and the front of the ramus of the mandible
4 Lowest fibres of temporalis, lying horizontally and responsible for pulling the head of the mandible backwards after it has been pulled forwards (in wide opening of the mouth) by the lateral pterygoid (13)
5 Capsule of temporomandibular joint and lateral temporomandibular ligament
6 Deepest fibres of masseter
7 Masseter, running from the zygomatic arch to the lateral surface of the ramus of the mandible
8 Sternocleidomastoid
9 External acoustic meatus
10 Mandibular fossa of skull, in the squamous part of the temporal bone
11 Interarticular disc
12 Head of mandible
13 Lateral pterygoid muscle, whose fibres pass backwards from the lateral pterygoid plate of the skull from which most of its fibres arise, to the neck of the mandible and the capsule and disc of the joint
14 Maxillary artery, from the external carotid
15 Buccal branch of mandibular nerve
16 Medial pterygoid, whose fibres pass downwards from the deep surface of the lateral pterygoid plate to the inside of the angle of the mandible
17 Lingual nerve, supplying the mucous membrane of the anterior part of the tongue
18 Inferior alveolar nerve, entering the mandibular foramen to supply the pulp cavities of the lower teeth
19 Inferior alveolar artery, behind the nerve (18) and also entering the foramen to supply the teeth
20 Nerve to mylohyoid, from the inferior alveolar (18)

emerging between the two pterygoid muscles: the **inferior alveolar nerve** which runs down to enter the mandibular foramen in the mandible and supply all the lower teeth of its own half of the jaw (p.152), and the **lingual nerve** which enters the side of the tongue to supply the mucous membrane (but *not* the muscle) of its own half (p.150). The **maxillary artery** (from the external carotid) also passes across the fossa between or through the pterygoids on its way to enter the nasal cavity (p.155).

NERVE SUPPLIES

All four mastication muscles are supplied by the **mandibular branch** of the **trigeminal nerve** (the fifth cranial nerve). Note that the buccinator muscle (p.142), which assists in chewing by helping to keep food between the upper and lower teeth and away from the cheeks, is not classified as a muscle of mastication since it does not move the mandible. It belongs to the *facial muscle* group and so is supplied by the *facial nerve*. Facial paralysis (p.142) interferes with chewing since food collects against the cheek on the paralyzed side and the buccinator can no longer force it inwards between the teeth.

MOUTH

Consult the introductions to the Respiratory System and Digestive System (pp.73 and 79).

The **mouth** (**16.14**) is the beginning of the digestive tract and is guarded at the front by the **lips**, with the **cheeks** at the sides. It contains the **teeth** and the **tongue**, and at the back it opens into the middle (oral) part of the **pharynx** (p.182), the muscular tube that extends down from the base of the skull. The **roof** of the mouth is formed by the **palate** – mostly by the **hard palate** which is bony, with the **soft palate** which is muscular (skeletal muscle) hanging down at the back. The hard palate separates the mouth from the nasal cavity which, like the mouth, opens into the pharynx. The nose and the uppermost part of the pharynx (the nasopharynx) are part of the respiratory tract, but the mouth and rest of the pharynx are shared by both the digestive and respiratory tracts; the mouth can be used for breathing as well as feeding. When swallowing (p.185), the soft palate is raised to close off the nasopharynx from the oral part, so preventing food and drink from passing upwards. The **floor** of the mouth is formed largely by the pair of mylohyoid muscles, which run between the hyoid bone and the mandible and join together in the midline. The smaller geniohyoids are in the floor just above the mylohyoids.

LIPS AND CHEEKS

The **lips** consist of the **orbicularis oris muscle** (p.142) which is covered on the outer side by skin (mostly keratinized epidermis with the usual hair follicles and sweat and sebaceous glands) and on the inside by the mucous membrane of the mouth (see below). The red margin at the opening is covered by modified skin, very thinly keratinized, with no follicles or glands. It appears red because the many capillaries in the connective tissue show through the thin epithelium. The muscle is supplied by the facial nerve; in facial nerve paralysis (p.142), the lips cannot be shut together on the affected side, allowing saliva to drip from the corner of the mouth.

The main cheek muscle is the **buccinator** (p.142), which is also supplied by the facial nerve. It helps to manipulate food, and also provides the resistance necessary for blowing actions; in facial paralysis, the cheek puffs out when attempting to whistle or blow.

VESTIBULE OF THE MOUTH

The **vestibule of the mouth** is the part inside the lips and cheeks and outside the teeth and gums. The parotid duct (p.144) opens into it on each side – on the inside of the cheek opposite the second upper molar tooth. The minor salivary glands on the inside of the lips and cheeks also open into the vestibule.

ORAL CAVITY

The main part of the mouth, inside the teeth, is often called the **mouth cavity proper** (**oral cavity, buccal cavity**), and its most obvious feature is the mobile **tongue** (**16.14**). On the floor of the front of the oral cavity in the midline is the **frenulum** of the tongue, a small fold of mucous membrane helping to anchor the undersurface of the tongue to the floor; an unusually tight frenulum (tongue-tie) may interfere with movement. On the floor just beside the frenulum is the opening of the **submandibular duct** (see below), and farther to the side is a ridge of mucous membrane formed by the underlying almond-shaped **sublingual gland**, whose secretions either enter the submandibular duct or reach the floor of the mouth through several minute ducts whose openings are too small to be seen with the naked eye.

Mucous Membrane and Salivary Secretion

The mouth in general is lined by *stratified squamous non-keratinizing epithelium*. The continual replacement of the cells ensures a suitably resistant surface to combat the 'wear and tear' of chewing food. In certain areas, the epithelium is partly or completely *keratinized* (rather like the epidermis of skin, p.17) for added protection, as on the upper surface (dorsum) of the tongue, on the gums (gingivae, the part covering the bony jaws), and on the hard palate.

The mouth is kept moist by its own secretion – *saliva* – which comes not only from the three major pairs of salivary glands – parotid (already described, p.144), submandibular and sublingual (see below) – but also from many minor glands in the mucous membrane of the cheeks, lips, palate and back of the tongue (the molar, labial, palatal and lingual glands). Although saliva contains an enzyme (*ptyalin* or *salivary amylase*) that begins the breakdown of starch, its overall effect on digestion is negligible, and its main function is to provide the necessary moisture for chewing and swallowing.

Submandibular Gland

Although the **submandibular gland** is, strictly speaking, in the neck, it is convenient to study it here. It lies in the angle between the lower, inner surface of the body of the mandible and the mylohyoid muscle (**16.35a**) (i.e. below the floor of

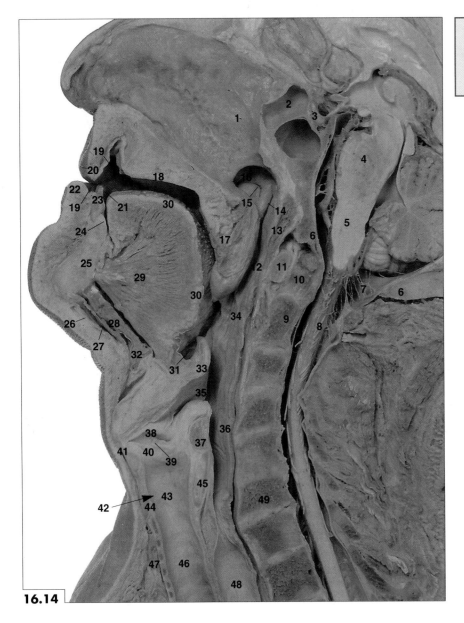

16.14

the mouth), and can be palpated about halfway along the lower border of the mandible (**16.34a**). It is roughly round, and about 2.5 cm (1 inch) in diameter. The **submandibular duct** (5 cm or 2 inches long, the same length as the parotid duct) leaves the posterior part of the gland and runs deep to mylohyoid to open into the floor of the mouth beside the midline frenulum of the tongue (see above). Its secretory (parasympathetic) nerve fibres run with the facial nerve's chorda tympani branch, which joins the lingual nerve and so leads the secretory fibres to the submandibular ganglion (on the side of the tongue) whose postganglionic fibres run into the gland.

Sublingual Gland

The almond-shaped **sublingual gland** lies beneath the mucous membrane of the floor of the mouth; it raises an elongated swelling, easily seen when the front of the tongue is raised. It secretes through about a dozen minute **ducts**; some open directly into the floor of the mouth and others open into the submandibular duct which lies beside it. It receives the same nerve supply as the submandibular gland.

TONGUE

The **tongue** (**16.14** and **16.15**) consists of a mass of skeletal muscle which is covered by a mucous membrane that is

1 Nasal septum
2 Sphenoidal sinuses
3 Pituitary gland
4 Pons
5 Medulla oblongata
6 Margin of foramen magnum
7 Filaments of arachnoid mater crossing subarachnoid space (cisterna magna)
8 Spinal cord and emerging nerve roots
9 Body   of
10 Dens   axis
11 Anterior arch of atlas
12 Nasal part of pharynx
13 Position of pharyngeal tonsil
14 Pharyngeal recess
15 Opening of auditory tube
16 Posterior nasal aperture (choana)
17 Soft palate
18 Hard palate
19 Vestibule of mouth, between lip (and cheek) and gum (and teeth)
20 Upper lip
21 Oral cavity, internal to gums (gingivae) and teeth, with the tongue in the floor of the cavity
22 Lower lip
23 Lower central incisior tooth
24 Lower gingiva (gum)

25 Mandible
26 Platysma
27 Mylohyoid, with overlying geniohyoid (28) forming the floor of the mouth
28 Geniohyoid
29 Genioglossus, the largest tongue muscle
30 Dorsum of tongue
31 Vallecula
32 Hyoid bone
33 Epiglottis
34 Oral part of pharynx
35 Inlet of larynx
36 Laryngeal part of pharynx
37 Transverse arytenoid muscle
38 Vestibular fold (false vocal cord)
39 Sinus (ventricle) of larynx
40 Vocal fold (vocal cord)
41 Laryngeal prominence (Adam's apple) and lamina of thyroid cartilage
42 Position of incision for laryngotomy
43 Lower part of larynx
44 Arch   of cricoid
45 Lamina   cartilage
46 Trachea, showing tracheal cartilages in wall
47 Isthmus of thyroid gland
48 Oesophagus
49 Body of sixth cervical vertebra

rough on the upper surface (dorsum) but smooth underneath, where it becomes continuous with the lining of the floor of the oral cavity. Internally, there is a thin, midline fibrous septum passing from front to back, with muscles on each side. Most of the **dorsum** faces upwards towards the hard palate, but the back part faces backwards towards the pharynx and contains lymphoid follicles (p.68). The **root** of the tongue attaches the organ to the mandible and the hyoid bone, and the main vessels and nerves enter through this part. In an unconscious patient lying on the back, the tongue can fall backwards and obstruct the airway through the pharynx (pp.126 and 182, and **15.29**).

Papillae and Taste Buds

The dorsum is roughened by many **papillae** (projections). The most numerous are the **filiform papillae**, which consist of narrow cones of keratinized cells (but no taste buds – see below) and give the general velvety appearance to this surface. **Fungiform papillae** are less common; they appear in the living tongue as bright red pinheads (whitish in dissecting room specimens, **16.15**), and are rather mushroom-like structures with a connective tissue core and a covering of non-keratinizing epithelium with usually a few taste buds. The **vallate papillae** (**16.15**) are the largest but least numerous, with about 8–12 situated in front of the surface

'V'-shaped line (the sulcus terminalis, with the apex of the 'V' pointing backwards) which divides the anterior two-thirds of the tongue from the posterior one-third. They have a connective tissue core and a deep, epithelial-lined cleft surrounding them (from the Latin 'vallum', for the Roman ditch), with many taste buds.

Taste buds are the receptor organs for the special sense of taste. They are microscopic barrel-shaped structures containing the neuroepithelial taste cells. They occupy the full thickness of the epithelium and, apart from being found on fungiform and vallate papillae, are scattered on other parts of the dorsum.

Muscles

The muscle fibres are arranged in various directions, which allow the subtle changes in position and shape needed for manipulating and swallowing food and also for speech. The largest muscle is **genioglossus** (**16.14**), which is best appreciated in sagittal sections where it can be seen to fan out from the back of the mandible into the tongue and down to the hyoid bone. The small **palatoglossus**, coming down from the hard palate, forms the **palatoglossal arch** which separates the mouth from the oropharynx and has the tonsil immediately behind it (p.182).

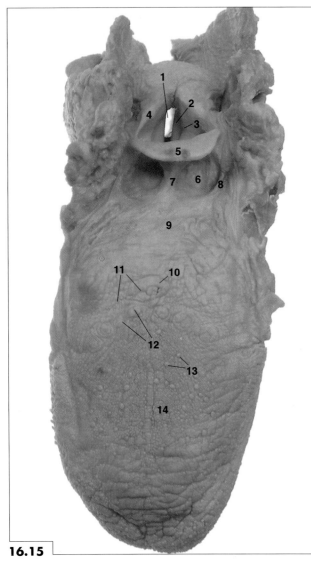

Fig. 16.15 Tongue and the inlet of the larynx, from above.

1 Rima of glottis, the gap between the two vocal folds (2)
2 Vocal fold (vocal cord)
3 Vestibular fold (false vocal cord)
4 Aryepiglottic fold, forming the lateral boundary of the laryngeal inlet
5 Epiglottis, at the front of the laryngeal inlet
6 Vallecula
7 Median glossoepiglottic fold, separating the bases of the two valleculae
8 Lateral glossoepiglottic fold, at the lateral edge of the vallecula
9 Pharyngeal or posterior part of dorsum of tongue, supplied by the glossopharyngeal nerve
10 Foramen caecum, the site of the embryonic thyroid downgrowth
11 Sulcus terminalis, not well shown in this tongue
12 Vallate papillae, whose margins contain the greatest concentration of taste buds, and which are supplied by the glossopharyngeal nerve from the posterior part of the tongue
13 Fungiform papillae, like whitish pinheads in the dissecting room tongue but red in life
14 Anterior part of dorsum of tongue, supplied by the lingual nerve

Blood Supply and Lymph Drainage

The main artery on each side is the **lingual branch** of the **external carotid artery** (**16.35b**); various veins unite to form the **lingual vein** which drains into the internal jugular. One of the veins can be seen easily beneath the mucous membrane on the under surface of the tongue when the tip is raised to the roof of the mouth.

Lymph drains to submandibular and deep cervical nodes. The essential feature is that lymph can *cross* within the tongue from one side to the other; carcinoma may thus spread to involve nodes on *both* sides of the neck.

Nerve Supply

The **motor nerve supply** of the muscles is by the **hypoglossal nerves** (the twelfth cranial nerves, **16.35b**) – each to its own half of the tongue. In hypoglossal nerve paralysis (a rare event), the tongue deviates towards the paralyzed side when trying to put it out, owing to the unopposed action of the muscles on the normal side.

The **sensory supply** for ordinary sensation (touch, pain and temperature) from the *anterior* part of the tongue is by the **lingual nerve**, from the mandibular part of the trigeminal nerve (the fifth cranial nerve – **16.13b**). The fibres for the special sense of taste run with a small branch of the **facial nerve** (seventh cranial nerve), the **chorda tympani**, which joins the lingual nerve. The posterior part of the tongue is supplied by the **glossopharyngeal nerve** (the ninth cranial nerve), both for ordinary and special sensations; this supply includes that of the taste buds of the vallate papillae.

All of the **taste fibres** pass in their respective nerves to the medulla of the brainstem. Here they synapse with neurons that reach the thalamus, from which the sensations are relayed to the sensory cortex. The basic tastes are sweet, salt, sour and bitter, and their appreciation is closely linked to the sense of smell (see p.155).

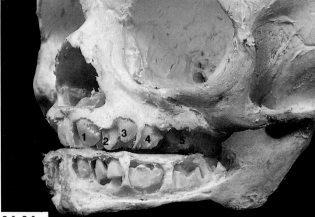

16.16a

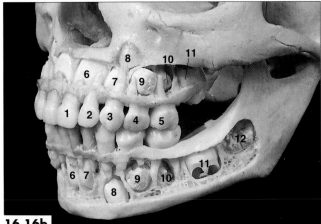

16.16b

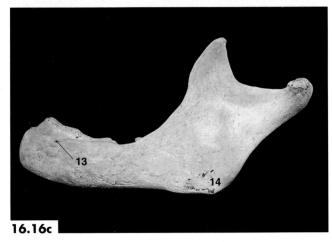

16.16c

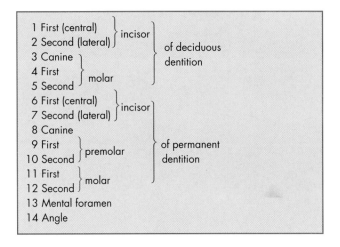

Fig. 16.16 Teeth and jaws in childhood and old age.
(a) In the newborn, with unerupted deciduous teeth.
(b) In a child of 4 years, with erupted deciduous teeth and unerupted permanent teeth. Developing third molars are not present.
(c) Edentulous mandible in old age. Without teeth the alveolar bone is absorbed, bringing the mental foramen to lie near the upper margin, and the angle between body and ramus becoming more obtuse like the infantile mandible in **(b)**. Compare with **16.12**.

1 First (central) ⎫ incisor ⎫
2 Second (lateral) ⎭   ⎬ of deciduous dentition
3 Canine   ⎫   ⎭
4 First   ⎬ molar
5 Second   ⎭
6 First (central) ⎫ incisor
7 Second (lateral) ⎭
8 Canine   ⎫ premolar ⎫ of permanent dentition
9 First   ⎬   ⎭
10 Second   ⎭
11 First   ⎫ molar
12 Second   ⎭
13 Mental foramen
14 Angle

TEETH

No teeth are visible in the mouth of the newborn infant (**16.16a**). Between the ages of approximately six months and three years, 20 teeth should have erupted (**16.16b**) – five in each half jaw or quadrant, and named from the centre backwards, as the central incisor, lateral incisor, canine, first molar and second molar. These teeth form the **deciduous dentition, primary dentition** or '**milk teeth**', which are gradually shed and, from the age of six years onwards, are replaced by the 32 teeth of the **secondary** or **permanent dentition** (**16.17**). The latter are named in each quadrant as central incisor, lateral incisor, canine, first premolar, second premolar, first molar, second molar and third molar. Note that the first and second milk molars are replaced by the first and second premolars, and that the three permanent molars have no forerunners among the milk teeth. In clinical dentistry, the milk teeth are often referred to by the letters A–E and the permanent teeth by the numbers 1–8 (both groups beginning with the central incisor and working laterally), and these letters and numbers are included in *Table* **16.1**.

The approximate dates of *tooth eruption* (when they become visible within the mouth) are also given in *Table* **16.1**.

Among the permanent teeth, those of the lower jaw erupt slightly before their corresponding fellows of the upper jaw. The first permanent molar usually erupts before any deciduous teeth have been shed, at about 6 years, and the other molars appear at 12–18 years, although the eruption of the third molar may be delayed for years and may even not erupt at all. Because it is the last tooth to appear, after the adolescent years have passed, it it commonly called the '*wisdom tooth*'.

Table 16.1 Deciduous and permanent teeth

Deciduous Teeth		
6 months	Lower central incisors	A
7 months	Upper central incisors	A
8 months	Upper lateral incisors	B
9 months	Lower lateral incisors	B
1 year	First molars	D
1.5 years	Canines	C
2 years	Second molars	E
Permanent Teeth		
6 years	First molars	6
7 years	Central incisors	1
8 years	Lateral incisors	2
9 years	First premolars	4
10 years	Second premolars	5
11 years	Canines	3
12 years	Second molars	7
18 years	Third molars	8

Tooth Structure

The main parts of a **tooth** (**16.17**) are the **crown, neck** and **root**, and the principal component is **dentine**, a hard calcified tissue. (In elephants' tusks, which are modified incisor teeth, dentine is called ivory.) The **crown** of the tooth is the part seen in the mouth and is covered by a thin layer of the hardest of all calcified tissues, **enamel**. The **root** of the tooth is buried in the jaw and covered by another specialized tissue, **cementum**, which helps to anchor the tooth to the surrounding bone. Enamel and cementum meet at the **neck** of the tooth (at the gum margin) so that no part of the dentine is exposed on the surface. Incisors, canines and premolars each have one root, lower molars have two and upper molars have three roots (often popularly called 'fangs'). In the centre of the dentine is the **pulp cavity** which contains loose tissue (**dental pulp**) and which communicates with the tissues outside the root through the root canal and apical foramen at the apex of each root. The pulp contains the vessels and sensory nerves of the tooth; although dentine is penetrated by minute canals (**dentinal tubules**), nerve filaments only enter the tubules to a limited extent and neither enamel nor cementum has any nerve fibres.

GINGIVAE (GUMS) AND PERIODONTAL LIGAMENT

The gum (properly known as the **gingiva**) is the part of the mouth's lining (its mucous membrane) that adheres firmly to the bone of the jaw, adjacent to the teeth. It consists of firm connective tissue covered by stratified squamous keratinizing epithelium. Round the neck of each tooth, it is attached to the junction of the enamel and cementum, but it has a free margin forming a 'collar' which projects upwards for a millimeter or two round the lowest part of the crown; there is thus a crevice (**gingival sulcus**) which is difficult to get into with a toothbrush and where 'plaque' may persist and set up gum disease (*gingivitis*). *Plaque* is a mixture of tissue and food debris with bacteria, and the main object of brushing teeth is to clear it away. Persistent plaque undermines the gum attachment, leading to bleeding gums and bacterial invasion of the tissues surrounding the teeth (the **periodontal ligament** or **periodontium**); in time, this leads to loosening of the teeth.

NERVE SUPPLY

The teeth of the *upper jaw* are supplied by the **dental branches** of the **superior alveolar branches** of the **maxillary nerve** or its continuation, the **infraorbital nerve**. Those of the *lower jaw* are supplied by the **dental branches** of the **inferior alveolar branch** of the **mandibular nerve** (**16.13b**). Gingival branches of all these nerves spread out to innervate the adjacent gums, supplemented in the upper jaw by some palatine nerves and in the lower jaw by the buccal and lingual nerves. All of these nerves come ultimately from the **trigeminal nerve** (the fifth cranial nerve), which is the important sensory nerve for ordinary sensations (touch, pain and temperature) in facial skin (p.143), the tongue (p.130) and other structures in the head.

DENTAL ANAESTHESIA

The bone surrounding the teeth in the upper jaw is porous, and *local anaesthetic* injected into the gum penetrates round the roots of the adjacent teeth readily – anaesthetizing the dental nerves and allowing painless dental procedures. However, the bone of the lower jaw is much less porous, especially towards the back, around the molar teeth, and while local infiltration anaesthesia may suffice for front teeth, the molars cannot be anaesthetized in this way. Here a '*nerve block*' is required – infiltration of the tissues surrounding the inferior alveolar nerve as it enters the mandibular foramen (**16.12** and **16.13b**). This can be achieved through the mouth by inserting the needle above the lower third molar tooth.

DENTAL DISEASE

Tooth decay (*dental caries*), like the common cold and malaria, is one of the most common human diseases. It is due to a combination of microorganisms and sugars reacting with the tooth surface, and may progress to involve the pulp

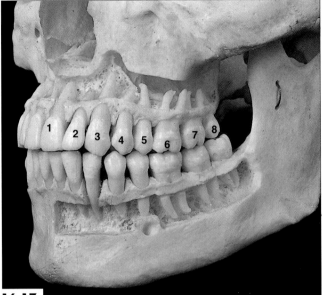

16.17

Fig. 16.17 Adult teeth (permanent dentition) and jaws, with bone dissected away to show tooth roots, which in life are covered by the cementum.
The crowns of the teeth are covered by white enamel; the junctional zone between enamel and cementum is the neck of the tooth.

1 First (central) ⎫
2 Second (lateral) ⎭ incisor
3 Canine ⎫
4 First ⎫
5 Second ⎭ premolar
6 First ⎫
7 Second ⎬ molar
8 Third ⎭

cavity and lead to abscess formation; *toothache* is essentially due to involvement of the pulp nerves.

Dental drilling enables damaged and decayed parts of a tooth to be drilled away, and also gives access to the pulp cavity. The deficiencies can be made good by *fillings*; nowadays, these are mainly plastic materials that do not react to the mouth's tissues or contents and which resist the stresses and strains of use. *Root treatment* involves destroying the nerves so that the tooth becomes insensitive. Artificial crowns can be fixed on to a sound root, but extensive disease may require teeth to be extracted and replaced by a *dental prosthesis* (i.e. *false teeth*, or a '*plate*').

NOSE AND PARANASAL SINUSES

The **nose** is for breathing (*respiration*), and part of its lining contains the special nerve cells concerned with smell (*olfaction*). The nose consists of the **external nose**, the part that projects on the face (**16.10**), and the **nasal cavity**, which lies above the mouth, below the front of the brain. At the back, the cavity opens into the upper part of the throat (the nasopharynx – **16.14**); the hard palate forms its floor.

The skeleton of the external nose is formed by the two **nasal bones** at the top (**16.8**), but the rest is cartilaginous (**16.20a**). The nasal cavity is divided into right and left halves by the **nasal septum**, and the two openings on the face are the **nostrils** (the **anterior nares**). Their rather small size limits the amount of air that can enter, so that when there is a need for increased intake (as during exercise) the mouth has to be opened as an extra airway. Any kind of nasal obstruction (whether temporary, as from swelling of the mucous membrane with a cold or hay fever, or more permanent as from a nasal polyp – a small benign tumour) will lead to mouth breathing (which can also just be a bad habit!). The nose and pharynx are often called the **upper respiratory tract**, and being so widely connected with one another, it is common for infections to involve both of them – *upper respiratory infection* (URI).

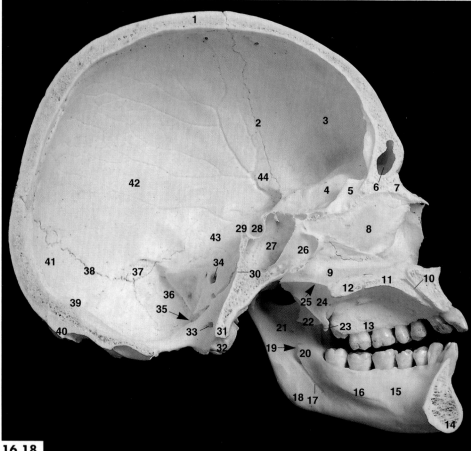

16.18

Fig. 16.18 Inner surface of the left half of the skull, with the bony nasal septum intact.

1 Diplöe, between outer and inner layers of dense bone
2 Coronal suture
3 Squamous part ⎫ of frontal
4 Orbital part ⎭ bone
5 Crista galli
6 Frontal sinus
7 Nasal bone
8 Perpendicular plate of ethmoid bone, forming the upper part of the bony nasal septum
9 Vomer, forming the posterior and lower part of the bony nasal septum. The front part of the septum is of cartilage, not bone, and is shown in **16.20b**
10 Incisive canal, for the nasopalatine nerves and greater palatine vessels
11 Palatine process of maxilla
12 Horizontal plate of palatine bone, forming the hard palate with the palatine process of the maxilla (11)
13 Alveolar process of maxilla, bearing the upper teeth
14 Mental protuberance
15 Body of mandible
16 Mylohyoid line, for attachment of the mylohyoid muscle (floor of the mouth)
17 Groove for mylohyoid nerve
18 Angle of mandible
19 Mandibular foramen, for inferior alveolar nerve and vessels
20 Lingula

21 Ramus of mandible
22 Lateral pterygoid plate
23 Pterygoid hamulus
24 Medial pterygoid plate
25 Posterior nasal aperture (choana)
26 Right sphenoidal sinus
27 Left sphenoidal sinus
28 Pituitary fossa
29 Dorsum sellae
30 Clivus
31 Margin of foramen magnum
32 Occipital condyle
33 Hypoglossal canal, for the hypoglossal nerve
34 Internal acoustic meatus, in the petrous part of the temporal bone, for the facial and vestibulocochlear nerves
35 Jugular foramen
36 Groove for sigmoid sinus
37 Groove for transverse sinus
38 Lambdoid suture
39 Internal occipital protuberance
40 External occipital protuberance
41 Occipital bone
42 Parietal bone
43 Squamous part of temporal bone
44 Grooves for middle meningeal vessels, in the region of the pterion (p.134)

NASAL SEPTUM

The **nasal septum** forms a smooth partition between the two halves of the nasal cavity. It is covered on both sides by mucous membrane (which is of the olfactory type in the uppermost part) and its framework consists of thin bone in its upper back part (**16.18**), but cartilage in its lower front part (**16.20b**). If the septum is so far deviated from the midline that it obstructs breathing or prevents drainage from the sinuses (e.g. as a congenital defect or after injury), its cartilaginous or bony framework can be removed, leaving intact the mucous membrane on either side – *submucous resection* (SMR).

NASAL CAVITY

The **roof** of the cavity on each side of the septum is only a millimeter or two wide (**16.22**); the front part of the cranial cavity (the anterior cranial fossa) lies above it. The **floor** on each side (formed by the hard palate) is more than a centimeter wide and is immediately above the mouth (**16.22b**). The openings at the back, into the nasopharynx, are the **posterior nares** or **choanae** (**16.14** and **16.19**). Nasal secretions can either escape through the nostrils at the front or pass backwards into the nasopharynx, from which they run down into the lower parts of the throat (as postnasal discharge) to be got rid of by swallowing or coughing.

The **lateral wall** of the nasal cavity is not smooth like the septum but has three scroll-like folds of bone (covered by mucous membrane) projecting from it – the **superior, middle** and **inferior nasal conchae** (**16.21a** and **16.21c**), which ENT surgeons still often call by their old names, the **turbinate bones**. They are considered to increase the surface area of the very vascular (and therefore warm) mucous membrane and so help to warm inspired air. The space under each concha is the **superior, middle** or **inferior meatus**, named according to the concha under which each meatus lies (**16.21b**). The superior and middle meatuses receive the openings of certain air sinuses (see below); the **nasolacrimal duct** (p.164) from the eye drains into the inferior meatus. Crying produces an accumulation of tears which overflow on to the face, but some pass down this duct into the nose, so giving the 'snuffly nose' associated with crying.

MUCOUS MEMBRANE

The lining of most of the cavity (the **respiratory mucous membrane**) is highly vascular, so helping to warm the air that passes over it. It is covered by epithelium that secretes *mucus* (from glands and individual mucous cells) to keep the cavity moist and trap dust and other small particles in the inspired air. **Cilia** on the surface of the epithelial cells beat in a rhythmic fashion towards the pharynx and help to clear away mucus with entrapped particles of debris. Stiff hairs grow just inside the nostril (in the vestibular part of the cavity, lined by skin); they become more prominent usually in the elderly. Constant irritation by such things as smoking and repeated infection can lead to changes in mucus production and ciliary activity, with complaints of a 'runny nose' or nasal catarrh.

BLOOD SUPPLY AND LYMPH DRAINAGE

The main artery of the nasal cavity is the **sphenopalatine artery**, which is the end of the maxillary artery that has changed its name on entering the back of the nose. It sends branches to both the septum and lateral wall, and forms anastomoses with other smaller vessels, particularly on the septum. The highly vascular mucous membrane, particularly over the conchae, readily becomes swollen and congested and can easily block the airway. Lymph drains to pharyngeal and deep cervical nodes.

NERVE SUPPLY AND SMELL

The **mucous membrane** of most of the nasal cavity receives ordinary **sensory** nerve fibres from branches of the **ophthalmic** and **maxillary divisions** of the **trigeminal nerve** (the fifth cranial nerve). Some of the nerves contain secretory fibres for the nasal glands (from one of the parasympathetic ganglia, **7.8**). The part of the nasal lining that contains the nerve receptor cells for the special sense of smell (the **olfactory mucous membrane**) is confined to the uppermost part of the cavity – the roof and the upper 2 cm or so of the septum and lateral wall. For any substance to be smelt, it has to be water-soluble and dissolved in the moisture on the nasal lining before it can be detected by the specialized olfactory cells that are scattered among the other epithelial cells of the olfactory area. This is one of the important reasons why the whole lining is kept moist, and not just the olfactory part. The **olfactory nerve** fibres pass straight up through the roof of the nose (the cribriform plate of the ethmoid bone, **16.20b**) to enter the brain via the olfactory bulb (**17.4a** and p.195). Fractures of the skull that involve the roof of the nose may tear the fibres and destroy the sense of smell, causing *anosmia*.

The sense of smell can be tested by closing each nostril in turn and sniffing familiar substances such as coffee or oranges (i.e. not very strong substances, which may be irritants). Compared with many animals, the human sense of smell is relatively unimportant but it is a necessary part of taste, and many complaints about loss of taste are in fact due to loss of smell. Most alterations in the sense of smell are due to affections of the nasal mucous membrane rather than nerve lesions.

PARANASAL SINUSES

The **paranasal sinuses** (**air sinuses**) are cavities within certain parts of the skull. There are four on each side, named after the skull bones within which they lie – giving the **frontal, ethmoidal, sphenoidal** and **maxillary sinuses** – and they contain air because they all communicate with the nasal cavity. (They must *not* be confused with venous sinuses,

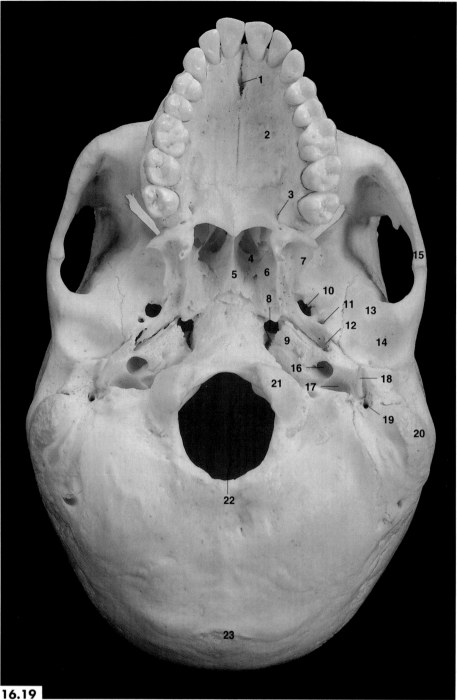

Fig. 16.19 External surface of the base of the skull.

16.19

which are mostly inside the skull, and which are blood vessels containing venous blood, p.133).

Their main purpose may be to help in shaping the front part of the skull, in particular to position the orbits for binocular vision, though they are commonly said to give a certain amount of resonance to the voice. They are lined by the same kind of mucous membrane as in most of the nasal cavity. Small holes allow for communication with the nasal cavity but, since they are not always at the lowest part of the

sinus, drainage depends largely on the activity of **cilia** lining the sinus. It is not possible to see the sinuses when looking into the nasal cavity, and they are usually examined radiologically. Because of their connections with the nasal cavity, infections of the sinuses are possible complications of colds and sore throats, and they can also affect neighbouring structures. Treatment with antibiotics is usually successful in sinus infections but occasionally surgery may be required to drain them.

1 Incisive foramen
2 Hard palate
3 Greater palatine foramen
4 Posterior nasal aperture (choana)
5 Vomer
6 Medial pterygoid plate, with pterygoid hamulus at its lower end
7 Lateral pterygoid plate
8 Foramen lacerum
9 Apex of petrous part of temporal bone
10 Foramen ovale, for the mandibular nerve
11 Foramen spinosum, for the middle meningeal vessels
12 Spine of sphenoid bone
13 Articular tubercle, on to which moves the head of the mandible (separated by the articular disc) when the mouth is
opened wide
14 Mandibular fossa, in the squamous part of the temporal bone, for the temporomandibular joint
15 Zygomatic arch
16 Carotid canal, in the petrous part of the temporal bone, for the internal carotid artery
17 Jugular foramen, for the internal jugular vein and the glossopharyngeal, vagus and accessory nerves
18 Styloid process, part of the temporal bone
19 Stylomastoid foramen, for the facial nerve
20 Mastoid process, part of the petrous part of the temporal bone
21 Occipital condyle, for the atlantooccipital joint
22 Foramen magnum
23 External occipital protuberance

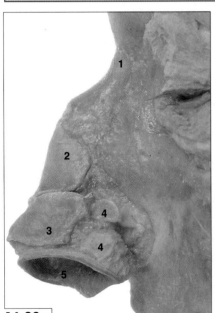

16.20a

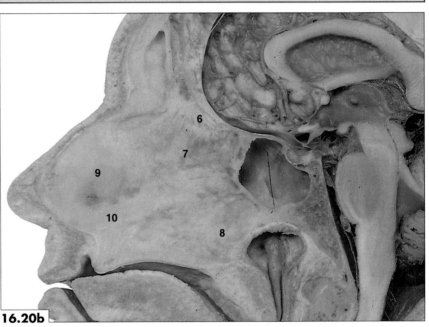

16.20b

Fig. 16.20 External nose and nasal septum.
(a) Cartilages of the external nose, left side.
(b) Nasal septum, from the left in a midline sagittal section. Compare with **16.18**.

1 Nasal bone, the part of the nose that supports a spectacle frame
2 Lateral nasal cartilage
3 Greater nasal cartilage
4 Lesser alar cartilages
5 Nostril
6 Cribriform plate of ethmoid bone and filaments of olfactory nerve
7 Perpendicular plate of ethmoid bone
8 Vomer
9 Septal cartilage
10 Common site for nosebleed, at the lower front part of the septum

Frontal Sinus

The **frontal sinus** (**16.18**, **16.21c** and **16.23**) is above the front of the orbit and drains into the **middle meatus**. The pair (one on each side) do not communicate with one another. Since they are adjacent to the front of the cranial cavity, severe infection in them could lead to such conditions as meningitis or brain abscess. If necessary, they can be drained surgically by making a hole in the bone (a trephine, p.134) above the eyebrow.

Ethmoidal Sinus

The **ethmoidal sinus** (**16.21c** and **16.22a**) forms part of the inner wall of the orbit and the outer wall of the nose. It is not a single cavity, but is divided by thin bony partitions into a number of air-filled spaces (**ethmoidal air cells**), each with its own opening; some drain into the **superior meatus** but most open into the **middle meatus**. Infection in them, which is more common in children than adults, can easily spread

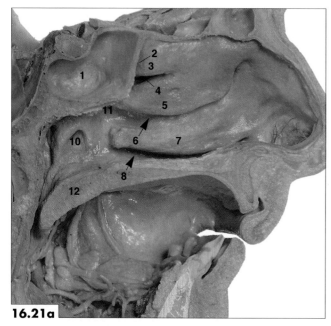

16.21a

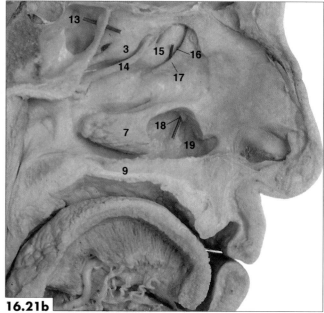

16.21b

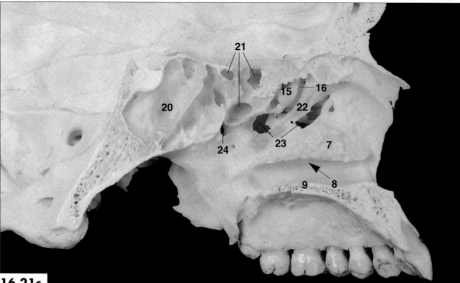

16.21c

Fig. 16.21 Lateral wall of the left nasal cavity.
(a) Nasal cavity, sphenoidal sinus and nasopharynx.
(b) Nasal cavity with the middle concha and part of the inferior concha removed, to show the semilunar hiatus and the opening of the nasolacrimal duct.
(c) Bony wall after removal of the superior and middle conchae.

1 Left sphenoidal sinus
2 Sphenoethmoidal recess, into which the sphenoidal sinus drains
3 Superior concha
4 Superior meatus, into which posterior ethmoidal air cells drain
5 Middle concha
6 Middle meatus, in which lies the semilunar hiatus (16)
7 Inferior concha
8 Inferior meatus
9 Hard palate
10 Opening of auditory tube in nasopharynx
11 Site of sphenopalatine foramen (24)
12 Soft palate
13 Marker in opening of left sphenoidal sinus
14 Cut edge of middle concha
15 Ethmoidal bulla, a bulge due to an ethmoidal air cell, forming the upper boundary of the semilunar hiatus (16)
16 Semilunar hiatus, a furrow below the ethmoidal bulla (15), into which the frontal sinus, maxillary sinus and some ethmoidal air cells drain. A marker is in the (hidden) opening of the maxillary sinus
17 Lower boundary of semilunar hiatus, formed by the uncinate process of the ethmoid bone (22)
18 Opening of nasolacrimal duct, with marker
19 Site for making artificial opening into maxillary sinus
20 Right sphenoidal sinus
21 Ethmoidal air cells, collectively forming the ethmoidal sinus
22 Uncinate process of ethmoid bone
23 Openings into maxillary sinus, closed in life by mucous membrane and usually leaving one small opening towards the back of the semilunar hiatus (16)
24 Sphenopalatine foramen, through which the sphenopalatine artery (end of maxillary artery) enters the nasal cavity. It lies immediately behind the posterior end of the middle concha, and in severe nosebleeds this area may have to be tightly packed to compress the vessel

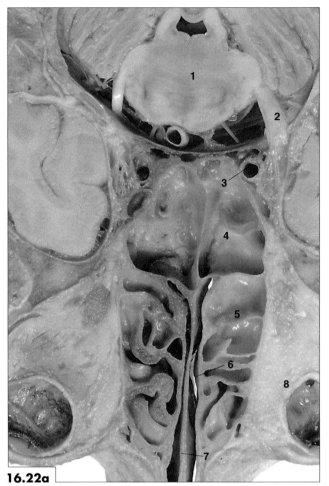

16.22a

Fig. 16.22 Sections through the nasal cavities.
(a) Horizontal section of the head through the upper part of the nose, about 1 cm below the roof, looking down from above.
(b) Coronal (vertical) section through the nose and eyes, from behind looking forwards and slighty upwards to show the opening of the right maxillary sinus.

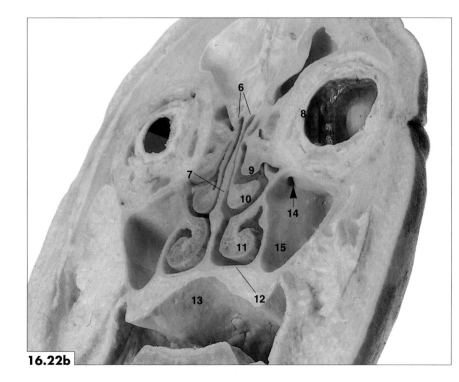

16.22b

1 Pons
2 Trigeminal nerve
3 Internal carotid artery, within the cavernous sinus
4 Sphenoidal sinus
5 Ethmoidal air cells
6 Upper part of nasal cavity, only a millimeter or two wide
7 Nasal septum
8 Orbital fat and eye
9 Superior concha
10 Middle concha
11 Inferior concha
12 Floor of nasal cavity, more than 1 cm wide
13 Hard palate
14 Right maxillary sinus, with opening (arrow) high on the medial wall
15 Site for artficial opening into sinus, near the floor and thus giving better drainage than the normal opening

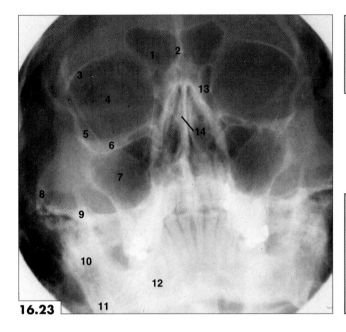

16.23

Fig. 16.23 Radiograph of the skull.
This view of a skull is taken with the chin tilted upwards (the occipitomental view), a position used to emphasize the frontal sinuses.

1 Frontal sinus	8 Zygomatic arch
2 Septum of frontal sinuses	9 Coronoid process
3 Supraorbital margin	10 Ramus
4 Lesser wing of sphenoid	11 Angle
5 Greater wing of sphenoid	12 Body
6 Infraorbital margin	13 Ethmoidal sinus
7 Maxillary sinus	14 Nasal septum

(8–12: of mandible)

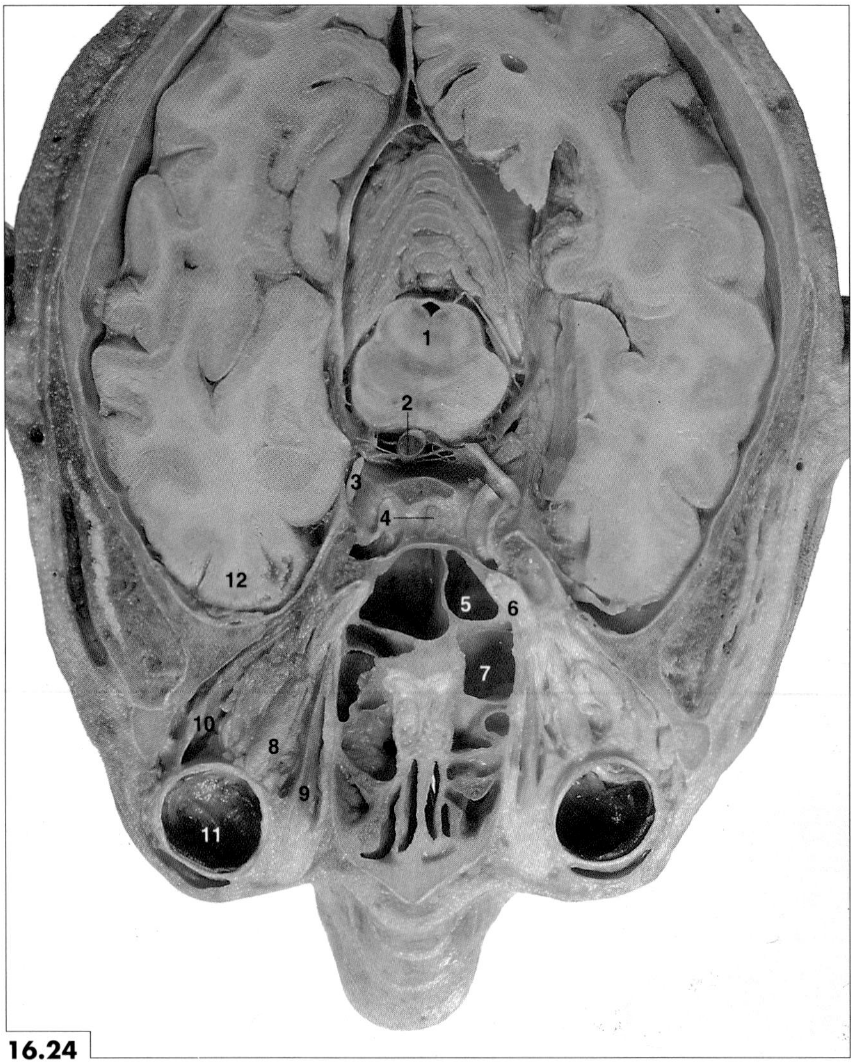

16.24

Fig. 16.24 Horizontal section of the head through the upper parts of the orbits and nose (at a slightly higher level than the section in 16.22a), looking down from above, to show the optic nerve beside the sphenoidal and ethmoidal sinuses.

1 Pons
2 Basilar artery
3 Oculomotor nerve, entering the roof of the cavernous sinus
4 Pituitary stalk
5 Left sphenoidal sinus
6 Optic nerve, lying against the wall of the sphenoidal and ethmoidal sinuses (5 and 7)
7 Posterior ethmoidal air cell
8 Right optic nerve
9 Medial rectus muscle
10 Lateral rectus muscle
11 Eye, with dark lining due to the retinal and choroidal pigment
12 Front of temporal lobe of cerebral hemisphere, lying in the lateral part of the middle cranial fossa

into the orbit (causing *orbital cellulitis* or abscess). At the back of the orbit, infection may damage the optic nerve (in *optic neuritis*) which lies right beside the most posterior ethmoidal air cell (**16.24**).

Sphenoidal Sinus

The **sphenoidal sinuses** (**16.21**, **16.22** and **16.24**) are in the sphenoid bone in the centre of the base of the skull and, unless they are very small, are usually indented from above by the bulge of bone (the pituitary fossa) which contains the pituitary gland. Each drains by an opening in its front wall into the part of the nasal cavity immediately behind the superior concha (at the *sphenoethmoidal recess*). Of all the sinuses, they are the ones least affected by disease. Surgery on the pituitary gland can be carried out by approaching it through the sphenoidal sinus, either via the nasal cavity or through the orbit and the ethmoidal sinus.

Maxillary Sinus

The **maxillary sinus** (**maxillary antrum, 16.21c, 16.22b** and **16.23**) – the sinus most commonly diseased in adults – occupies a variable part of the maxilla below the orbit, at the side of the nose and above the teeth. Its opening into the **middle meatus** is *very high up* on the inner wall of the sinus, so that drainage is entirely dependent on ciliary activity. The roots of upper molar teeth sometimes project into the sinus, becoming covered by mucous membrane with little or no bone; infection in the sinus may stimulate dental nerves, giving rise to a toothache which has nothing to do with the teeth themselves. If surgical drainage is required, an artificial opening (an *antrostomy*, **16.21b**) can be made near the floor of the sinus into the inferior meatus by perforating the bone with a trocar and cannula that are introduced through the nostril and passed under the inferior concha. This opening is used for washing out the sinus (*antral lavage*). A more extensive approach to the sinus can be gained through the vestibule of the mouth, elevating the upper lip and cutting away bone from the front wall of the sinus (the *Caldwell–Luc operation*).

EXAMINATION OF THE NOSE AND SINUSES

The front part of the nasal cavity can be examined by inserting a *nasal speculum* through a nostril (in *anterior rhinoscopy*), when the floor, much of the septum and the inferior and middle conchae and meatuses can be seen. In *posterior rhinoscopy* a *postnasal mirror* is introduced through the open mouth to behind the soft palate and directed upwards so that the choanae and the posterior part of the cavity can be viewed. The sinuses can be examined by various radiological methods.

COMMON UPPER RESPIRATORY DISEASES

The *common cold* (*coryza*) is a virus infection causing excessive secretion from the nasal mucous membrane, so giving a 'runny nose' (*rhinorrhoea*), sneezing and sore throat. If complicated, as it often is, by bacterial infection, the initial watery discharge becomes purulent (greenish yellow) and the infection may spread to any of the structures communicating with the nose or pharynx – the sinuses, middle ear (through the auditory tube), pharynx, larynx, trachea or bronchi. The very vascular nasal mucous membrane swells and the nose feels 'stuffed up'; breathing through it becomes difficult or impossible.

Swelling of the nasal mucous membrane with excessive production of watery fluid is a principal feature of *hay fever* (*seasonal allergic rhinitis* or *pollenosis*). This is a hyper-sensitivity disorder (antigen–antibody reaction, p.70) occurring in those whose nasal-tissue mast cells and blood basophils react to foreign protein (in this case, certain plant pollens) by releasing substances such as histamine which cause vascular dilatation. Bouts of sneezing and itchy, watery eyes are other features of this common condition. Anti-histaminic drugs usually form the basis of treatment, but where skin tests show that a particular allergen is responsible, an appropriate course of desensitizing injections can be given to stimulate the build-up of an immunity for the next season.

The nasal septum is the common site for *nosebleed* (*epistaxis*) which, although having many possible causes including injury, hypertension, tumours and blood diseases, often occurs for no known reason. The region where the vessels usually burst is at the lower front part. Squeezing the lower nose for 10 minutes to compress each side against the septum will usually stop the bleeding, but it may be necessary to pack the affected side of the nose with gauze in order to apply more prolonged pressure to the bleeding site. In occasional severe cases, it may be necessary to ligate the sphenopalatine artery as it comes into the back of the nasal cavity.

EYE

The **eye** is the organ of vision, and lies in the front part of the **orbit**, the bony cavity at the front of the skull (**16.8**). The back part of the orbit is traversed by muscles, vessels and nerves, and contains fat (as the orbital fat pad). The word 'eye' is often used in a more general sense to include adjacent structures such as the eyelids; thus, 'black eye' refers not usually to the eye itself, but to eyelids that are discoloured and swollen by haemorrhage, usually due to trauma. The most obvious features of the eye itself (**16.25a**) are the 'white of the eye' (the **sclera**), the central transparent area (the **cornea**) through which are seen the **iris**, which gives the eye its colour, and the **pupil**, the dark central area. Light enters the eye through the pupil, passes through the **lens**, and reaches the light-sensitive **retina** at the back. The eye is moved within its bony socket by six small skeletal muscles (the **extraocular muscles** or **eye muscles**).

EYEBROW

The **eyebrow** is a curved line of hairs at the upper margin of the orbit (though sometimes the word is taken to mean the upper bony margin itself). Its function is to help prevent sweat from the forehead running down into the eye. The inner end of the hairy line is usually level with the bony margin, but the outer end is above it (**16.10**).

EYELIDS AND CONJUNCTIVA

The **eyelids** protect the front of the eyeball and form an opening of variable size (a **palpebral opening, fissure** or **aperture**) which helps to control the amount of light entering the eye. The lids are folds of tissue covered on their outer surfaces by thin skin and on their inner surfaces by a thin membrane, the **conjunctiva**, which is reflected off the lids (as the **palpebral conjunctiva**) on to the front surface of the eye (as the **bulbar conjunctiva**). The free margins of the lids have two or three rows of hairs (**eyelashes**) which help to prevent dust and other particles from reaching the eye. The central area of each lid is strengthened by a plaque of dense connective tissue (the **tarsal plate**) which is best appreciated in the upper lid when it is everted, as when looking for a foreign body (see below). Each end of the palpebral opening forms an angle of the eye (the inner or outer **canthus**, **16.25a**). At the inner canthus there is a small vertical fold of conjunctiva (the **semilunar fold** or **plica semilunaris**; this may correspond to the third eyelid or **nictitating membrane** of some animals). Medial to the fold is a very small reddish elevation of tissue, the **lacrimal caruncle**.

On the insides of the lids, under the conjunctiva, are some large sebaceous glands (the **Meibomian glands**) which secrete an oily fluid that lubricates the lid margins. The dried secretion forms the gritty particles often noticed round the lids after a period of sleep. Infection of a gland may lead to the formation of a small abscess, commonly called a **sty** (a *hordeolum*). Blockage of a gland's duct leads to the formation of a *Meibomian cyst* (a *chalazion*) which can be removed by everting the lid and incising the overlying conjunctiva.

The upper lid is much more mobile than the lower, and opening and closing the eye depends mostly on movement of the upper lid. In the newborn child with eyes open, the lower lid lies level with the lower margin of the cornea, but the upper lid margin is above the cornea, so that some white sclera is visible above the cornea (as a **scleral rim**) and the child appears to have 'big eyes'. In adults, the upper lid normally overlaps the upper part of the cornea. A protuberant or 'staring' eye with a retracted upper lid showing sclera above the cornea suggests *toxic goitre* (p.192), a condition in which the eye is pushed forwards by an increase in the volume of the tissues behind it. A small muscle in the roof of the orbit (the **levator palpebrae superioris**) is responsible for elevating the upper lid, and is unusual because it contains some smooth muscle as well as skeletal muscle fibres. Closure of the eye is produced by the facial muscle that encircles the lids (the **orbicularis oculi, 16.25b**) and brings both lids together. These muscles are supplied by different nerves: the **levator** by the **oculomotor nerve** (the third cranial nerve, see p.168) and by **sympathetic** fibres (for the smooth muscle part) and the **orbicularis** by the **facial nerve** (the seventh cranial nerve, p.142). Drooping of the upper lid (*ptosis*) can thus be caused by paralysis of the oculomotor or sympathetic nerves, but *not* by facial nerve paralysis (p.142) which prevents the eye from being closed properly or 'screwed up'.

In the elderly, when tissues round the eye become somewhat lax, the lower lid may fall away from the eyeball (*ectropion*), and ointment may needed to prevent the conjunctiva from drying up. The opposite condition (*entropion*) leads to turning in of the margin of a lid and constant irritation by the eyelashes. Inflammation of the lid margins is known as *blepharitis marginalis*.

'Something in the eye' (any kind of *foreign body* such as a shed eyelash or dust particle) is the commonest cause of irritation and pain in the eye, and usually affects some part of the conjunctiva or cornea. The lower part of the conjunctiva can be inspected by placing a fingertip below the lid margin and gently pulling downwards while asking the patient to look upwards. To see the upper part properly, the upper lid must be everted while getting the patient to look downwards; the margin of the upper lid is made to protrude slightly by putting, say, the tip of the right forefinger on the upper part of the lid and pulling upwards, and the eyelashes are then held between the left thumb and forefinger so that the lid can be rotated round the right forefinger. (This manoeuvre, eversion of the lid, makes the outline of the tarsal plate obvious.) Foreign bodies can often be gently removed with the corner of a clean tissue, but if they are adherent to conjunctiva or cornea, local anaesthetic drops will have to be used, and the eye must be covered afterwards to protect the anaesthetized surface.

Conjunctivitis has many causes, ranging from simple irritation by dust to severe forms due to viruses and bacteria. In many parts of the world it is a legal requirement to instil silver nitrate drops into the eyes of the newborn to prevent *ophthalmia neonatorum*, a conjunctivitis which is due to gonorrhoeal infection in the mother's genitalia that may be conveyed to the infant during birth. *Trachoma* is a chronic infective conjunctivitis common in tropical parts of the world where hygiene is poor, and is due to the intracellular parasite *Chlamydia trachomatis*. It is dangerous not only because it spreads by direct contact and by such infected items as handkerchiefs, but because it may involve the cornea as well, with scarring and loss of vision. Early treatment with antibiotic ointment such as tetracycline can be curative.

LACRIMAL APPARATUS

The surface of the conjunctiva and cornea is kept moist by the secretion of the **lacrimal gland** (as tears). The gland lies in the upper outer corner of the orbit (**16.25c**). About 12

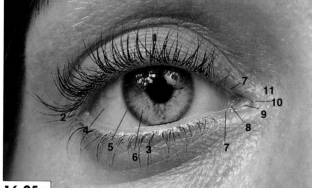

16.25a

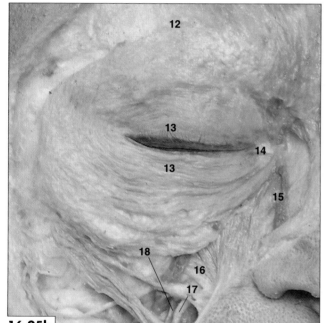

16.25b

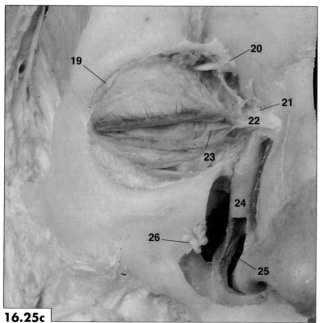

16.25c

Fig. 16.25 Right eye.
(a) Surface features.
(b) Orbicularis oculi muscle and adjacent structures, after removal of skin.
(c) Lacrimal apparatus, with part of the maxilla dissected away to show the nasolacrimal duct.

1 Upper eyelid
2 Outer canthus, the outer angle where the eyelids meet
3 Lower eyelid
4 Sclera, the white of the eye, with transparent overlying conjunctiva
5 Sclerocorneal junction (limbus)
6 Iris, the pigmented structure with a central hole, the pupil, seen through the transparent overlying cornea which is continuous with the sclera (4) at the sclerocorneal junction (5)
7 Lacrimal papilla, with the opening of the lacrimal canaliculus on its surface
8 Plica semilunaris, a small conjunctival fold
9 Lacrimal caruncle, belonging to the lower eyelid
10 Inner canthus, the inner angle where the eyelids meet
11 Skin overlying medial palpebral ligament and lacrimal sac (14 and 21)
12 Frontalis part of occipitofrontalis
13 Orbicularis oculi
14 Medial palpebral ligament, overlying lacrimal sac (21)
15 Angular vein, the upper end of the facial vein (18)
16 Levator labii superioris
17 Facial artery
18 Facial vein
19 Edge of lacrimal gland, which lies in a hollow at the upper outer part of the orbit
20 Trochlea, the pulley for the tendon of the superior oblique muscle which hooks backwards and laterally to reach the eye
21 Upper end of lacrimal sac
22 Medial palpebral ligament, overlying lacrimal sac (21)
23 Lower lacrimal canaliculus, passing from the lacrimal papilla (7) to the lacrimal sac (21). (The upper canaliculus is hidden behind the medial palpebral ligament, 22)
24 Nasolacrimal duct, with the lower half centimeter of its anterior wall opened to show the opening into the inferior meatus
25 Inferior meatus of nasal cavity
26 Infraorbital nerve, emerging from its foramen

minute ducts lead the secretion on to the surface of the eye. Blinking and any other closure of the eye spreads the fluid over the eye from the outer to the inner side; it is normally an imperceptible film, some of which evaporates and the rest is drained away by the lacrimal apparatus (see below). If secretion becomes excessive, e.g. as a reflex to get rid of irritation or with emotional crying, the overflow becomes noticeable and spills on to the face.

The lacrimal apparatus includes not only the lacrimal

gland but also a series of channels which eventually drain tears into the nose: the **lacrimal canaliculi**, **lacrimal sac** and the **nasolacrimal duct** (**16.25c**). There is a minute opening (the **lacrimal punctum**) on the inner end of the margin of each lid, leading into a **lacrimal canaliculus** that runs through the lid to join the **lacrimal sac**. This is the blind, upper end of the **nasolacrimal duct**; the sac lies in the lacrimal groove at the lower inner corner of the orbit, and the duct, which is about 2 cm long with an internal diameter of 3 mm, runs in the nasolacrimal canal in the maxilla to open into the **inferior meatus** of the nasal cavity under cover of the inferior concha (p.155; **16.21b**). The opening cannot be seen when looking into the nostril.

STRUCTURE OF THE EYE

The eye is a fluid-filled, almost completely circular structure, with a diameter of almost 25 mm (1 inch). It has **three coats** or layers (**16.26a**). The **sclera**, partly visible at the front as the white of the eye, forms most of the outer coat; at the front, however, this coat becomes modified to form the **cornea**, a transparent central area that bulges slightly forwards. Inside the sclera is a vascular and pigmented layer, the **choroid**, whose front part is modified with smooth muscle to become the **ciliary body** and the **iris**; the ciliary body adjusts the shape of the lens and the iris adjusts the size of the pupil. The inner layer is the nervous coat, the **retina**, containing the light-sensitive receptors.

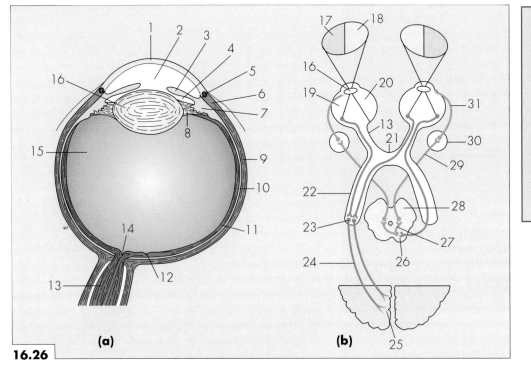

(a)

(b)

16.26

Fig. 16.26 Structure of the eye and the visual pathway.
(a) Structure of the eye, seen in a horizontal section through the middle of the right eye, viewed from above.
(b) Diagram of the visual pathway, from the fields of vision to the visual cortex (for details see p.195).

1 Cornea
2 Anterior chamber, from which aqueous humour drains into the canal of Schlemm
3 Iris, containing smooth muscle fibres controlling the size of the pupil
4 Posterior chamber, filled with aqueous humour communicating through the pupillary gap with the anterior chamber
5 Canal of Schlemm (sinus venosus sclerae), draining aqueous humour into ciliary veins
6 Sclerocorneal junction (limbus)
7 Ciliary body, continuous with the iris (3) and containing smooth muscle controlling the thickness of the lens (16) by tension on the suspensory ligament (8)
8 Suspensory ligament of the lens
9 Sclera, the fibrous outer coat, the visible part of which forms the white of the eye
10 Choroid, the vascular middle coat, continuous at the front with the ciliary body (7)
11 Retina, the inner nervous coat

12 Macula lutea, containing a concentration of cones, at the posterior pole of the eye
13 Optic nerve
14 Optic disc, on the medial (nasal) side of the macula (12), where fibres of the optic nerve and central retinal veins leave and the central artery of the retina enters eye
15 Vitreous humour, filling the space behind the lens (16)
16 Lens
17 Temporal half of visual field
18 Nasal half of visual field
19 Temporal half of retina, receiving light from the nasal half of the visual field (18)
20 Nasal half of retina, receiving light from the temporal half of the visual field
21 Optic chiasma, where fibres from the nasal halves of each retina cross (only one set of fibres is shown here)
22 Optic tract, containing fibres from the temporal half of one retina and from the

nasal half of the other
23 Lateral geniculate body, where fibres from the ganglion cells of the retina synapse
24 Optic radiation, formed by axons of cell bodies in the lateral geniculate body (23) passing to the visual area of the cortex
25 Visual cortex
26 Pretectal nucleus, taking part in light reflex pathways (see text)
27 Accessory oculomotor nucleus, consisting of parasympathetic cell bodies giving rise to preganglionic fibres (29)
28 Midbrain
29 Preganglionic fibre
30 Ciliary ganglion, whose cell bodies give rise to the postganglionic fibres (31), which innervate the ciliary muscle and sphincter pupillae
31 Postganglionic fibre

Cornea

The **cornea** is the central transparent part of the outer coat of the eye (**16.25a**). It is covered on its outer surface by a thin stratified epithelium (the **corneal epithelium**) which is continuous at the corneal margin with the **conjunctival epithelium** which overlies the sclera; its internal surface has a single layer of **corneal endothelium**. The cornea has no blood vessels within it; it obtains oxygen and other nutritive substances by diffusion from the air or surrounding tissues. Its transparency is due to the very regular way in which its component connective tissue fibres are arranged and embedded in a ground substance or matrix. If disease or injury disturbs this pattern (e.g. a corneal ulcer due to a scratch on the surface becoming infected and leading to invasion by blood vessels), it loses its transparency in the affected area, so interfering with vision. A narrow ring-shaped opacity (an **arcus senilis**) often develops at the edge of the cornea in older people but is of no significance. In corneal transplantation (*keratoplasty*) the whole diseased cornea is removed by cutting it out round the junction with the sclera, and a healthy cornea (from a recently dead body, or a cornea suitably preserved by freezing) is stitched in its place.

Foreign bodies or scratches on the cornea must receive rapid attention to prevent *corneal ulceration* and the later development of *opacities* which interfere with vision. A corneal ulcer may be the starting point of a more generalized infection of the cornea (*keratitis*), which is typically characterized by a ring of enlarged blood vessels round the edge of the cornea (as *ciliary* or *circumcorneal injection*). Injuries of the cornea by fragments of metal are particularly dangerous because rusty pigmentation occurs rapidly.

Sclera

The outer edge of the cornea is continuous with the 'white of the eye' – the **sclera** – at the **sclerocorneal junction** (the **limbus, 16.26a**). The sclera is the thickest of the three layers of the eye and consists of tough fibrous tissue. The visible part of the sclera and the parts under the eyelids are covered by the thin and transparent **conjunctiva** (see above), whose surface epithelium is continuous with the epithelium on the surface of the cornea. Seen against the white scleral background, the blood vessels of the conjunctiva become readily visible when injured or inflamed (as in *conjunctivitis*), giving the common sort of red or 'bloodshot' eye.

Choroid, Ciliary Body, Iris and Pupil

Adhering to the inside of the sclera is a thin, very vascular layer, the **choroid**, containing **dark pigment** whose purpose (like the black inside of a camera) is to prevent internal reflection of light. Towards the front of the eye, the choroid becomes modified to form the **ciliary body (16.26a)**, which contains smooth muscle and from which the **lens** is suspended. In front of the lens is a further muscular modification of the choroid, the **iris,** with its central hole (the **pupil**), which acts like a camera diaphragm to vary the amount of light passing through the lens to the retina. The pupil is not a structure, but is simply a space in the centre of the iris; its control is described on p.168.

The choroid, ciliary body and iris are sometimes known collectively as the **uveal tract** (from the Latin for 'grape', since it resembles the colour of a black grape; hence *uveitis*, meaning inflammation of this part of the eye). *Iritis* means affection of the iris only, and *iridocyclitis* includes involvement of the ciliary body as well. The pigment in the iris gives the eye its characteristic colour – basically blue or brown, or various combinations of these – which depends on genetic factors.

Retina

The **retina** is the innermost layer of the eye, containing not only more pigment, but also the light-sensitive receptors – the **rods** and **cones**. The retina of each eye contains about 6 million cones and 120 million rods; they are not evenly distributed, and the two types have different functions. Cones are most numerous in the most central part of the retina, the **macula lutea** (the 'yellow spot') at the posterior pole of the eye (**16.26a**), and are responsible for the perception of colour and for daylight vision (*photopic vision*). The central part of the macula is the **fovea centralis**, where the retina is thinnest and contains only cones; it is the part of the retina where *visual acuity* (its sharpness or clearness) is greatest. Rods, which are concentrated in more peripheral parts, are concerned with twilight or *scotopic vision* (i.e. 'seeing in the dark').

The rods and cones form junctions with other specialized cells of the retina – the **bipolar cells**. These, in turn, form synapses with a final layer of the neurons, the **ganglion cells**, whose axons become collected together to leave the back of the eye as the **optic nerve** (the second cranial nerve, **16.26a** and **16.26b**; pp.168 and 195). The point of exit of the fibres, where they pierce the sclera, is a little to the medial (nasal) side of the macula lutea, and is known as the **optic disc**. There are no receptor cells here, so the area is a blind spot.

By means of an *ophthalmoscope*, which shines a light into the eye through the pupil, the surface of much of the retina can be examined (this is commonly called examining the **fundus** of the eye). The retina is orange–red in colour, but the optic disc appears as a whitish circular area, from the centre of which branches of the **central artery** and **vein** of the retina can be seen fanning out over the retinal surface. The retinal arteries are *end-arteries*, without significant anastomosis with other eye vessels, so areas of retina that have lost their blood supply because of arterial disease (such as arteriosclerosis, or rupture – *retinal haemorrhage*) become functionless, producing a blind spot over the affected area without the possibility of a compensatory supply from other vessels.

The **macula**, which is about two disc widths to the temporal (lateral) side of the disc, has no vessels overlying it. Changes in the shape and colour of the disc, its emerging vessels, and the retina itself can provide much useful information, and no routine examination of a patient is complete without ophthalmoscopy. Not only diseases of the eye itself, but conditions such as hypertension and diabetes can cause characteristic changes in retinal vessels. Swelling of the optic disc (*papilloedema*) indicates increased intracranial pressure. *Macular degeneration* is a common cause of failing vision in the elderly, giving serious loss of visual acuity.

Detachment of the retina, beginning as a hole, and progressing to a tear leading to elevation of a flap of retina, is often, but not always, due to a blow on the eye (e.g. by a tennis ball or champagne cork!). The patient often complains of a visual 'shower of sparks' with later loss or blurring of vision (like a curtain moving across the eye or looking through a veil), and the condition (which is not itself painful) requires urgent expert attention to prevent the whole retina becoming involved. Modern laser treatment can 'stick' the retina back in place.

Aqueous Humour and the Anterior and Posterior Chambers

The space between the cornea and the lens is filled with a watery fluid – the **aqueous humour**. This space is divided into two by the projection of the iris into it; the space in front of the iris (between it and the cornea) is the **anterior chamber**, and the one behind the iris (between it and the lens) is the **posterior chamber (16.26a)**. These two chambers are in continuity with one another through the pupil. The aqueous humour is derived from blood plasma, and undergoes constant production, circulation and absorption. It filters out of the blood vessels of the ciliary body and iris into the posterior chamber. From here, it circulates through the pupil into the anterior chamber, to be absorbed through the angle between the iris and cornea (the **iridocorneal angle**) into tissue spaces – including a small channel commonly called the **canal of Schlemm** (whose proper name is the **sinus venosus sclerae**) – and so into ciliary veins.

Aqueous humour is responsible for maintaining the normal *intraocular pressure*. If the canal of Schlemm or other tissue spaces of the iridocorneal angle become obstructed, the intraocular pressure rises. This is a serious condition called *glaucoma*, which may occur quickly or slowly (ranging from hours to months) as a complication of other eye diseases but is often of unknown cause. The rise in pressure is not limited to the anterior and posterior chambers, but is transmitted throughout the eye, so causing damage to retinal vessels and nerves that may lead to blindness. On palpating the eye with the fingertips, through a closed upper lid, the eye feels hard. The pupil is dilated and often oval, and the cornea may be oedematous because fluid has been forced into it. The iris

may be pushed towards the cornea, so obliterating the iridocorneal angle. Acute glaucoma can cause pain of exceptional severity, but the chronic variety may be painless and the accompanying gradual loss of vision may be mistaken for the visual loss due to cataract (see below). The treatment of glaucoma aims at increasing the drainage of aqueous humour, e.g. by drugs such as pilocarpine drops or by surgery, to compensate for a blocked iridocorneal angle. *Iridectomy*, which involves cutting out a segment of the iris, re-establishes free communication between the anterior and posterior chambers.

Lens

The purpose of the **lens**, which is behind the iris and is attached all round its edge to the ciliary body (**16.26a**), is to focus light rays on the retina (**16.27a**). Unlike a solid camera lens, which focuses by being moved backwards and forwards, the human lens is flexible and focuses by being altered in thickness by contraction and relaxation of the ciliary muscle. The lens is not the only structure that can alter the direction of the light rays, i.e. alter *refraction*; the cornea (p.165), aqueous humour (see above) and vitreous body (see below) act as *refractory media* also, and in fact the interface between air and the cornea is where the greatest amount of refraction occurs. However, the lens is the body's only **adjustable** refractory medium. Variations in the uniform curvature of the cornea lead to *astigmatism*, a common cause of blurring of the vision, due to the light rays not all being brought to the same focus point.

Those who have blurred vision because their eyes bring images to a focus too far **behind** the retina are said to be *long-sighted* (the eyeball is too short – *hypermetropia, hyperopia*, **16.27b**), whereas if the focus point is in **front** of the retina they are *short-sighted* (the eyeball is too long – *myopia*, **16.27d**). Spectacles (glasses) and contact lenses make the necessary alterations in refraction to bring the focus point correctly on to the retina (**16.27c** and **16.27e**).

When focussing at a **distance**, the lens is relatively thin and is held under slight tension (because of its peripheral attachment to the ciliary body); the muscle of the ciliary body is **relaxed**. When looking at something **nearer** (less than 6 m away) and especially when close, as when reading, the ciliary muscle **contracts**, the tension on the lens decreases and so the lens becomes thicker (because of its own elasticity) and changes the focus. This adjustment of the lens, which alters the curvatures of its front and back surfaces, is called *accommodation*, and is accompanied by slight inward-turning of both eyes so that they can both look at the same near point. The nerve pathway involved is described on p.169. With age, the elasticity of the lens decreases so that its ability to accommodate diminishes; this is what happens in *presbyopia* ('old sight'), where a book or newspaper has to be held further and further away in order to get it in focus.

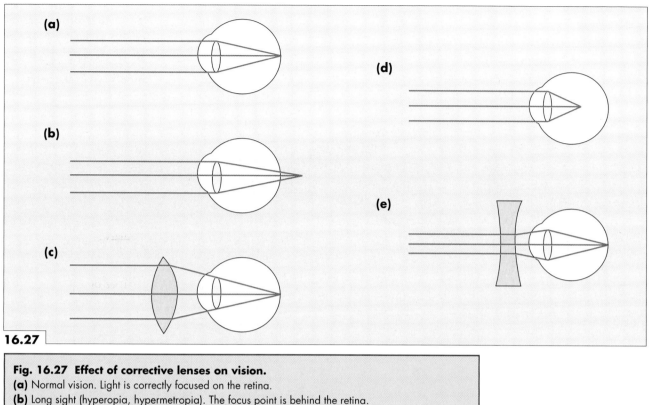

Fig. 16.27 Effect of corrective lenses on vision.
(a) Normal vision. Light is correctly focused on the retina.
(b) Long sight (hyperopia, hypermetropia). The focus point is behind the retina.
(c) Long sight corrected by a convex lens, bringing the focus point on to the retina.
(d) Short sight (myopia). The focus point is in front of the retina.
(e) Short sight corrected by a concave lens, bringing the focus point on to the retina.

Cataract is the name given to an increasing opacity of the lens (giving it a milky white colour), and is the commonest cause of progressive painless blindness. The lens can be removed and replaced by a plastic one, or removed and suitable glasses used to compensate for its loss.

Vitreous Humour

The space within the eye behind the lens (about 80% of the whole eyeball, **16.26a**) is filled with a transparent jelly-like material – the **vitreous humour** or **vitreous body**. It acts like a filled balloon, helping to keep the eyeball in its rounded shape. Unlike the aqueous humour, the vitreous body does not undergo continuous absorption and replacement, and is rarely the site of disease. Like the cornea and lens, it has no blood vessels to diminish its transparency.

Seeing 'spots before the eyes' is a common complaint, and they are often due to *floaters* – fragments of tissue debris that from time to time move about in the vitreous. They are of no significance, but the complaint must always be carefully investigated to exclude retinal or other diseases.

EXTRAOCULAR MUSCLES

Normal *movements* of the two eyes depend on the coordinated actions of 12 small skeletal muscles – six for each eye. Disturbance of one or more of them results in varying degrees of squint (*strabismus*) and double vision (*diplopia*).

The six muscles are like short narrow straps (**16.24** and **16.28**). There are four **rectus** muscles, named from their positions as the **superior, inferior, medial** and **lateral recti**; they arise from the back of the orbit and are attached to the eye in front of the equator (the imaginary circular line midway between the front and back of the eye). The other two muscles are the **obliques – superior** and **inferior**. The superior oblique comes from the back of the orbit and has a tendon that hooks round a fibrous pulley (the **trochlea**) and runs back to be inserted behind the equator. The inferior oblique is the only muscle to arise from the *front* of the orbit, near the nasolacrimal canal, and runs back to the eye behind the equator.

The **nerve supplies** are by three of the **cranial nerves**: the **superior oblique** by the **trochlear nerve** (the fourth cranial nerve), the **lateral rectus** by the **abducent** (the sixth cranial nerve) and all the **others** by the **oculomotor** (the third cranial nerve).

Muscle Actions

While it is customary to imagine what each individual muscle might do if acting alone (which means guessing its action from the position of its origin and insertion), eye movements are the result of combined actions. For the normal eye, it is

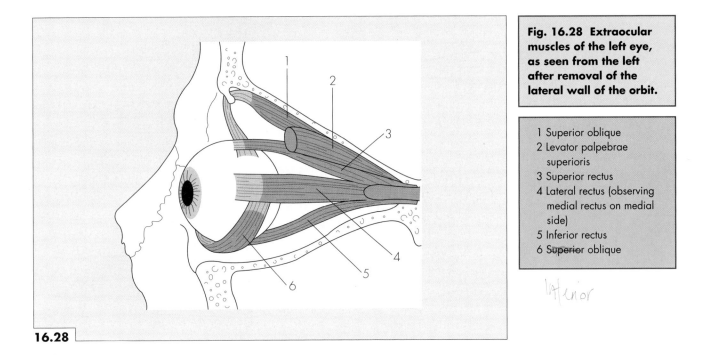

16.28

Fig. 16.28 Extraocular muscles of the left eye, as seen from the left after removal of the lateral wall of the orbit.

1 Superior oblique
2 Levator palpebrae superioris
3 Superior rectus
4 Lateral rectus (observing medial rectus on medial side)
5 Inferior rectus
6 Superior oblique

more useful to remember the following sets of muscles acting together:

- The lateral, superior and inferior recti turn the eye out.
- The medial rectus and the two obliques turn the eye in.
- The superior rectus and the inferior oblique turn the eye up.
- The inferior rectus and superior oblique turn the eye down.

Complete *paralysis* of each eye-muscle nerve causes characteristic features. The commonest paralysis is that involving the *abducent nerve* (i.e. the sixth cranial nerve) which paralyzes the lateral rectus – the eye cannot turn outwards. In fact, it tends to turn inwards, due to the unopposed action of the 'inward-turning' muscles. In an *oculomotor nerve* (third cranial nerve) paralysis, the eye is closed because the upper lid muscle (the levator palpebrae superioris, p.162) is also supplied by this nerve; if the lid is lifted up, the eye is seen to be looking down and out (because of the unopposed action of the superior oblique and lateral rectus which are supplied by the trochlear and abducent nerves). In a *trochlear nerve* (fourth cranial nerve) paralysis (which is rare), the eye cannot look as far down as it should, due to lack of the turn-down action of the superior oblique muscle.

NERVE SUPPLIES

The *motor* nerve supplies of the extraocular muscles have been described above.

The *sensory* nerve supply of the eye is quite different. General sensations like touch and pain are conveyed by branches of the **ophthalmic division** of the **trigeminal nerve** (the fifth cranial nerve).

The **optic nerve** (second cranial nerve) is concerned solely with the special sense of vision. The neurons involved in conveying the sensation of light from the retina to the visual area of the cerebral cortex constitute the *visual pathway* (**16.26b**), the details of which are described on p.195.

The surface of the **cornea** (p.165) is the most important of any part of the body surface, and is supplied by branches (**ciliary nerves**) from the **ophthalmic division** of the **trigeminal nerve**. These form the afferent part of the *corneal reflex*: anything touching the cornea causes protective blinking. The nerve pathway runs from the cornea into the brainstem where there are connections with the facial nerve nucleus which is stimulated to cause the orbicularis oculi muscle to contract and close the eye.

The **conjunctiva** is supplied by the same branches of the **ophthalmic** and **maxillary divisions** of the **trigeminal** nerve that supply the skin of the eyelids.

Pupil

The **smooth muscle** of the iris and ciliary body has a *parasympathetic supply* which causes *constriction* of the pupil and *releases tension* on the lens so that it can thicken and focus for near vision. The **preganglionic nerve** fibres arise from a special part of the oculomotor nucleus in the midbrain (the **Edinger–Westphal** or **accessory oculomotor nucleus**), and run in the **oculomotor nerve** to the tiny **ciliary ganglion**, which lies at the outer side of the optic nerve at the back of the orbit (**16.26b**). From there, the postganglionic fibres reach the eye by branches from the ganglion – the **short ciliary nerves**.

Sympathetic fibres (running with blood vessels and branches of the ophthalmic nerve) cause dilatation of the pupil and increased tension in the lens, thinning it for distant vision.

Light Reflexes

Shining a light into one eye causes the pupil of that eye to constrict – this is the *direct pupillary light reflex*. However, it also causes the pupil of the *other* eye to constrict; this is the *indirect* or *consensual pupillary light reflex*. The neural pathway involved is as follows: some of the fibres of the optic tract do not end in the lateral geniculate body, but pass into the midbrain where there are various synaptic connections with the accessory oculomotor nuclei of both sides (**16.26b**); hence, both ciliary ganglia are stimulated to constrict both pupils. The crossover of fibres in the optic chiasma is another reason for both pupils constricting.

The other important light reflex is the *accommodation–convergence reflex* (sometimes called the *near reflex*), which adjusts the eyes for near vision, as for reading (p.166). This depends on fibres passing from the visual cortex to another part of the cortex, the frontal eye field, in the frontal lobe (**17.1**). From here, further fibres run into the midbrain to the oculomotor nuclei, so causing the eyes to converge slightly (because of stimulation of the cell bodies whose axons supply the medial rectus muscles of each eye) and the lens to thicken (because of stimulation of the accessory part of the nuclei, whose fibres supply the ciliary body and pupil via the ciliary ganglia).

DISEASES OF THE EYE

Because each element of the eye has its own characteristic diseases, it has been considered more useful to include reference to the commoner eye conditions in the textual descriptions of each part, rather than collecting them together at the end of the chapter as has been the case for most other major organs.

EAR

The **ear** serves as the organ for the special sense of **hearing** and also of **balance** (i.e. equilibrium). Most of it is in the temporal bone of the skull. It consists of three parts: the **external ear**, the **middle ear** and the **inner ear**. All three are concerned with hearing, but only the inner ear is concerned with balance. The nerve concerned with both of these special sensations is the **eighth cranial** nerve or **vestibulocochlear nerve**; it is really two distinct nerves bound together – the vestibular part dealing with balance, and the cochlear part with hearing.

EXTERNAL EAR

The **external ear** (**16.29a**) is an obvious feature at the side of the head, and is composed of the **auricle** (the **pinna**) and the external acoustic meatus (the **ear canal** or **ear hole**). The auricle has a framework of elastic cartilage (**16.29b**) that gives the overlying skin its characteristic ridges and grooves; all have their own names (which are irrelevant for most students), but one important landmark is the **tragus**, which guards the front of the meatus. The lowest part of the auricle is the **lobule**; it has no cartilage, being simply a mass of tough connective tissue. Its only known function is to provide an attachment point for earrings!

The **external acoustic meatus** is a tubular passage about 4 cm long, with a **cartilaginous** framework at the *outer* end and part of the temporal **bone** at the *deeper* end (**16.29c**). The passage is not straight, but is slightly curved to give protection to the **tympanic membrane** (the eardrum, see below) which separates it from the middle ear (**16.30c**). The skin of the meatus, which is thin but firmly attached to the cartilage and bone of the meatus, contains **ceruminous glands**, which produce wax (*cerumen*) that helps to trap dust particles. Wax production is a normal process; it may become troublesome if the wax becomes hardened against the eardrum and interferes with sound conduction.

MIDDLE EAR

The **middle ear** (the **tympanic cavity**) is an air-filled space within the temporal bone (**16.30a** and **16.30b**). It contains three very small bones, the **auditory ossicles**, and is lined by a thin **mucous membrane**. The air in the cavity communicates with the nasopharynx through the **auditory tube** (the **Eustachian tube** or **pharyngotympanic tube**). Although the tube is closed most of the time, swallowing causes its cartilaginous part to open up slightly (by the contraction of tensor palati which is attached to it), allowing for exchange of air between the middle ear and the pharynx. Thus, the pressure of air in the middle ear should remain about the same as that of the outside air. This explains why swallowing is helpful in equalizing the pressures in the middle ear cavities and aircraft cabins as the cabin pressures change with ascent and descent (p.77); this is often recognized by 'popping of the ears' as the tympanic membrane suddenly moves inwards or outwards.

The **tympanic membrane**, commonly called the **eardrum**, forms the lateral wall of the middle ear (**16.30a**), and acts as a partition separating the middle ear from the external acoustic meatus. The membrane consists of very thin connective tissue, covered on its outer side by modified thin skin and on its inner surface by the mucous membrane that lines the middle ear cavity.

The **auditory ossicles**, called the **malleus, incus** and **stapes** (the Latin for 'hammer', 'anvil' and 'stirrup') are connected to one another by tiny joints to form a bony bridge across the middle ear cavity (**16.30a** and **16.31a**). The malleus is connected to the eardrum and the stapes to the oval window of the inner ear (see below).

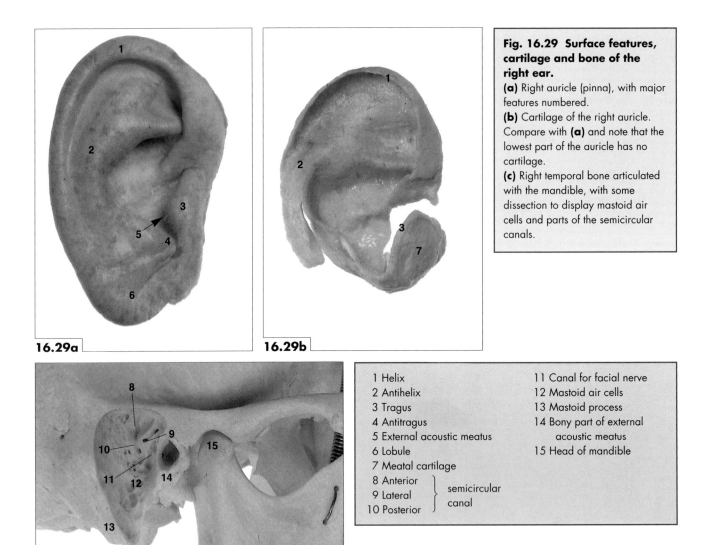

16.29a

16.29b

16.29c

Fig. 16.29 Surface features, cartilage and bone of the right ear.
(a) Right auricle (pinna), with major features numbered.
(b) Cartilage of the right auricle. Compare with **(a)** and note that the lowest part of the auricle has no cartilage.
(c) Right temporal bone articulated with the mandible, with some dissection to display mastoid air cells and parts of the semicircular canals.

1 Helix	11 Canal for facial nerve
2 Antihelix	12 Mastoid air cells
3 Tragus	13 Mastoid process
4 Antitragus	14 Bony part of external
5 External acoustic meatus	acoustic meatus
6 Lobule	15 Head of mandible
7 Meatal cartilage	
8 Anterior ⎫	
9 Lateral ⎬ semicircular canal	
10 Posterior ⎭	

INNER EAR

The **inner ear**, like the middle ear, is also within the temporal bone. At first sight it is a complicated structure with many unfamiliar names, but it is not difficult to understand, provided that two sets of fundamental facts are remembered:

• It consists of an irregularly shaped bony cavity, the **bony labyrinth**, within which lies a similarly shaped sac, the **membranous labyrinth**, containing a fluid called **endolymph**.

• The membranous labyrinth is not pressed tightly against the walls of the bony labyrinth but is separated from it by a fluid called **perilymph**.

The parts of the **bony labyrinth** (in order from front to back, **16.31a** and **16.31b**) are the **cochlea** (sometimes called the **cochlear canal**), the **vestibule**, and the **semicircular canals**. The parts of the **membranous labyrinth** (**16.31c**) are the **cochlear duct** (within the cochlea), the **utricle** and

saccule (within the vestibule), and the **semicircular ducts** (within the semicircular canals). Do not confuse the *membranous* semicircular *ducts* with the *bony* semicircular *canals* within which the ducts lie, nor the *membranous cochlear duct* with the *bony cochlea*. Also, do not confuse *endolymph* which is *inside* the ducts and other parts of the membranous labyrinth, with *perilymph* which is *outside* the membranous labyrinth, separating it from the bony labyrinth. The endolymph and perilymph do not communicate with one another.

Cochlea and Cochlear Duct

The **cochlea** is spiral-shaped, like a small snail shell (**16.31a** and **16.31b**), so that sections through the 'shell' show a number of sections through the spiral, i.e. through the (bony) cochlear canal (**16.31d**). The canal is roughly circular, and its contained (membranous) **cochlear duct** is triangular in section.

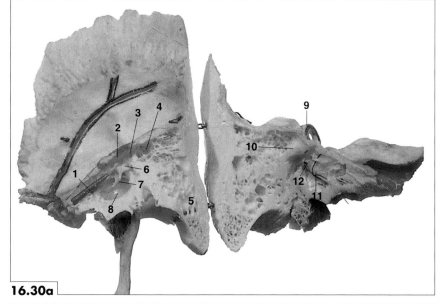

16.30a

Fig. 16.30 Right temporal bone and ear.

(a) Right temporal bone, cut in two through the middle ear cavity and the rest of the petrous part of the bone and opened out like a book. The part on the left of the picture shows the lateral wall of the middle ear which includes the tympanic membrane, seen from the medial side; the part on the right shows the promontory and other features of the medial wall of the middle ear, seen from the lateral side. Compare with **16.31a** and **16.31b**.

(b) Diagrams of the skull, from above, to show the relative positions of the parts of the right ear in relation to the skull. The inset indicates the part of the skull seen in the larger drawing.

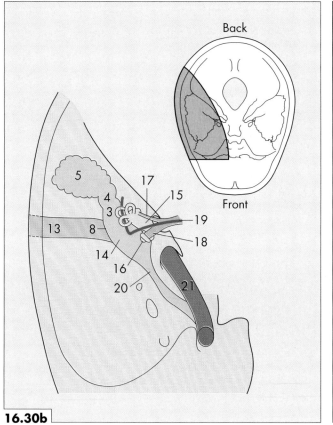

16.30b

1 Tensor tympani muscle, attached to the malleus (7)
2 Epitympanic recess, the part of the middle ear cavity above the tympanic membrane, communicating with the mastoid air cells (5) through the aditus (3)
3 Aditus to the antrum (4)
4 Mastoid antrum, the largest mastoid air cell, adjoining the aditus (3)
5 Mastoid air cells within the mastoid process
6 Incus, the middle of the three auditory ossicles
7 Malleus, with its handle attached to the tympanic membrane (8)
8 Tympanic membrane, separating the middle ear from the external ear
9 Anterior ⎫ semicircular
10 Lateral ⎭ canal
11 Promontory, the bulge on the medial wall of the middle ear produced by the first turn of the cochlea (see **16.31b**)
12 Stapes in oval window (see **16.31a**)
13 External acoustic meatus
14 Middle ear cavity
15 Vestibular ⎫ part of inner
16 Cochlear ⎭ ear
17 Vestibular nerve
18 Cochlear nerve
19 Facial nerve
20 Auditory tube
21 Internal carotid artery

Inside the cochlear duct (the triangle) is **endolymph**. *Outside* the cochlear duct, in the spaces of the cochlear canal above and below the duct (and known as the **scala vestibuli** and **scala tympani**), is **perilymph**. The most important 'side of the triangle' is the **basilar membrane**, because it supports the **spiral organ** (the **organ of Corti**), which contains the specialized **auditory receptors**.

On the *medial* wall of the middle ear, just above the bulge (the **promontory**) produced by the beginning of the first turn of the cochlea, the **scala vestibuli** of the cochlear canal is 'plugged' by the foot-piece of the **stapes**. The bony hole into which the stapes fits is commonly called, from its shape, the **oval window** (**16.30a** and **16.31a**); its proper name is the **fenestra vestibuli** (the Latin for 'window of the vestibule').

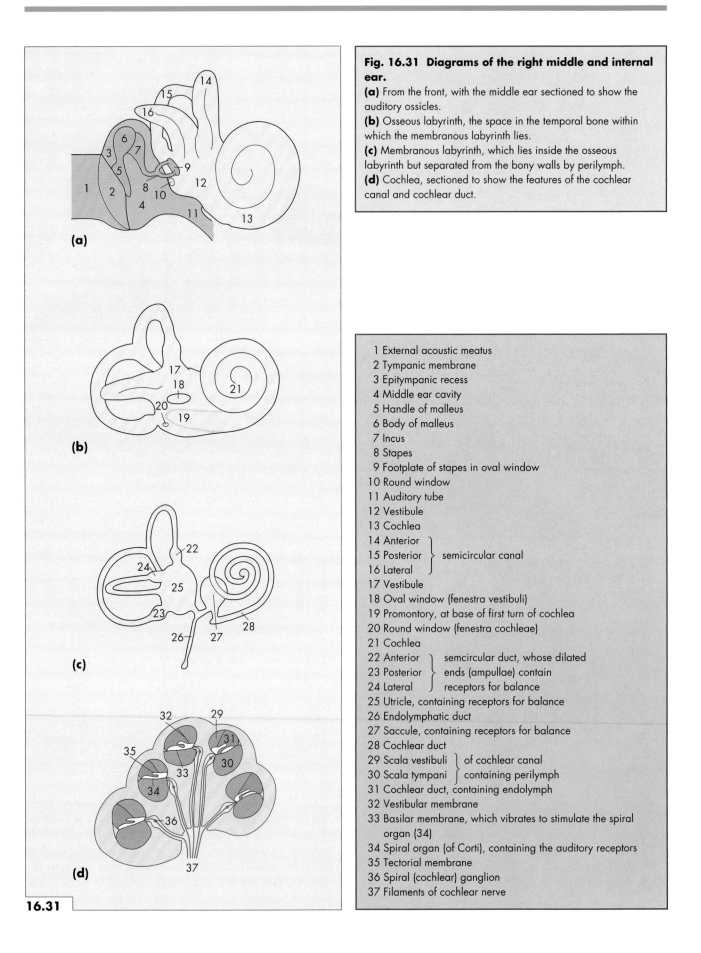

(a)

(b)

(c)

(d)

Fig. 16.31 Diagrams of the right middle and internal ear.
(a) From the front, with the middle ear sectioned to show the auditory ossicles.
(b) Osseous labyrinth, the space in the temporal bone within which the membranous labyrinth lies.
(c) Membranous labyrinth, which lies inside the osseous labyrinth but separated from the bony walls by perilymph.
(d) Cochlea, sectioned to show the features of the cochlear canal and cochlear duct.

1 External acoustic meatus
2 Tympanic membrane
3 Epitympanic recess
4 Middle ear cavity
5 Handle of malleus
6 Body of malleus
7 Incus
8 Stapes
9 Footplate of stapes in oval window
10 Round window
11 Auditory tube
12 Vestibule
13 Cochlea
14 Anterior ⎫
15 Posterior ⎬ semicircular canal
16 Lateral ⎭
17 Vestibule
18 Oval window (fenestra vestibuli)
19 Promontory, at base of first turn of cochlea
20 Round window (fenestra cochleae)
21 Cochlea
22 Anterior ⎫ semcircular duct, whose dilated
23 Posterior ⎬ ends (ampullae) contain
24 Lateral ⎭ receptors for balance
25 Utricle, containing receptors for balance
26 Endolymphatic duct
27 Saccule, containing receptors for balance
28 Cochlear duct
29 Scala vestibuli ⎫ of cochlear canal
30 Scala tympani ⎬ containing perilymph
31 Cochlear duct, containing endolymph
32 Vestibular membrane
33 Basilar membrane, which vibrates to stimulate the spiral organ (34)
34 Spiral organ (of Corti), containing the auditory receptors
35 Tectorial membrane
36 Spiral (cochlear) ganglion
37 Filaments of cochlear nerve

16.31

The **scala tympani** is similarly closed off just below the promontory, not by bone, but by a piece of connective tissue; this is the **secondary tympanic membrane**, filling the **round window** (the **fenestra cochleae**, **16.30a** and **16.31a**) and preventing perilymph from flowing out into the middle ear.

Semicircular Canals and Ducts

The **semicircular canals** with their contained **ducts** form the most posterior part of the inner ear, projecting backwards from the (bony) vestibule and its contained (membranous) utricle. The canals lie at right angles to one another, approximately in the vertical, transverse and coronal planes, so that head movements in any direction can be detected (see *Balance*, below).

HEARING

The **cochlear part** of the inner ear is concerned with *hearing*. Sound waves in the air in the external meatus cause the tympanic membrane to vibrate, which in turn causes the auditory ossicles to vibrate. The movement of the foot-piece of the stapes causes movement of perilymph which sets up vibrations in the basilar membrane. This in turn leads to stimulation of the nerve receptors of the spiral organ. The fibres of the cochlear part of the vestibulocochlear nerve that supplies the receptors run into the brainstem, within which there are connections leading to the thalamus and so to the auditory area of the cerebral cortex (p.193).

BALANCE

The **semicircular ducts**, the **utricle** and the **saccule** (**16.31c**) comprise what is known as the **vestibular system** or **vestibular apparatus**, and are concerned with *balance*. Specialized nerve receptors in parts of their linings can detect changes in the movement of the endolymph that occur with rapid head movements. The nerve impulses travel in the **vestibular part** of the vestibulocochlear nerve to the brainstem, where there are multiple connections with tracts helping to control body movements in response to the equilibrium sensations. There are also connections with the cranial nerves that control eye movements so that, if there is a sudden or rapid change in head position, the eyes can remain fixed on the same point. (If this did not happen, important visual 'clues' about the outside world would be lost as the head moved.)

EXAMINATION

The external acoustic meatus and the tympanic membrane can be examined through an *auroscope* (or *otoscope*); as the meatus is slightly curved, the pinna is pulled **upwards** and **backwards** to make it straighter and therefore to give the best possible view.

Simple *tests of hearing* include asking the patient (whose eyes should be shut) to detect whispers or the ticking of a watch; each ear is tested with the opposite ear occluded by pressing on the tragus with a finger. Clinicians use certain tuning fork tests to distinguish between *conductive* and *sensorineural deafness* (see below); the vibrations of a tuning fork can normally be heard via the external meatus (in *air conduction*) and by placing it in contact with the top of the skull or mastoid processes (in *bone conduction*). More precise information may be obtained by *audiometry*, which assesses the hearing of different sound frequencies.

The assessment of *vestibular function* includes the *caloric test* – irrigation of the external meatus with water that is hotter or colder than body temperature. The difference in temperature causes convection currents in the endolymph, and the vestibular receptors are artificially stimulated. Among the observable results of such a test is *nystagmus* – oscillating movements of the eyes, due in part to the connections between the vestibular system and the cranial nerves controlling eye movements. Results of stimulating the two ears can be compared.

DISEASES

The commonest feature of ear dysfunction is *deafness* (hearing loss). There are two types: *conductive deafness* is due to interference with the transmission of vibrations from the tympanic membrane to the inner ear via the auditory ossicles, i.e. the causal conditions are in the external or middle ears; the other type is *sensorineural deafness* (sometimes called *nerve deafness*), due to lesions of the inner ear or the cochlear nerve.

Excessive wax in the external ear is not a disease but is the commonest cause of deafness, preventing the tympanic membrane from vibrating properly. The wax can be gently syringed out with warm water.

Inflammation of the skin of the meatus (*otitis externa* – like a septic spot in any other part of the skin) can be extremely painful because of the tension in the tissues that are tightly bound to the cartilage and bone of the meatus.

Infection of the middle ear (*otitis media*), usually following upper respiratory tract infections, leads to a collection of pus in the middle ear cavity that causes deafness (because the ossicles cannot vibrate), pain and fever. It occurs particularly in young children, and may cause the tympanic membrane to burst (*perforation of the eardrum*); sometimes the eardrum can be deliberately incised (*myringotomy*, from the Latin for 'drum membrane') to prevent an uncontrolled perforation. The chronic variety of the condition is commonly known as *glue ear* (*serous otitis media*). Antibiotics should cure the acute type; glue ear is more difficult to eradicate but it is important to do so to prevent permanent impairment of hearing. It may be necessary to insert a *grommet* (a very short plastic tube) into the tympanic membrane, to provide an artificial opening into the middle ear so that the cavity can become re-aerated; an infected and swollen lining of the auditory tube does not allow efficient aeration. In the days before antibiotics, infection spreading to the mastoid air cells (*mastoiditis*) was a common complication of otitis media, but has now become rare. Incisions and perforations of the eardrum usually heal well, but a graft of skin or vein (*myringoplasty*) may be necessary to close an unhealed hole.

A common cause of deafness with increasing age is *otosclerosis*, where the stapes becomes fixed in the oval window and so cannot stimulate the inner ear. Hearing aids can improve this type of deafness, and microsurgical techniques can be used to replace the stapes with a plastic prosthesis (*stapedectomy*).

The causes of *sensorineural deafness* include the degenerative changes of old age, drug toxicity, tumours of the eighth nerve, and over-exposure to excessively loud noise (e.g. in factories; shooting). Hearing aids are usually of little help.

The commonest disorder involving the inner ear is *motion sickness* which, in susceptible individuals, occurs because of what, for them, is excessive stimulation of the vestibular apparatus, and is due to as yet undefined connections in the brainstem between the vestibular nerves and the vomiting centre. There are wide individual variations, and each affected person must learn by experience how best to avoid or minimize the aggravating factors. Specific treatment is centred on hyoscine or similar drugs which depress the vomiting centre.

Other disorders of equilibrium are much less common than those of the cochlear part of the ear, and *vertigo* (giddiness) is a particular feature. Diseases include infections of the labyrinth (*labyrinthitis*) and *Menière's disease*, a condition of unkown cause where attacks of vertigo are associated with nausea and vomiting, and also with progressive deafness.

NECK BONES, MUSCLES, VESSELS AND NERVES

The **neck** joins the head to the rest of the body, and contains, at the back, the cervical part of the **vertebral column** (the **cervical spine**). The most prominent feature in the front of the neck is the **Adam's apple** (**16.34a**) – properly called the **laryngeal prominence** – and due to the rather 'V'-shaped thyroid cartilage which forms part of the skeleton of the larynx (p.186). Between it and the mandible is the palpable, 'U'-shaped **hyoid bone** (**16.37a**), to which are attached some of the tongue muscles and the mylohyoid muscles that form most of the floor of the mouth. In manual strangulation, one side of the hyoid bone is invariably broken – a valuable clue for the forensic scientist. Below the thyroid cartilage and at the level of C6 vertebra is the **cricoid cartilage**, another part of the larynx which here becomes continuous with the **trachea**. The trachea runs down in the midline into the thorax, passing behind the jugular notch of the sternum.

The prominent muscle running obliquely at each side of the neck is the **sternocleidomastoid** (**16.34**). The region in front of each muscle, as far as the midline, is the **anterior triangle** of the neck, while behind it, as far as the **trapezius muscle** (attached to the outer part of the clavicle), is the **posterior triangle**. (Enlarged lymph nodes may be felt in either triangle.) The **great vessels** of the neck are largely under cover of the sternocleidomastoid, but the **external jugular vein** may be seen easily on its surface. The *carotid pulse* (p.178) can be felt by pressing between the larynx and the front edge of the muscle.

In the midline of the neck at the back is a slight furrow with a bulge on each side due to the upper part of the **erector spinae muscle**.

CERVICAL SPINE

The **cervical spine** is not straight but is curved into a slight forward convexity, and consists of **seven cervical vertebrae** – a number that is characteristic of mammals, so such diverse creatures as mice, humans and giraffes all have seven. The first two vertebrae are very different from the others (p.26). The first, the **atlas** (C1 vertebra, **16.32a**), is ring-like, having no body, and makes a joint on each side with the skull (the **atlantooccipital joints** – so called because they are with the occipital condyles of the skull). Nodding movements between the skull and atlas can occur at these joints, but there is no rotation possible here. The second, C2 or **axis** (**16.32c**), articulates with the atlas at three **atlantoaxial joints** – one in the midline by its **dens** (the **odontoid process**), and one on each side (**16.32d** and **16.33b**). Some rotation *does* occur at these joints – hence the name 'axis', about which the atlas rotates.

The axis and the other cervical vertebrae are joined together, like the rest of the vertebral column (p.27), with **intervertebral discs, ligaments** and **facet joints** (**16.33a**). When rotating the head from side to side, it is difficult to tell how much of the movement is purely cervical and how much is at the atlantooccipital joints. With the neck bent forwards (flexed), the *uppermost* of the prominent vertebral *spines* that can be seen or palpated easily is usually that of **C7 vertebra**, and this can be used as a landmark for identifying lower spines by counting downwards from it.

A **slipped disc** in the cervical region is much less common than in the lumbar region (p.27); when it does occur, it is likely to be the one between C6 and C7 vertebrae – i.e. the sixth cervical disc. Discs are named according to the number of the vertebra *directly above it*; the second cervical disc, between the axis and C3 vertebra is the highest since there is no disc between atlas and axis.

MUSCLES OF THE NECK

The uppermost parts of the **erector spinae** and **trapezius muscles** (see **6.2a**) help to *extend* the head and neck (i.e. to pull the head backwards and upwards); the deep muscles on the front of the vertebrae *flex* the neck (by pulling the head down towards the front of the chest). Some very short

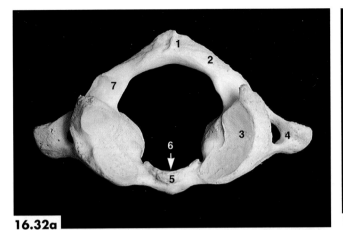

16.32a

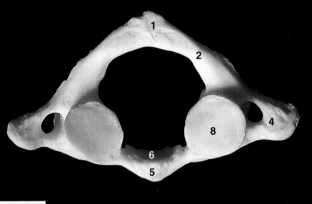

16.32b

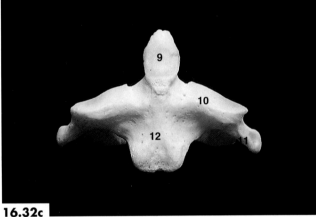

16.32c

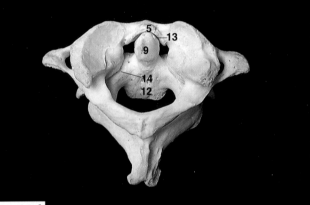

16.32d

Fig. 16.32 Atlas and axis.
(a) Atlas, from above.
(b) Atlas, from below.
(c) Axis, from the front.
(d) Atlas and axis articulated, from above and behind.

1 Posterior tubercle of atlas, replacing the usual vertebral spine
2 Posterior arch, much longer than the anterior arch (5)
3 Lateral mass with superior articular facet, concave and kidney-shaped, to articulate with the occipital condyle of the skull (**16.19**) as the atlantooccipital joint, for flexion/extension movements between the skull and the atlas
4 Transverse process with foramen for the vertebral artery
5 Anterior arch
6 Facet on its posterior surface (arrow), to articulate with the dens of the axis (9, 13)
7 Groove for vertebral artery, which leaves the foramen in the transverse process and lies here before turning up to enter the skull through the foramen magnum
8 Facet on lower surface of lateral mass, flat and round (compare with the upper surface; 3) to articulate with the superior articular facet of the axis (10) as the lateral atlanto-axial joint (14)
9 Dens (odontoid process) of axis, continuous with the body (12)
10 Superior articular facet, for articulation with the lateral mass of the atlas (8, 14)
11 Transverse process (foramen not seen in this front view)
12 Body of axis
13 Median atlantoaxial joint $\Big\}$ for rotation movements
14 Lateral atlantoaxial joint $\Big\}$ between atlas and axis

muscles, collectively called **suboccipital muscles**, connect the back of the atlas and axis to the occipital part of the skull, to assist in head movements.

At the side and front of the neck, the **sterno-cleidomastoid muscle** (still called commonly by its old name **sternomastoid**, **16.34a** and **16.35a**) is a prominent landmark and easy to see in most people, especially when it contracts (see below). It runs from the manubrium of the sternum and the inner end of the clavicle (hence the 'cleido' part of its name) to the mastoid process of the skull. It is supplied by the **accessory nerve** (p.181), which runs through the upper part of the muscle. When acting with its fellow of the opposite side, sternocleidomastoid moves the head straight forwards (as when peering forwards over someone's shoulder), but when one alone acts it tilts the face upwards and to the opposite side, i.e. the *right* muscle makes the face turn upwards and to the *left*.

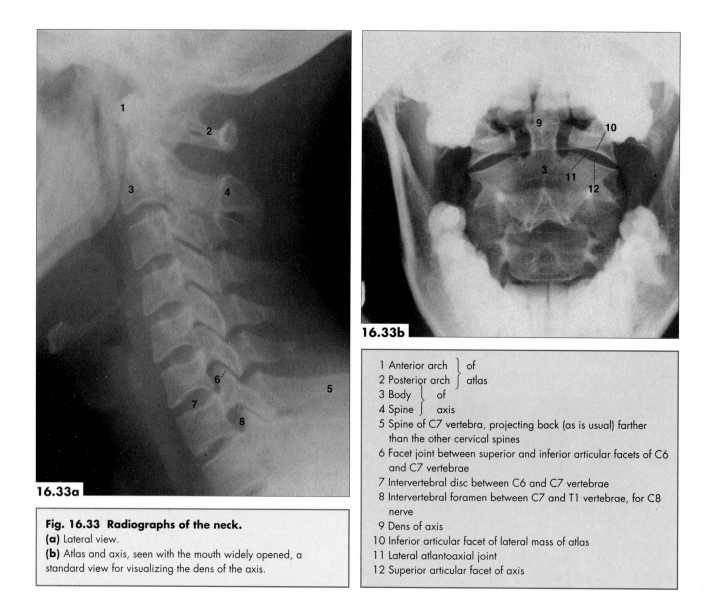

16.33a

16.33b

1 Anterior arch ⎱ of
2 Posterior arch ⎰ atlas
3 Body ⎱ of
4 Spine ⎰ axis
5 Spine of C7 vertebra, projecting back (as is usual) farther than the other cervical spines
6 Facet joint between superior and inferior articular facets of C6 and C7 vertebrae
7 Intervertebral disc between C6 and C7 vertebrae
8 Intervertebral foramen between C7 and T1 vertebrae, for C8 nerve
9 Dens of axis
10 Inferior articular facet of lateral mass of atlas
11 Lateral atlantoaxial joint
12 Superior articular facet of axis

Fig. 16.33 Radiographs of the neck.
(a) Lateral view.
(b) Atlas and axis, seen with the mouth widely opened, a standard view for visualizing the dens of the axis.

Some small muscles that are attached to the front of the hyoid bone (the **sternothyroid, sternohyoid, omohyoid** and **thyrohyoid muscles, 16.35b**) are often collectively called the **strap muscles** because of their narrow shape.

Of the deeper muscles at the front, **scalenus anterior** is particularly important as a landmark (**16.35b**). It runs between the first rib and the transverse processes of the C3–C6 vertebrae. The **phrenic nerve** (which supplies the diaphragm, p.101) passes downwards on the *front* of the muscle, and the roots of the **brachial plexus** (p.182) emerge *behind* it. The **subclavian vein** crosses the rib in *front* of the muscle, with the **subclavian artery** *behind* the muscle but at a higher level than the vein (because of the downward tilt of the rib). The artery is behind the medial end of the clavicle; its *pulsation* can be felt by pressing downwards and backwards from above the medial third of the bone. On the

right side, the **recurrent laryngeal branch** of the **vagus nerve** hooks under the artery (**15.27a**) and then runs upwards in the groove between the trachea and the oesophagus to supply the larynx (p.188). (On the left, the recurrent laryngeal nerve comes off the vagus in the thorax and hooks under the arch of the aorta, **15.26a**.)

VESSELS OF THE NECK

The main vessels of the neck – the **carotid arteries** and the **internal jugular vein** (see below) – are largely under cover of sternocleidomastoid; in cut-throat accidents or suicide attempts this can protect them. The common and internal carotid arteries and the internal jugular vein, together with the vagus nerve, are surrounded by a condensation of connective tissue, the **carotid sheath**.

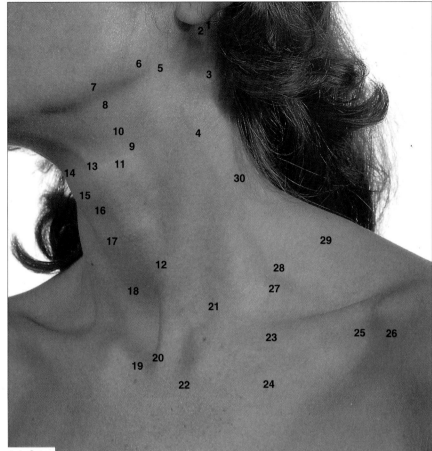

16.34a

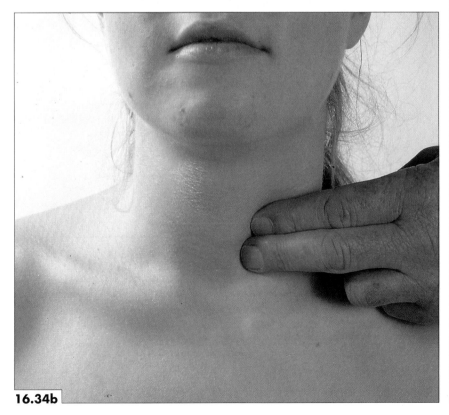

16.34b

Fig. 16.34 Surface features of the neck. Compare with the dissections in 16.35.
(a) From the front and the left.
(b) Palpation of the carotid pulse, in the angle between the sternocleidomastoid muscle and the larynx.

1 Mastoid process
2 Tip of transverse process of atlas, palpable when pressing deeply (and slightly painfully) in front of the mastoid process (1)
3 Sternocleidomastoid
4 External jugular vein
5 Lowest part of parotid gland
6 Angle of mandible
7 Facial artery and anterior border of masseter
8 Submandibular gland
9 Tip of greater horn of hyoid bone
10 Hypoglossal nerve
11 Internal laryngeal nerve
12 Site for palpation of common carotid artery (as in **b**)
13 Anterior jugular vein
14 Body of hyoid bone, at the level of C3 vertebra
15 Laryngeal prominence (Adam's apple) of thyroid cartilage
16 Vocal fold, halfway between the laryngeal prominence and the lower border of the thyroid cartilage
17 Arch of cricoid cartilage, at the level of C6 vertebra
18 Isthmus of thyroid gland
19 Jugular notch of sternum, with trachea behind it
20 Sternal head ⎫ of sternocleido-
21 Clavicular head ⎭ mastoid
22 Sternoclavicular joint, with behind it the union of the internal jugular and subclavian veins, forming the brachiocephalic vein
23 Clavicle
24 Pectoralis major
25 Infraclavicular fossa and cephalic vein
26 Deltoid
27 Inferior belly of omohyoid
28 Upper trunk of brachial plexus
29 Accessory nerve passing under anterior border of trapezius
30 Accessory nerve emerging from sternocleidomastoid

Carotid Arteries

The **common carotid artery**, arising on the right from the brachiocephalic trunk and on the left directly from the arch of the aorta (see **8.3**), runs up in the neck under cover of sternocleidomastoid to the level of the upper border of the thyroid cartilage or the hyoid bone, where it divides into the **internal** and **external carotid** (**16.35**). The common carotid itself gives off no branches, nor does the internal carotid while it is in the neck (it gives off its branches when inside the skull, p.196). The lower branches of the external carotid artery (the **superior thyroid**, **lingual** and **facial arteries**) are easily seen in dissections (**16.35b** and **16.35c**) and enable the internal and external carotids to be instantly distinguished from one another: the external is the one with the branches. The external carotid runs up into the parotid gland (p.144), wherein it divides into its terminal branches – the **maxillary** and **superficial temporal arteries**.

A slight swelling of the wall of the internal carotid artery, at the junction with the common carotid, is the **carotid sinus**. In the adjacent connective tissue is a small group of nerve cells, the **carotid body**. Both the carotid sinus and body and similar aortic tissues (p.116) are concerned with the reflex control of the heart rate (p.54).

Of those arteries whose pulsation can be felt easily, the common carotid is the nearest to the heart; in suspected cardiac arrest (p.126) the detection or absence of this pulse is a vital feature. Although the artery is under cover of sternocleidomastoid, its pulsation – the *carotid pulse* – can be felt by pressing backwards in the angle between the lower front border of the muscle and the midline larynx and trachea, below and lateral to the Adam's apple (**16.34a** and **16.34b**). Pressure here pushes the artery against the transverse processes of the lower cervical vertebrae and their attached muscles. It may be convenient to use the thumb for feeling this pulse, although many teachers advise using the fingertips as they believe that pulsation of the examiner's own thumb vessels may be confused with the patient's carotid pulse.

With the vertebral arteries, the internal carotid arteries supply the brain (p.144). Disease such as atheroma and arteriosclerosis causing narrowing may restrict the cerebral blood supply, and it may be possible to remove surgically the thickened internal lining of the carotid vessels (in *carotid endarterectomy*) to improve the circulation.

1 Body of mandible
2 Submandibular gland
3 Posterior belly of digastric
4 Lower part of parotid gland
5 External jugular vein
6 Great auricular nerve
7 Sternocleidomastoid
8 Lymph node
9 Facial vein, draining to internal jugular vein (32), in **(a)** hidden behind sternocleidomastoid (7)
10 Internal carotid artery
11 External carotid artery
12 Hypoglossal nerve
13 Hyoid bone, greater horn in **(a)** and body in **(b)** and **(c)**
14 Internal laryngeal nerve
15 Superior thyroid artery
16 Common carotid artery ⎫
17 Thyrohyoid ⎬
18 Superior belly of omohyoid ⎬ 'strap muscles'
19 Sternohyoid ⎬
20 Sternothyroid ⎭
21 Laryngeal prominence (Adam's apple)
22 Isthmus of thyroid gland
23 Sternoclavicular joint
24 Clavicle
25 Inferior belly of omohyoid
26 Upper trunk of brachial plexus
27 Suprascapular nerve

28 Accessory nerve
29 Trapezius, anterior border
30 Facial artery
31 Lingual artery
32 Internal jugular vein, double at upper end in **(b)**
33 Branches of cervical plexus
34 Levator scapulae
35 Scalenus medius
36 Scalenus anterior. The roots of the brachial plexus emerge behind it and the phrenic nerve (37) runs down in front of it
37 Phrenic nerve, the motor nerve to the diaphragm
38 Ansa cervicalis
39 Inferior thyroid artery
40 Suprascapular artery
41 Superficial cervical artery
42 Thoracic duct, curling from behind the internal jugular vein to enter the junction with it and the subclavian vein
43 Subclavian vein
44 Thyrohyoid membrane
45 Cricothyroid membrane
46 Cricothyroid, the only laryngeal muscle visible on the outer surface of the larynx
47 Pyramidal lobe of thyroid gland, an occasional upward extension (sometimes containing muscle, levator of the thyroid gland) but usually on the left side
48 Lateral lobe of thyroid gland
49 Inferior thyroid veins overlying trachea

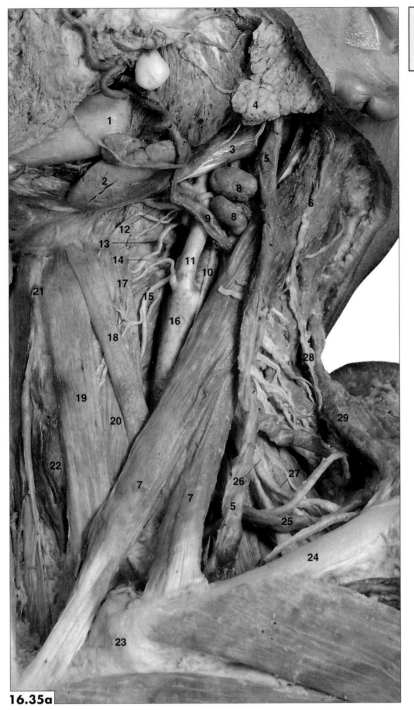

Fig. 16.35 Side and front of the neck.
(a) Superficial dissection of the left side.
See p.178 for key

16.35a

Internal Jugular Vein

The **internal jugular vein** (there is one on each side) is the largest vein of the neck. Beginning at the **jugular foramen** in the skull (as the continuation of the **sigmoid sinus, 16.18**), it runs down the neck on the lateral side of the internal and common carotid arteries (**16.35b**), to end by joining the **subclavian vein** behind the sternoclavicular joint to form the **brachiocephalic vein** (**8.4** and **16.35b**). In its course down the neck it receives several tributaries, including veins from the pharynx, tongue and face. Its junction with the subclavian vein is joined on the left by the thoracic duct (**16.35b**) and on the right by the right lymphatic duct (**9.2**).

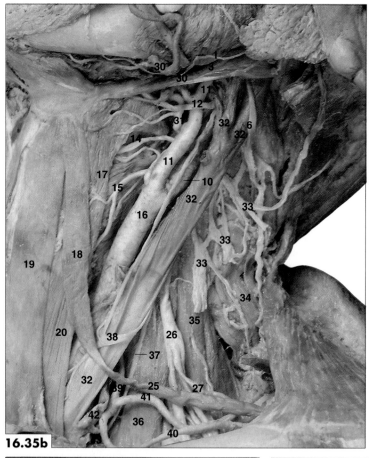

16.35 (b) Left side after removal of sternocleidomastoid, to show the great vessels.
See p.178 for key

16.35b

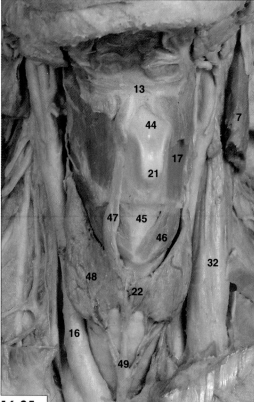

16.35 (c) Central part of the front of the neck, after removal of sternocleidomastoids, strap muscles and the right internal jugular vein, to show the larynx, trachea and thyroid gland.
See p.178 for key

16.35c

The vein is under cover of the sternocleidomastoid; a needle passed backwards and slightly laterally above the clavicle between the two heads of origin of the muscle (**16.35a**) will enter the vein. A venous catheter can also be inserted here, in a downward direction (to enter the superior vena cava and the right atrium); an alternative approach is 3 cm above the clavicle at the posterior border of sternocleidomastoid, in the direction of the jugular notch of the sternum. The vein may be used as an alternative to the subclavian vein for determinations of the central venous pressure (see below and p.60).

Although under cover of the muscle, the vein is the source of the *jugular venous pulse*; this is a slight pulsation which is transmitted to the overlying skin and should be visible just above the clavicle in a patient lying back at an angle of 45° (**8.7**). The pulsation is due to the contraction of the right atrium and the corresponding pressure changes in the column of blood above the level of the atrium. Unlike arterial (carotid) pulsation, the venous pulse is too weak to be felt. The venous pulsation becomes more obvious and rises to a higher level when the right atrial pressure (the central venous pressure, p.60) is unusually high.

External Jugular Vein

The **external jugular vein** is the largest superficial vein of the neck. It begins near the angle of the mandible and runs obliquely downwards over the surface of sternocleidomastoid (**16.34a** and **16.35a**) to the lowest part of the neck, where it slips off the back border of the muscle and then disappears behind the clavicle to drain into the **subclavian vein** (which is too far below the clavicle to be seen). In many people, the external jugular vein is easily seen; the lighting in films and television often displays it well. It becomes unduly distended (like the internal jugular vein, see above) by increased venous pressure. Despite its prominence as a superficial vein, it is not often used for taking blood specimens or for injections or transfusions, since the neck is an uncomfortable site for an indwelling needle.

CERVICAL LYMPH NODES

The numerous **deep cervical lymph nodes** are situated alongside the internal jugular vein (**16.35a**). These, together with more **superficial nodes** that may lie over or in front of or behind the sternocleidomastoid, form one of the most readily palpable groups of nodes in the body (**9.1**; the others are the axillary and inguinal nodes, pp.220 and 247). They receive the lymph drainage from all of the head and neck structures, and some of them may become affected by infections such as tonsillitis (p.186), by cancerous spread from the tongue (p.150), pharynx (p.186), larynx (p.189) and thyroid gland (p.192), or in generalized lymphoid conditions such as Hodgkin's disease (p.71). They drain to the thoracic duct (p.103) or the right lymphatic duct (p.69).

NERVES OF THE NECK

The main nerves of the neck are the **last four cranial nerves** (the ninth to the twelfth cranial nerves), the **cervical plexus**, the beginning of the **brachial plexus** and the cervical part of the **sympathetic trunk**.

Glossopharyngeal Nerve

The **glossopharyngeal nerve** (the ninth cranial nerve), after emerging from the skull through the jugular foramen, stays high in the neck and supplies sensory fibres to the **pharynx**, the posterior part of the **tongue**, and the **carotid sinus** and **carotid body**, which are of great importance in controlling the heart rate (p.54).

Vagus Nerve

The **vagus nerve** (the tenth cranial nerve) emerges from the jugular foramen and runs down the neck between the internal jugular vein and the internal or common carotid arteries (depending upon the level, **16.35c**), within the fibrous-tissue carotid sheath that surrounds these vessels. It gives branches to the **pharynx** (both motor and sensory), the **larynx** (mainly sensory), and the heart (again, both motor and sensory). On the right in the lowest part of the neck, it gives off the **right recurrent laryngeal nerve**, which hooks under the subclavian artery and then runs upwards in the groove between the trachea and oesophagus to reach the larynx as its all-important motor supply (p.188). (On the left, the recurrent laryngeal comes off the vagus in the *thorax* and hooks under the arch of the aorta, **15.26a**.)

Accessory Nerve

The **cranial part** of the **accessory nerve** (the eleventh cranial nerve) emerges from the jugular foramen and joins the vagus nerve high in the neck to supply the **pharynx**, the **larynx** and the **palate**.

The **spinal part** of the **accessory nerve** (usually called simply '**the accessory nerve**') emerges with the cranial part from the jugular foramen and then runs down *through* **sternocleidomastoid** (which it supplies). Leaving the posterior border of the muscle about halfway down its length (**16.35a** and **16.35b**), it passes across the posterior triangle of the neck (between sternocleidomastoid and trapezius) to enter **trapezius** at a point 5 cm (2 in) above the clavicle. In operations to remove cervical lymph nodes, the nerve must be preserved if possible, since it supplies trapezius which, if paralyzed, diminishes abduction movements at the shoulder (p.278).

Hypoglossal Nerve

The **hypoglossal nerve** (the twelfth cranial nerve) is the motor nerve to **tongue** muscles (p.150). It leaves the skull through the hypoglossal canal and runs down to the level of the hyoid bone before curling up into the tongue (**16.35b**).

Cervical Plexus

The **cervical plexus** is formed behind sternocleidomastoid from the ventral rami of the upper four cervical nerves. The various **cutaneous branches** of the plexus emerge behind the posterior border of the muscle, to supply the skin of the front and side of the neck and the clavicular region (**16.35a** and **16.35b**). The **phrenic nerve**, one of the most important in the whole body because it supplies its own half of the diaphragm, arises from C3–C5 nerves (mainly C4), and runs down on the surface of the scalenus anterior muscle (**16.35b** and **15.22**) before entering the thorax (p.101). Other motor branches of the plexus supply neck muscles.

Brachial Plexus

The ventral rami of the nerves that form the **brachial plexus** (C5–C8 and T1, p.42) emerge between the scalenus anterior and scalenus medius muscles in the lower part of the neck (**16.35b**). The uppermost parts of the plexus (the upper roots and trunk) can be felt in the angle between the clavicle and sternocleidomastoid. The largest branch of the plexus in the neck is the **suprascapular nerve**, which supplies the supraspinatus and infraspinatus muscles of the shoulder (p.217).

Cervical Sympathetic Trunk

The **cervical part** of the **sympathetic trunk** lies outside the carotid sheath behind the internal and common carotid arteries (depending on the level), and includes the superior, middle and inferior **sympathetic ganglia** which give branches (the **gray rami communicantes**) to the cervical nerves and to adjacent blood vessels, supplying them with their postganglionic fibres (p.47). The branches of the superior ganglion that enter the skull with the internal carotid artery are mainly distributed to the vessels of the eye and to the smooth muscle of the iris and ciliary body (p.169). Other branches from the superior ganglion and the other two ganglia provide the sympathetic supply for all other head structures such as blood vessels, sweat glands and arrector pili muscles, and give branches to the cardiac plexus (p.115).

PHARYNX

The **pharynx**, whose lower part in conjunction with the larynx is commonly called the **throat**, is a muscular tube (of skeletal muscle) about 12 cm (5 in) long, extending from the base of the skull to the level of C6 vertebra (**16.36**). Its anterior wall is largely deficient, with large openings into the nose, mouth and larynx (**16.14**); hence the division of the pharynx into nasal, oral and laryngeal parts, often called the **nasopharynx**, **oropharynx** and **laryngopharynx** respectively. The nasopharynx is part of the respiratory tract, but the other two parts belong both to the respiratory and digestive tracts; during swallowing, the nasal part becomes cut off from the rest by the raising of the soft palate.

NASOPHARYNX

The **nasopharynx** (**16.14**) is the part from the base of the skull to the lower border of the soft palate. It contains in its side wall the opening of the **auditory tube** (p.169), and on its posterior wall a collection of lymphoid tissue, the **pharyngeal tonsil** which, when enlarged, is commonly called the **adenoids**. At the front, above the soft palate which forms the lower anterior wall, are the **choanae** (the **posterior nasal apertures** – the openings into the nasal cavity, see p.155).

OROPHARYNX

The **oropharynx** (**16.14**) is the part between the soft palate and the upper border of the epiglottis. It extends forwards below the soft palate through the **palatopharyngeal arch** to the **palatoglossal arch**, which is the dividing line between the mouth and pharynx. Included in the oropharynx are the **tonsils** (the **palatine tonsils,** see below) which lie between the two arches, and the **valleculae** – hollows at the lower part of the base of the tongue and in front of the epiglottis (**16.14** and **16.15**).

It is of the utmost importance to appreciate that in an unconscious patient lying on the back, the tongue falls backwards, obstructing the pharynx and therefore obstructing the airway (see **15.29a**). Extending the neck and holding the mandible forwards and the chin up brings the tongue forwards (because of its attachments to the mandible, see p.149), and so opens up the airway; this is the essential first step of cardiopulmonary resuscitation (p.126).

Tonsils

The **tonsils**, properly called the **palatine tonsils** (because they lie immediately below the palate), are a pair of lymphoid tissue masses (p.68), each lying in the **tonsillar fossa** (or **tonsillar bed, 16.2**). This is a triangular area at the side of the front part of the oropharynx; it is between the palatoglossal and palatopharyngeal arches which run downwards from the soft palate to the tongue and lower pharynx respectively. In the old days, these arches were called 'the pillars of the fauces' – 'fauces' being a Latin name for the space between the mouth and the pharynx (now properly called the **oropharyngeal isthmus**). When looking into the open mouth, the tonsils appear to be at the back of the side of the mouth but, strictly speaking, the dividing line between mouth and pharynx is the palatoglossal arch (the more anterior of the two), hence the tonsils are in the oropharynx and not in the mouth.

The tonsils consist of numerous **lymphoid follicles** that are embedded in a connective tissue framework and are covered on their superficial surface by the same kind of stratified epithelium that lines the mouth and oropharynx. The epithelium dips down into the underlying tissue to form narrow but deep depressions – the **tonsillar crypts** – which can trap bacteria and other microorganisms and thus become sites for infection.

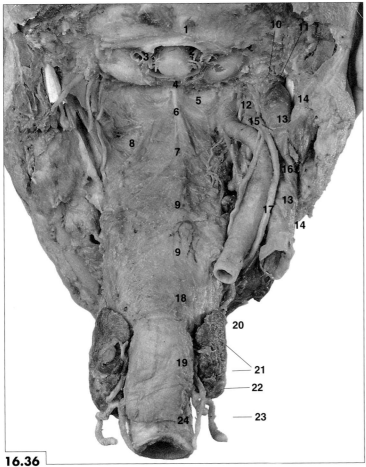

16.36

Fig. 16.36. Pharynx, seen from behind after removal of the vertebral column, prevertebral muscles and the great vessels of the left side.

1 Margin of foramen magnum
2 Spinal cord
3 Occipital condyle
4 Pharyngobasilar fascia, a thick area of connective tissue between the upper margin, the superior constrictor (6) and the skull
5 Pharyngeal raphe, midline connective tissue upon which the constrictor muscles converge (6, 7 and 9)
6 Superior constrictor
7 Middle constrictor
8 Stylopharyngeus, passing down between the superior and middle constrictors (6 and 7) and with the glossopharyngeal nerve on its surface
9 Inferior constrictor
10 Hypoglossal nerve
11 Accessory nerve
12 Internal carotid artery, usually straight but here rather tortuous
13 Vagus nerve
14 Internal jugular vein
15 External laryngeal nerve, the motor nerve to cricothyroid
16 Internal laryngeal nerve, sensory to the upper part of the larynx
17 Common carotid artery
18 Lower part of inferior constrictor (cricopharyngeus), forming a sphincter at the junction with the oesophagus (19)
19 Oesophagus
20 Posterior surface of lateral lobe of thyroid gland
21 Superior and inferior parathyroid glands, both supplied by the inferior thyroid artery (23)
22 Recurrent laryngeal nerve, the main motor nerve of the larynx
23 Inferior thyroid artery
24 Trachea

The tonsils in the young tend to be large; together with the lymphoid tissue at the back of the tongue (p.149) and on the posterior wall of the nasopharynx (the pharyngeal tonsil or adenoids – see above), they form part of a protective 'ring' of lymphoid tissue at the beginning of the respiratory and digestive tracts, and their lymphocytes take part in the many immune responses (p.69) that develop in early life.

LARYNGOPHARYNX

The **laryngopharynx** (**16.14**) is the part from the top of the epiglottis to the level of C6 vertebra, where the pharynx becomes the oesophagus. The **larynx** bulges backwards into this part of the pharynx, forming a deep groove on either side – the **piriform recess**. These two recesses are the pathways for fluid, which thus passes down on either side of the larynx rather than down the midline behind the larynx. The constant irritation of the lower part of the pharynx by the passage of food is no doubt a contributory factor to the high incidence of cancerous changes here (called *postcricoid carcinoma* by pathologists).

MUCOUS MEMBRANE

The **mucous membrane** lining the nasopharynx is, as might be expected, the same as that in the nose – respiratory epithelium with cilia (p.9) – but the rest of the pharynx is lined by stratified squamous epithelium similar to that in the mouth (p.147).

MUSCLES

The main muscles of the pharynx are the three pairs of **constrictor muscles** – the **superior**, **middle** and **inferior** (**16.36**) – which are rather like three glasses or flowerpots stacked one inside the other, but with large gaps in the front. The origins of the constrictor fibres on each side run from the **medial pterygoid plate** of the skull, the **pterygomandibular raphe** (a fibrous band stretching from the plate to the mandible behind the last molar tooth, **16.12**), the **hyoid bone**, and the sides of the **thyroid** and **cricoid** cartilages (**16.37**). The fibres converge at the back on to the **midline pharyngeal raphe** (a vertical fibrous band) attached to the pharyngeal tubercle on the base of the skull (**16.6**). There are three smaller pairs of muscles which blend with the constrictors: **palatopharyngeus** from the soft palate (see below), **stylopharyngeus** from the styloid process of the skull (**16.6**), and **salpingopharyngeus** from the auditory tube (p.169).

The *lowest* muscle fibres of the pharynx (the parts of the inferior constrictors arising from the cricoid cartilage) form the circular **cricopharyngeal sphincter**, at the junction of the pharynx and oesophagus (**16.36**). This is the *narrowest* part of the whole alimentary tract (apart from the appendix); if something that has been swallowed manages to pass through this sphincter, it is usually capable of passing through the

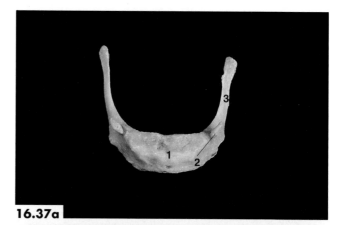

16.37a

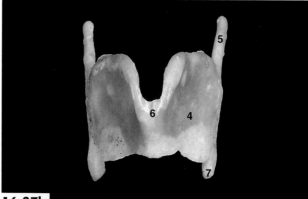

16.37b

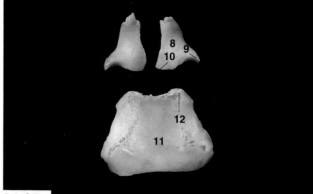

16.37c

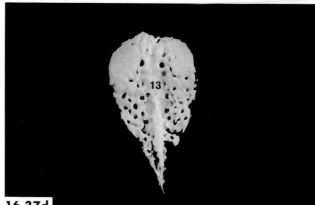

16.37d

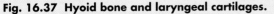

Fig. 16.37 Hyoid bone and laryngeal cartilages.
(a) Hyoid bone, from above and in front.
(b) Thyroid cartilage, from the front.
(c) Cricoid cartilage and the two arytenoid cartilages, from behind.
(d) Epiglottic cartilage, from behind.

1 Body of hyoid bone, a palpable landmark in the midline of the neck (**16.34a**)
2 Lesser horn
3 Greater horn, a palpable landmark at the side of the neck (**16.34a**)
4 Lamina of thyroid cartilage
5 Superior horn
6 Laryngeal prominence (Adam's apple) below thyroid notch
7 Inferior horn, forming cricothyroid joint with the side of the cricoid cartilage
8 Posterior surface of arytenoid cartilage
9 Muscular process, at the lateral side for some muscle attachments
10 Vocal process, at the anterior end for attachment of the vocal fold
11 Posterior surface of lamina of cricoid cartilage
12 Upper border of lamina, forming cricoarytenoid joint with base of arytenoid cartilage
13 Epiglottic cartilage, whose upper part when covered by mucous membrane forms the epiglottis

whole length of the gut and out through the anus (although a dangerous object may have to be removed surgically).

SOFT PALATE

This hangs down as a muscular curtain from the back of the hard palate (**16.14**). Its central feature, the **uvula**, is easily seen through the open mouth, and at each side it extends downwards to form the **palatoglossal** and **palatopharyngeal arches** in front of and behind the tonsils respectively (named after the underlying palatoglossus and palatopharyngeus muscles). Its most important muscles (causing no visible surface features) are the **tensor palati** and **levator palati muscles** (properly called **tensor veli palatini** and **levator veli palatini**). These two pairs are responsible for tensing and raising the soft palate, as in swallowing (described below); the tensor also opens the auditory tube (p.169).

NERVE SUPPLIES

The *muscles* of the pharynx and soft palate are mostly supplied by branches of the **vagus** nerve. Most of the nasopharynx receives its *sensory* innervation from the maxillary branch of the **trigeminal nerve**, but the rest of the pharynx is supplied by a mixture of **glossopharyngeal** and **vagal fibres**. The soft palate receives sensory fibres from the glossopharyngeal nerve and the maxillary part of the trigeminal nerve.

SWALLOWING

A bolus of food can be manipulated in the mouth by the tongue, cheeks and teeth until a *conscious* decision is made that it can be swallowed. The tongue then squeezes the bolus upwards and backwards against the hard palate and into the oral part of the pharynx. From now on, the rest of the swallowing process is an *involuntary* act. The soft palate is raised to meet the posterior pharyngeal wall, part of which momentarily projects forwards slightly to make contact with the palate, so closing off the nasopharynx and preventing the swallowed material from passing upwards. The pharyngeal constrictor muscles then contract in sequence from above downwards, the larynx rises (p.188) and the bolus is squeezed downwards through the cricopharyngeal sphincter (which relaxes) and into the oesophagus, where the wave of contraction (*peristalsis*) continues to drive the food into the stomach.

After food has left the pharynx, the larynx returns to its normal position, largely because it is pulled down by the elasticity of the trachea and by the attachment of the oesophagus to the cricoid cartilage (p.103). On its way through the laryngeal part of the pharynx, the food is prevented from entering the larynx by closure of the laryngeal inlet (p.188). Liquids are dealt with in a similar way to solid food, except that in the laryngeal part of the pharynx the fluid separates into two streams which pass through the piriform recesses on either side of the larynx.

Occasionally, especially when swallowing fluid, the normal process of muscular coordination may be 'caught unawares' and some fluid may escape past the soft palate into the nasopharynx and nose, causing a bout of spluttering and coughing. Because the first part of swallowing is a voluntary act, it is not possible to swallow when unconscious; fluid must *never* be given by mouth to an *unconscious* patient. Stimulating the soft palate or back of the pharynx by an unfamilar object such as a finger will induce retching or vomiting (the *gag reflex*), but the passage of food and drink against exactly the same areas does not – familiarity breeds contempt! The gag reflex involves the glossopharyngeal and vagus nerves and their central connections in the medulla of the brainstem, and is one of the tests for *brainstem death* (p.196).

EXAMINATION

Much of the oral pharynx and the tonsils are easily seen through the open mouth. Asking a patient to say 'Ah' with the mouth open enables the examiner to see the soft palate rise upwards – the usual way of making more of the posterior pharyngeal wall available for inspection. Inspection of the upper and lower parts of the pharynx requires the use of a postnasal mirror (p.161), directed upwards and downwards. Swallowing can be examined radiologically using a radio-opaque medium.

DISEASES

As part of the upper respiratory tract, the pharynx is subject to infections (called *pharyngitis*) that spread from the nose; in the common 'sore throat', the posterior pharyngeal wall can be seen through the mouth to be reddened with congested blood vessels.

Removal of the tonsils (*tonsillectomy*) is now carried out much less frequently than in earlier decades; mere size is not usually an indication for their removal, but repeated bouts of infection (*tonsillitis*) may be a valid reason. Postoperative haemorrhage from veins in the tonsillar bed is sometimes troublesome.

Cancerous change is commonest in the ***lower*** part of the pharynx (the food channel), and will in time cause difficulty in swallowing (*dysphagia*). Rarely, a pouch of mucous membrane (*pharyngeal pouch*) balloons out just above the junction with the oesophagus and causes swallowing difficulties because food accumulates in it and it cannot become emptied. Surgical removal is necessary.

LARYNX

The **larynx** (or **voicebox**) is situated in the part of the respiratory tract that lies between the pharynx and trachea in the front of the neck (**16.14** and **16.35c**). It is responsible for voice production (also called *phonation* or *vocalization*), and also plays a part in *swallowing* and in *abdominal straining*. It consists of various cartilages, connective tissue membranes and skeletal muscles. The most important feature is the pair of **vocal folds** (the **vocal cords**). The 'V'-shaped gap between the folds (properly called the **rima of the glottis** – 'rima' meaning 'cleft' and 'glottis' meaning 'the vocal part of the larynx') is the narrowest part of the respiratory tract, being about the same size as the opening of one nostril. It can be varied in size by some of the laryngeal muscles, so helping to control the amount of air passing between the folds and the way they vibrate to produce sounds.

CARTILAGES AND MEMBRANES

The main **cartilages** of the larynx are the *single* thyroid, **cricoid** and **epiglottic cartilages**, and the *pair* of small **arytenoid cartilages**. All but one are composed of hyaline cartilage (p.12); the exception, the epiglottic cartilage, is made up of elastic cartilage.

The **thyroid cartilage** (**16.37b**) consists of two plates (or **laminae**) that are fused together in a 'V'-shape at the front, with upward and downward projections (the **superior** and **inferior horns**) at the back. It lies in the middle of the front of the neck, at the level of C4 and C5 vertebrae. The upper part of the cartilage forms the **laryngeal prominence**, commonly called the **Adam's apple** (**16.14**, **16.35c** and **16.37c**) – the most obvious structure to be seen and felt in the front of the neck. It is more prominent in males because the angle between the laminae is more acute than in females. The thyroid cartilage is connected above by muscles and ligaments to the **hyoid bone** (at the level of C3 vertebra) and, at the sides, some muscles of the pharynx are attached to it. The inferior horn on each side makes a joint with the cricoid cartilage (the **cricothyroid joint**), allowing the thyroid cartilage to tilt backwards and forwards slightly on the cricoid.

The **cricoid cartilage** (**16.37c**) is like a signet ring, with the broad part (the **lamina**) at the back. It lies at the level of C6 vertebra, below the thyroid cartilage and connected with it by various ligaments and muscles. It can be felt below the thyroid cartilage, and the **trachea** (also palpable) continues downwards from it. The beginning of the oesophagus (which is continuous with the pharynx) is immediately behind it; and backward pressure on the cricoid can obstruct the oesophagus and so prevent vomiting, e.g. in an unconscious patient.

The **epiglottic cartilage** (**16.37d**) is leaf-shaped, with the upper end of the leaf covered by mucous membrane on both sides and forming the epiglottis, which guards the opening into the larynx (laryngeal inlet) from the laryngeal part of the pharynx.

Each of the pair of **arytenoid cartilages** (**16.37c**) is like a small three-sided pyramid, making a joint with the top of the lamina of the cricoid cartilage (the **cricoarytenoid joint**). At its base are two small projections: a **vocal process** pointing forwards (for the attachment of the cricothyroid ligament, see below), and a **muscular process** pointing laterally (for some muscle attachments).

VOCAL FOLDS

The **vocal folds** (or **vocal cords**, **16.14**, **16.15**, **16.38a**, **16.38b** and **16.39a**) are formed partly by connective tissue and partly by cartilage. The connective tissue part (i.e. the front part) is the 'V'-shaped upper, free edge of the **cricothyroid membrane** – a connective tissue sheet (sometimes called the **conus elasticus**) which is attached to the (round) upper margin of the cricoid cartilage. It has an apex (the pointed end of the 'V', at the front) which is attached to the back of the thyroid cartilage below the Adam's apple. Each limb of the 'V' (at the back) is attached to the vocal process of an arytenoid cartilage. Covered by mucous membrane, the upper edges of the cricothyroid membrane (here known as the **cricothyroid ligaments**) and the **vocal processes** of the **arytenoid cartilages** together form the pair of vocal folds. The anterior 60% of the fold is ligament, and can vibrate as air passes over it; the posterior 40% is cartilage.

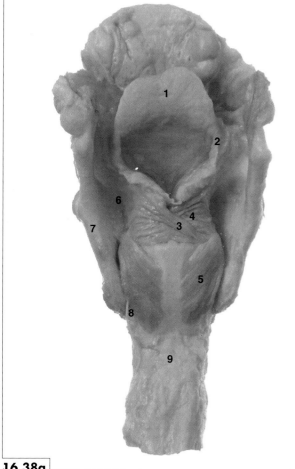

16.38a

Fig. 16.38 Larynx.
(a) Dissected from behind, to show muscles.
(b) Diagram of cartilages and the cricothyroid membrane, seen from above, to show how the upper free margin of the membrane, with the attached arytenoid cartilages, forms the framework for the vocal folds.

1 Epiglottis and laryngeal inlet
2 Aryepiglottic fold, forming the lateral boundary of the inlet
3 Oblique arytenoid muscle
4 Transverse arytenoid muscle
5 Posterior cricoarytenoid muscle, one of the most important in the body – the only abductor of the vocal folds
6 Piriform recess
7 Posterior border of thyroid lamina
8 Cricothyroid joint, with adjacent recurrent laryngeal nerve
9 Trachea
10 Laryngeal prominence, at the base of the laryngeal notch
11 Attachment of vocal folds, below laryngeal prominence (10)
12 Cricoid cartilage
13 Cricothyroid membrane, passing upwards from the cricoid cartilage (12), and with upper free margins (cricovocal ligaments) attached at the front to the thyroid cartilage (11) and at the back to the arytenoid cartilages (14), so forming (when covered by mucous membrane) the vocal folds
14 Vocal process of arytenoid cartilage
15 Cricoarytenoid joint

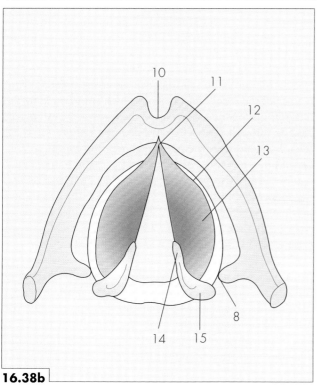

16.38b

The *surface marking* of the vocal folds (**16.34a**) is a transverse line on the lamina of the thyroid cartilage at a level halfway between the Adam's apple and the lower border of the thyroid cartilage.

The 'V'-shaped space between the two vocal folds, the **rima of the glottis**, changes in size because the arytenoid cartilages can be moved by muscles for a short distance up and down the sloping upper margin of the cricoid cartilage, at the cricoarytenoid joints. (In many animals, the arytenoid cartilages rotate on the cricoid, making the space between the vocal folds diamond-shaped rather than 'V'-shaped, but in the human larynx there is very little rotation.)

Just above the vocal folds is another pair of folds, the **vestibular folds** (**16.14** and **16.15**); unlike the vocal folds they are not mobile, and hence are often called the **false vocal folds**. The small transverse furrow between the vocal and vestibular folds is the **laryngeal ventricle** (also sometimes called the **laryngeal sinus**). Stretching from the sides of the epiglottis to the arytenoid cartilages are the **aryepiglottic folds**, forming the lateral boundaries of the **laryngeal inlet**. The vestibular and aryepiglottic folds are really the upper and lower borders of a thin sheet of connective tissue (the **quadrangular membrane**) which stretches between the epiglottic and arytenoid cartilages and is reinforced by some muscles.

MUSCLES

The most important **muscle** of the larynx is the **posterior cricoarytenoid** (**16.38a**), passing from the back of the cricoid lamina to the muscular process of the arytenoid cartilage. It is so important because it is the *only* muscle capable of *abducting* the vocal folds, i.e. moving them apart, so increasing the gap between them. Other laryngeal muscles are concerned with adducting the vocal folds, i.e. closing the gap (closing the glottis), and with decreasing the size of the laryngeal inlet.

Most laryngeal muscles can only be seen by internal dissection, but there is one (on each side) that is on the outside of the larynx – the **cricothyroid** (**16.35c**). This can pull the thyroid cartilage forwards slightly by tilting it at the cricothyroid joints, so increasing the tension and the length of the vocal folds.

BLOOD SUPPLY AND LYMPH DRAINAGE

Superior and **inferior laryngeal arteries** arise as branches from the superior and inferior thyroid arteries respectively, and with their corresponding veins provide the blood supply to the larynx. Lymph drains to the deep cervical nodes.

NERVE SUPPLY

All but one of the laryngeal muscles (of each side) are supplied by the **recurrent laryngeal nerve**, from the vagus. (The one exception is the **cricothyroid**, which is supplied by a small vagal branch, the **external laryngeal nerve**.) Thus,

the *two recurrent laryngeal nerves control the size of the airway through the larynx* and, with the phrenic nerves (supplying the diaphragm – the main respiratory muscle), must be considered among the most important in the body. Arising on the right in the root of the neck and hooking under the subclavian artery (**15.27a**), and on the left in the thorax and hooking under the arch of the aorta (**15.26a**), each nerve runs up on its own side in the groove between the trachea and oesophagus and enters the lower part of the *pharynx* (medial to the lateral lobe of the thyroid gland) before spreading out within the *larynx*. Its position behind the lower part of the thyroid gland (**16.36**) makes it the most *important hazard* in surgery of the thyroid gland (p.191). The nerve is also sensory to the mucous membrane below the level of the vocal folds; above this level, the mucosa is supplied by the internal laryngeal branch of the vagus (**16.35b**); this branch does not contain any motor fibres.

FUNCTION

In the vertebrate animal world, the *primary* purpose of the larynx is to act as a sphincter to protect the respiratory tract and allow only air to enter the bronchial tree; its modification in humans to produce *speech* is a secondary development. Obviously, the glottis must remain open in order to allow breathing, but there are moments when it is completely closed. This sphincteric action of the vocal folds is necessary when any prevention of air escape or build-up of air pressure is required; before speaking, singing or coughing, for example, there is a build-up of air in the trachea and lower larynx that is then released to 'explode' the cords open, with accompanying noise. The glottis is also closed during swallowing – it is not possible to breath and swallow at the same time. Although control of the vocal folds may appear as automatic as, say, the size of the pupil, all the laryngeal muscles are skeletal in type, not smooth.

The pitch of a sound depends upon the positions and tension of the vocal folds, both of which are adjusted by the muscles; the loudness depends on the force of the expired air passing through. The whole volume of air above the vocal folds is involved in the eventual sound produced, and so depends not only on the larynx itself, but also on the upper part of the pharynx, the soft palate, the nasal cavity including the paranasal sinuses, and the mouth, where the tongue and lips make specially subtle contributions. The degree of coordination required is complex, and the speech therapist is expert in advising how to overcome difficulties.

During *swallowing* (p.185), the whole larynx is raised by the suprahyoid and pharyngeal muscles that are attached to it – observe the rise and fall of the Adam's apple. The inlet becomes much narrowed by muscles that approximate the arytenoid cartilages to the epiglottis, and although the top part of the epiglottis momentarily flips backwards like a lid over the inlet, this 'trapdoor' is not necessary to prevent material entering the larynx. It is perhaps surprising that swallowing can take place perfectly well when the epiglottis has been removed. Material swallowed that 'goes down the wrong way' and sets up a reflex bout of coughing has not entered the larynx but has usually lodged in the vallecula at the base of the tongue (p.182); the coughing aims to dislodge it. It is rare for anything to actually enter the larynx, but peanuts given to small children are a dangerous hazard (as are teeth during dental extraction); if a peanut does enter, it falls through the glottis and trachea into one of the main bronchi (usually the right, p.120), requiring bronchoscopy to extract it (p.124).

In abdominal straining, e.g. when lifting a heavy weight, or during defaecation and childbirth, the glottis is closed to prevent air escaping from the lungs. This helps to keep the diaphragm from rising and therefore increases intra-abdominal pressure.

EXAMINATION

The laryngeal inlet and vocal folds can be inspected with a postnasal mirror (p.161), but a more efficient view is obtained with a *laryngoscope* (**16.38a**). One variety, used by ENT surgeons, has a **straight** blade (**16.39b**) which is placed **behind the epiglottis** so that it can be held forwards to obtain a complete view of the interior of the larynx and the vocal folds. Another type, used in anaesthesia to assist in the proper placement of an endotracheal tube, has a **curved** blade (**16.38c**) whose tip is placed **in a vallecula** at the base of the tongue and pulled forwards to give sufficient view of the vocal folds for guiding the tube into the trachea (**16.39d**).

DISEASES

Any laryngeal condition may cause some transient *hoarseness* of the voice, for which there may be a simple and obvious cause. Any persistent hoarseness must always be thoroughly investigated to exclude the possibility of cancerous change.

Laryngitis (inflammation of the larynx) with pain and coughing is a common accompaniment of any upper respiratory tract infection (p.153), and may cause some degree of hoarseness or even complete loss of the voice for a short time. Severe laryngeal infections such as *diphtheria* or even *severe allergic conditions* can be dangerous because they may cause excessive swelling of the laryngeal mucous membrane (*laryngeal oedema*) above vocal fold level; the mucosa at the folds is firmly attached to underlying tissues, but higher up the attachment is loose and can readily become congested, even blocking the airway and requiring *laryngotomy* (see below).

Small *polyps* (nodules on a tiny stalk) which are not cancerous can develop on the vocal folds, often in those accustomed to singing or shouting; they may make their presence felt because of hoarseness, and can be removed easily.

Damage to a **recurrent laryngeal nerve** results in *paralysis* of the *vocal fold* of that side. The fold is lax, lying midway between full abduction and adduction (it is often, but wrongly, called the 'cadaveric position'), and 'waves in the breeze', giving a hoarseness to the voice. A common cause of recurrent laryngeal paralysis is, regrettably, surgery of the thyroid gland, but it may also be damaged by disease (especially on the left side, where the nerve has a longer thoracic course than on the right, see p.188) such as carcinoma of the lung which presses on the nerve. For reasons that have not been fully explained, a *partial* cutting of the nerve (say during thyroidectomy, without cutting it across completely) results in the fold taking up a ***fully adducted*** position, with no abduction being possible. If this should happen on both sides, there is serious respiratory embarrassment because the airway is almost completely obstructed.

The larynx is one of the less common sites for *carcinoma*, ranging from a small nodule on a vocal fold to more extensive lesions that may require complete removal of the larynx (*total laryngectomy*) and its replacement by a length of intestine. By swallowing air and with suitable training, such patients can achieve remarkable degrees of *oesophageal speech*.

LARYNGOTOMY

Obstruction of the airway above the level of the vocal folds may require an artificial opening to be made below that level. As an emergency procedure, *laryngotomy* (*incising the larynx*) is now usually preferred to *tracheotomy* (p.120). A vertical incision is made in the midline of the neck between the thyroid and cricoid cartilages (both of which are palpable), going through the centre of the cricothyroid membrane (**16.14**) to enter the laryngeal cavity. The margins of the incision can be held open until a breathing tube is inserted.

THYROID GLAND

The **thyroid gland**, one of the endocrine glands whose primary (or chief) secretion is controlled by the anterior pituitary, lies in the front of the neck (**16.35a** and **16.35c**), wrapping round the front and sides of the larynx and upper trachea. It is approximately 'H'-shaped, and consists of a central part, the **isthmus**, and a **lateral lobe** on each side.

ISTHMUS AND LATERAL LOBES

The **isthmus** is about 1 cm broad and deep, and overlies the second, third and fourth cartilaginous rings of the trachea. On each side, it joins the **lateral lobe** which is about 6 cm long. Each lateral lobe lies against the side of the upper part of the trachea and the lower end of the larynx, extending up to near the middle of the thyroid cartilage and down as far as the sixth tracheal ring. An occasional small **pyramidal lobe** extends for a variable distance upwards from the isthmus; it represents the embryological remains of part of the **thyroglossal duct**, the downgrowth from the tongue from

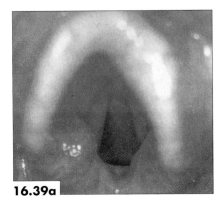

16.39a

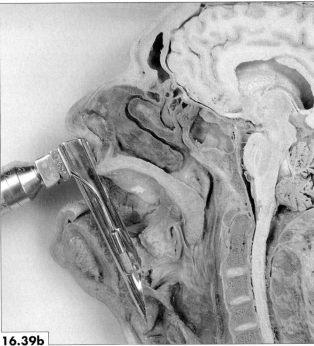

16.39b

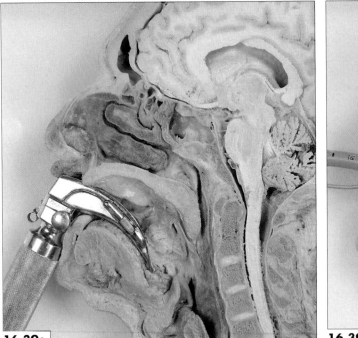

16.39c

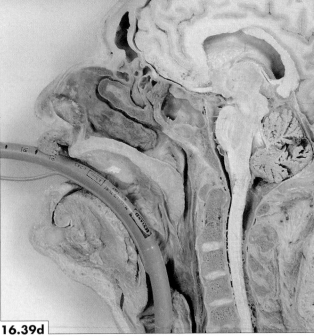

16.39d

Fig. 16.39 Laryngoscopy and tracheal intubation.
(a) Vocal folds, as seen during laryngoscopy.
(b) Straight laryngoscope, as used by ENT surgeons, with the tip behind the epiglottis, in position in a midline sagittal section of the head.
(c) Curved laryngoscope, as used in anaesthesia with the tip in the vallecula.

(d) Intubation of the trachea. The endotracheal tube has been introduced through a laryngoscope (now withdrawn); the tip of the tube has just passed the vocal folds and will be pushed further down into the trachea before inflating the cuff of the tube.

which the thyroid gland is developed. Other remnants of the duct may form a fibrous band or a swelling (a **thyroglossal cyst**) in the middle of the neck which, because it is attached to the base of the tongue, moves upwards on putting the tongue out.

At the front, the isthmus is covered only by fascia and skin, but the lobes are covered by the strap muscles and overlapped by sternocleidomastoid (**16.35a** and **16.35c**). At the back, the lobe overlaps the common carotid artery, and the pharynx and oesophagus are behind the larynx and trachea. Through its connective tissue capsule, the gland *adheres to the larynx*, so that when the larynx rises during swallowing the gland rises with it.

The **recurrent laryngeal nerve** (a branch of the vagus, see p.188) runs upwards in the groove between the oesophagus and trachea (**16.36**), and then lies behind the lower part of the lateral lobe before entering the pharynx and larynx (p.188). It has nothing to do with innervating the thyroid gland (whose blood vessels receive sympathetic nerve fibres), but is one of the most important structures associated with the gland because it may be damaged during thyroid surgery (see below).

BLOOD SUPPLY AND LYMPH DRAINAGE

The thyroid receives a blood supply from the **superior** and **inferior thyroid arteries** (**16.35b** and **16.35c**); they arise respectively from the external carotid and the thyrocervical trunk of the subclavian artery. **Superior** and **middle thyroid veins** drain to the internal jugular vein, but there are also **inferior thyroid veins** that pass straight downwards in front of the trachea (**16.35c**) to reach the left brachiocephalic vein; they are a hazard in tracheotomy (p.120). Lymph drainage is to deep cervical nodes.

THYROID HORMONES

The thyroid gland is unique in being the only endocrine gland to store secretion outside the cells, and it is also unique in its ability to extract and concentrate iodide ions from the blood. *Iodine* and the amino acid *tyrosine* (both derived from food and reaching the gland in the bloodstream) are both essential for the formation of the main thyroid hormone, *thyroxine*. A small number of special cells produce a second hormone, *calcitonin*.

Thyroxine

The gland consists of **epithelial (follicular) cells** which are arranged as single-layered, rounded follicles that contain *colloid*, the storage form of thyroid secretion. Colloid consists largely of *thyroglobulin*, a protein molecule to which is attached *T4* (*tetraiodothyronine*) – the main thyroid hormone, commonly called *thyroxine*. A similar compound, *T3* (*triiodothyronine*), is also produced and may be derived from T4. Under the influence of *TSH* (*thyroid-stimulating hormone*) from the anterior pituitary, thyroxine is released

from thyroglobulin and moves across the follicular cells to enter the bloodstream. Here it combines with plasma proteins, forming a compound known clinically as *PBI* (*protein-bound iodide*).

The main action of thyroxine, which is absorbed by cells in all parts of the body, is to *regulate cell metabolism* and *control growth*. It not only affects the amount of tissue formed, but also its further development and differentiation.

Calcitonin

A small number of thyroid cells (called **parafollicular** or **C cells**) produce the hormone *calcitonin* (*thyrocalcitonin*), which is unrelated to thyroxine. Calcitonin *lowers* the level of *calcium* in the blood, by depositing calcium in bone and inhibiting bone resorption.

EXAMINATION

Unless enlarged, the thyroid gland is not easily seen. To feel the gland, it is easiest for the examiner to be behind the patient so that the hands can be passed round to the front of the neck. A general enlargement of the gland is called a *goitre* and forms an obvious swelling (**16.40**); a localized enlargement is a *nodular goitre*. Both deficient and excessive secretion can cause enlargement.

Apart from inspection and palpation, laboratory measurements of T4 and TSH in the blood and studies of the uptake of radioactive iodine are commonly used for assessing thyroid activity. Needle biopsy of the gland can also be carried out, for microscopic examination.

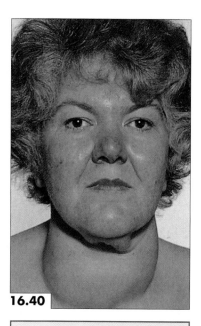

16.40

Fig. 16.40 Enlarged thyroid gland.

DISEASES

Infants who have thyroid *deficiency* develop *cretinism*, characterized by stunted growth and mental retardation. The condition can be corrected by giving thyroid hormone, but it must be recognized and treated quickly (within a few days of birth) before any changes from the normal have become irreversible.

Thyroid *deficiency* in *adults* causes *myxoedema* (probably an autoimmune disease, p.70), in which there is a slowly progressive lessening of physical and mental activity, loss of hair and an increase in weight with an accumulation of fluid in subcutaneous tissues which gives rise to the **non-pitting** form of oedema (in contrast to the pitting oedema of heart failure, p.119). Treatment with thyroid hormone can reverse the condition.

The *excessive* production of thyroid hormone (*hyperthyroidism*) gives rise to *toxic goitre* (*exophthalmic goitre* or *Grave's disease*). The cause is not certain; some patients have in the blood an immunoglobulin known as *TSI* (*thyroid-stimulating immunoglobulin*, formerly called *LATS* or *long-acting thyroid stimulator*) but in others it is not present. However, it is known that an excess of TSH from the anterior pituitary is not the cause. The patient becomes unusually active and nervous with an increase of appetite but loss of weight. The connective tissue in the orbit increases in volume and pushes the eyes slightly forwards (*exophthalmos*), giving a rather staring appearance. Treatment with antithyroid preparations such as thiouracil can be effective, but some patients may require removal of most of the gland (*partial thyroidectomy*). The isthmus and the front parts of the lateral lobes are removed, leaving intact a small part of each lobe (and the parathyroids, see below) beside the trachea. In any thyroid surgery, the greatest care must be taken to avoid damage to the recurrent laryngeal nerves (see above and p.188).

Cancer of the thyroid may occur, but is not common.

PARATHYROID GLANDS

The **parathyroid glands**, usually four in number – a **superior** and **inferior pair** – are very small seed-like structures that lie at the back of the lateral lobes of the thyroid gland (two behind each lobe, **16.36**). The total weight of all four is usually no more than 250 mg. They can be distinguished from thyroid tissue because of their slightly different colour (brownish-yellow rather than reddish), although if enlarged they will clearly be more obvious. Both glands of one side are supplied by the **inferior thyroid artery**; tracing branches of this vessel into the thyroid gland is the way to find the parathyroids. Occasionally, one or more may be found in unusual positions, such as in the mediastinum near the thymus; this is due to the similar developmental origins. Each gland consists of a mass of small cells, looking rather like lymphocytes, but with a network of many blood capillaries.

PARATHYROID HORMONE

Unlike the thyroid, the glands are **not** under the control of the anterior pituitary. Parathyroid hormone (*parathormone*, *PTH*) acts on bone and on the intestine and kidney tubules to **increase blood calcium** and to **decrease blood phosphate**. Low blood calcium (*hypocalcaemia*) will stimulate the secretion of PTH to remove calcium from bone (via the process of bone resorption, p.12) and so restore the normal blood level. Similarly, a high blood calcium (*hypercalcaemia*) will depress PTH secretion. The presence of vitamin D is necessary for the normal function of PTH; the vitamin is required for the absorption of calcium from the gut.

EXAMINATION

Being so small and behind the thyroid, the normal parathyroids are quite impalpable. A tumour in one of them may cause a local enlargement, but overactivity is not necessarily accompanied by an increase in size. Levels of calcium and of PTH in blood plasma, when considered with other signs and symptoms, will help to differentiate between the various disorders associated with calcium.

DISEASES

Too much hormone (*hyperparathyroidism*), usually due to parathyroid tumours, causes decalcification of bones which are thus easily fractured, and sometimes bone cysts are formed (*osteitis fibrosa cystica*). Treatment is by the surgical removal of some glandular tissue (*parathyroidectomy*), but there must **not** be **total removal** since a small amount of parathyroid tissue is essential to life. If all parathyroid tissue is removed accidentally or deliberately, as in *total thyroidectomy*, a small piece of one of the parathyroids is implanted into the forearm; being a ductless gland it does not really matter whereabouts in the body it is situated, and if later surgical treatment is necessary, it is easier to deal with a forearm than the neck. Too much blood calcium, as a consequence of hyperparathyroidism, may lead to an excess of calcium in the urine, so giving rise to *renal stones*.

Too little hormone (*hypoparathyroidism*), a rare condition, usually due to inadvertent removal of the parathyroids during partial thyroidectomy, produces *hypocalcaemia*. This causes the nerves that supply skeletal muscles to become unusually excitable, leading to muscle twitches and spasms called *hypocalcaemic tetany*. Spasms of the hands and/or feet (*carpal* and/or *pedal spasms* – collectively called *carpopedal spasms*) are characteristic, and if brain cells are affected there may be *convulsions*. (Tetany must not be confused with epilepsy, nor with **tetanus**, which is a term that can mean either a bacterial infection or the normal response of muscle fibres to repeated stimulation.) Treatment is by the administration of calcium salts, intravenously or orally, depending on the urgency of the condition.

CHAPTER 17

BRAIN AND SPINAL CORD

BRAIN

The **brain** is the part of the **central nervous system** that lies within the skull. The largest part of it is the **cerebrum**, consisting of right and left halves or **cerebral hemispheres**. Extending down from the under surface of the brain is the **brainstem**, to which most of the **cranial nerves** are attached, and sticking out from the back of the brainstem is the **cerebellum** (**7.1**, **7.2**, **17.1** and **17.2**).

The brain is protected not only by the bony skull, but also by being enclosed in a bath of fluid – the **cerebrospinal fluid** (p.132) – within a series of bag-like membranes, the **meninges** (p.130).

CEREBRAL HEMISPHERES

The surface of the **cerebral hemisphere** is the **cerebral cortex**. It is about 3–4 mm thick, consisting of **gray matter**, which is predominantly **neuronal cell bodies**. In the early embryo, the cortex is completely smooth, but during development it becomes thrown into folds and furrows – the **gyri** and **sulci** (**17.1a**) – in order to increase its surface area within its fixed-size box, the skull.

Beneath the cortex is the **white matter** of the hemisphere, which is predominantly **nerve fibres**, and buried in the white matter are various groups of nerve cell bodies (the **subcortical gray matter**, **17.3**). The most important are the **thalamus** (see below), which collects and distributes sensory input, and the **basal nuclei** (still often called by their old name – **basal ganglia**). The largest of the basal nuclei are the **caudate nucleus** and the **lentiform nucleus**; they assist in the coordination of muscular activity as part of the extrapyramidal system (p.206).

Cerebral Cortex

The gyri and sulci (singular – **gyrus** and **sulcus**) are not absolutely identical in every brain, but their pattern is sufficiently constant for each gyrus and sulcus to have a name (most of which need not be learned!). Some gyri (mentioned below) are of supreme clinical importance because they are concerned with the control of skeletal muscles or with various kinds of sensation; disease or damage in these areas leads to paralysis and loss of sensation. Other parts of the cortex may be equally important in their own way, but with functions that are less well defined and more difficult to examine, being concerned with thought, memory, emotion and all the other cerebral activities that contribute to human beaviour.

One of the most important sulci is the **central sulcus** which passes obliquely downwards and forwards on the outer surface of the hemisphere. It serves as the dividing line between the **frontal** and **parietal lobes** of the brain, but its real importance is that the gyrus immediately *in front* of it – the **precentral gyrus** – contains nerve cells which control skeletal muscles. The common name of this gyrus is thus the **motor cortex**.

The gyrus *behind* the central sulcus, the **postcentral gyrus**, is where *sensations* such as touch, heat and cold and pain reach consciousness (the **sensory cortex**). These **motor** and **sensory areas** (sometimes collectively known now as the **sensorimotor cortex**) extend beyond the top of the lateral surface of the hemisphere on to its *medial* surface.

In the motor and sensory areas of the cortex, each part of the body is represented in a definite position (**17.1b** and **17.1c**). Thus, the **leg area** is at the top (extending down on to the medial surface of the hemisphere), with the **trunk** and **arm areas** lower down (i.e. the body can be said to be represented 'upside down'). Below them are the areas concerned with the **face** and other **head** and **neck structures** such as the lips, tongue, pharynx and larynx. These areas, as well as that devoted to the hand, occupy particularly large parts of the cortex, in keeping with their importance in human life.

Below the lower end of the central sulcus is the **lateral sulcus** (or **lateral fissure**), with the **temporal lobe** below it. On the upper part of the temporal lobe is the **auditory area** of the cortex where hearing is appreciated (p.173).

At the back of the cerebral hemisphere, mainly on the medial surface of the occipital lobe, is the **visual area**, where impulses from the retina are perceived (p.195).

Thalamus

The role of the **thalamus** in the general sensory pathways from the spinal cord is described on p.208. Parts of the

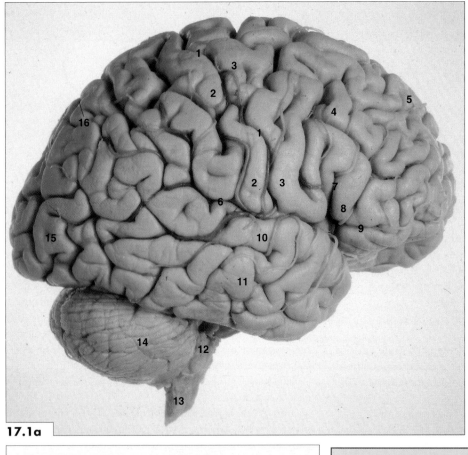

17.1a

Fig. 17.1 Right side of the brain.
(a) After removal of arachnoid mater but with branches of the middle and anterior cerebral arteries preserved.
(b) Diagram of the cerebral hemisphere, indicating the areas of the cortex associated with motor and sensory activities.

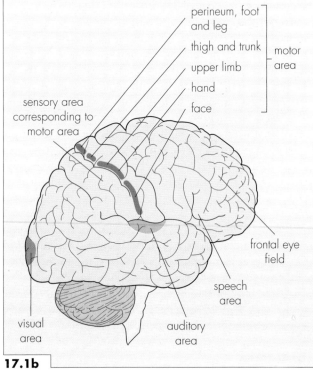

17.1b

1 Central sulcus, dividing frontal from parietal lobe
2 Post-central gyrus, the main sensory area of the cerebral cortex
3 Precentral gyrus, the main motor area
4 Various gyri and sulci of frontal lobe
5 Branches of anterior cerebral artery
6 Lateral sulcus (main part of posterior ramus), with branches of the middle cerebral artery emerging
7 Ascending ramus of lateral sulcus
8 Speech area (Broca's area)
9 Anterior ramus of lateral sulcus
10 Superior temporal gyrus, with the auditory area in its central part
11 Sulci and gyri of temporal lobe
12 Pons
13 Medulla oblongata
14 Cerebellar hemisphere, with folia (like miniature gyri)
15 Sulci and gyri of occiptal lobe
16 Parieto-occipital sulcus, separating parietal and occipital lobes

thalamus are also concerned with special senses. The most important of these is *vision*, and involves a special group of thalamic cells, the **lateral geniculate body**. The **visual pathway** (**16.26b**) conveys impulses from the ganglion cells of the retina to the visual cortex via the optic nerves, optic chiasma, optic tracts, lateral geniculate bodies and optic radiations. Each **optic nerve** is formed by the axons of the ganglion cells of the retina (p.164). At the **optic chiasma**, in the middle of the under surface of the brain (**17.4a**), the fibres from the nasal side of the retina (i.e. those conveying sensations from the temporal side of the visual field) cross to the opposite side (i.e. they *decussate*) and run back with fibres from the temporal side of the retina in the **optic tract** (**16.26b**). This is a band passing from the chiasma round the side of the midbrain to the **lateral geniculate body** which forms a small elevation on the under surface of the thalamus. Here, the retinal axons end by synapsing with cell bodies whose fibres run through the cerebrum as the **optic radiation** (**16.26b** and **17.3a**), so reaching the **visual cortex** on the medial surface of the occipital lobe (**17.2a**).

Pituitary tumours that press on the optic chiasma from below (p.134) interrupt the decussating fibres, so causing loss of vision in the temporal parts of the visual fields (i.e. *tunnel vision*, seeing only what is immediately in front). The biblical giant Goliath presumably had such a tumour – causing his gigantism (p.140) and visual defect, allowing the boy David to creep up unawares and slay him!

Another small group of thalamic cells, the **medial geniculate body**, is part of the **auditory pathway** to the temporal lobe (p.193), but this is much less important than the lateral geniculate body concerned with vision – do not confuse the two!

Other thalamic cells convey the sensations of *balance* and *taste* to regions of the sensory cortex near the face and tongue areas respectively. Fibres concerned with the sensation of *smell* (p.155) are unique in that they reach the cortex (of the **uncus** on the medial surface of the temporal lobe, **17.4a**) without passing through, or synapsing in, the thalamus – perhaps an indication of how 'old' smell is in terms of evolution.

Internal Capsule

The area of white matter between the thalamus and the caudate and lentiform nuclei is one of the most important anatomical regions in the whole body. Known as the **internal capsule** (**17.3a**), its main parts are the **anterior limb**, the **genu** and the **posterior limb** ('genu' is from the Latin for 'knee' – in transverse sections the three parts look like a bent knee). Many nerve fibres passing to and from the cerebral cortex pass through various parts of the internal capsule. In particular, masses of **sensory fibres** pass up from the thalamus to the cortex. Even more important, running down through the genu are the **corticonuclear fibres** passing to the **motor nuclei** of **cranial nerves**; and running through the

posterior limb are the **corticospinal fibres**, passing to the **anterior horn cells** of the spinal cord. Thus, running through these very few square centimeters of brain substance (on each side) are concentrated the motor nerve fibres controlling all the skeletal muscle in the body. Damage to the blood supply of this area is the common cause of a 'stroke' (p.199).

BRAINSTEM

The **brainstem** (**17.2**) is the part of the brain which connects the cerebrum (above), the spinal cord (below), and the cerebellum (at the back). It consists of three parts – the **midbrain**, **pons** and **medulla oblongata** (usually called simply the **medulla**, but do not confuse it with *spinal medulla*, which is the strictly proper name for the spinal cord). The midbrain is connected to the cerebral hemispheres, and below it is the pons which in turn runs into the medulla. It is the medulla that leaves the skull through the foramen magnum to become the spinal cord (**16.2** and **17.5a**).

In the different parts of the brainstem are situated **tracts** and **nuclei** (pp.14 and 40). Many of the tracts that run up and down through the brainstem form the principal communicating links between the brain and the spinal cord. Some of the nuclei give rise to the fibres of cranial nerves (see below). Other cells and fibres constitute the **reticular formation** (see below), including what are often called 'vital centres' for the control of the heart rate and respiration (pp.54 and 75), while others in the midbrain are usually classified for functional reasons as belonging to the basal nuclei (p.193).

Cranial Nerve Nuclei

The various cell groups that give origin to the motor fibres of cranial nerves, and groups with which the afferent fibres of cranial nerves make synaptic connections, constitute the **nuclei of the cranial nerves** (sometimes called the **central connections of cranial nerves**). The nuclei of the third to the twelfth cranial nerves lie approximately in numerical order from top to bottom of the brainstem (the first and second nerves – the olfactory and optic – are not attached to the brainstem). Thus, the nuclei of nerves III and IV are in the midbrain, those of V, VI and VII in the pons, those of VIII in the region where pons and medulla become continuous with one another, and those of IX to XII are in the medulla. The fibres constituting the individual nerves (summarized on p.41) are attached to the side of the brainstem in approximately the same order.

Reticular Formation

Apart from the cell groups that are associated with cranial nerves, there are enormous numbers of other nerve cells and fibres in the brainstem. Many of them form what is collectively called the **reticular formation**. This diffuse collection of cells and fibres, which is both difficult to define anatomically and to investigate physiologically, plays a part in many of the brain's activities. These include consciousness (by helping to determine the degree of 'alertness'), motor activity (as part of the extrapyramidal system, see p.206), sensory function (by controlling input to the thalamus, p.208), and autonomic activities (by controlling heart rate and respiration, pp.54 and 75).

Brainstem Death

The availability of machines that can maintain circulation and respiration in unconscious patients has led to the need for assessing whether or not *death* has occurred, i.e. whether there is *irreversible cessation of brainstem function*; the state of 'life' depends on the brainstem, not on the cerebrum. Such information is obviously of vital importance in helping to determine, for example, whether recovery is likely or whether organs may be legitimately removed for transplantation into a living patient. Clinicians must provide satisfactory answers to a number of criteria, and among the tests that are used are those to establish the absence of reflexes that normally depend on the proper functioning of different parts of the brainstem. Thus, to give just one example involving each of the three parts of the brainstem:

- Pupillary reflexes (p.169) involve the midbrain, where the oculomotor nerve nuclei are situated.
- The corneal reflex (p.168) involves the pons, where there are connections between the trigeminal and facial nerve nuclei.
- The gag reflex (p.185) involves the medulla, where the vagal nuclei are situated.

CEREBELLUM

The **cerebellum**, which consists mainly of two **cerebellar hemispheres**, sticks out from the back of the brainstem, being connected to it by three pairs of nerve fibre bundles: the **superior**, **middle** and **inferior cerebellar peduncles** (**17.2b**). One pair of peduncles goes to each of the three parts of the brainstem – the superior pair to the midbrain, the middle to the pons and the inferior to the medulla.

Like the cerebrum, the cerebellum has a **cortex** of **gray matter** on the surface but it is thrown into much smaller folds (**folia**) which are not individually named like the cerebral gyri. Below the cortex is the **white matter** within which lie groups of **nerve cell bodies**, the largest of which is the **dentate nucleus**. The cerebellum is concerned with the coordination of muscular activity, helping movements to be carried out in a smooth, controlled manner, rather than jerkily; it has nothing to do with conscious sensation.

VENTRICLES OF THE BRAIN

Within the brain, including the brainstem, there is a system of communicating cavities forming the **ventricular system**, which is filled with cerebrospinal fluid (CSF, p.132); in fact, the CSF is manufactured in certain parts of these cavities.

Within each cerebral hemisphere is a **lateral ventricle** (**17.3**), consisting of a central part, the **body**, and extensions passing forwards, backwards and downwards – the **anterior**, **posterior** and **inferior horns** respectively.

In the central part of the brain that is in continuity with the brainstem, there is a single narrow cavity, the **third ventricle** (**17.2a**), which has the **thalamus** and **hypothalamus** of each side in its lateral walls and the pineal body projecting backwards. Each lateral ventricle is in communication with the third ventricle through an **interventricular foramen**, situated just in front of the thalamus. (The two lateral ventricles were originally considered to be the first and second, hence the name 'third ventricle' for the midline cavity.)

At the back, the third ventricle joins a narrow passage passing through the midbrain – the **aqueduct of the midbrain** – and this connects the third ventricle with the **fourth ventricle**, which is the cavity within the pons and medulla.

Certain cell groups in the **hypothalamus** in the lateral wall of the third ventricle are the source of the *posterior pituitary hormones* (p.135) and of the *hypothalamic releasing hormones* controlling the release of anterior pituitary hormones (p.138).

The special bunches of blood capillaries that secrete CSF (the **choroid plexuses**, **17.2a**, **17.3a** and **17.3b**) are situated in the roof of the third ventricle and continue through the interventricular foramina into the body and inferior horn of each lateral ventricle. A separate choroid plexus lies in the roof of the fourth ventricle (**17.2a**). CSF produced in the lateral and third ventricles passes through the aqueduct into the fourth ventricle to mix with the CSF produced there, and then it escapes into the subarachnoid space (p.130) through three small apertures in the roof of the fourth ventricle; this is the only way CSF can get out of the ventricular system.

BLOOD SUPPLY

Three **cerebral arteries** – **anterior**, **middle** and **posterior** – supply the cerebral hemisphere of their own side (**17.4a** and **17.4b**). The anterior and middle cerebral vessels are terminal branches of the **internal carotid artery**. The posterior cerebrals are the terminal branches of the **basilar artery**, which is a midline vessel lying on the front of the pons and formed by the union of the two vertebral arteries. Another branch of each internal carotid, the **posterior communicating artery**, joins the posterior cerebral, and the two anterior cerebrals are joined by the very short **anterior communicating artery**. All of these anastomosing vessels form the **arterial circle** (the **circle of Willis**), which lies on the under surface of the brain in front of the brainstem.

Most of the cortex on the *lateral* surface of the hemisphere is supplied by branches of the middle cerebral artery, but a 1 cm strip at the very *top* is supplied by the anterior cerebral, whose branches creep over from the medial surface of the hemisphere. This means that the main motor

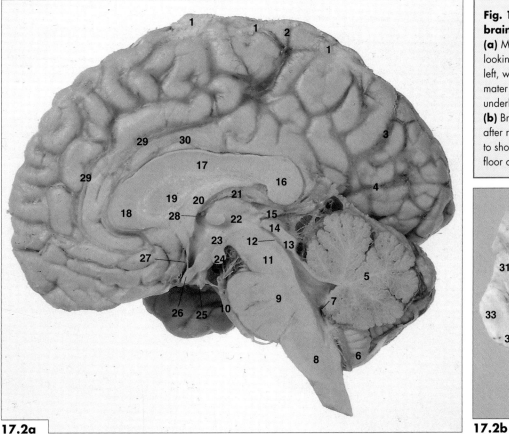

17.2a

Fig. 17.2 Brain and brainstem.
(a) Midline sagittal section, looking at the right half from the left, with most of the arachnoid mater preserved with the underlying vessels
(b) Brainstem, seen from behind after removal of the cerebellum, to show the diamond-shaped floor of the fourth ventricle

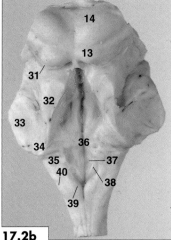

17.2b

1 Arachnoid granulations, through which cerebrospinal fluid escapes into the superior sagittal sinus
2 Central sulcus
3 Parieto-occipital sulcus
4 Calcarine sulcus, whose bordering gyri form the visual area of the cortex, with branches of posterior cerebral artery
5 Cerebellum
6 Tonsil of cerebellum, which overlies the foramen magnum and with increased intracranial pressure may sink down into it and block the flow of cerebrospinal fluid into the spinal subarachnoid space
7 Choroid plexus in posterior part of roof of fourth ventricle
8 Medulla oblongata
9 Pons
10 Basilar artery
11 Midbrain
12 Aqueduct of midbrain, connecting third and fourth ventricles
13 Inferior colliculus ⎱ of dorsum
14 Superior colliculus ⎰ of midbrain
15 Pineal body
16 Splenium ⎱
17 Body ⎬ of corpus callosum
18 Rostrum ⎰
19 Septum pellucidum, the partition between the right and left lateral ventricles

20 Fornix
21 Choroid plexus in roof of third ventricle
22 Thalamus ⎱ in lateral wall
23 Hypothalamus ⎰ of third ventricle
24 Mamillary body ⎱ in floor
25 Pituitary stalk ⎬ of third
26 Optic chiasma ⎰ ventricle
27 Lamina terminalis, the anterior wall of the third ventricle
28 Interventricular foramen, leading from the third ventricle to the lateral ventricle within the cerebral hemisphere (**17.3**)
29 Branches of anterior cerebral artery
30 Cingulate gyrus, the one immediately above the corpus callosum (17)
31 Trochlear (fourth cranial) nerve, emerging behind the inferior colliculus (13), the only cranial nerve to emerge from the dorsal surface of the brainstem
32 Superior ⎱ cerebellar
33 Middle ⎬ peduncles
34 Inferior ⎰ (cut edges)
35 Lateral recess ⎱ of fourth
36 Floor ⎰ ventricle
37 Hypoglossal trigone
38 Vagal trigone
39 Gracile tubercle
40 Cuneate tubercle

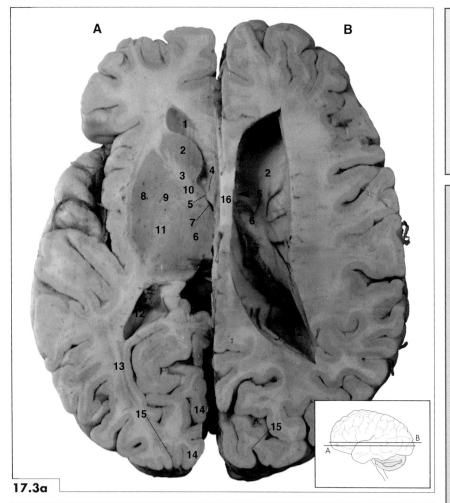

17.3a

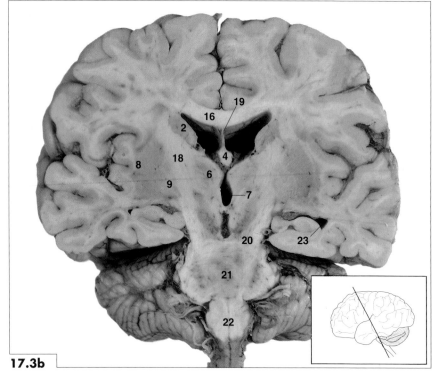

17.3b

Fig. 17.3 Brain sections.
(a) Horizontal sections, at the levels indicated in the inset and seen from above, to show on the left the structures bounding the internal capsule, and on the right the lateral ventricle.
(b) Oblique coronal section, at the level indicated in the inset and seen from behind, to show the internal capsule and the path of corticospinal fibres.

1 Anterior horn of lateral ventricle
2 Caudate nucleus
3 Anterior limb of internal capsule
4 Fornix
5 Interventricular foramen, joining lateral ventricle to third ventricle
6 Thalamus, in the lateral wall of the (central) third ventricle
7 Third ventricle
8 Putamen ⎫ forming the
9 Globus pallidus ⎬ lentiform nucleus
10 Genu of internal capsule, through which pass corticonuclear fibres from the cerebral cortex to the motor nuclei of cranial nerves
11 Anterior two-thirds of posterior limb of internal capsule, through which pass corticospinal fibres from the cerebral cortex to anterior horn cells of the spinal cord
12 Posterior horn of lateral ventricle
13 Optic radiation, passing from the lateral geniculate body (part of the thalamus) to the visual cortex (14)
14 Visual cortex
15 Lunate sulcus, the lateral limit of the visual cortex (14)
16 Corpus callosum
17 Choroid plexus of lateral ventricle, at the front passing through the interventricular foramen (5) and at the back continuing downwards and forwards into the inferior horn (within the temporal lobe, 23)
18 Path of corticospinal fibres, passing down through the internal capsule and brainstem to decussate in the lower medulla to form the lateral corticospinal tract of the spinal cord
19 Septum pellucidum, separating the two lateral ventricles
20 Cerebral peduncle (midbrain)
21 Pons
22 Medulla
23 Inferior horn of lateral ventricle

and sensory areas of the cortex have two supplies: the **perineal** and **leg areas** are supplied by the **anterior cerebral**, and the **trunk, arm** and **head areas** by the **middle cerebral**. The visual area on the medial surface of the hemisphere, at the back, is supplied by **posterior cerebral branches**.

Brain substance deep to the cortex is supplied by small branches of the cerebral vessels which penetrate deeply into the hemisphere through certain areas on the under surface of the brain – the **anterior** and **posterior perforated substance** (**17.4a** and **17.4c**). Some of these small vessels (usually called **striate arteries**) are among the most important in the whole body since (apart from nuclei of gray matter), they supply the parts of the internal capsule through which run the motor fibres controlling skeletal muscles (p.195, and below).

Branches from the **basilar** and **vertebral arteries** supply the **brainstem** and **cerebellum**. The largest (**17.4**) are the pair of **superior cerebellar** and **anterior inferior cerebellar arteries** from the basilar, and the **posterior inferior cerebellar** from each vertebral artery.

The **choroid plexuses** of the ventricles receive their own small branches – the **choroidal arteries** – usually from middle cerebral and posterior inferior cerebellar vessels.

Veins of the brain do not usually accompany the arteries, and they do not usually have corresponding names. Various veins from within the brain drain into the **great cerebral vein** which is behind the top of the brainstem; it runs back into the **straight sinus** (one of the venous sinuses of the dura mater, p.133). Numerous cortical veins, such as the **superior** and **inferior cerebral veins**, drain into nearby venous sinuses, such as the **superior sagittal** and **transverse sinuses**. From the point of view of disease, cerebral veins are much less important than the arteries.

Blood–Brain Barrier

Unlike capillaries in other tissues, those of the brain (and spinal cord) allow only selected substances, such as amino acids and sugars, to be transported through their walls. This **blood–brain barrier** thus has a protective effect on neural tissue. Only a few small areas of the brain have no such barrier; these include the posterior pituitary and parts of the hypothalamus and floor of the fourth ventricle. The barrier affects the rate at which drugs can enter the brain; some which enter the CSF via the bloodstream can then diffuse from the CSF into brain tissue.

Cerebral Haemorrhage and Thrombosis

Bursting or blockage of cerebral blood vessels (i.e. **cerebral haemorrhage, thrombosis** or 'stroke'), especially of the **striate vessels** that supply the parts of the **internal capsule** through which pass the fibres controlling motor activity (p.195), is one of the commonest diseases of later life. In a typical stroke involving, say, the *left* cerebral hemisphere, there is a *spastic paralysis* of the *right* arm and leg (*hemiplegia*)

and *increased stretch reflexes* (tendon jerks) with perhaps a paralysis of the left side of the face and an interference with speech.

Paralysis affects the limb muscles of the side *opposite* to that of the affected hemisphere because of the way most fibres from one side of the brain cross over in the brainstem to run down the opposite side of the spinal cord (i.e. in the lateral corticospinal tract, p.205). In most people (even those who are left-handed) the speech centre of the cerebral cortex is on the left side, so a right-sided haemorrhage will not usually affect speech. The outcome is very variable depending on the extent of the brain damage. Complete recovery suggests that the condition was due to arterial spasm rather than haemorrhage or blockage, but usually some degree of paralysis persists.

For other brain diseases, see p.211.

SPINAL CORD

The **spinal cord** is the continuation of the medulla oblongata of the brainstem (see **7.1a** and **17.5**), and lies within the **vertebral canal** of the vertebral column. The cord begins at the level of **C1 vertebra** (the atlas) and in the adult usually ends at the level of the lower border of **L1 vertebra**. The cord is surrounded by the same three **meninges** as the brain (**17.6**): pia mater adhering to the surface, with arachnoid mater separated from the pia in life by cerebrospinal fluid, and dura mater outside the arachnoid (p.130). The **roots** of the **spinal nerves** (p.40) emerge from the side of the cord (**17.5c** and **17.6**) to enter meningeal sheaths which fuse with the outer coverings of the spinal nerves just beyond the dorsal root ganglion. The *ventral* roots run *in front of*, and the *dorsal* roots *behind*, the **denticulate ligament** of pia mater which holds the cord in the middle of the spinal subarachnoid space.

LUMBAR PUNCTURE, AND SPINAL AND EPIDURAL ANAESTHESIA

Because the spinal cord usually ends at the level of L1 vertebra, a needle inserted into the subarachnoid space below this level will enable a specimen of CSF to be obtained without the danger of damaging the spinal cord. This procedure – *lumbar puncture* (**17.5e**) – is usually carried out by inserting the needle in the midline of the back between the spines of L3 and L4 vertebrae (counted up from L4 spine which is level with the highest points of the iliac crests).

Abdominal or lower limb operations can be carried out under either *spinal* or *epidural anaesthesia*. In *spinal anaesthesia*, the anaesthetic solution is introduced into the subarachnoid space (as for lumbar puncture), and it diffuses into the spinal nerve roots. In *epidural anaesthesia*, the solution is introduced into the **epidural space** (outside the dura mater; the space is sometimes called the **extradural**

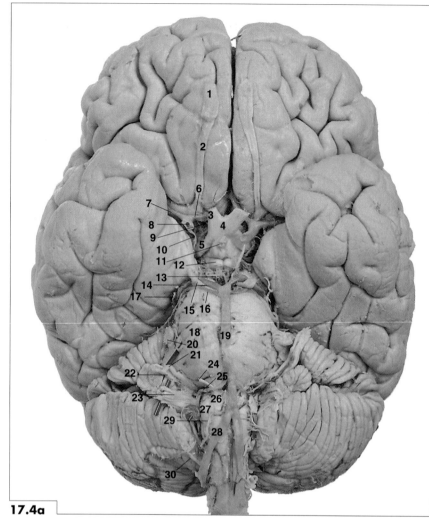

17.4a

Fig. 17.4 Brain and brainstem, from below
(a) With arteries in place.
(b) Arterial circle and basilar artery, dissected free and seen from below.
(c) With part of the brainstem and left cerebral hemisphere removed, to show the optic tract and the geniculate bodies.

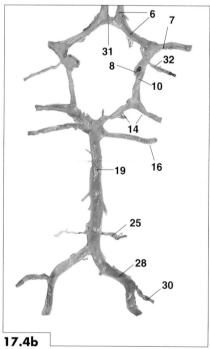

17.4b

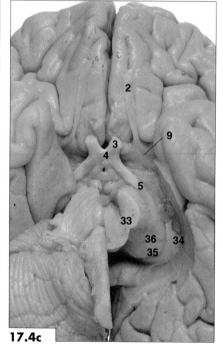

17.4c

1 Olfactory bulb, receiving filaments of olfactory nerve
2 Olfactory tract
3 Optic nerve
4 Optic chiasma
5 Optic tract, coursing back from the optic chiasma (4) round the side of the midbrain (c, 33) to the lateral geniculate body (c, 34)
6 Anterior cerebral artery, passing medially from the internal carotid (8) and joining its fellow of the opposite side by the anterior communicating artery (31)
7 Middle cerebral artery, passing into the lateral sulcus from the internal carotid (8)
8 Internal carotid artery, cut end
9 Anterior perforated substance, the region penetrated by striate arteries (from the anterior and middle cerebrals, 6 and 7) which supply the internal capsule (p.195) and are those commonly affected by thrombosis or haemorrhage, causing stroke
10 Posterior communicating artery, uniting the internal carotid (8) with the posterior cerebral (14)
11 Pituitary stalk
12 Mamillary body
13 Posterior perforated substance and branches of posterior cerebral artery (14)
14 Posterior cerebral artery, the terminal branch of the basilar (19) on each side
15 Oculomotor nerve, passing between the posterior cerebral and superior cerebellar arteries (14 and 16)
16 Superior cerebellar artery, arising from the basilar (19) just behind the posterior cerebral artery (14)
17 Trochlear nerve, passing forwards like the oculomotor nerve (15) between the posterior cerebral and superior cerebellar arteries (14 and 16)
18 Pons
19 Basilar artery, formed by the union of the two vertebrals (28)
20 Trigeminal nerve
21 Facial nerve, with blue marker at its upper border
22 Vestibulocochlear nerve
23 Filaments of glossopharyngeal, vagus and accessory nerves, in front of red marker
24 Abducent nerve
25 Anterior inferior cerebellar artery, arising from the basilar (19) shortly after the two vertebrals (28) have united
26 Pyramid of medulla oblongata
27 Olive, lateral to the pyramid (25)
28 Vertebral artery, joining its fellow to form the midline basilar artery (19)
29 Hypoglossal nerve
30 Posterior inferior cerebellar artery, arising from the vertebral (28)
31 Anterior communicating artery, joining the two anterior cerebrals (6)
32 Anterior choroidal artery, supplying the choroid plexus of the lateral and third ventricles (p.196)
33 Midbrain
34 Lateral geniculate body, where fibres from the retina synapse on the pathway to the visual cortex (p.195)
35 Posterior part of thalamus
36 Medial geniculate body, a site for synapses on the auditory pathway (p.195)

space) without entering the subarachnoid space (**17.5f**); it is still able to diffuse through the dural sheaths of the spinal nerve roots. This is a common method of anaesthesia for childbirth, providing pain relief for the whole of the lower part of the body but leaving the patient fully conscious.

INTERNAL STRUCTURE

On cross section (**17.6**) it can be seen (even with the naked eye) that the spinal cord consists of a slightly dark, central, 'H'-shaped region – the **gray matter** – which is composed mainly of **nerve cell bodies** (like the cerebral cortex), and a lighter peripheral area – the **white matter** – composed mainly of **nerve fibres** (with a whitish appearance, because many of the fibres are myelinated, p.47). A very narrow **central canal**, continuous with the cavity of the fourth ventricle at the lower end of the brainstem, extends down through the centre of the gray matter.

Horns of Gray Matter

The **gray matter** on each side is described as having **anterior, lateral** and **posterior horns** (**17.6**); the cells of each horn are functionally distinct. (In descriptions of the nervous system,

the terms *ventral* and *dorsal* are used just as frequently as *anterior* and *posterior*; thus it is common to see these areas of gray matter described as **ventral, lateral** and **dorsal horns** respectively.)

The **anterior (ventral) horn** contains **motor nerve cells**; these are actually the cell bodies of neurons whose fibres are the motor nerve fibres that run out in the spinal nerves to innervate **skeletal muscles**. The largest cells are the α (**alpha**) **motor neurons** supplying ordinary skeletal muscle fibres, and there are smaller γ (**gamma**) **motor neurons** supplying the fibres of the **muscle spindles** (p.35). The disease commonly called *polio* (*anterior poliomyelitis*) is a virus infection that specifically destroys anterior horn cells, hence the muscular paralysis of this condition.

The **lateral horn** contains **autonomic motor nerve cells**, supplying not skeletal muscle but **cardiac muscle, smooth muscle** and certain **glands**. This horn is small in comparison to the other two and is not present in the cervical region or in the lower lumbar and parts of the sacral regions. In all **thoracic segments** and the **first two lumbar segments**, the lateral horn contains the cell bodies of **sympathetic neurons**, while in the **second** to the **fourth sacral segments** it contains

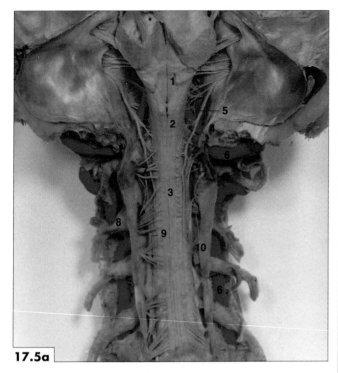

17.5a

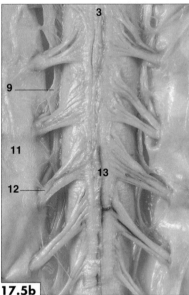

17.5b

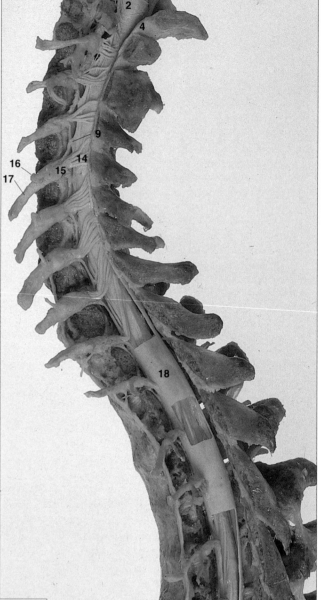

17.5c

Fig. 17.5 Spinal cord, and spinal and epidural anaesthesia.

(a) Cervical part, continuous with the brainstem, seen from behind after removing the posterior part of the skull and cerebellum, to show the emerging dorsal nerve roots.

(b) Cervical part, seen from the front, to show the emerging ventral nerve roots.

(c) Cervical and upper thoracic regions, from the left side

(d) Lower end and the cauda equina, with vertebral and sacral canals opened up.

(e) Sagittal section of lumbar vertebrae and subarachnoid space, with needle in position for spinal anaesthesia

(f) Similar section with needle in position for epidural anaesthesia.

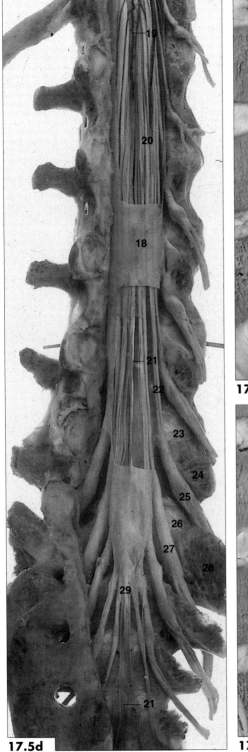

17.5d

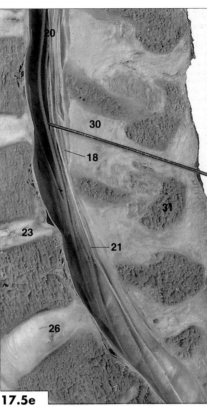

17.5e

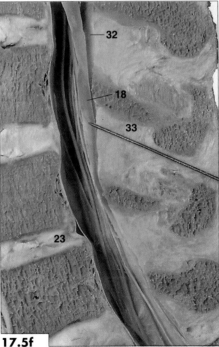

17.5f

1 Floor of fourth ventricle
2 Medulla oblongata
3 Spinal cord
4 Margin of foramen magnum
5 Spinal part of accessory nerve
6 Vertebral artery
7 Dorsal rootlets of left C2 nerve
8 Dorsal root ganglion of left C3 nerve
9 Denticulate ligament, formed of pia mater
10 Cut edge of dura and arachnoid mater
11 Arachnoid mater overlying dura mater, turned out to show ventral surface of the cord
12 Ventral root of C5 nerve entering meningeal sheath
13 Anterior spinal vessels
14 Dorsal roots ⎫
15 Dorsal root ganglion ⎬ of C5
16 Dorsal ramus ⎪ nerve
17 Ventral ramus ⎭
18 Dura mater
19 Conus medullaris, the lower end of the spinal cord
20 Nerve roots forming cauda equina
21 Filum terminale, the strand of pia mater extending from the conus medullaris (19) to the coccyx
22 Roots of L5 nerve
23 L4 intervertebral disc, between L4 and L5 vertebrae
24 Pedicle of L5 vertebra
25 Dorsal root ganglion of L5 nerve
26 L5 or lumbosacral disc, between L5 vertebra and sacrum
27 Meningeal sheath containing S1 nerve roots and dorsal root ganglion, passing behind L5 disc (26)
28 S1 piece of sacrum
29 Lower end of subarachnoid space, opposite S2 piece of sacrum
30 Needle penetrating interspinous tissue and dura mater (18) to enter subarachnoid space for spinal anaesthesia
31 Spine of L4 vertebra
32 Epidural space
33 Needle entering epidural space (32) but remaining outside dura mater (18) for epidural anaesthesia

the cell bodies of **parasympathetic neurons** (p.47). Do not be confused by the fact that most lateral horn cells are sympathetic, but in the sacral region cells in exactly the same positions are parasympathetic.

The **posterior (dorsal) horn** at all levels contains various

cell groups that are *sensory* (*afferent*) in function, in particular those that are concerned with the transmission of pain and temperature sensations (p.207).

Columns of White Matter

In contrast to the gray matter, the **white matter** of the cord contains no nerve cell bodies, but instead a large number of **nerve fibres** that run up or down the cord to provide connections between different levels of the cord, or between the cord and the brain. These nerve fibres tend to be divided into groups called **columns** by the horns of gray matter; on each side there is a **posterior (dorsal) column**, a **lateral column**, and an **anterior (ventral) column**. Do not confuse these *white columns*, which are *nerve fibres*, with the *gray horns*, which contain *cell bodies*.

The columns contain the important ascending and descending **tracts** that convey nerve impulses between the brain and the spinal nerves, and play an essential role in mediating sensations (p.207) or controlling muscle actions (see below). When looking at a cross section of a normal spinal cord with the naked eye, or even at a stained microscopic section of it, it is not possible to define the tracts. They are not like peripheral nerves which are made up of distinct bundles with a connective tissue covering. The position and function of the various tracts has only been discovered by applying the methods described on p.40.

The positions of the more important tracts are illustrated in **17.7**; they are described below.

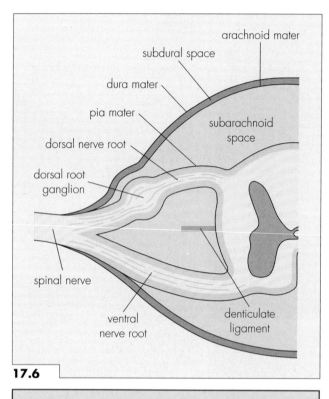

17.6

Fig. 17.6 Diagram of a transverse section of one half of the spinal cord with nerve roots and meninges

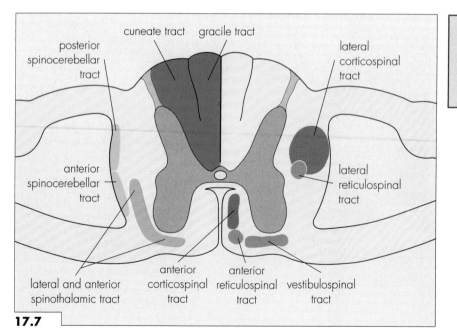

17.7

Fig. 17.7 Diagram of a transverse section of the spinal cord, showing positions of major tracts (sensory on the left of the diagram, motor on the right)

MOTOR PATHWAYS

For the normal functioning of the skeletal muscles that move the various parts of the body (head, trunk and limbs), the following elements must be working normally: upper motor neurons (otherwise known as the direct corticospinal or pyramidal neurons), neurons of the extrapyramidal (or indirect) corticospinal system, lower motor neurons, the neuromuscular junctions, and the muscle fibres themselves.

Upper Motor Neurons

The **upper motor neurons** are the nerve cells of the motor (and other) areas of the cerebral cortex; they leave the cortex to run down through the cerebral hemisphere and brainstem (p.195). Because of their origin from the cerebral cortex and destination in the spinal cord, they are called **corticospinal fibres**. In the lower part of the medulla most of the fibres (85% of them) *cross* to the *opposite side* to form the **lateral corticospinal tract** in the lateral white column. The criss-crossing of fibres from the two sides forms the *motor decussation* (**17.8**). The fibres of this tract end by making synaptic connections with the large motor cells (the lower motor neurons) in the anterior horn of gray matter. The small number of fibres that fail to cross in the medulla form the **anterior corticospinal tract** of the anterior white column. These fibres also end on anterior horn cells of the opposite side by crossing in the cord near their destination. Thus, all of the upper motor neurons arising on one side of the brain influence lower motor neurons of the *opposite* side of the cord.

The corticospinal fibres form a continuous, uninterrupted pathway from cortex to spinal cord (**17.7**) – hence the name **direct corticospinal pathway**. **Pyramidal tract** or **pathway** is another name used instead of **corticospinal**, because in the medulla the fibres are all collected together to form the swelling on the surface of the medulla called the **pyramid**. In each pyramid there are about 1 million corticospinal fibres. In the spinal cord, those tract fibres destined to synapse with anterior horn cells in the cervical part of the cord are the most deeply placed, while those descending as far as the sacral region are the most superficial, near the surface of the cord; thus the tract is said to be *laminated*, or *layered*. About 55% of all corticospinal fibres are concerned with controlling the upper limb – an indication of the importance of the hand in human activity.

Some muscles of the head and neck are supplied not by spinal nerves but by certain **cranial nerves**, with the cells of origin of these nerve fibres being activated by similar fibres from the cortex; these fibres are called **corticonuclear** (as they go to **cranial nerve nuclei** in the **brainstem**), in contrast to *corticospinal* fibres which pass to *anterior horn cells* in the *spinal cord*. (An older alternative name for corticonuclear fibres was **corticobulbar fibres**, because 'bulb' was an old name for part of the brainstem.) The term pyramidal fibres or pyramidal tract is usually taken to mean both corticospinal

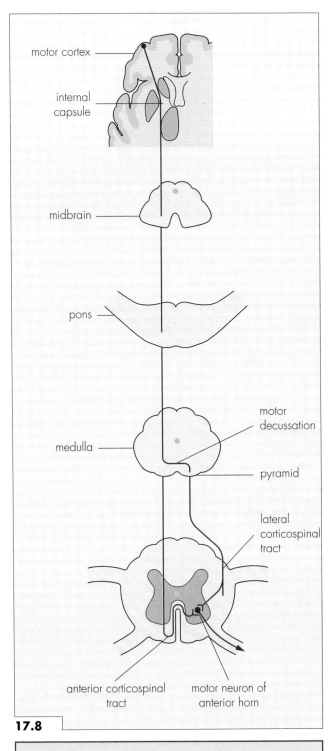

17.8

Fig. 17.8 Diagram of the main motor (corticospinal) pathway, from cerebral cortex to spinal cord

and corticonuclear fibres (this is a matter of convenience because of their similarity of function, but is not strictly correct since most corticonuclear fibres do not reach as low as the pyramid).

Extrapyramidal Fibres

Anterior horn cells (and the motor nuclei of cranial nerves) are not only influenced by fibres coming directly from the cerebral cortex but also by a large number of other fibres from cell groups in the cerebrum such as the basal nuclei (p.193) and brainstem. All of these fibres of non-cortical origin can be collectively called **extrapyramidal fibres** (because they do not pass through the pyramid in the medulla). They form several tracts in the spinal cord, the most important of which are the **reticulospinal tracts** (from the reticular formation) and the **vestibulospinal tract** (from one of the vestibular nuclei in the brainstem, **17.7**). Some of these fibres, especially the reticulospinal, are mixed up with corticospinal fibres in the lateral white column.

Lower Motor Neurons

The **lower motor neurons** are the α and γ **motor neurons** whose cell bodies are in the anterior horn of the spinal cord and whose fibres (axons) leave the cord in the ventral roots of the spinal nerves, to run in peripheral nerves and end as specialized motor nerve endings on skeletal muscle fibres (**neuromuscular junctions**). Because these anterior horn cells come under the influence of both pyramidal and extrapyramidal pathways, the lower motor neurons form what is sometimes called the 'final common path' to muscles.

Neuromuscular Junctions

The **neuromuscular junctions** (**7.11**) are where motor nerve fibres end on skeletal muscle fibres. Like synapses between neurons, there is a microscopic gap between the boundary membranes of nerve cell and muscle cell; acetylcholine is the transmitter that allows the stimulus for contraction to pass from nerve to muscle (as described on p.40). The condition called *myasthenia gravis* is a disease of neuromuscular junctions; there is muscular weakness, especially of the extraocular muscles, because for some unknown reason the acetylcholine fails to produce the usual contractile response in the muscles.

Motor Neuron Damage

It is of the greatest clinical importance to distinguish between damage to upper and lower motor neurons: *upper* motor neuron lesions produce **spastic** *paralysis*, and *lower* motor neuron lesions produce **flaccid** *paralysis*. In *flaccid paralysis* the muscles appear relaxed and flabby, and the tendon reflexes (p.50) are absent.

In the *spastic* type the muscles are tense and unrelaxed, with exaggerated reflexes and an *extensor plantar response* (*Babinski's sign*, **17.9**). This is seen as *dorsiflexion* (i.e. extension) of the great toe, and fanning of the other toes in response to firmly stroking the lateral part of the sole (the plantar surface) of the foot from the heel towards the toes (the sharp end of a key or the handle end of a tendon hammer is often a convenient instrument to use). The *normal* reaction to scratching the sole in this way is *plantarflexion* of the toes; the presence of an *extensor* type of response is **one of the most important signs in the whole of clinical medicine**, indicating some kind of damage to some part of the pyramidal pathway, i.e. *central nervous system damage*.

Injury or disease of any part of the **corticospinal pathway** (i.e. an upper motor neuron lesion) in the cerebral hemisphere or brainstem produces *spastic paralysis* of the muscles of the *opposite* side of the body (*hemiplegia*), because of the crossing over of most of the fibres (the motor decussation) in the medulla. The typical common example is a 'stroke', described on p.199.

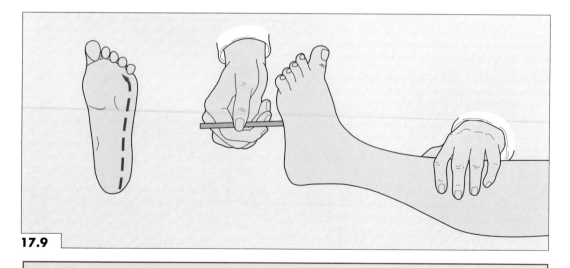

17.9

Fig. 17.9 Diagram of the extensor plantar response (Babinski reflex).
Scraping the lateral surface of the sole in the direction indicated normally produces flexion of the toes, but extension of the great toe and fanning of the other toes indicates upper motor neuron damage.

Damage to **anterior horn cells** (as in polio, mentioned above) or their fibres in peripheral nerves (as in wounds of the limbs) causes *flaccid paralysis*. Note that although the anterior horn cells are within the *central* nervous system, damage to them is like typical *peripheral* nerve damage and is not of the spastic type. Note also that *spinal cord damage* from a *fractured spine* in the *cervical* and *thoracic* regions is liable to cause pyramidal tract damage with *spasticity* (upper motor neuron damage), but fracture in the *lumbar* region, which is below the level of the end of the spinal cord, may only damage the *nerve roots* of the cauda equina, which are lower motor neurons, and therefore there will be *flaccidity* and *no spasticity*.

SENSORY PATHWAYS

Nerve impulses that are essential for **sensations** (*sensory impressions*) are conveyed along sensory (i.e. afferent) nerve fibres of peripheral nerves to the central nervous system, within which different kinds (*modalities*) of sensation have their own specific pathways to the appropriate region of the brain where they are consciously recognized. Sensations can be divided into *general* and *special*. *Special sensations* include vision (p.165), hearing (p.173), equilibration (maintenance of balance, p.173), taste (p.150) and smell (p.155). They travel by various cranial nerves and have been discussed on the pages indicated.

General sensations include *touch* (tactile sensation), *pressure*, *temperature* (appreciation of heat and cold), *pain*, and *proprioception* which means awareness of the position of joints and muscles and so is often called *muscle–joint sense* or *kinaesthetic sense*.

One of the most important facts to appreciate is that, in the spinal cord and brainstem, pain and temperature sensations travel by a *different pathway* from touch and the other types of sensation. This *dissociation* of the sensations into two groups, based on differences in their anatomical pathways, means that disease or injury may affect one group of sensations (pain and temperature, for example) and leave the others intact. Careful testing to determine which sensations are deficient and which are normal will help to localize the site of the damage.

Sensory Receptors

In order to conduct nerve impulses, sensory nerve fibres must be stimulated; for this purpose, the endings of the fibres are specialized as **receptors** which convert (or *transduce*, to use the technical term) the received stimulus into an electrical impulse. Microscopically, there are several different kinds of receptor, ranging from simple free nerve endings to more complicated types with connective tissue coverings (*encapsulated endings*, **3.1**) and even more specialized structures in the eye and ear. Each type of receptor is primarily associated with one type of sensation – e.g. free endings are associated with the sensation of pain, one kind of encapsu-lated ending with pressure, and special eye receptors with light. Each receptor responds easily to its own type of stimulus (it is said to have a *low threshold* for that stimulus), but it may also respond, though less easily, to other types of stimuli (for which it is said to have *high thresholds*). Thus receptors are not entirely limited to responding to a specific stimulus; excessive pressure, for example, on the skin could stimulate what is normally a pain receptor and the stimulus would be interpreted in the brain as pain, or excessive pressure on the eye could cause the perception of flashes of light even though there was no light shining into the eye.

Receptors are found all over the body. They are especially abundant in skin, allowing the individual to appreciate sensations such as touch, pressure, heat, cold and pain on the body surface. They are also found in joint capsules, ligaments, tendons and muscles, thus permitting proprio-ception (see above), as well as in the walls of many internal organs, where they signal pain or feelings of fullness (in the stomach or bladder, for example) or other sensations. Finally, they are of course present in the special sense organs that are found in the eye, ear, nose and tongue (see above).

Once impulses are generated by stimulation of a given receptor, they travel along the sensory nerve fibre attached to that receptor. **Sensory** (i.e. **afferent**) **neurons** are unusual in that they do not possess typical dendrites, their dendritic function having been taken over by the receptors on their peripheral ends. Thus, impulses generated at the receptor end of the neuron simply travel along the axon, or nerve fibre, all the way to the central nervous system. The **cell body** of such a sensory neuron seems, at least superficially, to be superfluous: it is located in the dorsal root ganglion (p.40) and appears to be an 'offshoot' of the axon just before the axon enters the central nervous system. The cell body is not in fact a superfluous appendage, for not only did it produce the axon during development, but it is essential for the axon's well-being throughout life. The peculiar anatomy of the sensory neuron has led many to describe its axon in two parts: the **peripheral process**, running from the receptor (in the periphery) to the cell body in the dorsal root ganglion, and the **central process**, leading from there into the spinal cord via the dorsal root.

Pathways for Touch and Associated Sensations

For all practical purposes, the *pathways* for ordinary sensations involve *three groups of neurons* in the transmission of the impulses from the periphery to the cerebral cortex. This principle is illustrated in two of the most important sensory pathways in the nervous system: that for touch and its associated sensations, and that for pain and temperature.

The pathway for *touch* begins (**17.10**) at tactile receptors in the periphery and continues along the peripheral processes of sensory neurons, which run through **spinal nerves** (and their branches) to the **dorsal root ganglia**. The **central**

processes of these neurons then enter the spinal cord, where they *divide*; some branches simply end locally by making synapses with anterior horn and other gray matter cells as part of **reflex arcs** (p.50), while others continue the touch pathway by entering the **posterior white column** and ascending in it towards the brain. Starting from the lower end of the cord, the fibres from sacral nerves lie nearest to the midline, and, progressing upwards, those from the lumbar, thoracic and cervical nerves are added more laterally in that order, so that the whole column can be said to be *laminated* (or *layered*). The column is roughly divided into two parts: a medial part forming the **gracile tract** containing sacral, lumbar and half the thoracic fibres, and a lateral part, the **cuneate tract**, containing the remaining thoracic and the cervical fibres. The gracile and cuneate tracts are sometimes collectively called the **posterior white columns**.

The columns ascend as far as the **medulla** of the brainstem, where the fibres end by synapsing with the cells of the **gracile** and **cuneate nuclei**. Note that there have been no synapses on the touch pathway up to this point. Some of the neurons concerned with touch sensation are the longest in the body; for example, a sacral nerve cell may have a peripheral process supplying skin on the sole of the foot and a central process entering the cord in the sacral region and running the whole way up the cord in the gracile tract to the medulla.

The touch pathway now continues upwards to the thalamus. The axons of cells in the gracile and cuneate nuclei cross to the opposite side of the brainstem (forming with their companions from the other side the **sensory decussation**), and then run up through the brainstem as the **medial lemniscus** to reach the **thalamus**. Here there is another synapse, and thalamic cells send their axons (the **thalamocortical fibres**) to the cerebral cortex.

Thus the three groups of neurons on the touch pathway are:
- Posterior root ganglion cells and their fibres which run peripherally in the spinal nerves and centrally in posterior nerve roots to enter the spinal cord and form the gracile and cuneate tracts.
- Cells of the gracile and cuneate nuclei and their axons which, after decussating, form the medial lemniscus of the opposite side.
- Thalamic cells and thalamocortical fibres.

To summarize one specific example of the pathway for touch, consider the case of touch from the skin of the pad of the right index finger – one of the most important sensory areas of the whole body (at least in right-handed people!). The impulses run in a branch of the median nerve (p.232) in fibres derived from C6 spinal nerve to C6 posterior root ganglion and then, by the dorsal nerve root, into the cuneate tract at the level of C6 segment of the spinal cord. From there, they run up in the cuneate tract to the cuneate nucleus in the medulla, where the fibres that started off in the skin now end by synapsing with cell bodies in the cuneate nucleus. Axons from cells of the cuneate nucleus cross from the right to the left side of the medulla in the sensory decussation, and then run up in the left medial lemniscus to the left thalamus. There they synapse with thalamic cells whose fibres pass to the hand area of the postcentral gyrus of the left cerebral cortex. Note that the touch pathway is a crossed pathway, the crossover occurring in the medulla (fibres of the second group of the three groups of neurons).

The touch pathway is not only for touch; some other important sensations are associated with this pathway as well, namely *proprioception* (p.207) and *vibration sense* (detecting the vibrations of a tuning-fork held against bony prominences such as those at the ankle). In addition, the pathway is used by impulses signalling *distension* of the **bladder** and **rectum**, thus indicating their fullness and the need to empty them. Because of its multiple functions, this pathway is commonly called the **posterior column** (or **dorsal column**) **pathway**.

Pain and Temperature Pathway

The second sensory pathway of major importance is that concerned with sensations of *pain* and *temperature* (i.e. heat or cold, **17.10**). The first group of neurons in this pathway consists of the fibres of the **peripheral nerves** and their **cell bodies** which are in the **dorsal root ganglia** of the spinal nerves – exactly the same as for the touch pathway. When pain and temperature fibres enter the spinal cord via the dorsal nerve roots, they end locally by synapsing (relaying) with various cells in the **posterior horn** of the same side that they entered; the impulses reach cells that give rise to fibres which *cross* to the opposite side of the cord and run up to the brain as the **spinothalamic tract**, known in the brainstem as the **spinal lemniscus**. This leads to the **thalamus**, where the fibres end by synapsing with cells that form the third group of neurons, with axons that pass to the **cerebral cortex**.

Thus, the three groups of nerve cells concerned on the pain and temperature pathway are:
- Dorsal root ganglion cells and their fibres which run peripherally in spinal nerves and centrally in the dorsal nerve roots to enter the spinal cord and its posterior horn.
- Posterior horn cells and their fibres which constitute the spinothalamic tract of the opposite side.
- Thalamic cells and their thalamocortical fibres – it is important to note that the crossing of fibres over to the opposite side does not take place transversely but in a *very oblique* manner, so that fibres from one segment may take up to four or five segments to complete the crossover.

To summarize one specific example of the pain and temperature pathway, consider the skin of the pad of the right index finger coming into contact with a hot object. The impulses pass in fibres of C6 nerve, as in the touch example given above, into the posterior horn of C6 segment of the cord, where they reach posterior horn cells whose axons cross

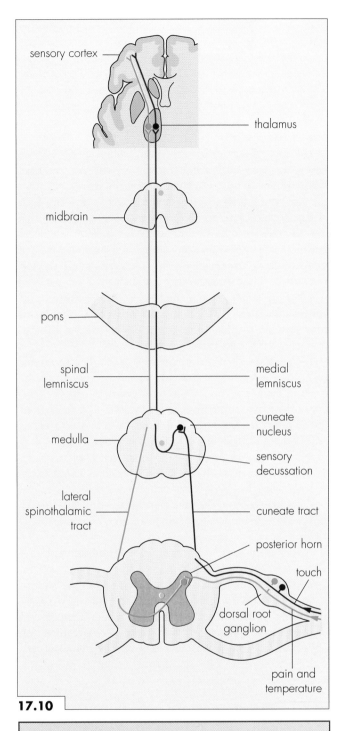

17.10

sensory cortex

thalamus

midbrain

pons

spinal lemniscus

medial lemniscus

cuneate nucleus

sensory decussation

medulla

lateral spinothalamic tract

cuneate tract

posterior horn

touch

dorsal root ganglion

pain and temperature

Fig. 17.10 Diagram of the pathways for touch and for pain and temperature.
The first synapses on the touch pathway (whose first neurons are represented here by the cuneate tract; the adjacent gracile tract, **17.7**, has been omitted for simplicity) are in the medulla, where the fibres of the second neuron cross to the opposite side (as the sensory decussation) to form the medial lemniscus. The first synapses on the pain and temperature pathway are in the spinal cord (in the posterior horn), where the fibres of the second neurons cross to the opposite side to form the lateral spinothalamic tract, which continues as the spinal lemniscus.

to the left side of the cord to form the left spinothalamic tract. This runs up through the brainstem to the left thalamus, where there is synaptic connection with thalamic cells whose fibres run to the hand area of the postcentral gyrus of the left cerebral cortex.

While the above three-neuron concept is sufficient for understanding the principles of the pain and temperature pathway, it has to be stated that in detail the pathway is somewhat more complicated. Firstly, in the posterior horn there may be several short **interneurons** between the incoming fibres from the posterior root ganglia and the cells of origin of the spinothalamic tract. Secondly, although it would be expected from the name that the fibres of the spinothalamic tract run from the spinal cord to the thalamus, only a small proportion actually reach the thalamus; most of the fibres end in the brainstem (before getting as far as the thalamus) by synapsing with cells of the reticular formation (p.195) which themselves may make many synaptic connections with one another before some send their axons eventually to the thalamus. This part of the pathway could therefore be called *spinoreticulothalamic*. Since there may be multiple synapses in the reticular formation and in the posterior horn, many more than just three neurons may be involved in the pathway, but nevertheless there are still just three long or main neurons.

There is an important reason for having to note the kind of detail just mentioned. The posterior horn and the reticular formation are sites where the *onward transmission* of the original pain impulse can be **modified** by other impulses arriving from other nerve fibres. The pain of, say, hitting the elbow against a hard object can be considerably relieved by vigorously rubbing the injured part; this stimulates other sensory receptors and fibres whose activity helps to modify (i.e. to *modulate*) the onward transmission of the pain impulse. Similarly, a severely wounded soldier may feel no pain at the time of injury because, in the stress of battle, various substances that are liberated within the central nervous system can suppress the pain by interfering with transmission along the pain pathway. The effect that some kinds of nerve fibre activity can have on others offers a general basis for the success of acupuncture in pain relief in some people, although it must be admitted that a full explanation is not yet possible.

The main differences between the touch pathway and the pain and temperature pathway must now be noted. In the **touch** pathway, the first synapse does not occur until the **medulla** is reached, where the **crossover** to the opposite side occurs. In the **pain** and **temperature pathway**, the first synapse occurs in the **posterior horn** of the spinal cord; the **crossover** to the opposite side occurs in the **cord**. Thus, both pathways are involved in a crossover of the **second** group of neurons, but the crossover **sites** are different; this has important implications in *spinal cord injury*. Imagine one side (one half) of the cord to be damaged, say the left side; as far as the sensory effects are concerned, *touch* sensation will be lost below the level of the injury on the *left* side of the body (because of damage to the left gracile and cuneate tracts which are composed of fibres from left-sided spinal nerves), but *pain* and *temperature* sensations will be lost on the *right* side (because of damage to the left spinothalamic tract which originated on the right side and received its afferent impulses from right-sided spinal nerves).

The pain pathway, like the touch pathway, conveys more than one kind of sensation. Apart from pain and temperature, the sensations of *itch* and *tickle*, and that of *sexual orgasms*, are known to be associated with this pathway. In addition, the pathway conveys sensations of *pressure* and what is usually called 'crude touch', to be distinguished from the 'light touch', with fine discrimination, which travels in the posterior columns. What is now called the spinothalamic tract was formerly divided into a *lateral* spinothalamic tract (in the lateral white column) concerned with pain and temperature, and an *anterior* spinothalamic tract (in the anterior white column) concerned with pressure and crude touch. Since these tracts really merge with one another, the single name is sufficient but, because of the combined position, some recent authorities use the name *anterolateral tract* instead of spinothalamic.

One further point to be made about this tract is that the fibres are so arranged that those from the sacral region are nearest to the surface of the cord, and those from the cervical region are the most deeply placed (similar to the laminated fibre arrangement in the lateral corticospinal tract, p.205).

Spinocerebellar Tracts

Other ascending tracts to be mentioned are the **anterior** and **posterior spinocerebellar tracts** (17.7). They begin from certain cell bodies in the posterior horn and run to the cerebellum, the anterior tract being crossed and the posterior uncrossed. They receive their afferent impulses from posterior root ganglia fibres supplying muscles and joints and, being destined for the cerebellum, they have nothing to do with conscious sensation but are concerned with the *unconscious*, smooth coordination of movements (p.196).

Sensory Pathways from Cranial Nerves

For those parts of the head and neck where spinal nerves are not involved, the fibres for general sensations run mostly in the **trigeminal nerves** (the fifth cranial nerves), with some others in the **glossopharyngeal** and **vagus nerves** (the ninth and tenth cranial nerves). The cell bodies are in the **ganglia** of those nerves (in the region of the base of the skull), corresponding to the dorsal root ganglia of spinal nerves. In the brainstem, the incoming fibres synapse with cell bodies in certain **sensory nuclei** associated with those cranial nerves. (Do not confuse cranial nerve *ganglia* with cranial nerve *nuclei*; ganglia are on the peripheral parts of the nerves, outside the CNS, and nuclei are within the CNS, in the

brainstem.) The **axons** from the cell bodies in these nuclei *cross* over to the opposite side of the brainstem and so run up to the **thalamus** beside the fibres from the spinal nerves. There are thus two groups of neurons as far as the thalamus, and a third goes from the thalamus to the **cerebral cortex** – three groups in all, just like the pathway for spinal nerves.

Visceral Pain

In the above description of the pain pathway, fibres of the first group of neurons subserving the sensation of pain have been assumed to be running with peripheral nerves, e.g. from the skin of the body surface. Pain fibres from **viscera**, such as the stomach, gall bladder, etc., and including the heart, use the same pathway within the CNS; how do these fibres get there? The answer is that they usually accompany the sympathetic fibres that supply the blood vessels of the viscus concerned. They pass through ganglia of the sympathetic trunk and enter spinal nerves via the **white rami communicantes** (7.2). Their cell bodies are in the **dorsal root ganglia**, just like those of the peripheral nerve fibres; from then on the pathways are the same.

In the **pelvis**, there are some exceptions to the general rule that pain fibres run with sympathetic nerves. Those from the *cervix* of the uterus run certainly with *parasympathetic* fibres, i.e. in the pelvic splanchnic nerves (p.290), and some from the bladder and rectum also appear to use this pathway as well as the sympathetic route (although those from the *body* of the uterus run with the usual sympathetic fibres).

In the head and neck, for structures such as the pharynx, larynx, trachea and oesophagus, which have glossopharyngeal or vagal innervation, the pain fibres run with those nerves (although some oesophageal pain seems to take a sympathetic pathway as well).

It is important to note that in the **abdomen**, a painful organ can cause *reflex contraction* of the overlying skeletal muscles of the abdominal wall (though the exact mechanism is not understood). This is detected by palpation of the abdominal wall, when the hand will recognize a certain amount of muscular rigidity or *guarding* – a feature that physicians and surgeons must look for in any suspected abdominal disease. The guarding has a protective effect, helping to keep the affected part at rest.

Referred Pain

Sometimes pain, especially visceral pain, may be felt in areas that are some distance from the actual site of origin of the pain. Ischaemic heart disease, for example, often causes pain in the left arm or neck. This phenomenon is known as *referred pain*. In the example given, fibres in the sympathetic nerves that supply the heart run into the same cervical or upper thoracic spinal nerves that supply skin in the arm or neck, and the pain is interpreted as coming from the skin rather than the heart. A less common but good example is pain at the tip of the shoulder due to irritation of peritoneum on the under surface of the diaphragm or over the gall bladder; the phrenic nerve, mainly from C4 nerve, supplies this part of the peritoneum, and the area of skin supplied by C4 nerve includes that over the shoulder tip. Pain from the intestinal tract, e.g. from the appendix, is felt in the central (umbilical) region of the abdomen, because the pain fibres run with the sympathetic nerves of the superior mesenteric artery which supplies much of the gut, and they enter spinal nerves T9–T11 which innervate the skin of this part of the abdomen. Other examples are pharyngeal or tonsillar pain referred to the middle ear (glossopharyngeal nerve), toothache referred to the orbit (from one branch of the trigeminal nerve to another), ureteral pain referred to the scrotum (via sympathetic fibres in L1 nerve), and pain from the hip referred to the knee (because both joints are supplied by the same main nerves).

EXAMINATION OF THE NERVOUS SYSTEM

The examination of the nervous system (often called *neurological examination*) includes the assessment of motor and sensory functions, and an appraisal of the patient's mental processes. Brain, spinal cord and peripheral nerves are all involved in motor and sensory activities, but mental processes such as thought and memory and general behaviour are a reflection of brain function, whose full assessment would involve psychiatric examination. The simple procedure of just observing the patient – general appearance, state of consciousness, respiratory rate, smell of the breath, signs of injury, etc. – may give important clues for diagnosis. Taking the blood pressure (p.59) is a part of neurological examination, to determine whether hypertension (and therefore vascular disease) is a possible factor in the condition being investigated.

Touch sensation is tested by seeing whether the patient can appreciate different areas of the skin surface being touched by a twist of cotton wool (or even the examiner's finger). *Pain* sensation is tested by the gauging appreciation of a pinprick. The extent of any defect is noted so that, coupled with other findings, an opinion can be formed on whether the defect is in a peripheral nerve or within the central nervous system (e.g. in the posterior columns, p.204). The ability to *move* different parts of the body, especially the limbs, and the observation and palpation of superficial muscles in action, is part of the examination of *motor activity*, which also includes testing the *stretch reflexes*, to help determine whether disturbances are of upper or lower motor neurons (p.206), or whether there is incoordination due to cerebellar disease.

There are specific tests for each cranial nerve, and in a full neurological examination each one must be examined. Usually those involving eye (p.167), pupil (p.168) and face (p.142) movements are the most important.

Modern *scanning* techniques have revolutionized the investigation of intracranial pathology, and can give accurate localization of such conditions as tumours and extradural haemorrhage (p.134). Examination of CSF by *lumbar puncture* may be required, especially in suspected infections, and *electroencephalography* (EEG) – recording 'brain waves' from electrodes placed on the scalp – is used for investigating epileptiform states (see below).

DISEASES OF THE NERVOUS SYSTEM

The diagnosis of the site of disease or injury in the nervous system is a prime example of the application of anatomical knowledge to a clinical problem; this is well illustrated by the effects of, say, haemorrhage in the internal capsule (p.195) or transection of the spinal cord (see below). Such organic conditions, whose pathological basis is well defined, can be broadly classified as *neurological disorders*, but the brain ('the mind') can also become the site of disturbances of behaviour which fall into the category of *psychiatric disorders* (mental diseases). It is not appropriate to discuss here conditions such as schizophrenia (whose symptoms include delusions and hallucinations), anxiety states, depression, psychosexual disorders and drug abuse, but they are all fields of intense research that will perhaps lead to full understanding of the biological background to these disturbed patterns of behaviour. Of the vast range of what may be broadly classified as *nervous diseases*, only a few are chosen here to illustrate the kind of disorders that can arise when specific parts of the nervous system are affected.

Among the commonest diseases of the brain are cerebral vascular conditions leading to *stroke*, already described (p.199). Similar damage to motor areas of the cerebral cortex during childbirth, or in childhood or adult life, constitutes *cerebral palsy*, giving rise to a patient commonly called 'spastic' (this is an upper motor neuron disease, p.206). Other types of demonstrable brain damage, including hereditary disorders such as *Down's syndrome* (*mongolism* – due to a chromosomal defect), may cause a wide range of physical and mental handicap. The gradual loss of mental faculties (memory, reason, thinking, etc.) in old age (in *senile dementia*) is usually due to cerebrovascular degeneration and some degree of cell loss in the brain, but *Alzheimer's disease*, which at least in some cases is due to genetic changes, is one variety of dementia where there is considerable loss of nerve cells in the cerebral cortex and other parts of the brain.

Parkinsonism (*paralysis agitans*) is an example of disease of the extrapyramidal system (p.206) occurring in later life, with tremors and uncoordinated jerky movements. It is now known to be due to a deficiency of the transmitter substance *dopamine* in the synaptic connections between some of the basal nuclei (pp.193 and 195).

Headache is not itself a disease but a symptom in a wide

variety of conditions, ranging from the harmless to dangerous intracranial disease. Most headaches do not originate in brain tissue itself but are due to the effects of vascular dilatation or constriction in pain-sensitive structures all over the head and neck, including blood vessels themselves in the scalp, meninges and brain. *Migraine* is a recurrent type of headache of unknown cause, more common in females; it is often associated with visual phenomena (such as flashes of light) which indicate the onset of an attack, and is accompanied by nausea and vomiting.

In such vital organs as the brain and spinal cord, and within the confines of the skull, the meninges and the vertebral canal, *infections* (usually blood-borne) are always serious. *Meningitis* may spread to the brain itself, where virus infections are called *encephalitis*. One of the dangers of meningitis is blockage of the outflow of CSF from the fourth ventricle, giving rise to one form of *hydrocephalus* (p.133), and for these, and other reasons, permanent brain damage may result. Early antibiotic therapy is necessary to prevent or minimize such complications.

Epilepsy (*epileptic fits* or *epileptiform convulsive seizure*) is characterized by convulsive movements accompanied by varying degrees of loss of consciousness. The cause is often unknown but some cases are due to minute scars in the cerebral cortex that periodically cause sudden electrical discharges to spread through parts of the cortex and so stimulate motor and other neurons. Anticonvulsant drugs can diminish the frequency and severity of the fits.

Cerebral tumours, commonly *gliomas*, usually occur in the cerebral hemispheres and eventually make their presence felt by causing a general increase in intracranial pressure (with headache, vomiting and papilloedema, see p.166). Specific signs and symptoms (including epilepsy) occur depending on the tumour's site, which also indicates whether surgery and/or radiotherapy may be possible. Tumours may also arise in any part of the brain as a result of blood-borne *metastatic spread* from malignant growths in other organs, most commonly the lung, breast and skin.

Diseases of the spinal cord are less common than those of the brain. Infections of the cord (*myelitis*) include the virus disease *poliomyelitis* (p.201). One of the commoner nervous diseases that affects both brain and spinal cord is *multiple sclerosis* (MS). There are scattered (*disseminated*) areas of loss of myelin (*demyelination*) and scarring in various parts of the brain and cord (hence the older name *disseminated sclerosis*). Tracts in the brainstem, the posterior and lateral columns of the cord, and the optic nerves are particularly affected, and the effects depend on the anatomical sites of the lesions. Thus, there may be disturbances of sensation if sensory tracts are involved, clumsy limb movements when motor tracts or cells are affected, or partial blindness with optic nerve lesions. The disease is subject to periods of remission (or 'getting better') and exacerbation ('getting worse'), and since the cause has not been defined (although it is now considered to be an autoimmune disease, p.70) there is no specific treatment.

Complete transection of the spinal cord, as in severe fracture of the vertebral column ('broken back'), results in loss of all voluntary movement and sensation below the level of the injured cord segment, because all the ascending and descending tracts have been interrupted. Control of bladder and anal sphincters is also lost. In transection of one half of the cord (*hemisection, Brown–Séquard syndrome*), there is loss of movement and of touch sensation below the level of the injury on the same side as the injury (because of interruption of the corticospinal tract and posterior column of that side), and the loss of pain and temperature sensation on the opposite side (due to interruption of the spinothalamic tract, which is a crossed tract, p.208).

Another condition that may be mentioned as a further example of the applied anatomy of the spinal cord is *syringomyelia*. Here, the minute central canal of the cord becomes enlarged in various places, and one of the prominent effects is *dissociated sensation* (p.207). The pain and temperature (*spinothalamic*) fibres that cross just in front of the canal from one side to the other are interrupted by the forward 'ballooning' of the canal in the affected region, so causing a loss of these sensations in skin areas where touch sensation remains intact (because the posterior columns have not been affected). Thus, the patient runs the risk of being burnt by touching hot objects – being aware of touching them, but unable to appreciate their heat.

The various rare but distressing types of *motor neuron disease* which lead to progressive muscular weakness (and are sometimes called *muscular atrophies*) are **neural** in origin, but the *muscular dystrophies* are degenerative disorders of skeletal *muscle fibres*, not of nerves.

CHAPTER 18

UPPER LIMB

PRINCIPAL FEATURES

Bones and Joints (see *Table* **18.1**)

Important Muscles (see *Table* **18.2**)

Important Nerves (see *Table* **18.3**)

Important Arteries (see *Table* **18.4**)

Important Superficial Veins (see *Table* **18.5**)

SHOULDER

The **shoulder** is the region at the upper end of the upper limb, and its principal feature is the **shoulder joint**. The **acromion of the scapula** is the highest point of the shoulder (positioned just above the joint, **18.1** and **18.3**), and here the acromion is attached to the clavicle at the **acromioclavicular joint** (see below).

SHOULDER GIRDLE

The bones of the **shoulder girdle** (p.29) are the **clavicle** and **scapula**, and the **acromioclavicular joint** is the only joint between these two bones (**4.1** and **18.1**). At its inner end, the clavicle forms the **sternoclavicular joint** with the manubrium of the sternum (**4.1** and **15.2**); this is the only bony connection between the shoulder girdle and the rest of the skeleton − the remaining attachments are purely muscular. Some of the body's more extensive muscles attach the girdle bones and the humerus to the rest of the skeleton.

At the front they include **pectoralis major** (from the Latin for 'chest', see **6.1a** and **18.4**), extending from the sternum and the medial half of the clavicle to the lateral lip of the humerus (**18.1a**). At the back, **trapezius** (**6.2a**, named from the shape it makes with its fellow of the opposite side − like an old-fashioned kite) has a wide origin from the skull down to T12 vertebra, and then converges on to the spine of the scapula, while **latissimus dorsi** (the 'flattest muscle of the back', **6.2a**) extends from fascia of the lower back and iliac crest to the floor of the intertubercular groove of the humerus (**18.1a**). At the side of the chest, **serratus anterior** (**6.1b**) runs back from its serrated or 'saw-toothed' origins

Table 18.1 Bones and joints of the upper limb		
Shoulder girdle	clavicle and scapula	Joined at the acromioclavicular joint, with the clavicle joined to the sternum at the sternoclavicular joint.
Bone of the arm	humerus	The head of the humerus makes the shoulder joint with the glenoid cavity of the scapula. Lower end − see below.
Bones of the forearm	radius and ulna	The lower end of the humerus makes the elbow joint with the ulna and the radius, and each end of the radius and ulna articulate with each other to form the proximal and distal radio-ulnar joints, enabling the lower end of the radius to rotate round the ulna (pronation and supination).
Bones of the wrist and hand	Eight carpal bones, five metacarpal bones, two phalanges for the thumb and three for each of the fingers	Three of the carpal bones make the wrist joint with the lower end of the radius. There are also carpometacarpal, metacarpo-phalangeal and interphalangeal joints.

Table 18.2 Important muscles of the upper limb

Trapezius	A muscle attaching the scapula to the trunk, and important in helping to raise the arm high.
Serratus anterior	A muscle attaching the scapula to the trunk, important in forward punching movements.
Deltoid	Covering the shoulder, important in raising the arm from the side.
Pectoralis major	The large muscle passing from the front of the chest to the humerus, important in bringing the raised arm towards the chest and moving the arm forwards.
Latissimus dorsi	The large muscle passing from the middle of the back to the humerus, important in bringing the raised arm towards the chest and moving the arm backwards.
Biceps	The prominent muscle on the front of the arm, important in bending the elbow and supinating the forearm.
Triceps	The only muscle of the back of the arm, important in straightening the elbow.
Brachioradialis	Passing from the lower end of the humerus to the lower end of the radius, important for holding the elbow at the desired angle.
Flexor carpi radialis	A landmark at the front of the wrist.
Interossei and lumbricals	For fine movements of the fingers.
Thenar muscles	Small muscles of the thumb, important for the movement of opposition of the thumb, allowing gripping.

Table 18.3 Important nerves of the upper limb

Axillary nerve	Supplying the deltoid muscle and skin overlying it.
Radial nerve	Supplying all the muscles on the back of the arm and forearm. Since these muscles are mainly extensors of the elbow, wrist and joints in the hand, the radial nerve is the nerve of extension in the upper limb.
Ulnar nerve	Supplying the small muscles of the hand that are responsible for intricate movements of the fingers, and skin on the ulnar side of the hand.
Median nerve	Supplying the muscles that enable the hand to grip between thumb and fingers, and skin on the radial side of the palm.
Musculocutaneous nerve	Supplying biceps and brachialis and skin of the lateral side of the forearm.

Table 18.4 Important arteries

Axillary artery	The main artery of the limb, the continuation of the subclavian artery into the axilla.
Brachial artery	The continuation of the axillary artery into the front of the arm, dividing at the front of the elbow into the radial and ulnar arteries, and used for taking the blood pressure.
Radial artery	The most 'used' artery in the body, for feeling the pulse at the front of the wrist.

Table 18.5 Important superficial veins of the upper limb

Cephalic vein	The main superficial vein on the lateral side of the limb.
Basilic vein	The main superficial vein on the medial side of the limb; the vein of choice for long venous catheters.

from the upper eight ribs to the whole length of the vertebral border of the scapula (**18.1a**). The smaller muscles attached to the scapula are **pectoralis minor** (the 'smaller chest muscle', **6.1b**, and an important landmark in the axilla, p.220), and **levator scapulae** (the 'elevator of the scapula') and the two

rhomboids (name from their shape, like oblique parallelo-grams) at the back (**6.2b**).

Movements in the shoulder region depend not only on movement at the shoulder joint itself but also on the way the scapula and clavicle can move. The great mobility of the shoulder girdle gives the upper limb a greater range of movement than the lower limb, where the hip or pelvic girdle is a solid bone (hip bone) firmly united to the vertebral column by a large and almost immobile joint (the sacroiliac joint, p.289).

CLAVICLE, STERNOCLAVICULAR AND ACROMIOCLAVICULAR JOINTS

The **clavicle** (**18.1a**) is approximately 'S'-shaped; its whole length is subcutaneous and is easily seen and felt. It acts as a strut holding the shoulder out at the side of the chest. (Animals such as cats and dogs have no clavicles, so their shoulder blades can lie further forward on the chest to bring the front limbs close together). The inner two-thirds of the clavicle bulges forwards in order to allow the subclavian

---

Fig. 18.1 Bones of the right shoulder.
(**a**) Scapula, clavicle and upper end of the humerus, from the front.
(**b**) Radiograph.

---

1 Acromioclavicular joint
2 Sternal end of clavicle, for articulation with the sternum at the sternoclavicular joint
3 Superior angle of scapula
4 Vertebral (medial) border. Serratus anterior is attached along its whole length
5 Inferior angle
6 Subscapular fossa, for the origin of subscapularis
7 Axillary (lateral) border
8 Margin of glenoid cavity, the very shallow 'socket' of the shoulder joint
9 Coracoid process
10 Head of humerus, forming the shoulder joint with the glenoid cavity of the scapula
11 Anatomical neck, the margin of the smooth head
12 Surgical neck, the upper part of the shaft below the head (10) and the tuberosities (13 and 14)
13 Lesser tuberosity, to which subscapularis is attached
14 Greater tuberosity. Supraspinatus is attached to the uppermost part shown here; farther back and lower down it receives infraspinatus and teres minor
15 Lateral lip of intertubercular (bicipital) groove, for the attachment of pectoralis major
16 Floor of intertubercular groove, for attachment of latissimus dorsi. The tendon of the long head of biceps is lodged in the groove
17 Medial lip of intertubercular groove, for attachment of teres major

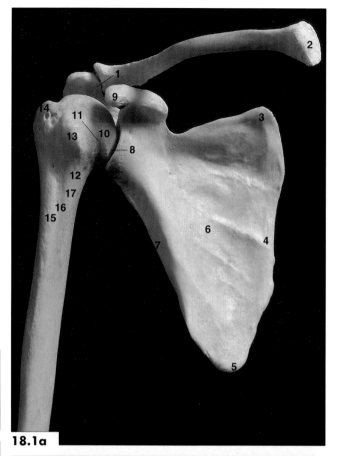

18.1a

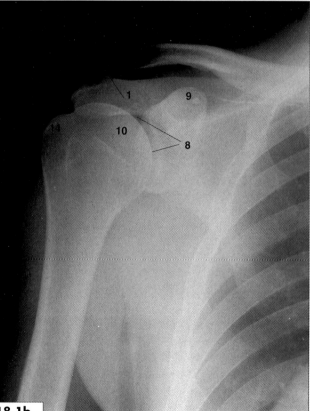

18.1b

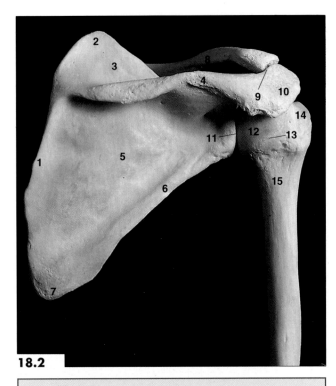

18.2

Fig. 18.2 Bones of the right shoulder, from behind.

1 Medial (vertebral) border of scapula
2 Superior angle
3 Supraspinous fossa, for origin of supraspinatus
4 Spine, for attachment of trapezius to its upper margin and deltoid to much of its lower margin
5 Infraspinous fossa, for origin of infraspinatus
6 Lateral (axillary) border, for origin of teres minor
7 Inferior angle, for origin of teres major
8 Clavicle
9 Acromioclavicular joint
10 Acromion, for attachment of deltoid to its outer margin
11 Rim of glenoid cavity
12 Head of humerus
13 Anatomical neck
14 Greater tuberosity, for insertions of supraspinatus, infraspinatus and teres major in that order from above downwards
15 Surgical neck

vessels and the nerves of the brachial plexus to pass from the side of the neck to the arm without being constricted (p.182). The bulbous inner end of the clavicle is at the side of the jugular notch at the top of the manubrium of the sternum where the two bones, together with the first costal cartilage, form the **sternoclavicular joint** (15.2). Part of the clavicle projects well above the manubrium, and the bones are held together not only by the joint capsule but by an **articular disc** of fibrocartilage which divides the joint cavity into two and,

by its firm attachment to the top of the clavicle, anchors the clavicle to the first costal cartilage. Another ligament – the **costoclavicular** – is highly important in holding the clavicle in its normal position by running from the under surface of the clavicle to the junction of the first rib and its costal cartilage (**18.5b**). This ligament forms a fulcrum about which a small amount of gliding and rotatory movement of the clavicle can take place. The disc and costoclavicular ligament form such strong connections that dislocation of the sternoclavicular joint is rare; fracture of the clavicle and dislocation of the acromioclavicular joint are much commoner.

The clavicle is among the bones most commonly *fractured*, usually by a fall on the outstretched hand when the clavicle has to take the strain between the arm and the rest of the bodyweight; the break occurs where the curve of the bone is greatest. The broken ends usually override one another as the weight of the arm pulls the outer fragment downwards, and sternocleidomastoid (**18.4**) tilts the inner fragment upwards. The shoulder may have to be braced back (e.g. by a figure-of-eight bandage across the back between both shoulders) to bring the bone ends back into line.

The **acromioclavicular joint** between the rather small and flat outer end of the clavicle and the acromion of the scapula (**18.1**–**18.4**) depends for its stability largely on the **coracoclavicular ligament**. This passes from the upper surface of the coracoid process of the scapula to the adjacent under surface of the clavicle (**18.5b**), so tethering the clavicle to the coracoid. A fall on to the side of the shoulder can dislocate the joint; its bony surfaces are slightly obliquely placed so that it is easy for the acromion to slip under the end of the clavicle, tearing the coracoclavicular ligament and causing an obvious step-like deformity beyond the end of the clavicle. Note that a small step down of about 2 mm is normal, with the end of the clavicle lying at a slightly lower level than the upper surface of the acromion (**18.3**).

DELTOID MUSCLE

Forming a cover for the whole shoulder region is the triangular-shaped **deltoid muscle** (named from the Greek capital letter delta, 'Δ', **6.1**, **6.2**, **18.3** and **18.4**), passing from the clavicle, the acromion and the spine of the scapula to its attachment halfway down the outer side of the shaft of the humerus. The tip or outermost part of the shoulder is formed by this muscle overlying the greater tuberosity of the humerus (not by the acromion, which does not extend so far out). The main function of deltoid is to *abduct* the humerus, but its anterior and posterior fibres can act as medial and lateral rotators respectively. (For a description of movements, see p.217.) The muscle is supplied by the axillary (circumflex) nerve.

The deltoid muscle has further importance as a possible site for *intramuscular injections*. The site selected should be the most lateral part of the muscle and no more than 4 cm

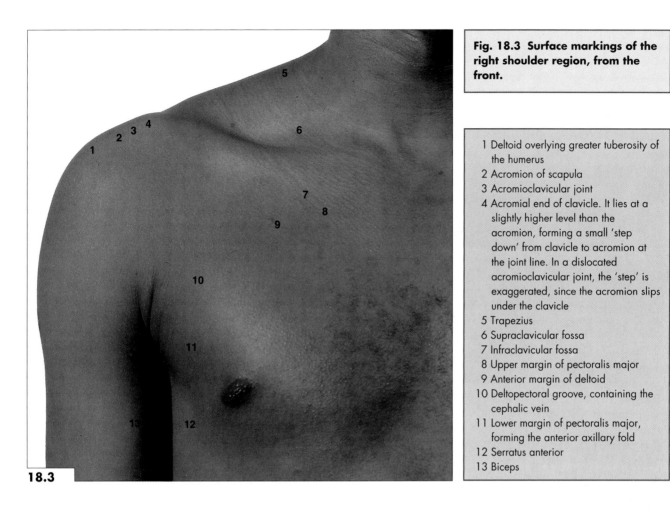

18.3

1 Deltoid overlying greater tuberosity of the humerus
2 Acromion of scapula
3 Acromioclavicular joint
4 Acromial end of clavicle. It lies at a slightly higher level than the acromion, forming a small 'step down' from clavicle to acromion at the joint line. In a dislocated acromioclavicular joint, the 'step' is exaggerated, since the acromion slips under the clavicle
5 Trapezius
6 Supraclavicular fossa
7 Infraclavicular fossa
8 Upper margin of pectoralis major
9 Anterior margin of deltoid
10 Deltopectoral groove, containing the cephalic vein
11 Lower margin of pectoralis major, forming the anterior axillary fold
12 Serratus anterior
13 Biceps

below the acromion, because the axillary nerve (which supplies the muscle) curls round the back of the humerus at a level 5–6 cm below the acromion.

SHOULDER JOINT

The **shoulder joint** is a ball-and-socket joint between the **glenoid cavity** of the **scapula** and the **head** of the **humerus** (**18.1** and **18.5a**). It is the *most mobile* joint in the body and the joint most commonly dislocated since the 'socket' formed by the glenoid cavity, although slightly deepened by a ring of fibrocartilage (the **glenoid labrum**) along its rim, is shallow and the capsule is very lax (**18.5b**). *Stability* depends entirely on the **muscles** surrounding the joint, and there are four that are particularly important in holding the head of the humerus against the glenoid cavity: **subscapularis** in front, **supraspinatus** across the top, and **infraspinatus** and **teres minor** at the back (**6.2b** and **18.5a**). All of them blend with the capsule of the joint before reaching their insertions. These four muscles are often called by clinicians the **rotator cuff muscles**, because they form a semicircular cuff round the upper end of the humerus and three of the four can rotate the humerus – subscapularis medially, and infraspinatus and teres minor laterally. The joint is further strengthened by a strong band of fibrous tissue – the **coracoacromial ligament**,

between the coracoid process and the acromion (**18.5b**) – which forms a protective arch above it. A bursa, variously known as the **subdeltoid** or **subacromial bursa** (**18.5b**) lies under the acromion and the upper part of deltoid and fuses with the outer part of supraspinatus tendon and its insertion.

Movements

As a reminder of the positions of the muscles to be mentioned here, refer to **6.1** and **6.2**.

Supraspinatus, being immediately above the middle of the joint, is not in a position to rotate the humerus, but is important in assisting deltoid in *abduction*; the two muscles work together. (The common view, that supraspinatus initiates abduction and then deltoid takes over, may not be correct.) The subacromial bursa (see above) helps to eliminate friction between the fixed acromion and the mobile muscles. If the bursa or tendon is diseased (as in *subacromial bursitis* or *supraspinatus tendinitis*) there is a 'painful arc' of movement from about 60° to 120° of abduction, when the bursa and tendon are subjected to pressure as they slip under the outer margin of the acromion. Beyond this point, when the bursa has moved completely under cover of the acromion, further movement is not painful.

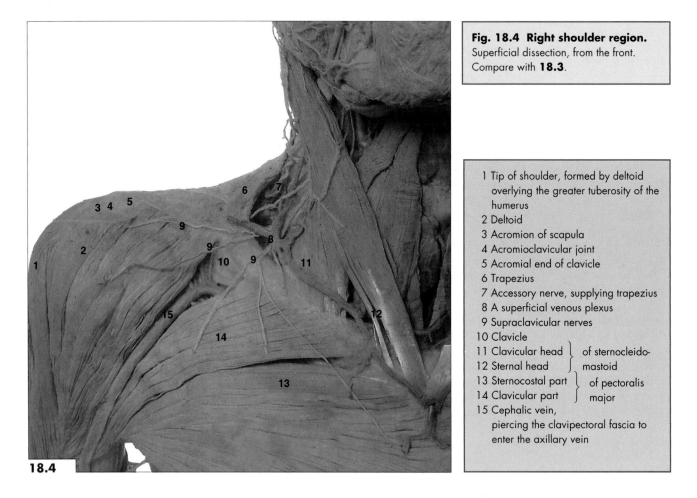

Fig. 18.4 Right shoulder region.
Superficial dissection, from the front.
Compare with **18.3**.

1 Tip of shoulder, formed by deltoid
  overlying the greater tuberosity of the
  humerus
2 Deltoid
3 Acromion of scapula
4 Acromioclavicular joint
5 Acromial end of clavicle
6 Trapezius
7 Accessory nerve, supplying trapezius
8 A superficial venous plexus
9 Supraclavicular nerves
10 Clavicle
11 Clavicular head ⎱ of sternocleido-
12 Sternal head ⎰ mastoid
13 Sternocostal part ⎱ of pectoralis
14 Clavicular part ⎰ major
15 Cephalic vein,
   piercing the clavipectoral fascia to
   enter the axillary vein

18.4

The amount of abduction possible at the shoulder joint itself is limited to about 120° or less, but the arm can be raised sideways right up to the side of the head; this further movement can occur partly because the **humerus** becomes *rotated laterally*, so getting the greater tuberosity out of the way of the acromion, and also because the scapula rotates on the chest wall to tilt the glenoid cavity upwards. The *scapular rotation* is brought about mainly by the *lower half* of **serratus anterior** which pulls the lower angle of the scapula forwards, and at the same time the *upper part* of **trapezius** pulls the acromion upwards (**18.5c**). A patient with a damaged accessory nerve (p.181), and hence a paralyzed trapezius, will have difficulty in reaching up to get something off a high shelf. The main *lateral rotator* of the humerus is **infraspinatus**.

When the *whole* of serratus anterior contracts, it pulls the scapula forwards on the chest wall (*protraction*), as in punching movements (the boxer's 'straight left'), without rotating it. *Retraction*, bringing it back to the normal position, depends on the middle part of trapezius and the underlying rhomboid muscles. Shrugging the shoulder (i.e. pulling the scapula upwards) depends on levator scapulae and the upper part of trapezius, while the lower part of the muscle helps to pull it down to its normal position (**6.2**).

Bringing the abducted arm back towards the chest wall (*adduction*) is carried out by the large pectoralis major, latissimus dorsi and teres major muscles, although in the usual upright position gravity plays a large part and the abductor muscles are important in controlling the adduction. *Flexion* at the shoulder (carrying the arm forwards) is brought about by the clavicular part of pectoralis major and the anterior part of deltoid, with some assistance from coracobrachialis and the long head of biceps. The opposite movement of *extension* (moving the arm backwards) is due to teres major, latissimus dorsi and the posterior part of deltoid, with assistance from the sternocostal part of pectoralis major when extension is being performed from the flexed position. Circumduction is the name given to the sequence of different movements at the shoulder joint occurring in such actions as serving at tennis or pitching a ball.

Because of its mobility and the shallowness of the glenoid cavity, the shoulder joint may be *dislocated* fairly easily, usually by a fall on the outstretched hand. The capsule is torn and the head of the humerus most often comes to lie in front of or below the glenoid cavity, being pulled inwards by subscapularis. The side of the shoulder has a flattened appearance because the greater tuberosity no longer causes the overlying deltoid to bulge outwards and the acromion

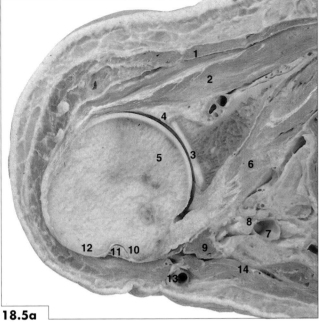

18.5a

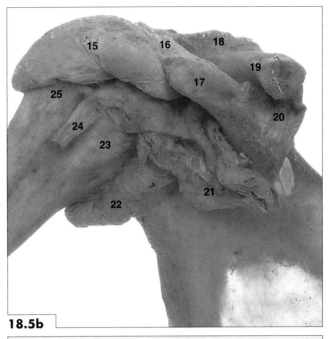

18.5b

Fig. 18.5 Right shoulder joint.

(a) Horizontal section through the centre of the joint, seen from above.

(b) From the front, with the joint cavity injected with resin, to show the bulge of the lower part of the capsule and the continuity of the cavity with subscapularis bursa. The subacromial bursa has also been injected separately; it does not communicate with the joint cavity.

(c) Diagram of scapular rotation. The acromion is pulled upwards by trapezius and the lower angle forwards by the lower half of serratus anterior, so tilting the glenoid cavity upwards.

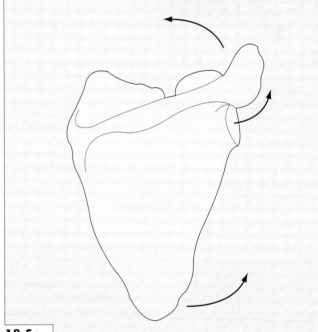

18.5c

1 Deltoid, embracing the whole region
2 Infraspinatus, passing behind the joint to the greater tuberosity (12)
3 Glenoid cavity of scapula, forming the very shallow socket of the joint
4 Glenoid labrum, forming a fibrocartilaginous rim which slightly deepens the socket
5 Head of humerus. Note the covering of hyaline cartilage on the articulating surfaces of the head and glenoid cavity (3).
6 Subscapularis, passing in front of the joint to the lesser tuberosity (10)
7 Axillary artery
8 Cords of brachial plexus, around the axillary artery (7)
9 Coracobrachialis and short head of biceps
10 Lesser tuberosity
11 Long head of biceps in intertubercular groove
12 Greater tuberosity, covered by deltoid (1)
13 Cephalic vein, in the groove between deltoid (1) and pectoralis major (14)
14 Pectoralis major
15 Subacromial bursa, distended by injected resin
16 Coracoacromial ligament
17 Coracoid process

18 Acromioclavicular joint
19 Clavicle
20 Coracoclavicular ligament, important for maintaining the stability of acromioclavicular joint (18)
21 Subscapularis bursa, communicating with the injected shoulder joint cavity (22)
22 Lowest part of shoulder joint capsule, distended by injection. The axillary nerve runs backwards immediately below this
23 Lesser tuberosity of humerus
24 Tendon of long head of triceps, emerging from the joint capsule into the intertubercular groove
25 Greater tuberosity

now becomes the most lateral part of the shoulder region. Since the axillary nerve is immediately beneath the capsule it may be damaged (in about 5% of dislocations), leading to paralysis of the deltoid and a small area of anaesthesia in the skin overlying the outer side of the muscle. With the joint dislocated it is obviously not possible to test the action of deltoid, but finding an area of anaesthesia in the skin over the muscle may give the clue to the nerve damage. There are several methods of reducing the dislocation. In one of the commonest (Kocher's method) the elbow is bent to a right angle and the forearm turned outwards (so laterally rotating the humerus and overcoming the tension in subscapularis), and then the elbow is moved medially across the chest so that the head of the humerus can slip back into place.

AXILLA

The **axilla** (**armpit**) is the space between the side of the chest and the arm; in addition to a mass of **fat** and **lymph nodes**, it contains the **axillary vessels** which become the main vessels of the upper limb, and the **cords** of the **brachial plexus** which give rise to all the main nerves of the limb (**18.6**).

BOUNDARIES

The **axilla** is roughly the shape of a pyramid whose base is the hairy skin easily seen when the arm is moved away from the side (abducted). The **apex** of the axilla is the triangular interval between the clavicle, scapula and first rib. Its **anterior wall** is formed by pectoralis major (p.213), with pectoralis minor under cover of it; the lower border of pectoralis major (**6.1a**) forms the lower anterior border (the **anterior axillary fold**) which can be felt easily between fingers and thumb. The **posterior wall** is mostly the subscapularis muscle on the front of the scapula (passing to the lesser tuberosity of the humerus), but the lower border (the **posterior axillary fold**, also easily felt) consists of teres major (**6.2b**) with the tendon of latissimus dorsi (p.213) curling round from below to end up in front of the teres muscle (**18.6**). The **lateral wall** is extremely narrow and is the floor of the intertubercular groove (the bicipital groove) of the humerus (**18.1a**) between the attachment of pectoralis major (to the lateral lip of the groove) and latissimus dorsi (to the floor itself, in front of the insertion of teres major into the medial lip of the groove). The **medial wall** is formed by the upper four ribs and the intercostal spaces, overlaid by the upper part of serratus anterior (**6.1b**).

The **skin** of the axillary floor is held up as the concavity of the armpit because it is attached by fascia to the lower border of pectoralis minor. Apart from many hair follicles and associated sebaceous glands, the skin contains **sweat glands** (p.18) which respond to emotional stimuli, so that this is an area to which deodorants are most commonly applied.

LYMPH NODES

The number of **lymph nodes** embedded in the axillary fat is variable, but averages about 35. They are traditionally classified as being in five groups, related to blood vessels of the anterior, posterior and lateral axillary walls and in the central and apical fat, but all eventually drain lymph to the apical group, which is continuous with the deep cervical nodes (p.181). Apart from draining lymph from the whole of the upper limb and from the trunk above the level of the umbilicus, they are of supreme importance because they also drain lymph from the **breast** – the commonest site for cancer in females (p.107).

Normal axillary lymph nodes are not usually palpable, but become so when affected by disease. Those draining lymph from, say, a septic finger may become enlarged and tender and perhaps the site of an axillary abscess which may have to be incised. However, when involved in cancerous spread, as from *carcinoma* of the breast, axillary nodes are painless but firm to the touch, as they are in *Hodgkin's disease* (*lymphadenoma*) and other lymphoid conditions. Damage to branches of the brachial plexus is a hazard of surgical removal of cancerous nodes.

BRACHIAL PLEXUS

The pectoralis minor muscle of the anterior wall of the axilla is unimportant as far as its effect on scapular movement is concerned, but in the anatomy and surgery of the axilla it is a most important landmark. It overlies the major blood vessels and nerves of the axilla (**18.6a** and **18.6b**), namely: the **axillary artery** and **vein**, and the three **cords** of the **brachial plexus** (which are grouped closely round the axillary artery). These brachial plexus cords (**7.4**) give rise to the major limb nerves: the **musculocutaneous nerve** from the lateral cord (on the lateral side of the artery), the **ulnar nerve** from the medial cord (medial to the artery), the **median nerve** from both medial and lateral cords, and the **radial** and **axillary nerves** from the posterior cord (behind the artery).

AXILLARY ARTERY AND VEIN

The **axillary artery** is the continuation of the subclavian artery at the outer border of the first rib (**8.3a**); at the lower border of the axilla it becomes the brachial artery. The **axillary vein** is on the medial side of the artery and the two vessels, together with the brachial plexus cords and their branches, are enclosed in a connective tissue sheath (the **axillary sheath**). This part of the brachial plexus can be *anaesthetized* by introducing local anaesthetic solution into the sheath so that it can percolate freely around the nerves; if the needle tip remains outside the sheath the result will be poor. The artery is used as the landmark and can be palpated with the arm abducted by pressing the fingertips up into the axilla and outwards towards the front of the humerus (as for palpating the upper end of the brachial artery, **18.7b**, but higher up); the artery lies *medial* to the humerus, not in front

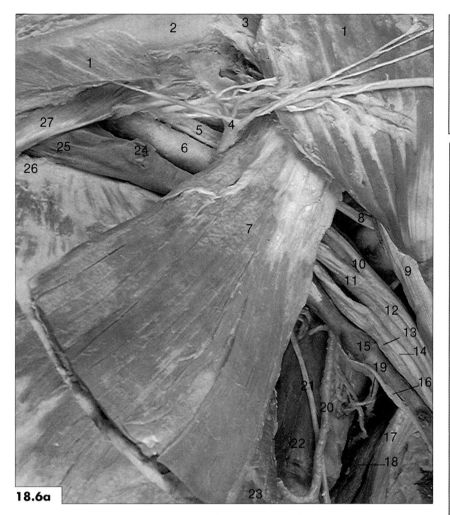

18.6a

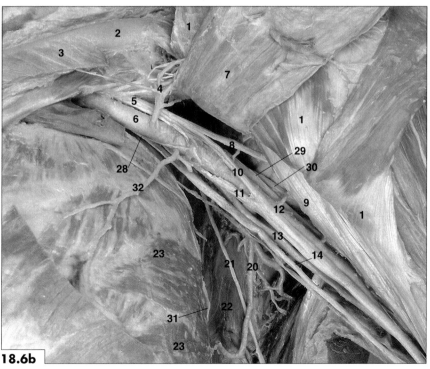

18.6b

Fig. 18.6 Left axilla and brachial plexus.
(a) Pectoralis major is reflected upwards and laterally to show pectoralis minor.
(b) Pectoralis minor is reflected upwards and laterally to show axillary artery and brachial plexus (with all veins removed)

1 Pectoralis major
2 Clavicle
3 Deltoid
4 Lateral pectoral nerve and thoracoacromial vessels
5 Lateral cord of brachial plexus, on the lateral side of the axillary artery (6)
6 Axillary artery, the continuation of the subclavian artery
7 Pectoralis minor, the landmark behind which lie the three cords of the brachial plexus around the axillary artery
8 Musculocutaneous nerve, arising from the lateral cord (**b**5) and entering coracobrachialis (9), a key identification feature
9 Coracobrachialis and short head of biceps
10 Lateral root ⎱
11 Medial root ⎰ of median nerve
12 Median nerve, with its roots (10 and 11) embracing the axillary artery (6)
13 Ulnar nerve, on the ulnar side of the axillary artery (6)
14 Medial cutaneous nerve of forearm, lying in front of the ulnar nerve (13)
15 Axillary vein, becoming the subclavian vein (25) as it crosses the first rib
16 Medial cutaneous nerve of arm, much smaller than the forearm nerve
17 Latissimus dorsi
18 Teres major
19 Circumflex scapular artery
20 Thoracodorsal artery
21 Thoracodorsal nerve, the supply for latissimus dorsi (17)
22 Subscapularis, forming with latissimus dorsi and teres major (17 and 18) the posterior wall of the axilla
23 Serratus anterior
24 Entry of cephalic vein into axillary vein
25 Subclavian vein
26 First rib
27 Subclavius
28 Medial cord of brachial plexus
29 Radial nerve ⎱ from posterior cord,
30 Axillary nerve ⎰ hidden behind axillary artery
31 Long thoracic nerve, the supply for serratus anterior (23)
32 Lateral thoracic artery

of it, so it will not be felt if pressing backwards. The needle is inserted just in front of the artery (pulsation transmitted to the needle suggests that it is in the right place), and the injection can be made after aspirating to ensure that the needle is not in a vessel.

ARM

The word 'arm' is commonly used to mean the whole upper limb, but strictly speaking it refers to the part of the limb between the shoulder and elbow, and to avoid confusion it can be called the **upper arm**. Its bone is the shaft of the **humerus** (see **4.1**) which is tubular but becomes flattened towards the lower end.

FRONT OF THE ARM
The front of the upper arm is made up mainly of three muscles – **biceps**, **brachialis** and **coracobrachialis** (**6.1**). Since the first two are large and both can cause flexion at the elbow (see below), this part of the arm is known as the *flexor compartment*.

Biceps – properly called **biceps brachii** (**6.1a**) meaning 'the two-headed muscle of the arm' to distinguish it from biceps femoris at the back of the thigh – is probably the best known muscle in the body; a 'bulging biceps' is the popular image of the strong man! Of its two heads of origin, the **long head** arises within the cavity of the shoulder joint from the upper margin of the glenoid cavity, by a tendon which is continuous with the glenoid labrum (p.217). The tendon runs over the top of the head of the humerus to reach the inter-tubercular groove (the bicipital groove) and emerges from the joint to become muscular. It is joined lower down the arm by the **short head** which arises with coracobrachialis from the tip of the coracoid process of the scapula. The insertion of the muscle is by a rounded tendon (**18.10d**) into the tuberosity of the radius (**18.9a**); the tendon is easily felt in front of the elbow where it is an important landmark (p.228; **18.10**). As it crosses the elbow joint the tendon gives off, on its medial side, a flat band of tissue (the **bicipital aponeurosis**, **18.10c**) which fuses with the deep fascia over the common flexor origin of the forearm muscles (p.228). The upper margin of the aponeurosis can be felt with the forearm partly flexed. Biceps is a powerful flexor of the elbow joint and a supinator (see pp.227–8).

Brachialis is under cover of biceps on the front of the humerus (**6.1b**) and is inserted into the tuberosity of the ulna in front of the coronoid process. It assists biceps as a flexor of the elbow joint. The much smaller **coracobrachialis** runs from the tip of the coracoid process of the scapula to halfway down the inner side of the shaft of the humerus. It plays a small part in flexion and adduction of the shoulder joint, but is most notable because the musculocutaneous nerve passes *through* the muscle – a useful identifying feature in

dissections of the axilla (**18.6b**). This nerve supplies all three flexor muscles.

BRACHIAL ARTERY, MEDIAN NERVE AND ULNAR NERVE
The **brachial artery** runs down the arm, just overlapped by the inner border of biceps (**18.7a**). The **median nerve** is in front of the artery, starting off as it leaves the axilla on the *lateral* side of the artery and slowly crossing as it goes down the arm so that in the cubital fossa at the front of the elbow, the nerve is *medial* to the artery (p.225). The **ulnar nerve** runs down *behind* the artery and enters the posterior compartment to lie in front of triceps so that at the elbow it is behind the medial epicondyle of the humerus (**18.11b** and **18.11c**). The **cephalic vein** passes up the arm near the outer border of biceps to reach the deltopectoral groove in front of the shoulder (**18.4**), but the **basilic vein** on the medial side pierces the deep fascia about halfway up the arm to become the **brachial vein** which runs beside the artery.

In the upper part of the upper arm, the brachial artery can be *palpated* (**18.7b**) by pressing with the fingertips *laterally* in the groove just behind biceps; here the artery lies not in front of the humerus but *medial* to it, so (like the axillary artery, see p.220) it will not be felt here if pressing backwards. When taking the blood pressure (p.59), the cuff of the sphygmomanometer is placed round the upper arm to occlude the artery here.

BACK OF THE ARM
The back of the upper arm is the *extensor* (or *posterior*) *compartment* and contains one muscle – **triceps (6.2)** – which is the extensor of the elbow joint. It has three origins or heads (hence its name, meaning 'three-headed'): from the lower margin of the glenoid cavity of the scapula (long head) and the upper and lower parts of the back of the humerus (lateral and medial heads). The three parts of the muscle join to form a single tendon which is inserted into the olecranon of the ulna. Triceps is supplied by the radial nerve.

RADIAL NERVE
After leaving the axilla the **radial nerve** passes *behind* the humerus (**18.8**), spiralling downwards from the medial to the lateral side to enter the flexor compartment. *Fractures* of the shaft of the humerus are liable to injure the nerve. A complete radial nerve *paralysis* is characterized by *wrist drop* – the inability to extend the wrist because all of the muscles on the back of the forearm are supplied by this nerve (p.230), and the flexor muscles of the wrist can now act unopposed to keep the wrist flexed. Triceps may not be affected because the branches that supply this muscle arise from the nerve very high up, before the usual level of injury. The area of skin anaesthesia in a radial nerve lesion is usually confined to a small coin-shaped area on the back of the hand beside the thumb (p.236).

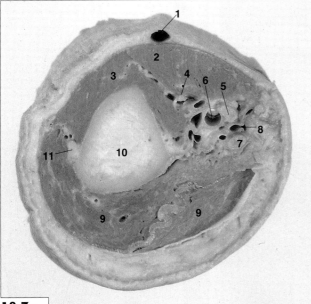

18.7a

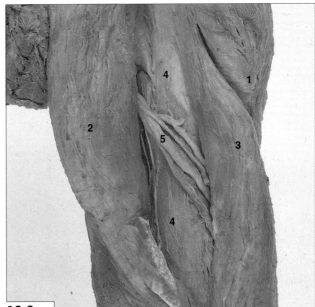

18.8

Fig. 18.8 Upper part of the right arm, from behind, with the long and lateral heads of triceps separated to show the radial nerve and branches.

1 Deltoid, lower end
2 Long head of triceps, on the medial side and displaced medially
3 Lateral head of triceps, on the lateral side and displaced laterally
4 Medial head of triceps, normally under cover of the other two heads (2 and 3) and crossed from medial to lateral by the radial nerve (5)
5 Radial nerve and branches to triceps, with branches of the profunda brachii vessels. At this level the upper fibres of the medial head of triceps (upper 4) intervene between the nerve and the humerus

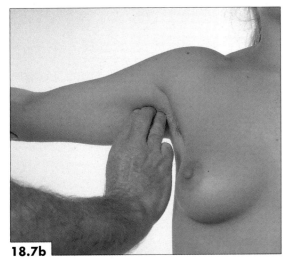

18.7b

Fig. 18.7 Right arm.
(a) Cross section of the middle of the arm, looking from below towards the shoulder.
(b) Palpation of the upper part of the brachial artery, pressing laterally (not backwards) because the artery at this level lies medial to the humerus, not in front of it.

1 Cephalic vein	7 Ulnar nerve
2 Biceps	8 Basilic vein
3 Brachialis	9 Triceps
4 Musculocutaneous nerve	10 Humerus
5 Median nerve	11 Radial nerve, at this high
6 Brachial artery. The	level in contact with the
accompanying veins will	humerus (10). Compare
join the basilic vein (8)	with the higher level in
to become the brachial	**18.8**.
vein at a higher level	

ELBOW

BONY PROMINENCES

At the sides of the elbow the **medial** and **lateral epicondyles** of the **humerus** (**18.9a**) are easily felt, especially the one on the medial side (the 'funny bone'). At the back, the junction of the **olecranon** with the **posterior border** of the **ulna** (**18.11a**) makes the bony 'point of the elbow' that is so easily knocked against things. With the elbow straight, there is a depression at the back on the outer side, and here can be felt the **capitulum** of the **humerus** and the **head** of the **radius** (**18.11b**). Any of the bony prominences are possible sites for pressure sores (**4.1c**), especially over the lateral epicondyle (when lying on the side with the arm under the body) and over the olecranon (when lying on the back).

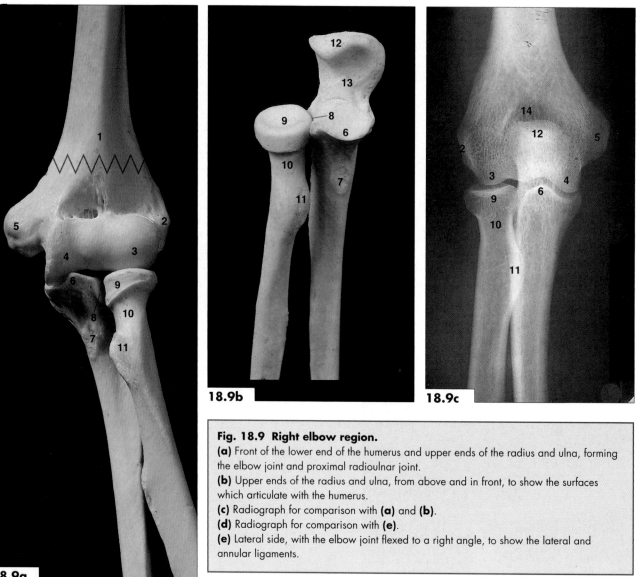

18.9b

18.9c

Fig. 18.9 Right elbow region.
(a) Front of the lower end of the humerus and upper ends of the radius and ulna, forming the elbow joint and proximal radioulnar joint.
(b) Upper ends of the radius and ulna, from above and in front, to show the surfaces which articulate with the humerus.
(c) Radiograph for comparison with **(a)** and **(b)**.
(d) Radiograph for comparison with **(e)**.
(e) Lateral side, with the elbow joint flexed to a right angle, to show the lateral and annular ligaments.

18.9a

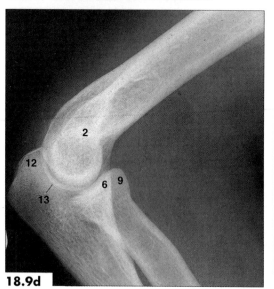

18.9d

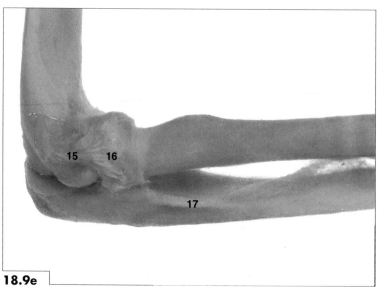

18.9e

1 Lower end of shaft of humerus, with the common site for supracondylar fracture indicated by the jagged line
2 Lateral epicondyle, the 'common extensor origin' for some extensor muscles of the forearm
3 Capitulum, the lateral part of the articular surface
4 Trochlea, the medial part of the articular surface which has a prominent medial margin. The capitulum (3) and trochlea of the humerus form the elbow joint by articulating with the trochlear notch of the ulna (13) and the head of the radius (9)
5 Medial epicondyle, the 'common flexor origin' of some flexor muscles of the forearm. It forms a more prominent 'knob' than the lateral epicondyle (2)
6 Coronoid process of ulna, at the front of the trochlear notch (13)
7 Tuberosity of ulna, below the coronoid process, for the attachment of brachialis
8 Radial notch of ulna. It articulates with the head of the radius (9) to form the proximal radioulnar joint
9 Head of radius
10 Neck of radius
11 Tuberosity of radius, on the ulnar side of the shaft below the neck for insertion of the tendon of biceps
12 Olecranon of ulna, at the back of the trochlear notch (13)
13 Trochlear notch of ulna, bounded behind by the olecranon (12) and in front by the coronoid process (6)
14 Olecranon fossa, on the posterior surface of the humerus (**18.11a**)
15 Lateral ligament, fusing with the annular ligament (16)
16 Annular ligament, embracing the head of the radius (9)
17 Supinator crest of ulna, for part of the origin of the supinator muscle

Falls on to the outstretched hand or on to the point of the elbow may fracture the lower end of the humerus a few centimeters above the joint (*supracondylar fracture*). Usually the upper part of the shaft of the humerus projects forwards and the small part remaining attached to the elbow region projects backwards. The forward projection of the upper part of the shaft, coupled with swelling of the damaged soft tissues, may constrict the **brachial artery** (see below) and interfere with the blood supply of the forearm muscles. If prolonged without correction for some weeks, a serious contraction of the flexor muscles of the forearm may occur (*Volkmann's ischaemic contracture*).

OLECRANON BURSA

There is a bursa under the loose skin over the posterior surface of the olecranon of the ulna – the **olecranon bursa** (**18.11b** and **18.11c**). Damage can cause an accumulation of fluid within it, producing a prominent swelling (*olecranon bursitis*) that may reach the size of a plum and, if infected, an abscess may form. If the bursa has to be aspirated (with a needle and syringe) to withdraw the fluid, or an abscess incised to let out pus, the presence of the **ulnar nerve** behind

the medial epicondyle must be remembered (**18.11b** and **18.11c**). The nerve can be felt easily here and rolled against the bone; its subcutaneous position in this area makes it the commonest site for injury. Since the effects of ulnar nerve injury chiefly involve the hand, they are discussed on p.238.

CUBITAL FOSSA

At the front of the elbow is the area known as the **cubital fossa** (**18.10**). It is triangular, with the base of the triangle being an imaginary line between the two epicondyles of the humerus. The sides which lead to the apex that points down the forearm are formed by **brachioradialis** laterally and **pronator teres** medially (**18.10c**). The fossa is a landmark for the three important structures which form its principal contents: the **tendon** of **biceps**, the **brachial artery** and the **median nerve**. They lie in that order from lateral to medial; the tendon is used as the guide to the position of the brachial artery. The **radial nerve** is under cover of brachioradialis and is not seen unless the muscle is displaced (**18.10d**). Just below the skin lie some important veins.

SUPERFICIAL VEINS

The **superficial veins** in front of the cubital fossa (**18.10a** and **18.10b**) commonly make an 'H' or 'M' pattern. The **cephalic vein** on the lateral side may be joined to the **basilic vein** on the medial side by an obliquely running **median cubital vein** (giving an 'H' pattern), or there may be a **median forearm vein** passing up the middle of the forearm to divide into a **median cephalic** and **median basilic vein** to join the cephalic and basilic veins respectively (the 'M' pattern). Other patterns may exist because like most veins these ones are variable and it is not necessary to be able to give a precise name to every one.

A light tourniquet round the upper arm usually makes these veins prominent, and together with the parts of them further down the forearm or on the back of the hand they are the ones most commonly used for taking *specimens* of venous blood and for giving *intravenous injections*. The same veins are used for blood transfusions and intravenous drips but preferably a little further down the forearm below the level of the skin crease at the bend of the elbow. This is so that the patient can still bend the elbow; it is uncomfortable to have to keep the elbow straight for prolonged periods.

The **basilic vein** just above the elbow is the vein of choice for *cardiac catheterization* (**15.24**). The catheter is pushed up the vein into the axillary and subclavian veins and so into the superior vena cava and the right atrium.

The veins are subcutaneous and lie superficial to the deep fascia. Thus the brachial artery and median nerve which lie *deep* to the fascia (**18.10c**) should not be damaged by a needle which only penetrates the subcutaneous tissues. Rarely the radial artery (normally a branch of the brachial artery in the cubital fossa) has an origin high in the arm, in which case it may lie subcutaneously in the fossa; its palpable or even

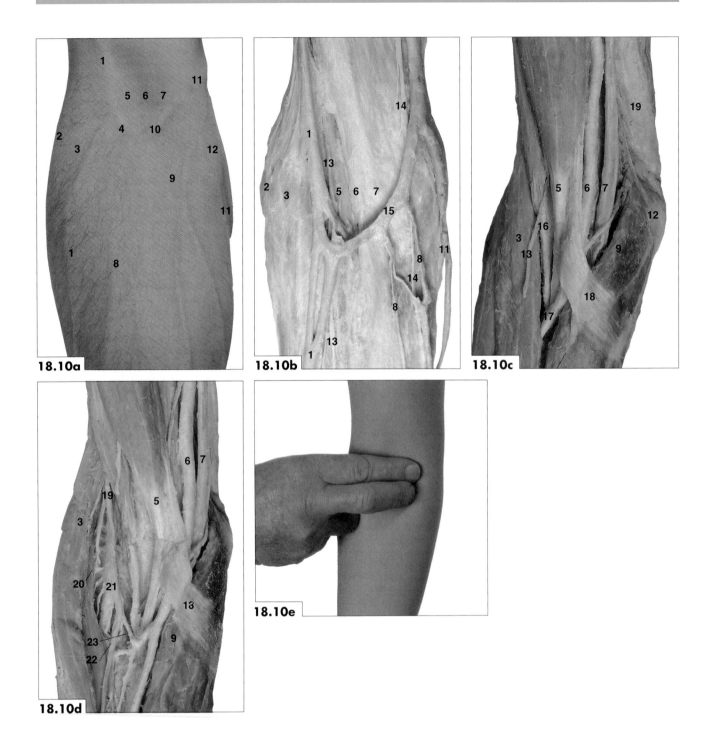

18.10a

18.10b

18.10c

18.10d

18.10e

visible pulsation distinguishes it from the veins.

BRACHIAL ARTERY

The **brachial artery** (see **8.3a**) is the one used for taking the *arterial blood pressure* (p.59). The vessel in the upper arm (**18.7a**) is occluded by a pneumatic cuff and, in order to listen for the pulsatile sounds as the air pressure in the cuff is slowly released, the stethoscope is placed over the artery as it lies in the cubital fossa (**18.10c** and **18.10d**). The precise position of the artery is found by *palpation* (**18.10e**): it lies **medial** to the biceps tendon which is easily felt. The median nerve is on the medial side of the artery; although it is near the surface here, the front of the elbow is not a common site for injury to the nerve compared with the wrist (p.232).

The brachial artery can be used as an alternative to the femoral artery for *catheterization* for *arteriography*, although it is not usually the first choice because it is smaller than the femoral and more liable to complications such as thrombosis. If the brachial artery has to be used, the catheter can be introduced into the artery in the cubital fossa and pushed

Fig. 18.10 Right elbow region, from the front.
(a) Surface markings and superficial veins.
(b) Dissection of superficial veins.
(c) Dissection of the cubital fossa, after removal of superficial veins and fascia but with the bicipital aponeurosis preserved.
(d) As in **(c)** but with brachioradialis displaced laterally to show the radial nerve.
(e) Palpation of the brachial artery.

1 Cephalic vein
2 Lateral epicondyle
3 Brachioradialis, forming the lateral boundary of the cubital fossa and displaced laterally in **(d)** to show the radial nerve (20) and its posterior interosseous branch (22)
4 Median cephalic vein
5 Biceps tendon, a palpable guide to the brachial artery (6) which is on the medial side of the tendon
6 Brachial artery, labelled where the stethoscope is placed for taking the blood pressure
7 Median nerve
8 Median forearm vein (double in **b**)
9 Pronator teres, the medial boundary of the cubital fossa
10 Median basilic vein
11 Basilic vein, often used for cardiac catheterization
12 Medial epicondyle
13 Lateral cutaneous nerve of forearm, the continuation of the musculocutaneous nerve
14 Medial cutaneous nerve of forearm
15 Median cubital vein
16 Brachialis, the floor of the cubital fossa
17 Radial artery, the superficial terminal branch of the brachial artery (6)
18 Bicipital aponeurosis, whose edges are sharply defined here because the deep fascia of the forearm has been removed
19 Radial nerve, dividing into a superficial branch (22) and deep (posterior interosseous) branch (21)
20 Extensor carpi radialis longus
21 Posterior interosseous nerve, passing through the supinator muscle (24) to supply the extensor muscles on the back of the forearm
22 Superficial branch of radial nerve, supplying skin but no muscles
23 Supinator

onwards into the aorta (checking its progress radiologically). On the left side, the catheter will pass through the left axillary and subclavian arteries to reach the aorta, while on the right it will traverse the right axillary and subclavian arteries and then the brachiocephalic (**8.3a**). Because of the

way the brachiocephalic, left common carotid and left subclavian arteries branch off the arch of the aorta, it is easier to get a catheter into the thoracic part of the aorta from the *left* brachial artery than from the right.

ELBOW JOINT
The **elbow joint** is the joint between the lower end of the humerus and the upper ends of the ulna and radius: the **trochlea of the humerus** articulates with the **trochlear notch of the ulna**, and the **capitulum of the humerus** articulates with the upper surface of the **head of the radius** (**18.9**). The head of the radius and the ulna also articulate with one another to form the **proximal radioulnar joint** (p.228) which shares the same joint cavity and capsule as the elbow joint. The radius and ulna are held together here by the **annular ligament** which fuses with the joint capsule. With the elbow straight (in full extension) the hook-like **olecranon of the ulna** fits into the **olecranon fossa** at the back of the **humerus**. This humeroulnar articulation is the main part of the elbow joint, and its pulley-like shape aids its stability. The humeroradial part of the joint is simply an apposition of slightly curved surfaces which hardly contribute to stability.

Movements
For all practical purposes the elbow acts as a hinge joint. *Flexion*, bringing the forearm up towards the arm, is carried out mainly by biceps and brachialis (supplied by the musculo-cutaneous nerve), with brachioradialis (supplied by the radial nerve) helping to keep the forearm in the required degree of flexion, usually in the midprone position (p.228). Triceps (which is also supplied by the radial nerve) is the extensor that straightens out the joint, although in the normal upright position gravity usually assists this movement. When testing for the action of triceps it is important to abduct the arm to 90° at the shoulder to eliminate the effect of gravity. (The movements of the radius on the ulna take place at the radio-ulnar joints and are discussed with the forearm, see p.228.)

Joint injuries at the elbow (such as fractures through the articular surface of the trochlea) are notorious for leading to diminution of the full range of movement when fully healed, and any attempts by the patient or medical attendants to increase mobility by *passive* movements, instead of by the use of the patient's own muscles, only makes things worse in the long run. *Dislocation* of the elbow joint may put tension on the structures in front of the joint, including the median nerve and brachial artery. Checking the radial pulse at the wrist and observing the colour and warmth of the fingers, to make sure that there is still good blood circulation, are important parts of the examination of these and other elbow injuries (such as supracondylar fractures, mentioned above).

FOREARM

RADIUS AND ULNA

The bones of the forearm are the **radius** and **ulna** (**4.1**). The **shafts** of the two bones are held together by a sheet of fibrous tissue – the **interosseous membrane** – whose fibres run obliquely downwards from radius to ulna so that pressure on the hand (which is attached mainly to the radius) is transmitted from the radius to the ulna, helping to equalize the strain. A unique feature of the forearm bones is that the lower end of the radius can be twisted round in front of the ulna (**4.1b**); since the hand is essentially attached to the radius, this means that the hand turns over as the radius rotates. The movement of turning the forearm and hand over (changing from looking at the palm to looking at the back of the hand) is *pronation*; turning it back to look at the palm again is *supination*. Twisting a door knob and using a screwdriver or corkscrew are typical examples of these alternating movements. In many everyday actions such as holding a cup, the forearm is held in the *midprone position*, halfway between full pronation and full supination. These movements take place at the superior and inferior radioulnar joints.

RADIOULNAR JOINTS, PRONATION AND SUPINATION

At the **proximal radioulnar joint**, the head of the radius rotates against the radial notch on the side of the ulna, being held in contact with it by the **annular ligament** which encircles the head (**18.9e**). Small children walking hand-in-hand with a tall adult can have the head of the radius dislocated by a sudden jerk pulling the radius out of the fibrous ring.

At the **distal radioulnar joint**, the lower end of the radius swings round the head of the ulna (**18.15**), the bones being kept in contact by a **triangular disc of fibrocartilage** which separates this joint from the wrist joint. The joint capsule is sufficiently lax to allow the radius to rotate forwards (pronate) almost 180° on the head of the ulna. (Note that the head of the ulna is at the lower end of the bone, whereas the head of the radius is at its upper end.)

In the position of *supination* with the elbow straight, the radius and ulna are parallel with one another but they are not quite in line with the humerus (**4.1a**); they make an angle with the humerus of about 170° (the *carrying angle*), which is due to the shape of the bones at the humeroulnar part of the elbow joint. In *pronation* the radius crosses over the ulna and so effectively brings the forearm into line with the humerus (**4.1b**). Note that only the radius rotates, not the ulna, but the ulna does move slightly outwards with pronation. When looking at the *back* of the hand with the forearm pronated, the *front* of the head of the ulna forms a prominent bulge above what is now the outer side of the wrist (**18.16a**).

The main supinators are the **supinator muscle** itself (**6.2b**), which is supplied by the radial nerve, and **biceps**, which is supplied by the musculocutaneous nerve. When the elbow is flexed, biceps is the most powerful supinator; it 'puts the corkscrew in and pulls the cork out'.

The main muscles concerned in pronation are pronator teres (**18.10d**) and pronator quadratus (both supplied by the median nerve). **Pronator quadratus**, a rectangular muscle (hence its name, quadrate or 'four-sided') passing between the lower ends of the ulna and radius under cover of the long flexor tendons above the front of the wrist (**18.13b**), is stronger than pronator teres because its fibres run straight across from the lower end of the ulna to the radius; **pronator teres** (from the Latin meaning 'long and rounded') runs very obliquely from the medial epicondyle of the humerus to halfway down the radius and so is working at less of a mechanical advantage than the transverse fibres of pronator quadratus.

FLEXOR AND EXTENSOR MUSCLES

The forearm muscles are divided into flexor and extensor groups, on the front and back of the forearm respectively (see **6.1** and **6.2**). Although a few act on the forearm only (like the pronators and supinator mentioned above), most have tendons which extend into the hand to move the thumb and fingers and/or the wrist. Some of the flexor muscles have a *common flexor origin* from the **medial epicondyle** of the humerus (**18.10c**), and some extensors from a *common extensor origin* from the **lateral epicondyle** (**18.11c**). Knowledge of the arrangement of their tendons at the wrist and in the hand (**18.13** and **18.17**) is more important than that of their bony origins.

Many of the muscle names indicate their positions. **Carpus** is the Latin for 'wrist' ('carpi' being the genitive of 'carpus' – 'of the wrist'), and there is a flexor muscle on the radial (lateral) and ulnar (medial) sides, hence the names **flexor carpi radialis** and **flexor carpi ulnaris**. It is quite easy to guess that **palmaris longus** is the long muscle of the palm. There are superficial and deep flexors of the digits or fingers – **flexor digitorum superficialis** and **flexor digitorum profundus** ('digitorum' being the genitive plural of 'digitus' – 'finger'). The reason for needing to know some of these names is because they are useful landmarks, as emphasized in the appropriate places in the text and figure legends.

Strain of some muscle fibres attached to the lateral epicondyle (i.e. to the common extensor origin) is commonly known as *tennis elbow*; its proper name is *lateral humeral epicondylitis*. It is caused by actions such as repeated extension of the pronated forearm, as in the backhand at tennis, or strenuous use of a screwdriver. Rest usually cures the condition, but incising the deep fascia over the muscles near the epicondyle is sometimes necessary to relieve the painful tension.

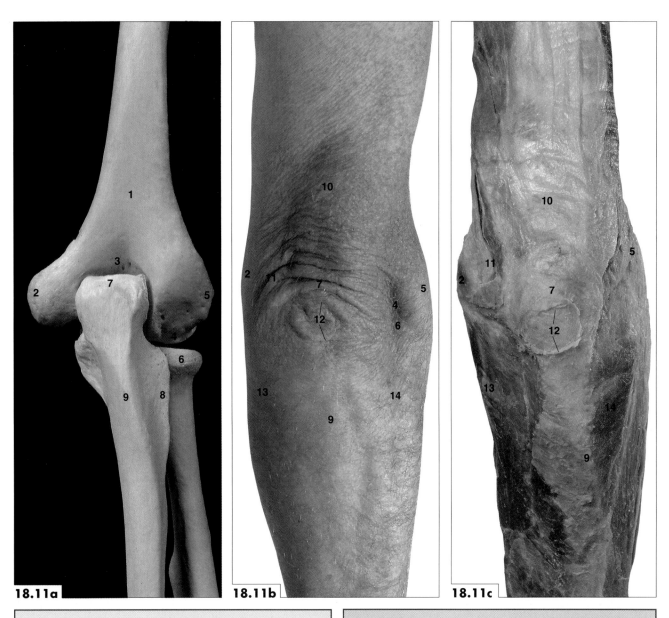

18.11a

18.11b

18.11c

Fig. 18.11 Right elbow region, from behind.
(a) Lower end of the humerus and upper ends of the radius and ulna.
(b) Surface markings.
(c) Superficial dissection, to show the olecranon bursa.

1 Shaft of humerus
2 Medial epicondyle
3 Olecranon fossa, occupied by olecranon of ulna (7)
4 Capitulum
5 Lateral epicondyle
6 Head of radius, articulating with capitulum of humerus (4)
7 Olecranon of ulna
8 Supinator crest of ulna
9 Posterior border of ulna, subcutaneous throughout its whole length
10 Triceps
11 Ulnar nerve; its most vulnerable position, behind the medial epicondyle (2)
12 Margins of olecranon bursa
13 Flexor carpi ulnaris
14 Extensor muscles

RADIAL AND ULNAR ARTERIES

The **radial** and **ulnar arteries** (into which the brachial artery divides in the cubital fossa, p.225) pass down the lateral and medial sides of the forearm respectively (**8.3a**). They are not subcutaneous until just above the wrist joint (p.231); the radial artery is under cover of brachioradialis, while the ulnar artery is mostly at a deeper level.

ULNAR, RADIAL AND MEDIAN NERVES

The **ulnar nerve** comes to lie on the medial side of the ulnar artery near the middle of the forearm, in which it supplies two flexor muscles (flexor carpi ulnaris and the medial half of flexor digitorum profundus). The **radial nerve** does not accompany the radial artery. It divides in the elbow region under cover of brachioradialis (**18.10d**) into an unimportant superficial branch which supplies skin on the back of the forearm and hand, and a highly important deep branch, usually called the **posterior interosseous nerve**, which penetrates the supinator muscle to reach the back of the forearm and supply the extensor group of muscles. The **median nerve** runs down the forearm between superficial and deep flexor muscles and supplies them. The positions of these major nerves at the wrist and in the hand are described below.

SUPERFICIAL VEINS

The largest **superficial veins** of the forearm, the **cephalic** and **basilic veins**, begin on the back of the hand and gradually move on to the flexor surface as they approach the elbow region (**18.10a**). On the front of the forearm they are used extensively for intravenous infusions and anaesthesia.

WRIST AND PALM OF THE HAND

BONES OF THE WRIST

The **wrist** is the region between the forearm and hand, but is often more loosely used to include the lowest part of the forearm. Bracelets and watches are said to be worn on the wrist but are often just above the wrist proper. The bones of the wrist – the **carpal bones** – consist of two rows of four bones each (**18.12**). A 'broken wrist' is the common term for fracture of the lower end of the radius, but could mean a fractured scaphoid or any other fracture in this region.

Fracture of the lower end of the radius (*Colles' fracture*) about an inch or so above the wrist joint is the commonest of all fractures, and is usually caused by a fall on the outstretched hand. It causes a characteristic 'dinner-fork' deformity because the lower fragment is displaced backwards and upwards by the force of the fall. Because of the upward displacement, the styloid process of the lower end of the radius comes to lie at the same level as the ulnar styloid; normally the radial styloid projects about a centimeter below the level of the ulnar styloid – a feature to note on a radiograph and on palpating the wrist (**18.12b**). The lower bone fragment must be forced forwards and downwards to restore the normal position.

WRIST JOINT AND MIDCARPAL JOINT

Three of the four of the first row of carpal bones (**scaphoid, lunate** and **triquetral**, **18.12a** and **18.12b**) make the wrist

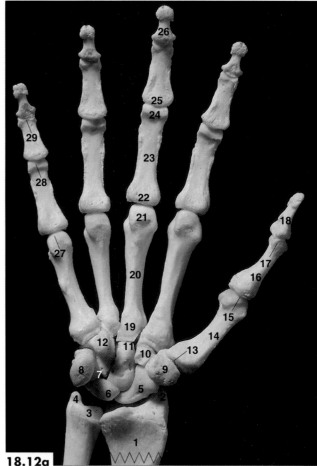

18.12a

joint by articulating with the **radius** and the triangular **disc** which joins the radius to the ulna. The ulna itself does not take part in the wrist joint (whose proper name is the **radiocarpal joint**) because the disc intervenes, separating the wrist joint from the distal radioulnar joint. The wrist joint capsule is reinforced at the sides by **collateral ligaments** attached to the radial and ulnar styloid processes, and at the front by the **radiocarpal ligament**.

Movements at the wrist take place not only at the wrist joint itself but also at the joint between the two rows of carpal bones (the **midcarpal joint**); pronation and supination (p.228) occur at the distal radioulnar joint, not at the wrist joint, but many activities using the hand involve a combination of these joints. *Flexion* and *extension* are produced by movement at both the wrist and midcarpal joints, but *adduction* and *abduction* (sometimes called *ulnar* and *radial deviation*, respectively) occur only at the wrist joint itself. The amount of possible ulnar deviation (about 45°) is much more than radial deviation, because the styloid process of the radius extends to a lower level than the ulnar styloid. Ulnar deviation is one of the characteristic features of rheumatoid arthritis of the wrist. At the flexor surface of the wrist there are usually three

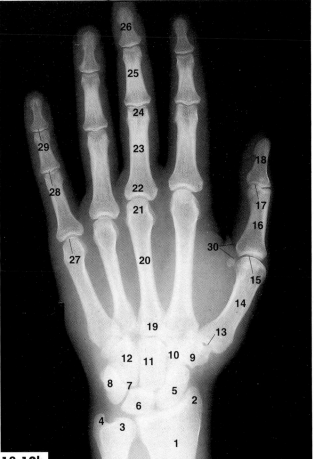

18.12b

Fig. 18.12 Right wrist and hand, from the front.
(a) Bones of the wrist and hand, palmar surface.
(b) Radiograph.

1 Lower end of radius, the most commonly fractured bone of the whole body, at the site indicated by the jagged line
2 Styloid process of radius, lying at a lower level than the ulnar styloid (4)
3 Head of ulna, at the lower end of the bone. Note that the head of the radius is at its upper end (**18.9**)
4 Styloid process of ulna
5 Scaphoid, the carpal bone most commonly fractured
6 Lunate, the carpal bone most commonly dislocated
7 Triquetral
8 Pisiform
9 Trapezium
10 Trapezoid
11 Capitate
12 Hamate
13 First carpometacarpal joint
14 First metacarpal
15 Metacarpophalangeal (MP) joint of the thumb
16 Proximal phalanx of thumb
17 Interphalangeal (IP) joint of the thumb
18 Distal phalanx of thumb
19 Base ⎫
20 Shaft ⎬ of third metacarpal
21 Head ⎭
22 Base ⎫
23 Shaft ⎬ of proximal phalanx of middle finger
24 Head ⎭
25 Middle phalanx ⎫ of middle
26 Distal phalanx ⎭ finger
27 Metacarpophalangeal (MP) joint ⎫
28 Proximal interphalangeal (IP) joint ⎬ of little finger
29 Distal interphalangeal (IP) joint ⎭
30 Sesamoid bones

transverse *skin creases* (**18.13a**); the middle one indicates the level of the wrist joint, but if there are only two creases the more proximal one overlies the joint line.

SCAPHOID AND LUNATE BONES AND THE TRAPEZIUM

Of all the carpal bones, the **scaphoid** (**18.12** and **18.15**) is the one most commonly *fractured*, usually transversely across the middle or 'waist' of the bone. Because of the way blood vessels penetrate the bone, fracture may deprive one fragment of its blood supply, leading to *avascular necrosis*. Fine hairline fractures are often not apparent on a radiograph taken at the time of injury, and only when some bone changes have occurred after two or three weeks may it be possible to confirm a suspected fracture. The poor vascularity prolongs healing, and this small bone may take longer to heal than any of the big limb bones.

The **lunate bone** (**18.12** and **18.15**), because of its half-moon shape, is the carpal bone most likely to be *dislocated*; such an injury is usually caused by the same kind of sudden stress that fractures the scaphoid. It may compress the flexor tendons and the median nerve in the carpal tunnel (see below).

The **trapezium**, at the radial end of the distal row, makes a saddle-shaped joint with the base of the first metacarpal (the **first carpometacarpal joint**, **18.12** and **18.15**), at which most of the unique movement of opposition of the thumb takes place (p.232).

RADIAL PULSE

The traditional site for 'feeling the pulse' is over the **radial artery** at the wrist (**18.13a–18.13c**). The artery lies under the skin in front of the lower end of the radius and on the lateral (radial) side of the tendon of flexor carpi radialis (a useful landmark for the pulse). The pulse is felt by pressing the artery backwards against the bone and the pronator quadratus muscle.

MEDIAN NERVE AND THE FLEXOR RETINACULUM

The **median nerve** at the level of the wrist joint (**18.13a** and **18.13b**) lies under the skin on the medial (ulnar) side of the tendon of flexor carpi radialis. In most people, another 'landmark' tendon, that of palmaris longus, lies on the medial side of the flexor carpi radialis tendon and slightly overlaps the median nerve. Bending the wrist slightly, with the fingers extended, will usually bring the palmaris longus tendon into prominence, but note that it is absent in 13% of arms. In the hand, the median nerve normally supplies the three small **muscles** of the **thenar eminence** at the base of the thumb (flexor pollicis brevis, abductor pollicis brevis and opponens pollicis), the **lumbrical muscles** of the index and middle fingers (p.238), and skin of the flexor surface of the thumb and the index and middle fingers (and perhaps part of the ring finger, **18.13d**). These thumb muscles have great importance since they help to carry out *opposition* of the thumb – carrying the thumb across the palm in the direction of the base of the little finger, so helping to grip things between thumb and fingers (**18.14**). This movement is largely possible because of the saddle-shaped surfaces of the first carpometacarpal joint. The cutaneous area of supply includes the skin over the pads of the thumb, index and middle fingers, which are in constant use for touching things and are therefore among the most important sensory areas in the whole body (p.45).

Being subcutaneous at the wrist, the median nerve is liable to damage by cuts on the front of the wrist, and this is the commonest site for *median nerve injury*. To check whether the median nerve is functioning normally, test for the action of abductor pollicis brevis by feeling the muscle contract under the skin when abducting the thumb. (Flexor pollicis brevis should not be chosen as the test muscle because it is frequently supplied by the ulnar nerve.) For the cutaneous supply by the median nerve, test sensation over the pulp of the index finger; despite the wide overlap possible from adjacent ulnar and radial nerves, this area of the index finger can be relied upon to have a median supply. Note that with a median nerve injury at the level of the wrist there will be no anaesthesia over the radial side of the palm of the hand, because the palmar branch of the median nerve which supplies this area arises several centimeters above the wrist.

After crossing the wrist joint, the median nerve enters the hand by passing underneath the **flexor retinaculum (18.13b)** – a dense band of fibrous tissue about the size of a small postage stamp, stretching between the scaphoid and trapezium on the radial side and the hamate and pisiform bones on the ulnar side. The space between the retinaculum and the carpal bones is commonly called the **carpal tunnel**, and the long flexor tendons and the median nerve pass through the tunnel. Here the nerve may be subject to *compression*, giving paraesthesia (a 'pins and needles' sensation) in the digits supplied by the nerve and weakness of the thumb muscles

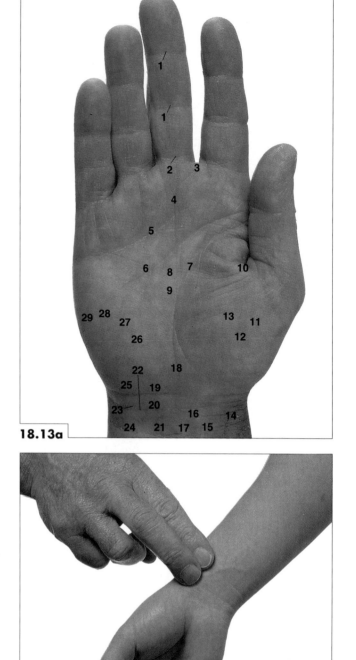

18.13a

18.13c

discussed above. This condition, the *carpal tunnel syndrome*, is often due to rheumatoid disease that causes swelling of the synovial membranes surrounding the flexor tendons. The retinaculum may have to be incised longitudinally to relieve the pressure, carefully avoiding damage to the median nerve

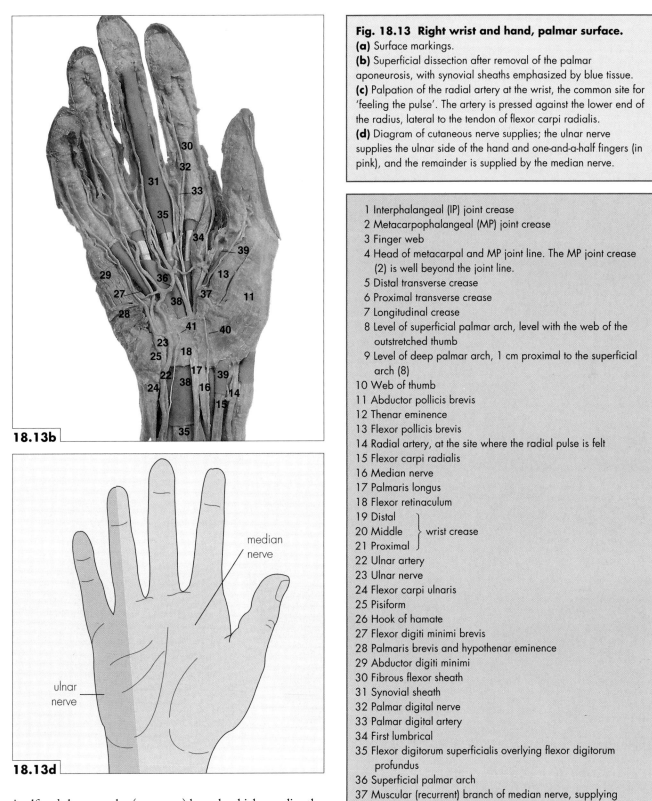

18.13b

18.13d

Fig. 18.13 Right wrist and hand, palmar surface.
(a) Surface markings.
(b) Superficial dissection after removal of the palmar aponeurosis, with synovial sheaths emphasized by blue tissue.
(c) Palpation of the radial artery at the wrist, the common site for 'feeling the pulse'. The artery is pressed against the lower end of the radius, lateral to the tendon of flexor carpi radialis.
(d) Diagram of cutaneous nerve supplies; the ulnar nerve supplies the ulnar side of the hand and one-and-a-half fingers (in pink), and the remainder is supplied by the median nerve.

1 Interphalangeal (IP) joint crease
2 Metacarpophalangeal (MP) joint crease
3 Finger web
4 Head of metacarpal and MP joint line. The MP joint crease (2) is well beyond the joint line.
5 Distal transverse crease
6 Proximal transverse crease
7 Longitudinal crease
8 Level of superficial palmar arch, level with the web of the outstretched thumb
9 Level of deep palmar arch, 1 cm proximal to the superficial arch (8)
10 Web of thumb
11 Abductor pollicis brevis
12 Thenar eminence
13 Flexor pollicis brevis
14 Radial artery, at the site where the radial pulse is felt
15 Flexor carpi radialis
16 Median nerve
17 Palmaris longus
18 Flexor retinaculum
19 Distal ⎫
20 Middle ⎬ wrist crease
21 Proximal ⎭
22 Ulnar artery
23 Ulnar nerve
24 Flexor carpi ulnaris
25 Pisiform
26 Hook of hamate
27 Flexor digiti minimi brevis
28 Palmaris brevis and hypothenar eminence
29 Abductor digiti minimi
30 Fibrous flexor sheath
31 Synovial sheath
32 Palmar digital nerve
33 Palmar digital artery
34 First lumbrical
35 Flexor digitorum superficialis overlying flexor digitorum profundus
36 Superficial palmar arch
37 Muscular (recurrent) branch of median nerve, supplying muscles of the thenar eminence
38 Ulnar bursa, enclosing flexor digitorum tendons
39 Radial bursa, enclosing flexor pollicis longus tendon
40 Palmar branch of median nerve
41 Palmar branch of ulnar nerve

itself and the muscular (recurrent) branch which supplies the thumb muscles and arises from the main nerve as soon as it emerges from under cover of the retinaculum. Note that, unlike the median nerve, the ulnar nerve (with its accompanying artery) passes into the hand *superficial* to the flexor retinaculum.

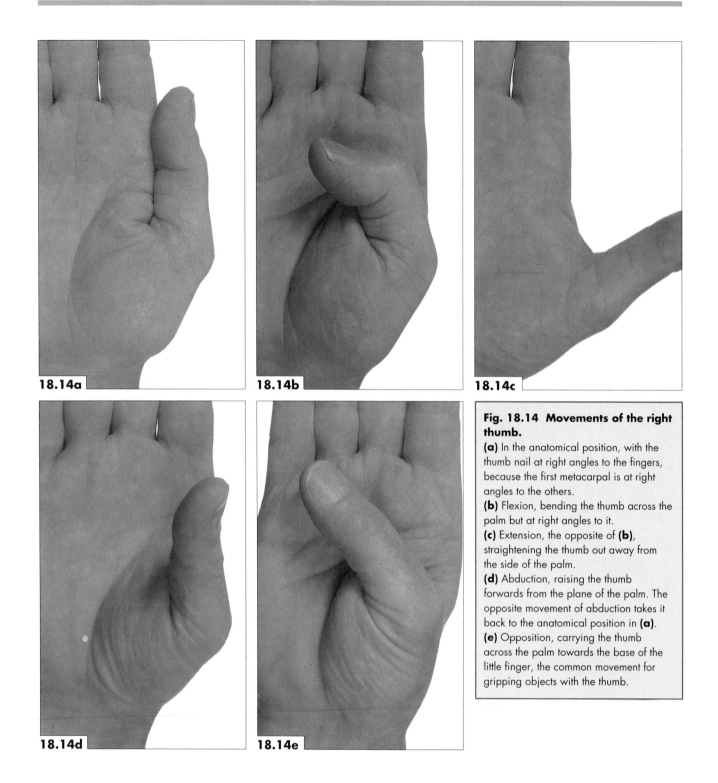

Fig. 18.14 Movements of the right thumb.

(a) In the anatomical position, with the thumb nail at right angles to the fingers, because the first metacarpal is at right angles to the others.

(b) Flexion, bending the thumb across the palm but at right angles to it.

(c) Extension, the opposite of **(b)**, straightening the thumb out away from the side of the palm.

(d) Abduction, raising the thumb forwards from the plane of the palm. The opposite movement of abduction takes it back to the anatomical position in **(a)**.

(e) Opposition, carrying the thumb across the palm towards the base of the little finger, the common movement for gripping objects with the thumb.

PALMAR APONEUROSIS

The **palmar aponeurosis** is a tough sheet of fibrous tissue underlying the skin of the palm, and its main part is roughly triangular. The 'apex' of the triangle is continuous with the flexor retinaculum, while the 'base' divides into slips that become attached to the skin of the proximal flexion creases of the fingers, and also to the sides of the metacarpophalangeal joint capsules. The overlying skin in the centre of the palm is firmly attached to the fascia; this gives a firm support for gripping and helps to protect underlying structures from undue pressure.

Dupuytren's contracture is a condition of unknown cause where there is an excessive production of fibrous tissue in the distal part of the aponeurosis leading to flexion deformity of

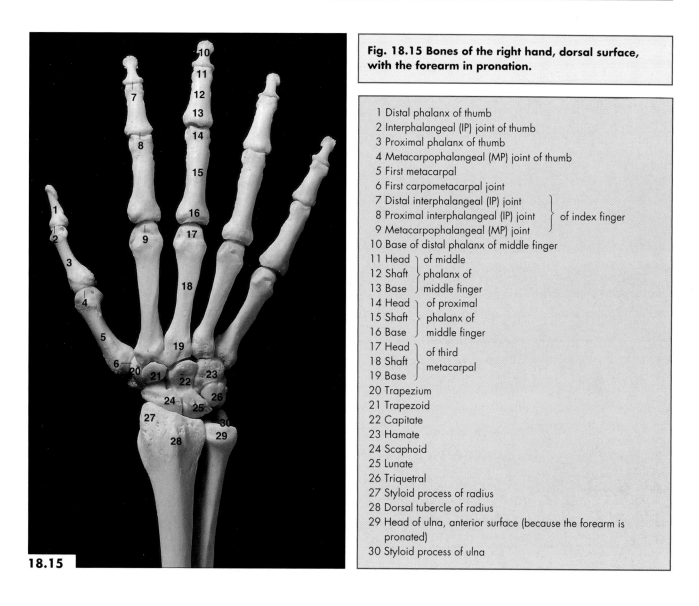

18.15

Fig. 18.15 Bones of the right hand, dorsal surface, with the forearm in pronation.

1 Distal phalanx of thumb
2 Interphalangeal (IP) joint of thumb
3 Proximal phalanx of thumb
4 Metacarpophalangeal (MP) joint of thumb
5 First metacarpal
6 First carpometacarpal joint
7 Distal interphalangeal (IP) joint ⎫
8 Proximal interphalangeal (IP) joint ⎬ of index finger
9 Metacarpophalangeal (MP) joint ⎭
10 Base of distal phalanx of middle finger
11 Head ⎫ of middle
12 Shaft ⎬ phalanx of
13 Base ⎭ middle finger
14 Head ⎫ of proximal
15 Shaft ⎬ phalanx of
16 Base ⎭ middle finger
17 Head ⎫
18 Shaft ⎬ of third
19 Base ⎭ metacarpal
20 Trapezium
21 Trapezoid
22 Capitate
23 Hamate
24 Scaphoid
25 Lunate
26 Triquetral
27 Styloid process of radius
28 Dorsal tubercle of radius
29 Head of ulna, anterior surface (because the forearm is pronated)
30 Styloid process of ulna

the fingers, usually beginning with the ring finger and spreading to involve the little and possibly other fingers. Nodules of tissue (not usually painful) can be felt under the skin. The condition is slowly progressive and requires surgery to remove the constricting tissue, but there is always the possibility of recurrence. Treatment by the injection of steroids or other drugs to control new connective tissue formation is not successful.

MIDPALMAR AND THENAR SPACES

The region in the ulnar side of the palm of the hand deep to the long flexor tendons of the middle, ring and little fingers is the **midpalmar space**. The similar area on the radial side under the tendons to the index finger is the **thenar space**. In the days before antibiotics, these spaces were important because penetrating injuries of the hand could cause infections which became 'walled off' in these spaces, but such infections are now rarely seen.

FLEXOR TENDONS AND TENDON SHEATHS

In their course along the fingers and thumb, the **long flexor tendons** are kept in place and prevented from bowing forwards by the **fibrous flexor sheaths** (18.13b). In order to prevent friction between the tendons and these sheaths, the tendons of each digit are enclosed by a **synovial sheath** which is inside the fibrous sheath. The synovial sheath of the long flexor muscle of the thumb (flexor pollicis longus – from 'pollex', the Latin for thumb) continues under the flexor retinaculum at the wrist, and here the sheath becomes known as the **radial bursa**. The synovial sheath of the little finger tendon not only continues under the retinaculum but also expands to include the other finger tendons and become known as the **ulnar bursa**. Injuries such as pinpricks, which happen to penetrate synovial sheaths, are possible sources of sheath infection; the sheaths are thinnest under the finger joint flexion creases, and these are the most dangerous places for penetrating injuries as far as synovial infection is concerned.

DIGITAL VESSELS

The main vessels of the fingers are the **palmar digital arteries** (**18.13b**), derived from the **superficial palmar arch** and running up the sides of the fingers immediately behind the corresponding nerves. Like vessels elsewhere, they have a sympathetic nerve supply to control the bloodflow through them and, in a cold environment for example, they will constrict to prevent heat loss, so contributing to the feeling of cold in the fingers. In some people, the hands and fingers seem to be unusually sensitive to cold, presumably due to sympathetic overactivity without an apparent cause, but in others arterial disease may restict bloodflow (as in *arterio-sclerosis* in diabetics). One of the more severe disturbances of finger bloodflow occurs in *Raynaud's disease*, where there are bouts of excessive vasospasm. Smoking must be avoided since it produces vasoconstriction of these vessels. In the severest cases, *sympathectomy* (p.47) may be required to eliminate the nervous impulses causing the constriction.

FINGER PADS AND PULP SPACES

The **skin** of the **finger** and **thumb pads** (supplied by the median and ulnar nerves, **18.13d**) is richly innervated to make the fingers and thumb the most highly discriminative parts of the body surface for touch, temperature and other sensations, in keeping with the importance of the hand in human life.

The pads of the tips of the fingers and thumb are made up of **pulp spaces** which contain fatty tissue divided into numerous compartments by connective tissue septa passing from the terminal phalanx to the skin. Terminal branches of the palmar digital arteries run through the pulp and some supply most of the bone of the phalanx, so that if the vessels are damaged or occluded the bone may undergo necrosis. The pulp space does not extend along the finger because the skin of the flexion crease of the distal interphalangeal joint adheres firmly to the underlying tissue. *Pulp infections*, commonly due to pinprick, become very painful due to the tension produced in a confined space, and abscesses may have to be drained, usually by incisions through the side of the pulp space (to avoid a scar on the tactile surface of the pad).

WRIST AND DORSUM OF THE HAND

SKIN AND SUBCUTANEOUS TISSUE

The **skin** on the back (dorsum) of the hand (**18.16a**) is very mobile, due to the **loose subcutaneous tissue**. Any injury or disease causing accumulation of tissue fluid causes obvious swelling here, even if the cause of the swelling is on the palmar surface; excess fluid cannot be accommodated on the palmar surface because the skin is firmly attached to the palmar aponeurosis, and so the fluid is forced to migrate to the dorsal surface. The skin over the thumb and finger joints has to be lax and has numerous creases to allow for flexion at these joints.

EXTENSOR RETINACULUM AND SYNOVIAL SHEATHS

The **extensor muscles** of the forearm often have names corresponding to those of the flexors (p.228). Their long tendons, which pass into the hand, are kept in place on the dorsal surface of the wrist by the various compartments of the **extensor retinaculum** (**18.17a**) – a band of fibrous tissue passing rather obliquely over the back of the wrist from the radius on the lateral side to the triquetral and pisiform bones on the medial (ulnar) side. As on the flexor surface of the wrist, the tendons are surrounded by **synovial sheaths** that prevent friction as they move beneath the retinaculum (**18.17b**). Doing a job that involves unaccustomed wrist movements can cause painful swelling of synovial sheaths (*tenosynovitis*). Note that there are no fibrous or synovial sheaths on the dorsum of the fingers since, unlike the flexor tendons, the extensor tendons do not have to be prevented from bowing forward. As on the flexor surface, some extensor muscles act only on the wrist while others continue on to the thumb or fingers.

RADIAL NERVE

All the **muscles** of the **back** of the **forearm** whose tendons cross over the wrist joint are supplied by the **radial nerve**, mostly by its (deep) **posterior interosseous branch** which passes through the supinator muscle to reach the posterior compartment of the forearm (p.230). The characteristic feature of paralysis of the radial nerve is 'wrist drop', with inability to extend the wrist because all of the extensor muscles are now out of action.

Although the superficial branch of the radial nerve can be seen, on dissection, to give numerous **cutaneous branches** on the dorsum of the hand, the thumb, the index and middle and part of the ring fingers (**18.16b** and **18.16c**), the *anaesthesia* occurring with a damaged radial nerve is usually confined to a coin-shaped area in the skin over the cleft between the thumb and index finger (overlying the slight bulge caused by the first dorsal interosseus muscle, **18.16c**). This is because there is so much overlap from cutaneous branches of adjacent nerves (i.e. the median, ulnar and lateral cutaneous of the forearm). As a cutaneous nerve the radial is unimportant, in contrast to its motor branches, which supply all the muscles of the extensor compartments of both the arm (p.222) and forearm.

ANATOMICAL SNUFFBOX

The most obvious tendons on the back of the wrist are those at the base of the thumb. With the thumb held out sideways (extended, **18.14c**), there is a depression over the base of the first metacarpal (the **anatomical snuffbox**) with tendons on either side (**18.16a** and **18.17a**). The lateral or radial

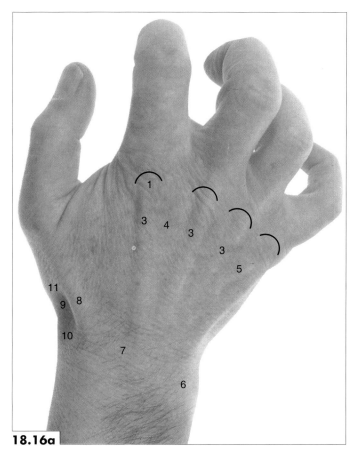

18.16a

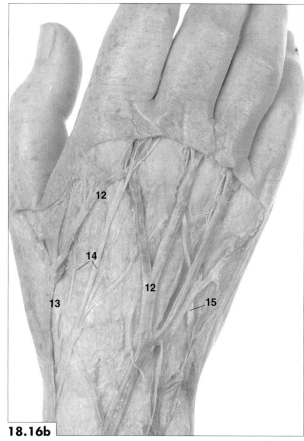

18.16b

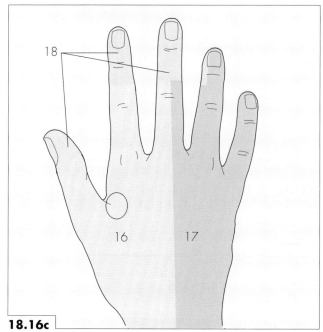

18.16c

Fig. 18.16 Right wrist and hand, dorsal surface.
(a) Surface markings, with the forearm in pronation. Compare
with the bones in **18.15** and the dissections in **18.17**
(b) Dissection of superficial veins and nerves
(c) Diagram of cutaneous nerve supplies

1 Head of metacarpal and line of MP joint
2 First dorsal interosseus muscle, causing the bulge between the
   thumb and the second metacarpal
3 Extensor digitorum
4 Extensor indicis
5 Extensor digiti minimi
6 Head of ulna. This is the anterior surface of the head; in
   pronation the lower end of the radius rotates round the lower
   end of the ulna but the ulna itself does not rotate (see **4.1b**)
7 Extensor retinaculum
8 Extensor pollicis longus, forming the ulnar boundary of the
   anatomical snuffbox (9)
9 Anatomical snuffbox
10 Styloid process of radius
11 Extensor pollicis brevis and abductor pollicis longus, forming
   the radial boundary of the snuffbox (9)
12 Dorsal venous network, draining the fingers and also the palm
   which does not contain a superficial plexus like this
13 Cephalic vein, beginning from the dorsal venous network in the
   snuffbox (9)
14 Branches of radial nerve
15 Dorsal branch of ulnar nerve
16 Skin area supplied by radial nerve, with (encircled) the area of
   anaesthesia in radial nerve injury; there is much overlap from
   adjacent nerves
17 Skin area supplied by ulnar nerve
18 Skin area supplied by median nerve, whose digital branches
   curl round from the palmar surface

boundary of the snuffbox is formed by the tendons of two muscles (though on palpation they usually feel like one tendon): **abductor pollicis longus**, passing to be attached to the base of the first metacarpal, and **extensor pollicis brevis** going to the base of the first phalanx of the thumb. The single tendon that forms the medial or ulnar boundary of the snuffbox is that of **extensor pollicis longus**, which passes to the base of the distal phalanx. The **scaphoid bone** and the **trapezium** are in the floor of the snuffbox, and there may be tenderness here when the scaphoid is fractured (p.231). The **radial artery** passes through the snuffbox (though it is not easy to feel its pulsation here), and this is also the place where the **cephalic vein** begins as a continuation of the dorsal venous network that lies in the subcutaneous tissue over the back of the hand. Any of the prominent veins here can be used for injections, and they are often chosen for intravenous anaesthesia.

EXTENSOR TENDONS AND EXTENSOR EXPANSIONS

Other tendons can be seen on the dorsum of the hand running to the bases of the fingers (**18.17a**). As they pass over the metacarpophalangeal joints these **extensor tendons** develop triangular-shaped expansions (**extensor** or **dorsal digital expansions, 18.17c**). The basal angles of the triangles wrap themselves round each side of the proximal phalanges to receive the attachments of the **lumbrical** and **interosseus muscles** (see below). The tendons then continue across the interphalangeal joints to be attached to the bases of the second and third phalanges. Unexpectedly, the long extensor tendons of the fingers can by themselves only extend the metacarpophalangeal joints; to extend the interphalangeal joints they need the assistance of the lumbricals and interossei (described below). Thus, while it is easy to understand how the flexor tendons in the palm of the hand can flex the finger joints, the way the fingers can be extended is not so simple and is described in the next paragraph.

LUMBRICAL AND INTEROSSEUS MUSCLES AND FINGER MOVEMENTS

The **lumbricals** are four small worm-like muscles (from lumbricus, the Latin for 'earthworm') which arise in the palm of the hand from the tendons of flexor digitorum profundus and are inserted into the radial side of the dorsal digital expansions of each finger. The **interosseus muscles** (four palmar and four dorsal) arise between the adjacent metacarpal bones and are inserted partly into the dorsal digital expansions and partly into the bases of the proximal phalanges (**18.17a** and **18.17c**). The actions of the interossei are traditionally learned and remembered by the words PAD and DAB; the Palmar interossei ADduct the fingers (bring them together) and the Dorsal interossei ABduct them (separate them), the normal position of the middle finger

being taken as the baseline for these movements. However, these actions are relatively unimportant compared with the fact that, assisted by the lumbricals, they pull on the extensor expansions and bring about *extension* of the **interphalangeal joints** (**18.18**), though the precise mechanism by which they do this has not been satisfactorily explained. At the same time, these muscles can flex the metacarpophalangeal joints; a long 'upstroke' in writing is an example of combined metacarpophalangeal joint flexion and interphalangeal joint extension. The **nerve supplies** of all eight interossei and two of the four lumbricals (those to the ring and little fingers) are from the **ulnar nerve**; the lumbricals of the index and middle fingers are supplied by the **median nerve**. The ulnar nerve, therefore, is the primary controller of these small muscles of the hand, and is the one mostly responsible for fine, intricate finger movements.

ULNAR NERVE

Study of what happens to finger movements when the ulnar nerve is paralyzed helps in understanding what the interossei and lumbricals do in the normal hand. There is a natural tendency in the resting hand for the fingers to be held in partial flexion. In *ulnar nerve paralysis* the fingers remain in flexion at the interphalangeal joints but they are extended at the metacarpophalangeal joints (by the extensor muscles, supplied by the radial nerve) to give the characteristic *claw hand* of an ulnar nerve lesion. The index and middle fingers are not flexed as much as the ring and little fingers because the lumbricals of the index and middle fingers are still working (since they have a median nerve supply). However, they cannot be completely straightened because their interossei are paralyzed and the lumbricals by themselves are not capable of extending the interphalangeal joints. In a long-standing ulnar nerve paralysis there is wasting of the interossei with a 'guttering' appearance on the back of the hand; the metacarpals seem to stand out because the wasted muscles form furrows or gutters between the bones.

The *sensory loss* in ulnar nerve lesions above wrist level includes anaesthesia along the ulnar side of the palm (**18.13d**), and on the ulnar one-and-a-half or two fingers. If the injury is at or below wrist level, only the fingers and not the palm will be affected, since the palmar branch of the ulnar nerve (like that of the median nerve) arises several centimeters above wrist level.

METACARPAL BONES

In a clenched fist, the knuckles are made by the heads of the metacarpal bones (**18.16a**). Blows with the fist can fracture parts of these bones, particularly the neck of the fifth metacarpal (a common boxing injury) and the base of the first metacarpal where it articulates with the trapezium, becoming partly displaced (*Bennett's fracture-dislocation*).

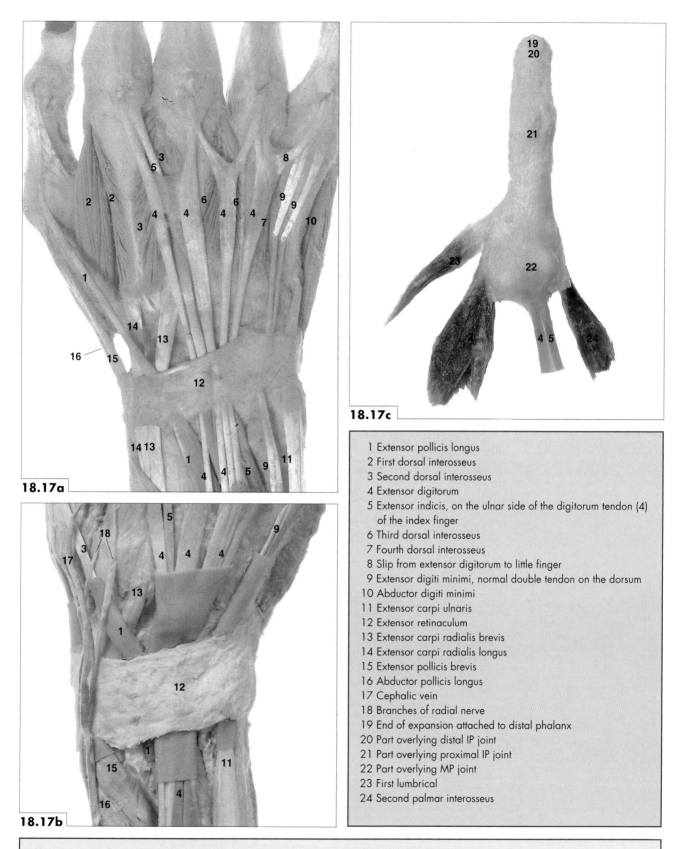

18.17a

18.17b

18.17c

1 Extensor pollicis longus
2 First dorsal interosseus
3 Second dorsal interosseus
4 Extensor digitorum
5 Extensor indicis, on the ulnar side of the digitorum tendon (4) of the index finger
6 Third dorsal interosseus
7 Fourth dorsal interosseus
8 Slip from extensor digitorum to little finger
9 Extensor digiti minimi, normal double tendon on the dorsum
10 Abductor digiti minimi
11 Extensor carpi ulnaris
12 Extensor retinaculum
13 Extensor carpi radialis brevis
14 Extensor carpi radialis longus
15 Extensor pollicis brevis
16 Abductor pollicis longus
17 Cephalic vein
18 Branches of radial nerve
19 End of expansion attached to distal phalanx
20 Part overlying distal IP joint
21 Part overlying proximal IP joint
22 Part overlying MP joint
23 First lumbrical
24 Second palmar interosseus

Fig. 18.17 Right wrist and hand, dorsal surface.
(a) Tendons of the dorsum of the wrist and hand.
(b) Tendons of the dorsum of the wrist and hand, with synovial sheaths emphasized by blue tissue.

(c) Dorsal expansion of the index finger, removed from the finger with lumbrical and interosseus muscles attached.

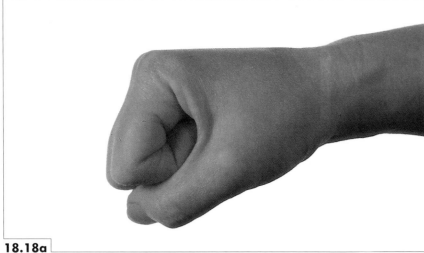

18.18a

Fig. 18.18 Finger movements of the right hand.

(a) With metacarpophalangeal (MP) and interphalangeal (IP) joints flexed. The heads of the metacarpals make the knuckles.

(b) With MP joints extended and IP joints flexed. The long extensor tendons act to extend the MP joints but cannot extend the IP joints.

(c) Extension of MP and IP joints. To extend the IP joints from **(b)** to **(c)** the action of the interossei and lumbricals is necessary.

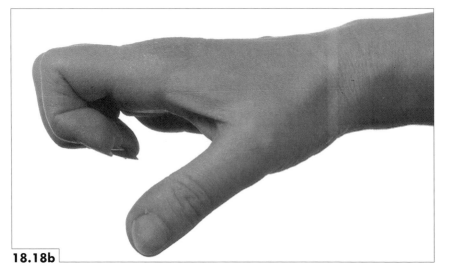

18.18b

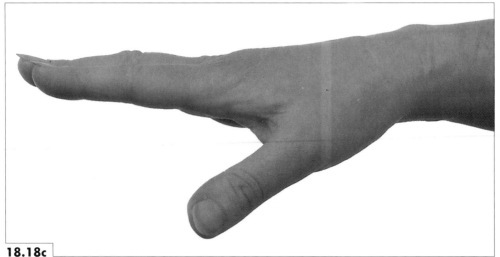

18.18c

NAILS

Infection at the side of a nail (variously known as *paronychia*, *whitlow* or *felon*) is commonest on the index finger because it is the most used finger. Part of the nail (p.19) may have to be removed if infection spreads underneath it. Bleeding into the nailbed (*subungual haematoma*) from trauma (such as a misdirected hammer blow) becomes painful because of the increasing tension, and can be relieved by making a small hole in the nail over the haematoma to let the blood out. A damaged nail that becomes loose and is about to fall off should be kept in place as long as possible to protect the sensitive nailbed while a new nail grows up.

The skin over the nailbed and the dorsal surface of the distal phalanx is supplied by branches of the nerves that supply the finger pad of the corresponding finger; the branches 'creep round' from the flexor surface on to the dorsum.

CHAPTER 19

ABDOMEN AND PELVIS

INTRODUCTION

The **abdomen** is the largest part of the trunk of the body. Its upper limit is the **diaphragm**, which separates it from the **thorax** (**15.5** and **15.6**), and its lower limit is another, but much smaller sheet of muscle, the **pelvic floor** or **pelvic diaphragm**. The tissues beneath the pelvic diaphragm, between it and the lower skin surface, make the most inferior region of the trunk, the **perineum**.

The upper and larger part of the abdomen is the **abdomen proper**, and the smaller lower part is the **pelvis**. The demarcation between the two is the **pelvic brim** (**4.1**a and **20.1a**), formed in the midline by the sacral promontory and the pubic symphysis, and on either side by the ala of the sacrum, the arcuate line of the ilium, and the pubic crest. While the abdominal cavity extends throughout the abdomen, from the diaphragm to the pelvic floor, the portion of it below the pelvic brim is known as the pelvic cavity.

The diaphragm forms the dome-shaped roof of the abdomen, and the lowest part of the diaphragm at the back is part of the posterior abdominal wall (p.252; **19.10**). The lumbar part of the vertebral column forms the central part of the posterior wall, with the psoas major muscle on either side, quadratus lumborum laterally, and then the transversus abdominis muscle which curls forwards as part of the anterolateral wall.

PERITONEUM

A smooth membrane, the **peritoneum**, lines the entire abdominal cavity and is reflected over the contained organs. The part that lines the walls of the cavity is the **parietal peritoneum**, while the part covering the abdominal organs to a greater or lesser extent is the **visceral peritoneum**. In the male, the peritoneum forms a closed cavity; in the female there is a theoretical communication with the outside world through the uterine tubes, uterus and vagina, but in reality the complex linings of the uterus and its tubes tend to close off any potential space and prohibit the entrance of air into the peritoneal cavity.

Many peritoneal details are only necessary for surgeons, but an understanding of the difference between the abdominal cavity and the peritoneal cavity is necessary for any student of anatomy. In order to appreciate the general arrangement of peritoneum and the way it is related to abdominal structures, visualize an empty box (the abdominal cavity) filled by an inflated balloon (the peritoenum, **19.1a**). With the box being empty, the balloon will be in contact with the walls of the box; in the same way the parietal peritoneum lies in contact with the abdominal wall. Now place some objects inside the box but outside the balloon (**19.1b**). When the walls of the balloon are inspected from within the balloon, the objects are seen to bulge into the cavity of the balloon. This is the same situation that exists in the abdomen with organs such as the kidneys and the ascending and descending colon which lie on the posterior abdominal wall; they bulge into the peritoneal cavity from behind, and so are said to be *retroperitoneal* (they are overlaid by visceral peritoneum). Now imagine some other object that bulges so far into the balloon that it loses contact with the box and becomes surrounded by a fold of balloon (**19.1c**). This is the situation that exists with most of the small intestine, the transverse colon and the sigmoid colon; they are suspended from the posterior abdominal wall by a double fold of peritoneum – the mesentery (p.260), transverse mesocolon (p.264) and sigmoid mesocolon (p.265) respectively. Each of these organs is ***surrounded*** by visceral peritoneum.

It can now be understood that a surgeon approaching, say, the small intestine through the anterior abdominal wall does so by opening not only into the abdominal cavity but into the peritoneal cavity as well. Similarly, approaching the kidney from behind through the posterior abdominal wall involves opening into the abdominal cavity ***without*** opening the peritoneal cavity. While the abdominal cavity can be said to be full of abdominal organs, ***the peritoneal cavity is empty*** (apart from a very small amount of lubricating fluid); organs simply bulge into it or are covered by it – they are ***not inside*** it (**19.1d**).

Greater Sac and Lesser Sac

The general peritoneal cavity is sometimes known as the **greater sac** of peritoneum. Because of the way the stomach

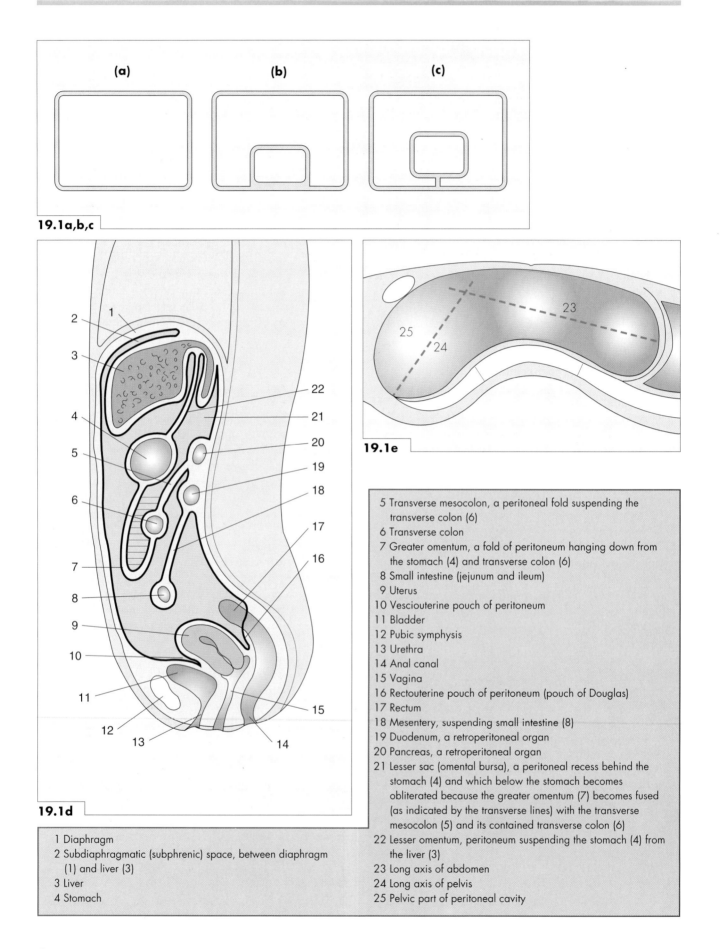

(a)　　　**(b)**　　　**(c)**

19.1a,b,c

19.1d

19.1e

1 Diaphragm
2 Subdiaphragmatic (subphrenic) space, between diaphragm (1) and liver (3)
3 Liver
4 Stomach

5 Transverse mesocolon, a peritoneal fold suspending the transverse colon (6)
6 Transverse colon
7 Greater omentum, a fold of peritoneum hanging down from the stomach (4) and transverse colon (6)
8 Small intestine (jejunum and ileum)
9 Uterus
10 Vesciouterine pouch of peritoneum
11 Bladder
12 Pubic symphysis
13 Urethra
14 Anal canal
15 Vagina
16 Rectouterine pouch of peritoneum (pouch of Douglas)
17 Rectum
18 Mesentery, suspending small intestine (8)
19 Duodenum, a retroperitoneal organ
20 Pancreas, a retroperitoneal organ
21 Lesser sac (omental bursa), a peritoneal recess behind the stomach (4) and which below the stomach becomes obliterated because the greater omentum (7) becomes fused (as indicated by the transverse lines) with the transverse mesocolon (5) and its contained transverse colon (6)
22 Lesser omentum, peritoneum suspending the stomach (4) from the liver (3)
23 Long axis of abdomen
24 Long axis of pelvis
25 Pelvic part of peritoneal cavity

and spleen develop in relation to the liver, there is a small peritoneal recess behind the stomach – the **lesser sac** (now properly called the **omental bursa**). It communicates with the greater sac through a small vertical opening (like the coin slot in a vending machine) variously known as the **epiploic foramen** or the **aditus to the lesser sac**, situated below the liver and above the first part of the duodenum, with the inferior vena cava behind the foramen and the portal vein in front of it (easily remembered, therefore, as lying between the two great veins of the abdomen, **19.15**).

Peritoneal Compartments

The attachments of the peritoneum to the abdominal walls and organs helps to determine the way pathological collections of fluid within the peritoneal cavity can collect or move. With a patient lying on the back in bed, the lowest part of the whole cavity is the pelvis (**19.1e**), forming the pelvic compartment of peritoneum (p.289). Other important peritoneal compartments are related to the way that the peritoneum is attached to the liver and intestines, and these are considered with the organs concerned (19.17a and b, p.261).

Lesser Omentum and Greater Omentum

Two other structural features of the peritoneum must be mentioned here. The **lesser omentum** (**19.1d** and **19.11**) is the double layer of peritoneum extending from the liver to the upper margin (lesser curvature) of the stomach (p.253). It acts as a sling for the stomach, suspending it from the liver.

The **greater omentum** is an apron-like fold of peritoneum hanging down from the lower margin (greater curvature) of the stomach (**19.1d** and **19.11**), lying free over coils of intestine but with its upper part fused with the transverse colon and mesocolon. It has the important function of being able to adhere to diseased organs and so help, for example, to prevent the spread of infected fluid by 'walling it off'. Because the greater omentum is the part of the peritoenum most profusely supplied with blood vessels (by the epiploic branches of the gatsroepiploic vessels), it can bring masses of blood phagocytes (polymorphs and macrophages) to areas to which it adheres and so help to combat infections. Having these protective functions, the greater omentum has been called 'the policeman of the abdomen'.

ANTERIOR ABDOMINAL WALL

The anterior abdominal wall extends from the costal margin to the iliac crest, inguinal ligament and pubic symphysis.

ABDOMINAL REGIONS

In order to help describe the position of pain, swellings, etc., within the abdomen, it is divided into regions or areas by imaginary lines drawn on the anterior abdominal wall (**19.2**). There are two vertical and two horizontal lines. The vertical lines correspond to the *midclavicular lines*, drawn down from the midpoint of the clavicle to the midinguinal point, midway between the anterior superior iliac spine and the pubic symphysis. The upper horizontal line is the *transpyloric plane*, which is properly defined as being midway between the jugular notch of the sternum and the pubic symphysis,

---

Fig. 19.1 Diagrams representing the abdominal and peritoneal cavities.
(a) A box (abdominal cavity) containing a balloon (peritoneum).
(b) An organ inside the abdomen and partly covered by peritoneum, such as the kidney which is said to be retroperitoneal (behind the peritoneum).
(c) An organ suspended from the abdominal wall by a fold of peritoneum, such as the small intestine suspended by its mesentery.
(d) A diagrammatic sagittal section through the female abdomen and pelvis, with the peritoneum (**19.1d**) in heavy line, indicating how various organs are covered or suspended by peritoneum.
(e) As shown when lying down, the backward tilt of the pelvis makes it the lowest part of the peritoneal cavity.

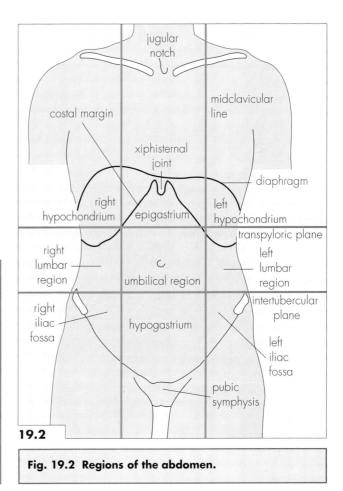

19.2

Fig. 19.2 Regions of the abdomen.

but is more easily considered as being a handsbreadth below the xiphisternal joint and on the same level as the point where the lateral border of the rectus sheath meets the costal margin. The pylorus lies at approximately this level, which corresponds to the lower part of the body of the first lumbar vertebra. (Some clinicians use the *subcostal plane* instead of the transpyloric; it is level with the lowest part of the costal margin, corresponding to the upper part of the body of the third lumbar vertebra.) The lower transverse line is the *intertubercular (transtubercular) plane*, level with the tubercles of the iliac crests and the fifth lumbar vertebra. Using these guidelines the abdomen is divided into nine *regions*. The three central regions from above downwards are the *epigastric*, *umbilical* and *hypogastric* (or *suprapubic*) *regions*, while at each side are the right or left *hypochondrial*, *lumbar* and *iliac regions* (the last often called the *iliac fossa*).

The positions of the principal abdominal organs in relation to these regions and to the surface of the anterior abdominal wall are illustrated in **19.3a** and **19.3b**, and described further with the individual organs.

ABDOMINAL MUSCLES

Underneath the skin and subcutaneous tissue, which, in the obese, contains a large amount of fat, there are four large muscles on each side (**6.1**): **rectus abdominis** on either side of the midline, and, lateral to it, the flat and sheet-like **external oblique**, **internal oblique** and **transversus abdominis** which lie in layers, in that order, from superficial to deep. The rectus muscle passes from the top of the pubis to the fifth, sixth and seventh costal cartilages. The other three extend from the iliac crest to various ribs. As it comes round from the side towards the rectus muscle, the middle one of these three (the internal oblique) loses its muscle fibres and continues as a fibrous tissue sheet (an aponeurosis) that splits to enclose the rectus muscle, so forming the **rectus sheath**. The external oblique and transversus also end in aponeuroses which fuse with the anterior and posterior layers of the sheath respectively, except over the lowest part of the rectus, where all three aponeuroses come to lie in front of the muscle.

The rectus muscle usually has three transverse **tendinous intersections** (6.1a): one just below the costal margin, one at umbilical level and the other between these two. In muscular individuals, their positions can be seen on the abdominal wall because they *adhere* to the *anterior layer* of the sheath (but not to its posterior layer) and appear to divide the muscle into segments. The lateral border of the rectus muscle and its sheath reach the costal margin at the **ninth costal cartilage** – a highly important landmark on the right side, since the tip (i.e. the fundus) of the gall bladder lies immediately beneath this point; this is the area of pain and tenderness in gall-bladder disease.

UMBILICUS

The **umbilicus** is a puckered scar in the midline of the anterior abdominal wall (**19.3**), normally level with the disc between the fourth and fifth lumbar vertebrae. The scar forms soon after birth at the site of detachment of the umbilical cord. Occasionally the tissues becomes stretched by intra-abdominal pressure to form an infantile umbilical hernia. Many such hernias disappear with a suitable supporting bandage but, if persistent, a surgical repair is necessary.

Converging on the umbilicus from below on the back of the abdominal wall (underneath the peritoneum) are the obliterated remains of **umbilical vessels** (two arteries and one vein). Rarely, another fibrous cord may be attached to the back of the umbilicus: the persistent remains of the embryonic **vitellointestinal duct** which connected the small intestine to the umbilical part of the developing abdominal wall.

ABDOMINAL INCISIONS

Most abdominal operations involve *incisions* through the anterior abdominal wall so that the surgeon can gain adequate exposure of the required organ. There are certain standard sites for incisions, as illustrated in **19.4**, the choice depending on the organ concerned. Thus, midline and paramedian incisions are used for approaches to the stomach and duodenum, Kocher's incision for the gall bladder, the gridiron incision for the appendix, and Pfannenstiel's incision for Caesarian section (childbirth by incision of the uterus).

Small incisions just above or below the umbilicus and near the lateral border of the rectus sheath can be made for the insertion of the instruments used in *laparoscopic surgery* which is coming increasingly into vogue. The laparoscope, which is essentially a tube with fibreoptic illumination, was formerly used for inspection of the abdominal and (especially) pelvic cavities, and for minor operations carried out through it (e.g. ligation of the uterine tubes for female sterlization); technological improvements now allow more extensive procedures such as operations on the gall bladder.

INGUINAL REGION AND SCROTUM

The **inguinal region** is the area just above, below and in front of the inguinal ligament (defined below). It therefore includes the lowest part of the anterior abdominal wall and the uppermost part of the front of the thigh (**19.5**). In the male, the scrotum (with its contained testis and epididymis) and penis hang down below the midline pubic symphysis. The **inguinal ligament** is the part of the aponeurosis of the external oblique muscle that stretches between the anterior superior iliac spine and the pubic tubercle (2.5 cm from the midline pubic symphysis). These bony points are all palpable but the ligament is usually not. In fat people, there is a skin

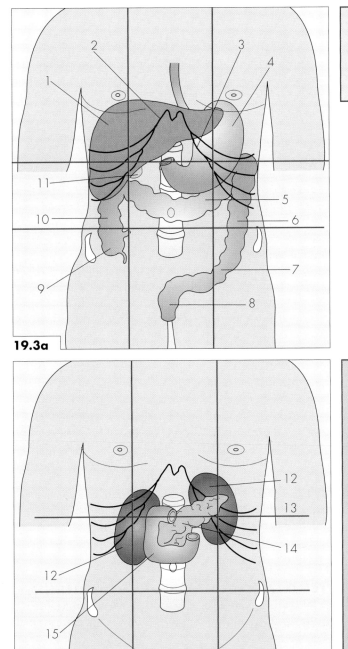

19.3a

19.3b

Fig. 19.3 Surface markings of abdominal viscera in relation to the abdominal regions in 19.2 and the five lumbar vertebrae.
(a) Liver, stomach and large intestine.
(b) Pancreas, duodenum and kidneys.

1 Liver
2 Seventh costal cartilage
3 Costal margin, formed by the seventh to tenth costal cartilages
4 Stomach
5 Transverse colon, whose level is extremely variable, sometimes reaching the pelvis
6 Descending colon
7 Sigmoid colon
8 Rectum
9 Caecum and appendix
10 Ascending colon
11 Fundus (tip) of gall bladder, at the level of the ninth costal cartilage (where the lateral border of the rectus sheath meets the costal margin, **6.1a**)
12 Kidney, slightly lower on the right than the left (due to mass of the liver on the right), with the hilum of the kidney (where the vessels and ureter enter or leave) on the left just above, and on the right just below, the transpyloric plane (13)
13 Transpyloric plane
14 Pancreas
15 Duodenum, embracing the head of the pancreas (14) at the level of L2 vertebra

fold in this region but it does not correspond to the inguinal ligament which is a little higher than the fold.

The scrotum is described here because of its association with inguinal hernia (see below); the testis, epididymis and penis are described with the pelvic male organs (p.307).

INGUINAL LYMPH NODES

The **inguinal lymph nodes** lie mostly in the subcutaneous tissue below the inguinal ligament and form roughly the pattern of a capital 'T', with some nodes parallel to the ligament and others alongside the great saphenous vein (**19.5**). All of these, about 15 or so, form the **superficial**

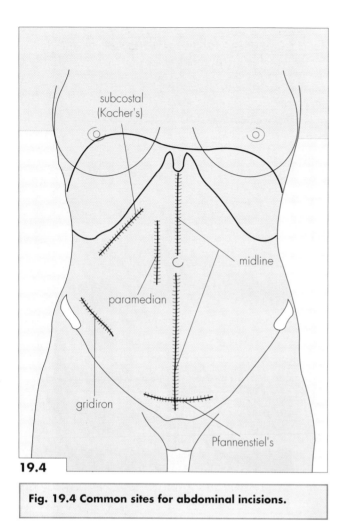

subcostal
(Kocher's)

midline

paramedian

gridiron

Pfannenstiel's

19.4

Fig. 19.4 Common sites for abdominal incisions.

inguinal nodes. The **deep inguinal nodes** are two or three that lie deep to the deep fascia beside the femoral vein.

Some of the larger nodes may be palpable in a normal person without any disease affecting them. The nodes are important not only because of their superficial position which makes them easily felt, but because of their wide drainage area. They receive lymph *not only* from the whole of the lower limb, including the gluteal region, but *also* from the lower anterior abdominal wall and back (below umbilical level), the perineum including the scrotum and penis (but *not* the testis which drains to aortic nodes in the abdomen) and the labia and vulva, the lower end of the anal canal and the lower vagina, and possibly also the body of the uterus and ovary. Enlarged inguinal nodes may therefore give a clue to disease over a wide area of the body, as well as being affected in lymphoid disorders such as Hodgkin's disease.

INGUINAL CANAL AND INGUINAL HERNIA

The **inguinal canal** in both sexes is a slit-like gap about 4 cm long in the lower anterior abdominal wall just above the medial half of the inguinal ligament (**19.6**). In the male, it contains the **spermatic cord** whose main constituents are the ductus deferens (vas deferens) and the blood vessels of the testis (p.307); the canal exists because, in the male fetus, the testis has to descend from the abdomen into the scrotum. In the female, the canal is occupied by the **round ligament** of the uterus (**19.5**). The canal is a potentially weak area of the abdominal wall and is the commonest site in males for hernia; the canal is smaller in females and, in them, inguinal hernia is uncommon.

An **abdominal hernia** is the protrusion of part of the abdominal contents through the abdominal wall, so causing an obvious swelling. An **inguinal hernia** (**19.7**) consists usually of a prolongation of peritoneum (the **hernial sac**) containing a loop of small intestine and causing a characteristic swelling in the inguinal canal; if large, the bulge extends into the scrotum. Infants may have a congenital type of inguinal hernia due to the persistence of a fetal sac of peritoneum (the **processus vaginalis**) which normally becomes obliterated. Coughing causes a sudden increase in abdominal pressure and momentarily increases the size of a hernial swelling; this is why the doctor may say 'Cough' when examining a patient for a suspected hernia. Because of the constant pressure of abdominal contents, hernias tend to gradually increase in size and have to be repaired (see below). Occasionally a painful and dangerous complication arises – a *strangulated hernia*. Here the contents of the hernial sac become constricted (usually at the neck of the sac), perhaps obstructing the intestine or cutting off its blood supply; the condition calls for emergency surgery to relieve the 'strangled' loop of intestine.

Operations to repair a hernia involve removing the hernial sac after returning its contents to the abdominal cavity, and strengthening the walls of the canal by suitably stitching together its muscular and fibrous tissue components to the inguinal ligament.

FEMORAL CANAL AND FEMORAL HERNIA

The **femoral canal** is a vertical space (not detectable on palpation) extending for about 3 cm below the inguinal ligament into the femoral region of the thigh (p.317), on the medial side of the femoral vein (**19.5**). It contains fat and a lymph node; its presence allows for expansion of the femoral vein and unrestricted passage for lymphatic channels from the inguinal nodes into the abdomen. The entrance to the canal is in the abdomen at the **femoral ring** (**19.8**), which is beneath the medial end of the inguinal ligament; the medial border of the ring is the sharp edge of the lacunar ligament. The peritoneum that covers the entrance may become pushed into the canal, so forming the sac of a **femoral hernia** (**19.9**). This is the commonest type of hernia in females but is never congenital. A femoral hernia (i.e. a loop of small intestine) may protrude through the saphenous opening in the deep fascia of the thigh (see below) and then bulge upwards under the skin of the abdominal wall; it does not

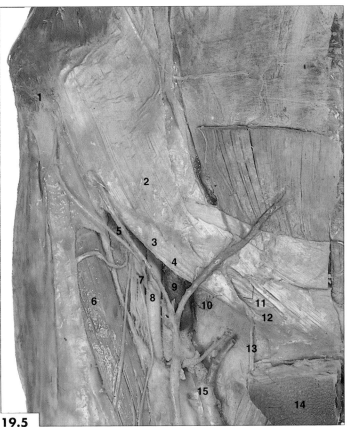

Fig. 19.5 Right inguinal and upper femoral regions, in the female.
Part of the deep fascia of the thigh has been removed to show the femoral vessels and nerve.

19.5

1 Anterior superior iliac spine, at the front end of the iliac crest
2 External oblique aponeurosis, whose lower end forms the inguinal ligament (3)
3 Inguinal ligament, stretching between the anterior superior iliac spine (1) and the pubic tubercle (12)
4 Position of deep inguinal ring, at the lateral end of the inguinal canal
5 Superficial circumflex iliac vessels
6 Sartorius
7 Femoral nerve, breaking up into a sheaf of branches after passing beneath the inguinal ligament (3)
8 Femoral artery, the continuation into the thigh of the external iliac artery

9 Femoral vein, on the medial side of the artery and receiving the great saphenous vein (15)
10 Position of femoral canal, the site for femoral hernia
11 Margins of superficial inguinal ring, defined by cutting away the fascia that closes it, at the medial end of the inguinal canal
12 Pubic tubercle
13 Round ligament of uterus, emerging through the superficial ring (11) after traversing the inguinal canal
14 Mons pubis
15 Great saphenous vein, receiving several tributaries immediately before joining the femoral vein (9)

extend further down the thigh because the subcutaneous tissues there are more firmly attached to the deep fascia. The narrowness of the abdominal opening of the canal may lead to strangulation of the hernia (see above). The lacunar ligament may need to be cut to free the loop of bowel.

FEMORAL ARTERY

The **femoral artery**, which is the continuation into the thigh of the external iliac artery, lies below the inguinal ligament, midway between the pubic symphysis and the anterior superior iliac spine (**19.5**); its *pulsation* can be felt here (**20.2b**). This is also where it can be cannulated (**15.24**),

being conveniently near the skin surface. The catheter can be pushed upwards through the external and common iliac arteries into the aorta to any desired level (under radiological control) for arteriography, e.g. of renal or coronary vessels. The femoral artery is flanked by the femoral vein (medially) and the femoral nerve (laterally).

GREAT SAPHENOUS VEIN AND FEMORAL VEIN

The **great saphenous vein**, returning blood from the medial side of the lower limb, ends by passing through the **saphenous opening** in the fascia lata of the thigh and joining

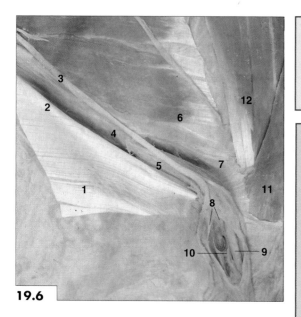

19.6

Fig. 19.6 Right inguinal canal, spermatic cord and testis.
The inguinal canal has been opened up by incising the external oblique aponeurosis and turning it downwards. The coverings of the spermatic cord have been incised just below the margin of the superficial inguinal ring, to show the ductus deferens.

1 External oblique aponeurosis, turned downwards
2 Inguinal ligament
3 Ilioinguinal nerve
4 Medial edge of internal oblique muscle, arising from the upper surface of the inguinal ligament (2) and labelled where it overlies the deep inguinal ring
5 Spermatic cord
6 Internal oblique
7 Conjoint tendon, formed by the lowest fibres of the internal oblique (6) and the transversus muscle (hidden behind the internal oblique)
8 Incised margins of coverings of spermatic cord (5)
9 Ductus deferens, labelled where it is cut for vasectomy
10 Bundle of vessels, including the pampiniform plexus of veins and testicular artery
11 Pyramidalis
12 Rectus abdominis

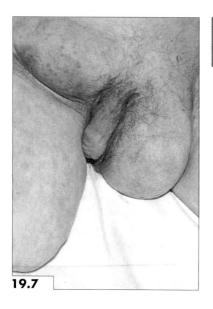

19.7

Fig. 19.7 Right inguinal hernia, causing a bulging enlargement of the inguinal canal.

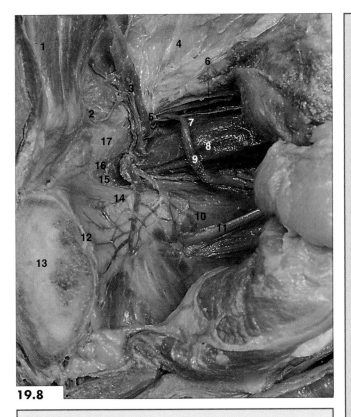

19.8

Fig. 19.8 Right femoral ring and deep inguinal ring, seen when looking into the right half of the male pelvis, showing the posterior surface of the lower part of the anterior abdominal wall and the region below the medial part of the inguinal ligament.

1 Rectus abdominis
2 Conjoint tendon
3 Inferior epigastric vessels, lying medial to the deep inguinal ring (5)
4 Transversalis fascia overlying transversus abdominis muscle
5 Deep inguinal ring, formed by transversalis fascia (4). An indirect inguinal hernia passes through this ring (lateral to the inferior epigastric vessels, 3) into the inguinal canal. A direct inguinal hernia forces its way into the canal medial to the vessels
6 Testicular vessels
7 External iliac artery
8 External iliac vein
9 Ductus deferens, leaving the deep inguinal ring to pass down into the pelvis
10 Superior ramus of pubis
11 Obturator nerve
12 Body of pubis
13 Pubic symphysis
14 Pectineal ligament, thickened periosteum along the pectineal line of the pubis and continuous with the lacunar ligament (15)
15 Lacunar ligament, a small triangular part of the inguinal ligament (17) forming the medial boundary of the femoral ring (16)
16 Femoral ring, the abdominal opening of the femoral canal, bounded by the lacunar ligament (15), inguinal ligament (17), pectineal ligament (14) and the external iliac vein (8) becoming the femoral vein as it passes under the inguinal ligament). A femoral hernia passes through this opening into the femoral canal
17 Medial end of inguinal ligament

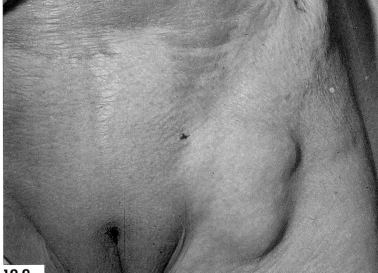

19.9

Fig. 19.9 Femoral hernia, causing a bulging enlargement of the femoral canal.

the **femoral vein** (**19.5**). The opening lies 3.5 cm below, and lateral to, the pubic tubercle (a palpable landmark 2.5 cm lateral to the top of the pubic symphysis), and is mentioned here (as well as in the section on the femoral region, see p.318) to emphasize that a femoral hernia may bulge through the opening (see above).

SCROTUM

The **scrotum** is a pouch of wrinkled, pigmented skin and connective tissue, which hangs down below the pubic symphysis and between the uppermost, anteromedial parts of the two thighs. It is divided into two compartments, each of which contains a testis and its associated structures (the epididymis and the end of the spermatic cord). There is no fat in the connective tissue but there are smooth muscle fibres (constituting the **dartos muscle**) which can cause additional wrinkling of the skin. An inguinal hernia (see above) may extend into its own side of the scrotum.

POSTERIOR ABDOMINAL WALL

The **posterior abdominal wall** (the back wall of the abdominal cavity) consists of the lumbar part of the vertebral column, the twelfth rib, the iliac fossa of the hip bone, part of the origin of the diaphragm, and some other muscles – psoas, quadratus lumborum and iliacus (**19.10**). The lumbar vertebrae with their intervening discs form a vertical ridge that projects forwards towards the anterior abdominal wall in the midline. On either side of the ridge is a depression, often called the **paravertebral gutter** which is partly filled in by psoas and quadratus lumborum. The kidney and adrenal gland lie in the upper part of this gutter.

POSTERIOR ABDOMINAL MUSCLES

The upper lumbar vertebrae give attachment to the **crura of the diaphragm** (p.101), with other diaphragmatic fibres coming from the twelfth (and higher) ribs. From these points of origin, the fibres arch upwards and centrally to reach the **central tendon** of the diaphragm (**15.5b**). Behind those fibres that arise from the lowest rib is the **costodiaphragmatic recess** of the pleural cavity (p.120; **15.5a**), a small part of the thoracic cavity is thus *behind* the upper part of the abdominal cavity.

The sides of the lumbar vertebrae give origin to the **psoas major** muscle (**19.10**), which slopes obliquely downwards to pass under the inguinal ligament and enter the upper thigh. Here it is attached to the lesser tuberosity of the femur and is a main flexor of the hip joint (p.321), as well as a lateral flexor of this part of the spine. The **lumbar plexus** of nerves

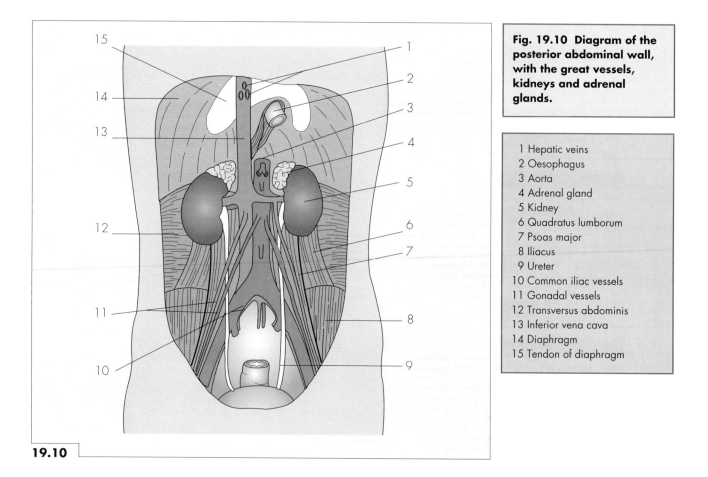

Fig. 19.10 Diagram of the posterior abdominal wall, with the great vessels, kidneys and adrenal glands.

1 Hepatic veins
2 Oesophagus
3 Aorta
4 Adrenal gland
5 Kidney
6 Quadratus lumborum
7 Psoas major
8 Iliacus
9 Ureter
10 Common iliac vessels
11 Gonadal vessels
12 Transversus abdominis
13 Inferior vena cava
14 Diaphragm
15 Tendon of diaphragm

19.10

(p.42) is within the psoas muscle, from which the branches of the plexus emerge (see below). **Quadratus lumborum** (**19.10**) stretches between part of the iliac crest and the twelfth rib, which it helps to stabilize. **Iliacus** (**19.10**) arises from the iliac fossa of the hip bone and passes into the thigh with psoas to assist in flexion of the hip.

AORTA AND INFERIOR VENA CAVA

Beneath the central arch between the two crura of the diaphragm, the **aorta** passes from the thorax into the abdomen (**19.10**). It runs down in front of the vertebral column and divides at the level of the fourth lumbar vertebra into the two **common iliac arteries**. The **inferior vena cava** is formed by the union of the two **common iliac veins** at a slightly lower level, opposite the fifth lumbar vertebra. It runs upwards on the right side of the aorta to enter the thorax through its foramen in the tendon of the diaphragm at the level of the eighth thoracic vertebra. The vena cava thus has a longer course in the abdomen than the aorta (though the upper part of the vein is hidden behind the liver, see p.270).

NERVES OF THE POSTERIOR ABDOMINAL WALL

The **femoral nerve**, the largest branch of the lumbar plexus (p.42), emerges from the *lateral* side of the psoas muscle about 5 cm (2 inches) above the inguinal ligament (**19.46**); stab wounds of the lower abdomen may injure it here. The **obturator nerve** leaves the *medial* edge of psoas at the pelvic brim (**19.46**), to pass along the side wall of the pelvis. Smaller branches of the plexus include: the **iliohypogastric** and **ilio-inguinal nerves** which first run behind the kidney (**19.31**) and then enter the anterior abdominal wall; the **lateral femoral cutaneous nerve** which crosses iliacus to enter the thigh under the lateral end of the inguinal ligament (see **20.2a**); and the **genitofemoral nerve** which runs down in front of psoas to the deep inguinal ring (**19.40**).

The lumbar part of the **left sympathetic trunk** lies level with the left margin of the aorta (**19.31**), and the **right trunk** is just under cover of the right margin of the inferior vena cava.

STOMACH

The **stomach** acts as a *reservoir* and *mixer* for swallowed food and drink, and is where the *digestion of protein* begins. It is the most dilated part of the alimentary canal; in the newborn it is the size of a hen's egg but in the adult it can comfortably contain 1–1.5 litres of contents. It is roughly 'J'-shaped and lies underneath the left dome of the diaphragm, partly under cover of the left costal margin (see **11.1**), and so is mainly in the left hypochondrial and epigastric regions of the abdomen. Although just behind the upper part of the abdominal wall, here the stomach is not usually palpable unless unduly

distended. (The Greek for stomach gives the adjective 'gastric'.)

The junction with the oesophagus is the **cardia** (the **cardio-oesophageal** or **gastro-oesophageal junction**, **19.11**), and lies just to the left of the midline at the level of T10 vertebra and about 10 cm (4 inches) behind the left seventh costal cartilage (**19.3a**). The small part that lies above the level of this opening is the **fundus** of the stomach. The main part is the **body**, and the end that becomes continuous with the small intestine (i.e. the duodenum) is the **pyloric part** (or **pyloric antrum**).

At the **gastroduodenal (pyloroduodenal) junction** there is a muscular thickening – the **pylorus** or **pyloric sphincter** (**19.11** and **19.12**). This lies just to the right of the midline, level with the lower part of L1 vertebra (**19.3a**); it is too deeply placed to be palpable. The right and left margins of the stomach are the **lesser** and **greater curvatures** respectively. The part of the peritoneum that forms the **lesser omentum** (p.245) suspends the lesser curvature from the liver, while, from the greater curvature, the apron-like **greater omentum** hangs down to overlie coils of intestine (**19.11**).

The stomach gets its blood supply from branches of the **coeliac trunk** of the aorta (**19.13** and **19.14**) and, like the rest of the gastrointestinal tract, the venous blood drains into the **portal vein** to reach the liver. Lymph drains to lymph nodes that are associated with the major vessels and with the aorta. Sympathetic nerves supply the blood vessels and, as with most viscera, pain fibres travel with these nerves (p.210); the most important nerve supply is from the **vagus nerves** which stimulate both movement and secretion (see below and p.260).

FUNCTION

The stomach receives ingested food from the oesophagus and, by contraction and relaxation of its wall, it helps to break down food and mix it with secretions that begin the digestion of *protein*. The pyloric part is particularly concerned with churning up the food (the 'pyloric mill') and, periodically, squirts some of the gastric contents through the pylorus into the duodenum. The amount of water absorbed by the stomach is negligible compared with the rest of the intestinal tract. The only significant substances to be absorbed directly from the stomach are aspirin and alcohol – a fact to be emphasized to all drivers of motor vehicles.

Motility

In the empty (fasting) stomach, the anterior and posterior walls are in apposition, and there is a small gas bubble in the fundus (due to swallowed air). Small wave-like contractions of the muscular wall (*peristalsis* or *peristaltic waves*) pass down from the cardia to the pylorus about three times a minute. When food passes into the stomach, the stomach distends to accommodate the increasing bulk without increasing the tension in the wall (this is called *receptive relaxation*). With

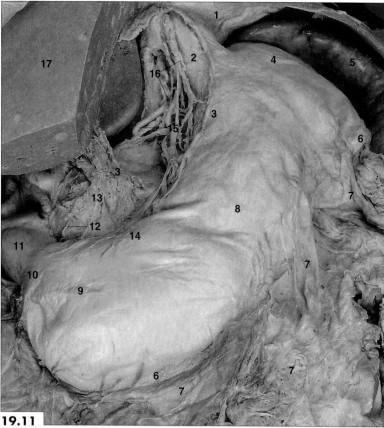

Fig. 19.11 Stomach and adjacent structures, from the front, after removal of the left lobe of the liver and part of the lesser omentum.

19.11

1 Diaphragm
2 Oesophagus
3 Cut edge of peritoneum that formed the lesser omentum (13)
4 Fundus of stomach, the part above the level of the oesophageal opening
5 Spleen
6 Greater curvature of stomach, along which run the left and right gastroepiploic vessels within the attached greater omentum (7)
7 Greater omentum, the fold of peritoneum hanging down from the greater curvature of the stomach (6)
8 Body of stomach, whose mucous membrane contains peptic and parietal cells, secreting pepsinogen and hydrochloric acid respectively
9 Pyloric part of stomach, whose mucous membrane contains G cells, the endocrine cells that control acid secretion by the parietal cells in the body of the stomach
10 Pylorus, the sphincter between stomach and duodenum (11)
11 First part of duodenum
12 Right gastric vessels
13 Lesser omentum, the peritoneum passing from the liver (17) to the lesser curvature of the stomach (14), labelled near the edge of the part removed; the cut edges at their attachment to the stomach are seen at 3
14 Lesser curvature of stomach, along which run the right and left gastric vessels (12 and 15) and the vagal trunks (16) between the layers of the lesser omentum
15 Left gastric vessels
16 Anterior and posterior vagal trunks, controlling the nervous phase of gastric secretion
17 Liver

increasing amounts of food, distension stimulates bigger peristaltic waves, especially in the pyloric part, which serve not only to mix the contents but also to squeeze 2–3 ml through the pylorus into the duodenum. The mixture of dissolved food and digestive juices is called **chyme**. The rate of gastric emptying is proportional to the volume of gastric contents. When a large meal is ingested, it causes more distension of the stomach, and therefore more forceful contractions and an increased rate of gastric emptying, than a small meal. As the volume of gastric contents decreases, however, the force of contraction decreases and the rate of emptying slows. After an average meal the stomach takes about 3 hours to empty; fatty foods tend to delay gastric emptying.

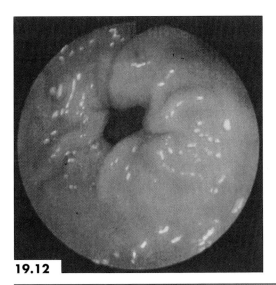

19.12

Fig. 19.12 Pylorus, seen through an endoscope within the stomach and looking towards the duodenum.

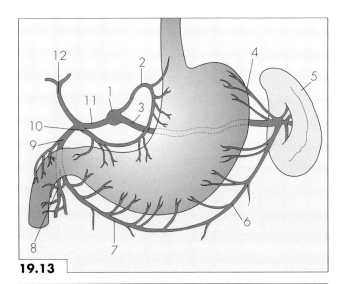

19.13

Fig. 19.13 Blood supply of the stomach.

1 Coeliac trunk, from the aorta and dividing into three arteries – left gastric (2), splenic (3) and common hepatic (11)
2 Left gastric artery, curling down to the lesser curvature of the stomach, and giving off an upward branch to the oesophagus
3 Splenic artery
4 Short gastric arteries, from the splenic (3) and running up to the fundus of the stomach
5 Spleen
6 Left gastroepiploic artery, from the splenic (3)
7 Right gastroepiploic artery, from the gastroduodenal (9)
8 Superior pancreaticoduodenal artery
9 Gastroduodenal artery, from the common hepatic (11)
10 Right gastric artery, from the common hepatic (11) or gastroduodenal
11 Common hepatic artery
12 Hepatic artery, the continuation of the common hepatic (11) after giving off the gastroduodenal (9)

Nausea and Vomiting

Vomiting (being sick) is the forceful expulsion of gastric contents through the mouth, and is usually preceded by *nausea* – the feeling of wanting to vomit. There are all kinds of causes varying from direct irritation of the gastric mucosa to psychic stimuli and substances circulating in the bloodstream. All stimulate the **vomiting centre** in the medulla of the brainstem, and this coordinates not only gastric contraction (which itself plays a surprisingly small part in vomiting) but also the contraction of the diaphragm and abdominal muscles (which supply the main expulsive force) and the elevation of the soft palate to prevent the regurgitated material from passing into the nose.

In vomiting that includes blood (*haematemesis*), the colour of the blood may give a clue to its origin – this may include swallowed blood, e.g. from a nosebleed. If bright red, it may have come from the oesophagus; it is often darker from a bleeding peptic ulcer, while if blackish it may have been in the stomach long enough for the gastric acid to have broken down the haemoglobin to a dark by-product.

Secretion and Digestion

Gastric secretion is the term for the release of water containing secretory products (*gastric juice*) from the epithelial cells of the mucous membrane to take part in digestion; about 3 litres a day is produced, and is usually divided into three stages or *phases*. The anticipation, the sight and the smell of food all help to prepare the stomach to get ready for digestion by causing the gland cells to secrete. This depends on the nerve supply from the vagus nerves and is the first or *cephalic phase* of secretion ('psychic secretion'). Apart from mucus that adheres to the surface of the mucous membrane (and is an

important factor in preventing the stomach from digesting itself), the main secretory products are *hydrochloric acid* and *pepsinogen*; the acid (from the **parietal cells**) is necessary to convert pepsinogen (from the **chief cells**) into *pepsin* which begins the breakdown of protein into small molecules. The secretion of acid also provides an acid environment in the lumen that helps to dissolve particulate matter in the food and release the polysaccharides and proteins. This is the second or *gastric phase* of secretion, and is due to the presence of food in the stomach which stimulates the release of the hormone *gastrin* from certain endocrine cells (the **G cells**) in the epithelium of the antral part. The hormone diffuses locally within the gastric wall and stimulates parietal-cell secretion, as do other substances such as histamine and acetylcholine. (This special type of secretion, whereby the

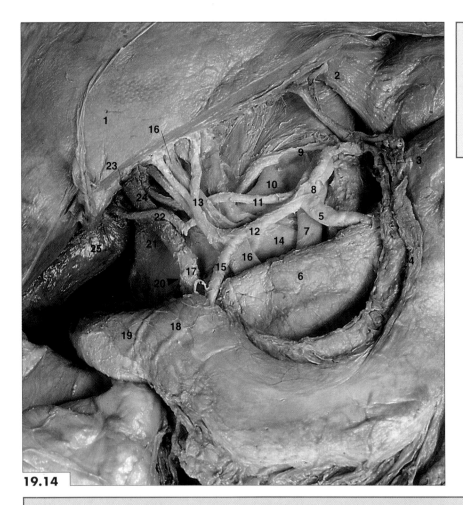

Fig. 19.14 Upper abdominal dissection with part of the left lobe of the liver and the lesser omentum removed, to show the coeliac trunk, portal vein, bile duct and related structures - one of the most important regions in the abdomen.

1 Liver

2 Oesophagus, having just passed through the diaphragm

3 Left gastric artery, curling towards the lesser curvature of the stomach (4)

4 Lesser curvature of the stomach, with the cut edge of the lesser omentum

5 Splenic artery, passing behind the upper border of the pancreas (6)

6 Pancreas

7 Superior mesenteric artery, arising from the aorta unusually high up near the coeliac trunk (8)

8 Coeliac trunk, arising from the aorta (10) just below the aortic opening of the diaphragm (9)

9 Margin of aortic opening of diaphragm

10 Abdominal aorta

11 An accessory hepatic artery, a common variation, arising from the left gastric (3)

12 Common hepatic artery, dividing into the hepatic (13) and gastroduodenal arteries (15)

13 Hepatic artery

14 Left renal vein, crossing in front of the aorta (10) and behind the superior mesenteric artery (7) to join the inferior vena cava (21)

15 Gastroduodenal artery, passing down behind the first part of the duodenum (19)

16 Portal vein, emerging from behind the pancreas (6) and passing up to the liver (1)

17 Bile duct, passing down behind the first part of the duodenum (19). When the peritoneum forming the lesser omentum is intact (here removed but see **19.11**), the bile duct, hepatic artery (13) and portal vein (16) lie in its right margin

18 Pylorus

19 First part of duodenum

20 Arrowhead indicating position of epiploic foramen, the opening into the lesser sac (peritoneal recess behind the stomach) bounded behind by the inferior vena cava (21) and in front by the bile duct (17) and portal vein (16)

21 Inferior vena cava

22 Cystic artery, from the hepatic (13) and passing to the gall bladder (25)

23 Cystic duct, from the gall bladder (25), joining the common hepatic duct (24) to form the bile duct (17)

24 Common hepatic duct, formed by the union of the right and left hepatic ducts that merge from the liver (1)

25 Gall bladder

active agent reaches its target cells by diffusion rather than by blood circulation, is called *paracrine secretion*.) Note that the G cells are concentrated in the **pyloric** part of the stomach, but the parietal cells that are stimulated by gastrin to produce hydrochloric acid are concentrated in the **body** of the stomach. A small amount of gastrin is released from G cells in the duodenum, forming the third or *intestinal phase* of gastric secretion, but this phase is relatively unimportant. .

The presence of chyme in the small intestine inhibits gastric secretion (as the *enterogastric reflex*), so that, as the stomach empties, gastric secretion ceases.

A highly important and perhaps unexpected function of the stomach is its role in normal blood formation. The parietal cells secrete a protein known as *intrinsic factor* into the lumen; upon reaching the small intestine it combines with *vitamin B$_{12}$* (in the ingested food), and the resulting complex is absorbed in the ileum. Vitamin B$_{12}$, an essential factor in normal erythropoiesis, is a very large, charged molecule, and would not be absorbed at all if it did not first bind to intrinsic factor (p.64).

EXAMINATION

Unless unduly distended or the site of an obvious tumour, the stomach is not normally palpable. Radiological investigation includes drinking a quantity of barium sulphate solution (i.e. a *barium meal*), which is radio-opaque and so outlines the stomach, enabling ulcers and tumours to be recognized and the motility pattern to be observed. *Gastroscopy* (passing an endoscope into the stomach through the mouth, pharynx and oesophagus), enables the interior to be examined directly.

The secretion of acid can be assessed by gastric analysis (via a *fractional test meal*). After passing a stomach tube and emptying the stomach, secretion is stimulated by a subcutaneous injection of histamine or an intravenous injection of a synthetic gastrin (pentagastrin). The secretion is sucked out at intervals so that its acid content can be measured chemically.

DISEASES

Medical attendants must appreciate that the general public often use the word 'stomach' to mean any part of the abdomen, and that 'stomach ache' can mean any sort of abdominal pain (or pain that may appear abdominal to the patient – even that of coronary artery disease).

The stomach itself is subject to many kinds of disorder, often minor and temporary and giving rise to the rather vague term *indigestion* which infers discomfort related to eating. Dietary indiscretions are an obvious cause of gastric disturbances, and gastrointestinal activity in general can also be affected by psychological stresses.

Among the most common pathological conditions are peptic ulcer and cancer. *Peptic ulcers* in the stomach (i.e. gastric ulcers – similar to duodenal ulcers, p.259) are usually single, small, rounded areas of localized destruction of the mucous membrane, occurring in the antral part and causing pain related to eating. An association with infection by the bacterium *Helicobacter pylori* is often present but may not be causal, although its eradication may be helpful in treatment. *Cancer* of the stomach is one of the commonest forms of malignant disease. Its danger lies in the fact that the tumour can grow surprisingly large before making its presence known by causing any significant symptoms, and by that time it may have spread extensively by lymphatics or the bloodstream (*metastatic spread*) to involve other organs such as the liver.

The blood disease *pernicious anaemia* (*Addisonian anaemia*) (p.64) is due to degeneration of the gastric parietal cells which thus fail to produce enough intrinsic factor (see above). The cause of the degeneration is unknown but it may be an autoimmune disease (p.70). Patients have little or no hydrochloric acid in their gastric juice (they are said to be *achlorhydric*).

Gastrectomy

Being near the anterior abdominal wall, the stomach is easy to approach surgically. Partial removal (*partial gastrectomy*) usually involves removing the pyloric part and a variable amount of the body, together with the first centimeter or two of the duodenum. The continuity of the gut is restored by anastomosing the cut end of the stomach to the side of a loop of jejunum just beyond the duodenum; the cut end of the first part of the duodenum is simply closed off. Complete removal (*total gastrectomy*) is quite compatible with life, provided vitamin B$_{12}$ is given to make up for the loss of intrinsic factor (p.64). The oesophagus is joined to the jejunum, and the patient has to take frequent small meals since the reservoir function of the stomach has been lost. The intestinal and pancreatic secretions are capable of dealing with the proteins whose breakdown normally begins in the stomach. The various kinds of *vagotomy* (cutting the vagus nerves) to cut down the nervous stimulation of gastric acid secretion are carried out for **duodenal** ulcer (not gastric ulcer) and are discussed on p.260.

DUODENUM

The **duodenum** is about 25 cm (10 inches) long, and lies behind the peritoneum of the posterior abdominal wall in a 'C'-shaped curve (**19.15**) which is often called the **duodenal loop** by radiologists. It is described as having four parts, which are respectively 2, 3, 4 and 1 inches long (**19.3b**). From the pylorus, the **first (superior) part** runs upwards, backwards and to the right, towards the neck of the gall bladder, and is at the level of L1 vertebra. The **second (descending) part** passes vertically downwards, overlapping the hilum of the right kidney, level with L2 vertebra. The **third (horizontal) part** runs transversely in front of the

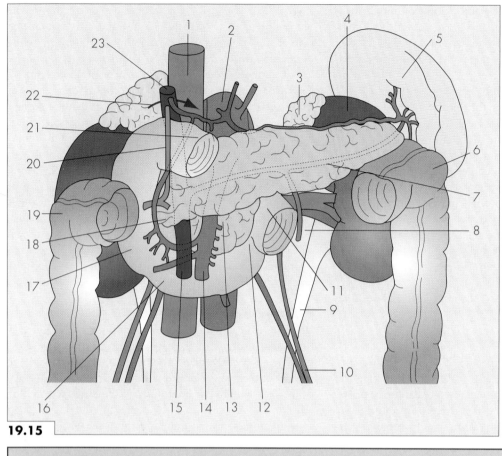

Fig. 19.15
Diagrammatic representation of upper abdominal viscera, showing the formation of the portal vein behind the pancreas.

1 Inferior vena cava
2 Abdominal aorta
3 Left adrenal gland
4 Left kidney
5 Spleen
6 Left colic flexure (splenic flexure)
7 Splenic vein, behind the pancreas and joining the superior mesenteric vein (15) to form the portal vein (23)
8 Inferior mesenteric vein, joining the splenic vein (7)
9 Left ureter
10 Left gonadal vessels
11 Duodenojejunal flexure
12 Fourth part of duodenum
13 Uncinate process of pancreas, with the superior mesenteric vessels (14 and 15) in front of it
14 Superior mesenteric artery
15 Superior mesenteric vein, continuing upwards as the portal vein (23) after being joined by the splenic vein (7)
16 Third part of duodenum
17 Second part of duodenum
18 Head of pancreas
19 Right colic flexure
20 Bile duct, joined at its lower end by the (unlabelled) main pancreatic duct
21 First part of duodenum
22 Arrow indicating position of epiploic foramen, between the inferior vena cava behind (1) and the portal vein in front (23)
23 Portal vein

inferior vena cava and aorta at the level of L3 vertebra. The **fourth (ascending) part** runs upwards at the level of L2 vertebra to become continuous with the jejunum at the **duodenojejunal** flexure. Thus, the first three parts can be conveniently remembered as lying at the levels of the first three lumbar vertebrae; this is the usual anatomical textbook description, but in life (and especially when standing up) the duodenum is commonly lower.

Most of the duodenal curve surrounds the head of the pancreas (**19.15** and **19.16**). The **main pancreatic duct** and the **bile duct** normally share a common opening into the second part of the duodenum, at the **major duodenal papilla** (p.276) which is situated on the posteromedial wall about 10 cm (4 inches) from the pylorus (**19.16**).

The blood supply is by branches from the coeliac trunk and the superior mesenteric artery, with corresponding veins. For the lymphatics and nerve supply of the small intestine see p.260.

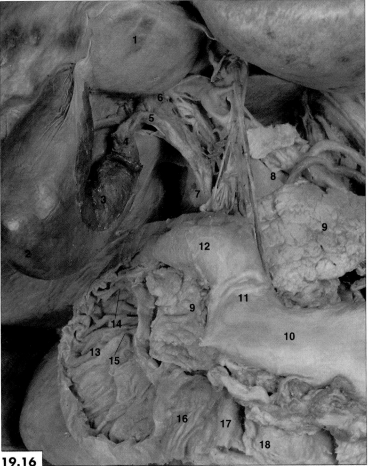

Fig. 19.16 Gall bladder, bile duct and related structures.

1 Liver
2 Fundus ⎫
3 Body ⎬ of gall bladder
4 Neck ⎭
5 Cystic duct, continuous with the neck of the gall bladder (4) and joining the common hepatic duct (6) to form the bile duct (7)
6 Common hepatic duct, formed in the porta hepatis of the liver by the union of the right and left hepatic ducts
7 Bile duct
8 Portal vein
9 Pancreas
10 Pyloric part of stomach
11 Pylorus
12 First part of duodenum
13 Second part of duodenum, with most of the anterior wall removed
14 Minor duodenal papilla, with the opening of the accessory pancreatic duct
15 Major duodenal papilla, with the common opening for the bile and main pancreatic ducts
16 Third part of duodenum
17 Superior mesenteric vein
18 Superior mesenteric artery

FUNCTION

Being the first part of the small intestine and in continuity with the stomach, the duodenum receives gastric contents that are squirted through the pylorus a few millilitres at a time and about three times a minute. The **mucus** secreted by **goblet cells** and by **Brunner's glands** in the submucosa (p.81) helps to protect the surface from damage by the *acid* chyme. Pancreatic juice and bile, both of which are *alkaline*, act to neutralize the acid. The digestive functions are considered with the rest of the small intestine (i.e. the jejunum and ileum, p.262).

EXAMINATION

No part of the duodenum is palpable, and investigations involve radiology and endoscopy. A *barium meal* (p.257) enables the duodenum as well as the stomach to be examined. *Duodenoscopy* is used not only for investigating the interior of the duodenum but also for cannulating the bile duct and the main pancreatic duct through the major duodenal papilla. Small pieces of mucous membrane can be removed (as biopsy samples) for microscopic examination; the biopsy sites heal rapidly.

DISEASES

The commonest disease of the duodenum is *peptic ulcer* (specifically a *duodenal ulcer* – the term *peptic ulcer* can refer to gastric or duodenal lesions). It occurs characteristically in the first part of the duodenum, where the acid gastric contents first come into contact with the duodenal mucosa after being squirted through from the pylorus. Most patients seem to have an unusually large amount of hydrochloric acid in their gastric juice, coming from an unusually large number of parietal cells. Since histamine is involved in the pathway of acid secretion (p.255), certain synthetic histamine antagonists (H_2 antagonists) can be used to keep secretion in check.

Vagotomy

If careful dieting and drugs are not successful in controlling the condition, the operation of *vagotomy* may be required. This provides a good example of the application of anatomy and physiology to the treatment of disease. Cutting the main trunks of the vagus nerves where the oesophagus joins the stomach (in a ***truncal*** *vagotomy*) or cutting their branches as they run along the lesser curvature (in a ***selective*** *vagotomy*) abolishes the cephalic phase of gastric secretion (p.255) and so cuts down acid production; however, this also diminishes gastric motility and leads to poor emptying. To combat this, these types of vagotomy are usually combined with a *gastroenterostomy*, anastomosing a loop of jejunum (with a transverse cut in its side) to the edges of a transverse cut in the stomach wall; this 'drainage procedure' provides an extra exit from the stomach into the small intestine as well as the normal route through the pylorus. An alternative method of vagotomy is the ***highly selective*** *vagotomy* which involves cutting only the branches to the body of the stomach, and leaving the branches to the antrum intact. This denervates the parietal cells (and is hence sometimes called *parietal-cell vagotomy*), but leaves the antral branches intact and so does not interfere with the propulsive effects of the pyloric part.

An earlier method of controlling the level of gastric-acid secretion in duodenal ulcer was by *partial gastrectomy* – removing the pyloric part of the stomach (but not the ulcer itself). This removes most of the G cells and deprives the parietal cells of their secretory stimulus; the ulcer is thus given a better chance to heal.

In contrast to the stomach, where cancer is common, malignant disease of the duodenum and the rest of the small intestine is very rare, an as yet unexplained phenomenon.

JEJUNUM AND ILEUM

Unlike the duodenum, the rest of the small intestine (the **jejunum** and **ileum**) is not plastered down on to the posterior abdominal wall but is suspended by a skirt-like fold of peritoneum – the **mesentery** – and lies in coils below the liver and stomach to fill much of the abdominal and pelvic cavities (**11.1**). The **root of the mesentery** (the 'waist' of the skirt) is attached to the posterior abdominal wall and passes downwards and to the right at an angle of about 45° from the duodenojejunal flexure towards the right iliac fossa, and is 15 cm (6 inches) long (**19.17** and **19.26b**). The border that supports the intestine (the **mesenteric border** – the elaborately frilled lower edge of the skirt) varies with the length of the intestine which, in the living body, is less than 3 m long (about 8 feet). In the cadaver, it is much longer due to postmortem relaxation of the muscular wall. The depth of the mesentery (the distance from the root on the posterior abdominal wall to the intestine) is about 15–20 cm (a micro-miniskirt in fact!).

There is no sharp distinction between the jejunum and the ileum, but there are two features that help in distinguishing whether a given loop of bowel belongs to the more proximal jejunum or more distal ileum: the pattern of **vascular arcades**, and the pattern of **fat** in the mesentery (**19.18**). Numerous branches of the **superior mesenteric artery** (and the accompanying veins) run in the mesentery to supply the whole length of the small bowel and, as they approach the gut, they form a series of anastomosing arcades; in the *jejunum* there are only one or two arcades which, in turn, give off rather *long* straight vessels that run into the gut wall, but in the *ileum* the vessels form several series of arcades before giving off rather *short* vessels to the gut wall. In the jejunum, the fat in the mesentery is not as copious as in the ileum, and there are frequent 'windows' of fat-free mesentery near the gut. In the ileum, the mesentery has more fat, and it extends right up to the gut wall without any fat-free areas. These facts are useful to the surgeon or pathologist who opens the abdomen and examines a loop of bowel. The jejunum also feels thicker than the ileum when rolling it between thumb and finger.

In about 2% of individuals, about 60cm (2 feet) from the ileocaecal junction, a short **ileal diverticulum (Meckel's diverticulum)** extends at right angles from the ileum, rather like a thick appendix. It represents the remains of the vitellointestinal duct (p.246) which, during development, connected the gut to the yolk sac via the future umbilical cord; its importance is that it may become the site of inflammatory disease and may mimic appendicitis (p.268).

The **superior mesenteric vein** has tributaries corresponding to the arterial branches, and the main vein lies on the right side of the artery as they both cross the third part of the duodenum (**19.15**). Behind the pancreas, the vein is joined by the splenic vein to form the portal vein (p.271).

The mesentery contains about 100 **lymph nodes**, which are concentrated in three positions: near the gut wall, along the blood vessels and at the root. Lymph drains to para-aortic nodes and from there into the cisterna chyli at the beginning of the thoracic duct (p.69).

The *extrinsic* **nerve supply** of the small intestine from the vagus and sympathetic nerves is of little importance when compared with the *intrinsic nerves*. These form two plexuses, one in the submucosa (the **submucosal plexus, Meissner's plexus**) and the other between the circular and longitudinal layers of smooth muscle (the **myenteric plexus, Auerbach's plexus**). They are responsible for coordinating peristalsis and other movements that mix and propel intestinal contents towards the large intestine (see below).

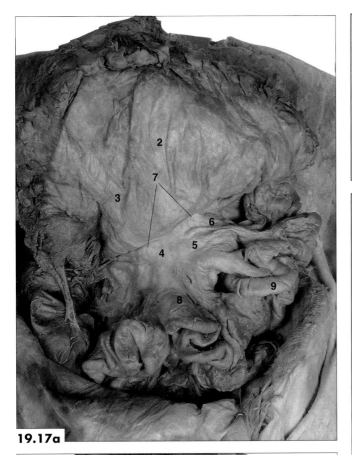

19.17a

Fig. 19.17 Root of the mesentery and the small intestine.
(a) With the transverse colon and mesocolon lifted upwards, to show the anterior surface of the mesentery and the upper (right) infracolic compartment, below and to the left of the root of the mesentery.
(b) With the transverse colon and mesocolon and the small intestine and its mesentery lifted upwards, to show the posterior surface of the mesentery and the lower (left) infracolic compartment, below and to the left of the root of the mesentery.

1 Transverse colon
2 Transverse mesocolon, posterior surface (because it has been lifted upwards)
3 Second part ⎫
4 Third part ⎬ of duodenum behind peritoneum
5 Fourth part ⎭
6 Duodenojejunal flexure
7 Root of messentery. The region above the root in **(a)** is the upper (right) infracolic compartment, and in **(b)** the region below the root is the lower (left) infracolic compartment. Compare with **19.26**
8 Mesentery, anterior surface
9 Coils of jejunum and ileum
10 Mesentery, posterior surface (because it has been lifted upwards)
11 Descending colon
12 Sigmoid colon

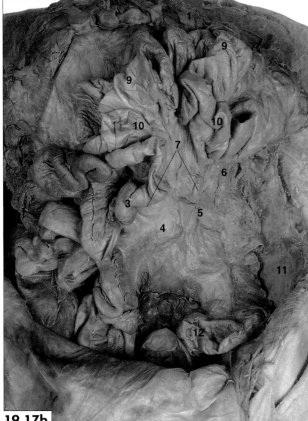

19.17b

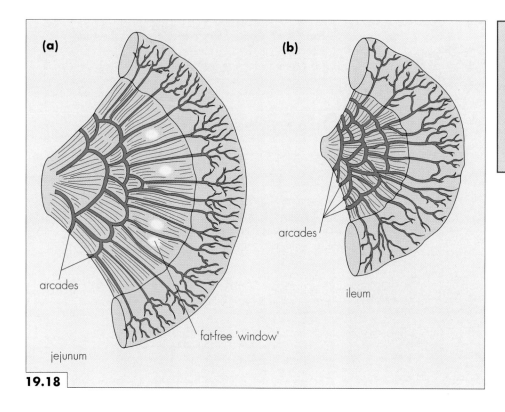

Fig. 19.18 Typical segments of jejunum and ileum with the mesentery.
(a) Jejunum, showing one or two arterial arcades and fat-free 'windows' in the mesentery.
(b) Ileum, showing several arterial arcades and no fat-free areas in the mesentery.

(a)

(b)

arcades

ileum

arcades

fat-free 'window'

jejunum

19.18

FUNCTION

The digestive process that began in the stomach (p.253) is continued and extended in the small intestine, which is also the main site of absorption of the products of digestion. *Tables* **11.1** and **11.2** (p.80) summarize the main enzymes and hormones.

Motility

Movements of the small intestine include *peristalsis* (which moves the contents onwards), and *segmentation movements* (like alternately squeezing and releasing a rubber hosepipe, which cause local mixing of contents). Segmentation predominates soon after a meal, ensuring that the luminal contents are well-mixed and brought into contact with the mucosa for efficient absorption. After most of the food is absorbed, peristalsis is the more common; short peristaltic waves tend to move the luminal contents towards the large intestine. In the first part of the duodenum, there appears to be a centre or 'pacemaker' from which peristalsis begins; peristaltic waves in the stomach do not necessarily pass on into the duodenum. After a meal, some products of digestion may reach the ileocaecal valve (the junction with the large intestine) in an hour, while others may take four to five hours.

Digestion

The breakdown of protein that began with peptic activity in the stomach is supplemented in the small intestine by carbohydrate and fat digestion, with each type of foodstuff having its own enzymes and hormones.

Protein digestion (i.e. breaking proteins down into peptides) is continued within the lumen of the gut by the enzyme *trypsin*, which is derived from the *trypsinogen* of pancreatic juice by the action of the enzyme *enterokinase* from the epithelial cells of the small intestine. Peptides are further broken down to amino acids by *peptidases* (sometimes collectively called *erepsin*); while some of these act on the peptides in the lumen of the gut, others appear to be associated with the epithelial-cell membranes and the interior of the cells, so that some breakdown continues after absorption. Enzymes themselves are proteins and, since the epithelial lining of the gastrointestinal tract which produces many of them is replaced every few days (p.82), almost half of the total protein in the lumen of the gut is derived from the gut itself (i.e. as *endogenous protein*).

Carbohydrate digestion, which may have been begun to a very minor extent by the enzyme amylase from the salivary glands in the mouth, involves *amylase* from pancreatic juice and various *disaccharidases* associated with intestinal epithelium. Starch and other carbohydrates are reduced to glucose and other sugars (mostly fructose and galactose) which can be absorbed.

Fat digestion depends on *lipases* from the pancreas and the intestinal epithelium, assisted by the emulsifying action of bile from the liver, which is delivered (like pancreatic juice) into the second part of the duodenum. The end-products are fatty acids and monoglycerides which are absorbed.

The presence of acid contents in the duodenum stimulates the epithelial cells to secrete the hormone *secretin*; this circulates in the blood and causes the pancreas to discharge secretion with a high bicarbonate content, thus neutralizing the acid. (While the **gastric** digestion of protein requires an **acid** environment, **intestinal** digestion requires an **alkaline** one.) The presence of proteins or fats in the lumen is the stimulus for the release of a second intestinal hormone, *CCK*, which also acts on the pancreas, causing it to discharge pancreatic juice with a high enzyme content (i.e. *trypsinogen*, *amylase* and *lipase*). Glucose and fat in the duodenum stimulate the release from intestinal epithelium of *GIP* (*gastric inhibitory peptide*), which helps to decrease digestive activity in the stomach now that its contents are leaving it. (Recent research suggests that this hormone should be renamed 'glucose insulinotropic peptide' since it may stimulate pancreatic islets to release insulin, p.279.)

Absorption

Absorption occurs throughout the small intestine, but mostly in the jejunum. Among the exceptions are bile salts (p.276) and vitamin B_{12} (p.64), both of which are only absorbed by the terminal ileum. *Table* **11.5** shows the amount of water entering the gastrointestinal tract from various sources, and the amount absorbed; a surprisingly large amount enters the gut with its secretions. The absorbed water enters the blood and lymphatic systems, and the kidneys play the largest role in determining how much remains in the body and how much is excreted as urine (p.284).

EXAMINATION

As in the duodenum (p.259), *radiology* and *endoscopy*, including *jejunal biopsy*, play a part in investigating function and disease in the jejunum and ileum. Among the commonest tests used for absorption is the analysis of *faecal fat* – an excess of fat (*steatorrhoea*) is a reliable indication of malabsorption. Other absorptive tests include measurements of the amount of the sugar xylose in the urine after the oral ingestion of a standard dose (in a *xylose absorption test*), and tests for the absorption of radioactively labelled vitamin B_{12}.

DISEASES

For reasons that have not yet been discovered, *cancer* of the small intestine is rare, and most intestinal diseases are due to infections or defects in absorption. *Infections*, with diarrhoea and vomiting ('D and V') of varying severity, are due to many kinds of organisms, of which the more serious are due to the *Salmonella* (causing gastroenteritis) and *Shigella* (causing bacillary dysentery) groups. *Cholera*, caused by the bacterium *Vibrio cholerae*, can be one of the most severe because of the excessive water and electrolyte loss. All can reach epidemic proportions under conditions of poor hygiene because they spread by contamination of water and food supplies. They usually respond well to the appropriate antibiotics and correction of fluid and electrolyte balance. *Typhoid fever* is another important infection; some people can become unrecognized *carriers* of the disease without suffering from

it themselves, and are often the unwitting source of an epidemic, especially when their job involves food handling. *Infestations* with tapeworms and other parasites are common in tropical climates.

The condition commonly called *Crohn's disease* (or *regional ileitis*, *inflammatory bowel disease – IBD*) is of unkown cause and often affects the colon as well (where it may be called *ulcerative colitis*, see p.269). There are many signs and symptoms, including diarrhoea and rectal bleeding, with various nutritional deficiencies and (perhaps surprisingly) arthritis. Prolonged treatment with antibiotics and steroids is usually required, though the response is variable.

One of the commonest disturbances of intestinal absorption is *coeliac disease* (*non-tropical sprue*), which is now known to be an allergic response to the gluten of wheat (and hence sometimes called *gluten enteropathy*). The passage of pale, foamy stools with a high fat content (*steatorrhoea*) is a characteristic feature, and the condition responds to a gluten-free diet which must be maintained for life.

LARGE INTESTINE

The end of the small intestine (the **terminal ileum**) does not join the large intestine as a direct continuation (i.e. in the way that the stomach enters the duodenum), but joins its *side* at the **ileocaecal junction** (**11.1**). The small part of the large intestine below the level of the junction is the **caecum**; opening off it is a small, blind-ending tube – the **appendix**. From here the large intestine continues upwards as the **colon** with ascending, transverse, descending and sigmoid parts. The sigmoid colon ends at the middle of the sacrum by continuing into the rectum, which in turn becomes the **anal canal**, ending at the **anus**.

CAECUM

The **caecum** (**19.19a**) lies in the right iliac fossa, and is held in place because the ascending colon (which extends upwards from it) is held on to the posterior abdominal wall by peritoneum. The caecum may be in contact with the anterior abdominal wall, but usually a coil of small intestine or greater omentum intervenes.

When the front of the caecum is opened up (**19.19b**), the two lips of the **ileocaecal valve** are seen lying transversely and protruding slightly into the lumen. Any increased pressure in the caecum sqeezes the two lips together, so preventing reflux of contents into the ileum. About 2 cm **below** the ileocaecal valve is the round **opening of the appendix** (without any valve-like mechanism at the entry).

APPENDIX

The **appendix** (properly called the **vermiform appendix**) is a worm-shaped tube, and is the narrowest part of the whole alimentary tract (usually less than 0.5 cm in internal diameter). It opens off the caecum (**19.19**) and is suspended

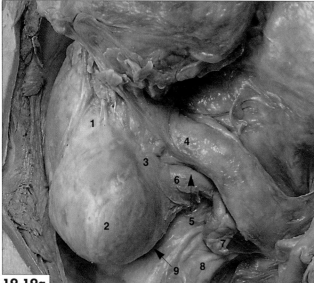

19.19a

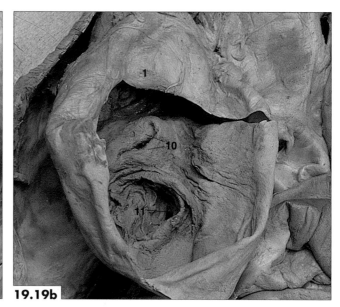

19.19b

Fig. 19.19 Caecum and appendix.
(a) From the front.
(b) From the front, with the anterior wall of the caecum cut open, to show the opening of the appendix below the lips of the ileocaecal valve.

1 Ascending colon, with fatty appendices epiploicae on the surface
2 Caecum
3 Anterior taenia coli, leading down to the base of the appendix (6)
4 Terminal ileum, joining the large intestine at the junction of the caecum (2) and ascending colon (1)
5 Inferior ileocaecal recess
6 Base of appendix
7 Tip of appendix, here lying over the pelvic brim
8 Mesoappendix, the small mesentery (peritoneal fold) attaching the appendix to the terminal ileum and within which runs the appendicular artery
9 Retrocaecal recess
10 Lips of ileocaecal valve
11 Opening of base of appendix (6)

from the terminal ileum by a small fold of peritoneum, the **mesoappendix**. The length of the appendix varies from 2 –20 cm, but is commonly about 8 cm (3 inches) long. Although the **base** of the appendix has a constant position where it opens into the caecum, the **tip** may lie in a variety of sites (**19.20**), such as over the brim of the pelvis, perhaps in contact with the ureter or some other pelvic organ, or tucked up behind the caecum or ascending colon.

The blood supply comes from the **appendicular artery**, a small branch from one of the caecal branches of the superior mesenteric. The vessel at first runs in the free edge of the mesoappendix and later approaches the appendix to lie close to it.

COLON

The **ascending colon** (which continues upwards on the right side of the abdomen from the caecum towards the liver), and the **descending colon** (which extends from near the spleen on the left side of the abdomen down to the left iliac fossa, **11.1**), are both *retroperitoneal* (like the duodenum) and are held in contact with the posterior abdominal wall by the overlying peritoneum. However, the **transverse colon** which joins the ascending and descending parts is suspended by a fold of peritoneum (the **transverse mesocolon, 19.1d**), largely from the lower border of the pancreas. (Despite the similarity of the names – colon and mesocolon – they are of course different structures: the *colon* is part of the large intestine and the *mesocolon* is part of the peritoneum.) The

transverse colon and mesocolon are behind the greater omentum (which hangs down from the stomach) and adhere to it, so that the transverse colon appears to be suspended from the stomach. Thus, when the greater omentum is lifted upwards, the transverse colon and mesocolon become lifted up with it. Although the ascending and descending parts are constant in position, the extent to which the transverse colon hangs downwards is very variable; it may be high up near the stomach or low enough down to lie partly in the pelvis.

From the lower end of the descending colon in the left iliac fossa, the **sigmoid colon** extends towards the middle of the sacrum in the pelvis and, like the transverse colon, it also is suspended by a peritoneal fold, the **sigmoid mesocolon**. The attachment of the sigmoid mesocolon to the body wall is in the shape of an inverted 'V' (**19.26b**), one limb of the 'V' running along the brim of the pelvis over the external iliac vessels, and the other passing down towards the middle of

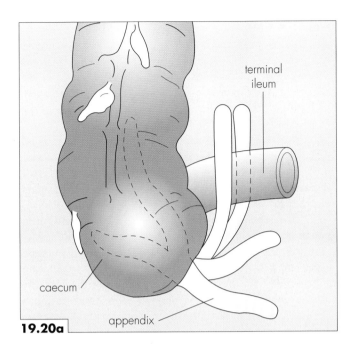

19.20a

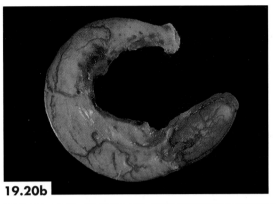

19.20b

Fig. 19.20 Positions of appendix, and appendicitis.
(a) Diagram of common positions for the appendix – behind the caecum or ascending colon, in front of or behind the terminal ileum, and over the pelvic brim.
(b) Appendicitis. A typical enlarged and inflamed organ, the commonest reason for emergency abdominal surgery.

the sacrum. The apex of the 'V' is an important landmark: the **left ureter** enters the pelvis from the abdomen by passing exactly beneath it. At operation, the position of the ureter can be pinpointed by lifting up the sigmoid colon with its mesocolon and feeling with a fingertip at the very apex of the attachment of the mesocolon. Do not confuse the two mesocolons: one is the *transverse*, the other the *sigmoid*.

The **hepatic flexure** of the colon (or **right colic flexure**) is the name given to the colon where it changes direction from ascending to transverse, at a point below the liver (**19.15**). Similarly, the **splenic flexure** (**left colic flexure**) is where the transverse becomes the descending colon, below the spleen. Because of the larger bulk of the liver on the right, the hepatic flexure is usually at a slightly lower level than the splenic flexure.

All parts of the colon are easily distinguished from small intestine by the presence on their outer surfaces of three longitudinal bands of muscle, the **taeniae coli**. There are also little tags of fat (**appendices epiploicae**) scattered over the surface (**19.15**). These features give immediate recognition of the colon at operation.

When full of faecal material, the descending and sigmoid parts of the colon may be palpable through the anterior abdominal wall (a 'loaded colon', **19.3a**), but the rest of the colon is not normally felt.

The colon from the caecum up to near the splenic flexure is supplied by branches of the **superior mesenteric artery** (the **ileocolic**, **right colic** and **middle colic** branches), but from there onwards the blood supply comes from the **inferior mesenteric artery** (through the **left colic** and **sigmoid** branches, **19.21**). There are corresponding veins, with all blood draining to the **portal system** (p.273). With

the vessels are associated lymph nodes and lymphatic channels, draining to para-aortic nodes.

The autonomic nerve supply of the large intestine has a similar 'watershed' to that of the blood supply. From the caecum to the splenic flexure, the parasympathetic supply is from the **vagus** (and is unimportant), but for the remainder it is from the **pelvic splanchnic nerves** (p.290), which are responsible for contraction at defaecation (p.267). Apart from supplying the blood vessels, **sympathetic nerves** contract the ileocolic and internal anal sphincters and relax the gut wall.

RECTUM

The **rectum** (see **11.1**) is continuous with the lower end of the sigmoid colon opposite the middle piece of the sacrum (the third sacral vertebra). It is about 15 cm (6 inches) long and internally shows three rather prominent folds of mucous membrane, one on the right and two on the left side – known jointly as **Houston's valves**. The rectum follows the forward curve of the lower sacrum and the coccyx (**19.1d**), and ends about 3 cm (1 inch) below and in front of the coccyx, where it becomes continuous with the **anal canal** at the **anorectal junction**. There is an angle of about 120° between the rectum and anal canal, and the forward bulge of the gut at this point is maintained by a muscular sling formed by the **puborectalis** parts of the **levator ani** muscles (p.290). The sling is a highly important element in maintaining *rectal continence*; clinicians call the site of the angle the **anorectal ring**, which is palpable on rectal examination (p.268).

In the pelvis (p.289), peritoneum covers the front and sides of the upper part of the rectum and the front of the middle part. The lower part is below the point where the peritoneum is reflected, in the male, on to the back of the

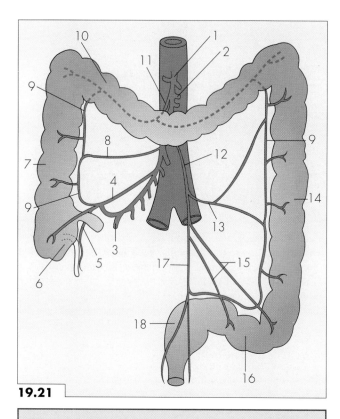

19.21

Fig. 19.21 Diagrammatic representation of the blood supply of the large intestine, from the superior and inferior mesenteric arteries.

1 Superior mesenteric artery
2 Jejunal and ileal branches
3 End of superior mesenteric artery, supplying the ileal (Meckel's) diverticulum (if present)
4 Ileocolic artery
5 Posterior caecal artery, giving off appendicular artery
6 Caecum and appendix
7 Ascending colon
8 Right colic artery
9 Anastomotic connections, forming the 'marginal artery'
10 Tranverse colon
11 Middle colic artery
12 Inferior mesenteric artery
13 Left colic artery
14 Descending colon
15 Sigmoid arteries
16 Sigmoid colon
17 Superior rectal artery
18 Rectum

bladder (the **rectovesical pouch**, **19.38**) and, in the female, on to the upper part of the vagina (the **rectouterine pouch**, **19.40**).

ANAL CANAL

The **anal canal** is the last 4 cm (1.5 in) of the alimentary tract, and from the **anorectal junction** it passes downwards and backwards to the **anus**, the opening at the lower end of the canal. The canal is important for several reasons, including the fact that it is a junctional zone between the embryological gut tube and the external surface of the body. For this developmental reason the *upper* part has a blood supply from the **superior rectal vessels** (from the inferior mesenteric, **19.21**) and the *lower* part from the **inferior rectal vessels** (from the internal pudendal,p.293). The upper part is thus one of the sites of *portal–systemic anastomosis* (p.273). Lymph from the *upper* part runs upwards into **pelvic nodes** (which are not palpable), but, from the *lower* part, it reaches the **superficial inguinal nodes** (which are easily felt, p.247).

Internally the most important feature is the way the mucous membrane in the upper part forms three cushion-like *swellings* which are normally in contact with one another and so keep the canal closed. The swellings are due to plexuses of **veins**, and when enlarged they form *haemorrhoids* (or *piles*) which may become troublesome when they bleed or project through the anus. Although the region where the swellings occur is the site where tributaries of the portal vein anastomose with systemic veins (p.273), the reason for haemorrhoid formation is not known; they are not more common in patients who have increased pressure in the portal venous system.

In the wall of the anal canal (**19.22**) the inner circular layer of muscle becomes thickened to form the **internal anal sphincter** (of smooth muscle supplied by autonomic nerves), while outside this and continuous with the puborectalis part of levator ani (p.290) is the **external anal sphincter** (of skeletal muscle, supplied by the inferior rectal branch of the pudendal nerve). The lower end of the external sphincter curls inwards to lie below the end of the internal sphincter; the slight gap between the two is the **intersphincteric groove** which is palpable on rectal examination (see below). (This probably corresponds to the old term 'Hilton's white line', which should not now be used.)

FUNCTION

The large intestine receives the fluid contents from the ileum and delays its onward progress so that further water can be absorbed; the contents are converted into a semisolid mass (*faeces*) that can be conveniently stored in the lowest part until they are discharged. The secretion of *mucus* from **goblet cells** has a lubricating function that counteracts the loss of fluid. Although most digestive processes occur in the small intestine, the large intestine is a site for *bacterial activity* that can also be considered to be digestive. The appendix appears to have no digestive function in man, but its high content of lymphoid tissue must mean that it contributes to the immune system (p.69).

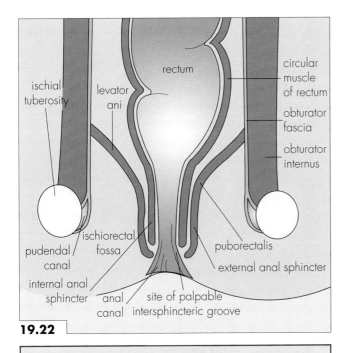

19.22

Fig. 19.22 Diagrammatic coronal section through the pelvic floor and anal canal, to show how the lower (puborectalis) part of levator ani becomes continuous with the external anal sphincter.

Motility

The ileocaecal valve is normally closed, and material passes through it into the caecum and ascending colon when a peristaltic wave reaches the terminal ileum. In the large intestine, peristalsis like that in the small intestine is not often observed, but there are *segmentation movements* (p.262) and occasional *mass movements*, especially in the descending and sigmoid colon and rectum, which move faecal material onwards. All of these movements are due to intrinsic nervous and muscular activity, and are little affected by the external nerve supply. However, defaecation (see below) is under extrinsic nervous control.

Defaecation

Defaecation is the release of faeces (also known as *stools*) through the anus; *bowel movement* is a common name for this process. Like the stomach, the rectum can accommodate itself to receive a certain amount of colonic contents without any increase in pressure, but there comes a time when the pressure causes some faeces to enter the upper anal canal; at this stage, the external sphincter contracts to force the contents back into the rectum. The feeling of distension is conveyed to the brain by the gracile tract (part of the posterior column, p.208). If defaecation is allowed to occur (by release of the cortical inhibition developed by childhood training), a combination of events occurs: abdominal pressure is increased by the diaphragm and by anterior abdominal

muscles, puborectalis relaxes to straighten out the anorectal angle, the sphincters relax; and the lower part of the colon and rectum undergo a *mass contraction* (by their parasympathetic nerves) to expel their contents. Distension of the stomach by taking a meal appears to cause reflex contraction of the lower colon and rectum (the *gastrocolic reflex*), so the desire to defaecate after food is common. Among the causes of *incontinence* are damage to the external sphincter (e.g. in obstetrics or perineal operations) and loss of cortical control (e.g. spinal cord lesions or cerebral vascular disease).

Diarrhoea

Diarrhoea refers to the passage of unusually frequent or unusually liquid stools. There are multiple causes, originating not only in the large bowel, but also in the small intestine and stomach. They include various gastrointestinal disturbances (e.g. gastroenteritis) ranging from mild and transient upsets to the severe infections with organisms such as *Salmonella* and typhoid. *Dehydration* and the accompanying *salt depletion* are the serious consequences, especially in the young, and may require intravenous therapy for the rapid restoration of body fluid and electrolytes. The severest water and electrolyte loss occurs in cholera, where there is massive small intestinal **secretion** of water and salts (and not just failure of absorption).

Constipation

Constipation refers to a decrease in the customary frequency of defaecation or the passage of unusually dry stools. Many people have a bowel movement once a day, some three times a day, some once every two or three days – there are wide variations among individuals, and all are perfectly normal for that individual. There is no such thing as the absorption of 'toxins' or noxious substances from prolonged distension of the rectum as a cause of ill-health, but any alteration in an individual's own pattern of bowel habits suggests the need for investigation to find the cause.

Digestion

The *digestion* of most foodstuffs into a form suitable for absorption occurs in the small intestine. In the large bowel, however, the normally resident bacteria are able to break down cellulose (e.g. from vegetables and beans) which is unaffected by intestinal enzymes. This bacterial digestion results in the formation of products such as ammonia, methane and indole which give rise to flatus ('wind') with its characteristic odour.

EXAMINATION

Although a 'loaded colon' (p.265) may be palpable in the lower left abdomen, it is not usual to be able to feel the rest of the large intestine through the anterior abdominal wall. The highly important *rectal examination* by the finger is described below. Endoscopy and radiology are the methods for examining the upper rectum and the colon. The *proctoscope* is a short instrument that is inserted through the anus into the anal canal and rectum; the longer *sigmoidoscope* reaches the sigmoid colon, and the *colonoscope* can reach the ileocaecal junction and even the terminal ileum. These instruments allow visual inspection of the gut wall and the taking of biopsy specimens. The *barium enema* corresponds to the barium meal (p.257) but is given by tube inserted into the rectum through the anus.

Rectal Examination

This implies feeling the inside of the anal canal and lower rectum with a lubricated, rubber-gloved index finger inserted through the anus (**19.23a**). The patient lies on one side with the knees drawn up. The structures that can be palpated in either sex are the coccyx and lower sacrum behind, the ischial spines and ischiorectal fossae at the sides, and the anorectal ring at the anorectal junction. In the male at the front, the prostate is palpable (but not usually the seminal vesicles). In the female (**19.23b**) the uterine cervix can be felt through the vaginal wall, with the uterosacral ligaments on each side of the rectum, and sometimes the ovaries.

No physical examination of any patient by any doctor is complete without rectal examination. Abnormalities in any of the structures mentioned above may be detected, especially prostatic and rectal tumours. The lowest parts of the peritoneal cavity, the rectovesical or rectouterine pouches, are just within reach of the tip of the finger at the front of the rectal wall and, though not normally recognizable, they may be the sites of cancerous deposits which have gravitated downwards and become detectable. (Compare with vaginal examination, p.302.)

DISEASES OF THE LARGE INTESTINE

Inflammatory disease of the appendix (*appendicitis*) is the commonest condition requiring emergency abdominal surgery. Although most frequently seen in teenagers and young adults, no age group is immune, and, despite its

frequency and the obvious fact that there is a bacterial infection, the precise cause remains unknown. The abdominal pain in the **early** stages of appendicitis is situated in the **umbilical** region of the abdomen (as referred pain, see p.210), but **later** when the peritoneum adjacent to the organ becomes involved the pain becomes localized to the **right iliac fossa**. This change in the location of the pain in the course of a few hours is one of the diagnostic features of the

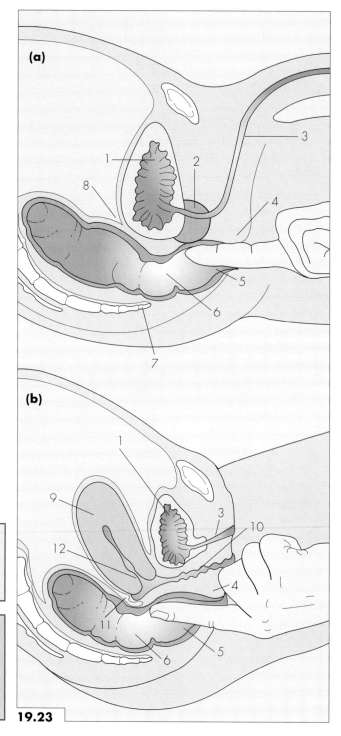

Fig. 19.23 Rectal examination, seen in diagrammatic midline sagittal sections.
(a) In the male.
(b) In the female.

1 Bladder	7 Coccyx	11 Rectouterine
2 Prostate	8 Rectovesical	pouch of
3 Urethra	pouch of	peritoneum
4 Perineal body	peritoneum	12 Cervix of
5 Anal canal	9 Body of uterus	uterus
6 Rectum	10 Vagina	

19.23

condition. Palpation over **McBurney's point** (a third of the way along a line from the anterior superior iliac spine to the umbilicus) presses on the caecum and over the base of the appendix (no matter where the tip lies); this perhaps forces caecal contents into the rest of the organ and momentarily increases the pain – another diagnostic feature.

Typical attacks require surgical removal (called *appendicectomy* in Britain and *appendectomy* in the US), otherwise the organ may burst and form an abscess or more general peritonitis. Although usually regarded as a simple operation (which it often is) with a successful recovery without complications, it can be one of the most difficult, especially when adherent to surrounding structures. Rupture of the appendix with peritonitis is a dangerous complication.

After the skin, lung and breast, the colon and rectum are the commonest sites for *cancer*, the sigmoid colon being more affected than other parts. The growths are usually slow-growing and painless in their early stages and so may have spread locally or by blood and lymph before making their presence felt. A changing bowel habit with alternating bouts of diarrhoea and constipation isa common symptom, and there will be eventual intestinal obstruction. Cancer of the rectum often gives rise to bleeding, and it is of the utmost importance in any case of rectal bleeding to distinguish this possible source from piles, which may be the patient's own diagnosis. Treatment is by surgical removal; the extent of the removal (e.g. *partial colectomy*, or *resection of the rectum*) depends upon the blood vessel and lymphatic patterns in the affected area, and must always include some normal adjacent bowel. With rectal lesions that involve the removal of the anal canal as well, an artifical opening (*colostomy*) must be made in the anterior abdominal wall.

Ulcerative colitis is a disease of unknown cause, with multiple ulcerated areas in the large bowel causing bouts of bloody diarrhoea, and having a predisposition to cancerous change. Treatment varies from intestinal antibiotics and steroids to control the inflammatory process, to colectomy in the severest cases.

The condition variously known as *mucous colitis* or *spastic colitis*, but more commonly now as the *irritable bowel syndrome*, is of psychological origin in those with an anxious, obsessive type of personality, and is an example of how emotional stress acting via the autonomic nervous system can cause organic disease – 'The sorrow that has no vent in tears can make other organs weep'. Tranquilizers and drugs that depress gut motility may be helpful, but the greatest asset may be an understanding physician.

In *congenital megacolon* (*Hirschprung's disease*) there is a congenital absence of ganglion cells in the myenteric and submucosal nerve plexuses, usually in the distal part of the colon. The affected part is widely dilated and the normal part beyond it is narrow and constricted, resulting in very infrequent defaecation (every two weeks or more). The affected part can be surgically removed.

In *intestinal obstruction* (which can affect the small intestine as well as the large), the onward passage of material through the gut may be hampered by various kinds of constriction, such as adhesions or fibrous band formation following surgical operations, strangulation of a hernia, or tumour growth, all of which may develop slowly, but may suddenly reach a critical stage of mechanical obstruction. Abdominal pain and distension ensue; vomiting is a late feature unless the site of obstruction is high in the gut. Operation is required to relieve the obstruction and deal with any complications such as an ischaemic loop of bowel. A non-mechanical variety of obstruction is *paralytic ileus* (*adynamic ileus*) – an uncommon but distressing complication of any abdominal operation. Peristalsis is normally absent for some hours after most abdominal operations, but with ileus there is prolonged absence, perhaps caused by the handling of loops of gut. When listening to the abdomen with a stethoscope, bowel sounds are completely absent.

LIVER

The **liver** is the largest gland in the body, weighing 1500 g and receiving 1500 ml of blood per minute. Like any other organ, it has an arterial blood supply (from the common hepatic artery – a branch of the coeliac trunk of the aorta) and a venous drainage (via hepatic veins draining into the inferior vena cava). However, it also receives blood from the gastrointestinal tract (portal venous blood, p.82), so that the absorbed products of digestion can be conveyed to the liver for processing by this vital organ. Blood from the spleen also drains into this portal system. About 20% of the blood reaching the liver is arterial, the rest being portal blood.

Among the many metabolic activities of the liver is the production of **bile**, which is delivered into the duodenum by a duct system which includes a storage and concentrating organ – the gall bladder (p.275).

The liver lies under the diaphragm, occupying the **right hypochondrial** and **epigastric regions** of the abdomen and extending into the **left hypochondrium** perhaps as far as the midclavicular line (**19.3a**). The upper limit of the surface marking of the liver is the same as that of the diaphragm and therefore extends surprisingly high into the thoracic cage – as high as the **fifth rib** in the right midclavicular line, level with the xiphisternal joint in the midline, and to the fifth intercostal space below the apex of the heart. Below the lower part of the **right costal margin**, the liver may just be palpable when the patient takes a deep breath (lowering the diaphragm and so pushing the liver down). Although part of the liver is immediately behind the anterior abdominal wall below the xiphisternum, it is not normally felt here because it is too soft and offers no resistance, unless, of course, it is hardened by disease. When enlarged, the liver can be felt easily below the costal margin, but even when of normal size it gives an area of dullness on percussion.

Viewed from the right side, the **right surface** of the liver extends from the **seventh** to the **eleventh ribs**, so that between the diaphragm and the ribs is interposed the **pleural cavity**, with the lower part of the lung included in the higher part of this area. Because the lower limit of the lung is about 5 cm above the lower limit of the pleura, the **eighth intercostal space** in the midaxillary line is chosen as the site for the insertion of the needle for **liver biopsy** (**19.24**); the needle passes through the empty part of the pleural cavity without damaging the lung.

An area of liver at the back (the **bare area**) is in direct contact with the diaphragm (**19.25**), but the rest is surrounded by a capsule of peritoneum which passes off the liver on to adjacent structures (**19.26**). These peritoneal reflexions form the so-called **peritoneal ligaments** (the **left**

and **right triangular ligaments**, and upper and lower layers of the **coronary ligament**), but despite their names they are not tough bundles of tissue like joint ligaments but simply peritoneal folds that play little part in holding the liver in its normal position. The liver is held up because at the back it clasps the **inferior vena cava** which lies in a deep **groove** of liver tissue; the **hepatic veins** (usually three large ones and perhaps one or two small accessory vessels) are *completely buried* within the liver and run into the vena cava while it is in its groove (**19.26b**), so that these veins can be said to have *no extrahepatic course*. The lowest reflection of peritoneum on the right side (the inferior layer of the coronary ligament) passes from the liver to the front of the right kidney, so forming a peritoneal recess (the **hepatorenal pouch** or **Morison's pouch**) where fluid may collect in a patient when lying on the back.

PORTA HEPATIS AND LESSER OMENTUM

The region where the hepatic artery, portal vein and biliary ducts enter or leave the liver is the **porta hepatis** (**19.25**), and passing from it to the lesser curvature of the stomach is the **lesser omentum** – the double fold of peritoneum that suspends the stomach from the liver. The **hepatic artery**, **portal vein** and **bile duct** are enclosed by this peritoneal fold, which has a *free margin* on its *right* side where it curls round to envelop these structures. Within this free margin of the lesser omentum, which forms the anterior boundary of the **epiploic foramen** (p.245), the portal vein is the most posterior structure, with the hepatic artery lying in front of the vein towards its left edge and the bile duct in front of the vein towards its right edge (**19.15**). This is one of the most important regions in the upper abdomen, because in all upper abdominal operations, especially those on the gall bladder, bile duct and stomach, the greatest care must be taken to avoid damaging these structures and to identify them correctly. From the point of view of surgery, it is perhaps fortunate that the bile duct is in front of the portal vein and towards its right, for this is the most accessible position for it.

LOBES AND SEGMENTS

The liver is descriptively divided into four named **lobes** – **right, caudate, quadrate** and **left** – but it is important to note that the *right* lobe (which is by far the largest) is supplied by the *right* branches of the hepatic artery and portal vein, while the *other three* are supplied by the *left* branches; thus the caudate and quadrate lobes belong *functionally* to the left lobe. Because of the way the main vessels divide within the liver, it is now customary to divide the liver into **segments**. Liver specialists (*hepatologists*) describe many segments based on vessel subdivisions, but there are four main segments which correspond to the lobes as follows:

left lateral segment = left lobe
left medial segment = caudate and quadrate lobes
right anterior segment = anterior part of right lobe
right posterior segment = posterior part of right lobe

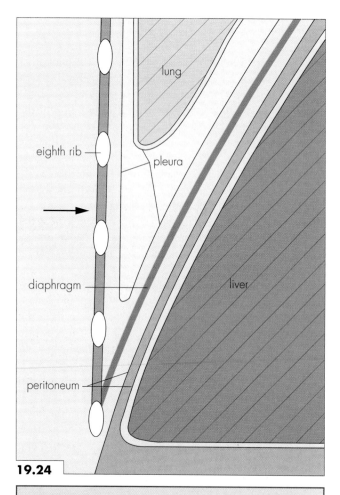

19.24

lung

eighth rib

pleura

diaphragm

liver

peritoneum

Fig. 19.24 Diagrammatic section through the right pleural cavity and liver, with the arrow indicating the path of the needle for liver biopsy.

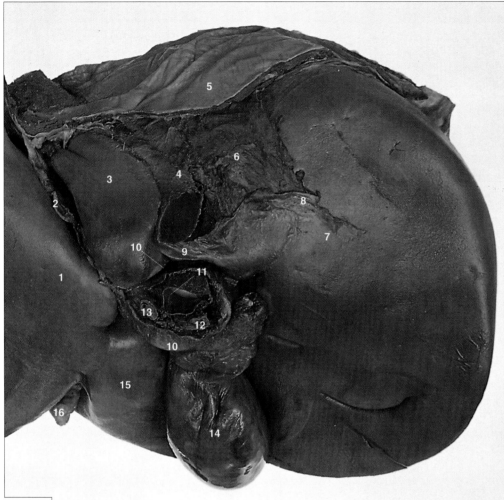

19.25

Fig. 19.25 Central part of the liver, looking down from above and behind, with part of the diaphragm in place.

BLOOD SUPPLY AND LYMPH DRAINAGE

The liver gets its arterial blood from the **common hepatic artery,** which is one of the three main branches of the coeliac trunk from the aorta (the other two are the left gastric and the splenic, **19.15**). The artery runs up in the free margin of the lesser omentum in front of the portal vein to the porta hepatis, where it divides into right and left branches that enter the liver.

The **portal vein** (**19.14**) is formed behind the neck of the pancreas by the union of the superior mesenteric and splenic veins (**19.15**); like the hepatic artery, it divides into right and left branches before entering the liver. For anastomoses between the portal and systemic veins, see below.

The **hepatic veins** (see above) drain into the inferior vena cava (**19.26b**).

The flow of lymph from the liver is greater than from any other organ and amounts to 0.75 ml per minute. It passes to

1 Left lobe
2 Fissure for ligamentum venosum, containing the lesser omentum
3 Caudate lobe
4 Inferior vena cava, lying in its deep groove of liver tissue and where the hepatic veins join it
5 Diaphragm
6 Bare area, with no peritoneal covering
7 Right lobe
8 Lower layer of coronary ligament, the part of the peritoneum reflected on to the right kidney forming the hepatorenal pouch
9 Caudate process, connecting the caudate lobe (3) to the right lobe (7) and forming the upper boundary of the epiploic foramen
10 Lesser omentum, surrounding the structures entering or leaving the porta hepatis - the portal vein (11), common hepatic duct (12) and hepatic artery (13)
11 Portal vein
12 Common hepatic duct, formed by the union of the right and left hepatic ducts
13 Hepatic artery
14 Gall bladder
15 Quadrate lobe
16 Falciform ligament containing ligamentum teres in fissure for the ligamentum teres

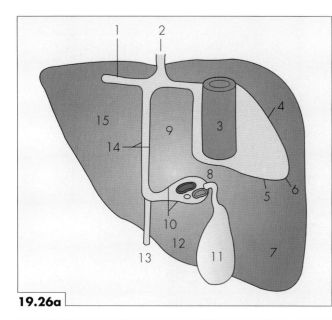

19.26a

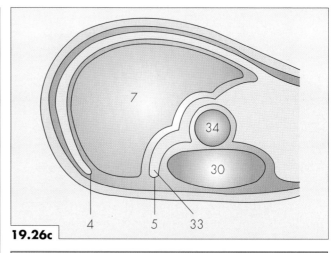

19.26c

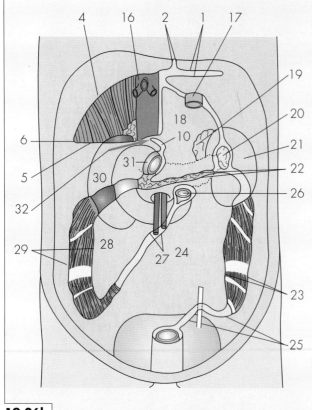

19.26b

Fig. 19.26 Diagrammatic representations of the peritoneal attachments on the liver and posterior abdominal wall.

(a) On the liver, seen from behind.

(b) On the posterior abdominal wall, seen from the front.

(c) Below the liver on the right, seen in a sagittal section through the right kidney.

1 Left triangular ligament
2 Falciform ligament (to diaphragm)
3 Inferior vena cava
4 Upper layer ⎫ of coronary
5 Lower layer ⎭ ligament
6 Right triangular ligament
7 Right lobe
8 Caudate process
9 Caudate lobe
10 Lesser omentum (in porta hepatis in **(a)**)
11 Gall bladder
12 Quadrate lobe
13 Falciform ligament (to anterior abdominal wall)
14 Lesser omentum
15 Left lobe
16 Hepatic veins entering inferior vena cava
17 Oesophagus
18 Lesser sac, the peritoneal recess behind the stomach
19 Left adrenal gland
20 Tail of pancreas in lienorenal ligament
21 Left kidney
22 Transverse mesocolon, the dividing line between the supracolic and infracolic compartments of peritoneum
23 Attachment of peritoneum to descending colon
24 Lower (left) part of infracolic compartment, below the root of the mesentery (27)
25 Sigmoid mesocolon, with the left ureter passing behind the apex of the inverted V-shaped attachment, a guide to the position of the ureter
26 Duodenojejunal flexure
27 Root of mesentery, with superior mesenteric vessels between its two peritoneal layers
28 Upper (right) part of infracolic compartment, above the root of the mesentery (27)
29 Attachment of peritoneum to ascending colon
30 Right kidney
31 Pylorus
32 Arrow in epiploic foramen, the entrance to the lesser sac
33 Hepatorenal pouch, where fluid may collect when laying down
34 Transverse colon

nodes in the porta hepatis and around the upper part of the inferior vena cava, and eventually reaches the thoracic duct (p.103).

NERVE SUPPLY

Sympathetic nerves enter the liver with the hepatic artery to control the calibre of the vessels, and, as with other viscera, pain fibres probably run with them, although the phrenic nerves (p.101) may also be involved. There are also some vagal (parasympathetic) fibres, but their function is not known for certain.

PORTAL–SYSTEMIC ANASTOMOSES

Certain diseases of the liver, in particular cirrhosis (which includes among its characteristic features the formation of new fibrous tissue), may cause an increase in the portal venous pressure (i.e. **portal hypertension**) to above the normal low value of 6–10 mmHg. When there is obstruction to the outflow of blood from the hepatic veins into the inferior vena cava, the backpressure that builds up in the portal system causes an increase in the size of the normally very small communications with vessels of the systemic system. These **portal–systemic anastomoses** allow some of the blood that would otherwise be dammed up in the portal system to escape into the general circulation.

There are *five sites* of portal–systemic anastomosis, but one is of particular importance because it may be dangerous to life; this is the wall (mainly the submucous layer) of the **lower end of the oesophagus** (p.103), where veins draining to the left gastric vein (which belongs to the portal system) anastomose with those draining to posterior intercostal vessels and the azygos vein (of the systemic system). In portal hypertension, these anastomotic connections may become dilated (leading to *oesophageal varices*, like varicose veins in the leg) and may burst, causing serious haemorrhage into the oesophagus and stomach which can be difficult to stop.

The other anastomotic sites are in the **upper end of the anal canal**, in the **periumbilical region of the anterior abdominal wall**, in **retroperitoneal areas of the abdomen** behind the ascending and descending colon, and at the **bare area of the liver**. Perhaps surprisingly, there is no increased incidence of haemorrhoids (p.266) in patients with portal hypertension.

STRUCTURE

Functionally, the liver consists of millions of hepatic **acini**, which in histological sections appear as diamond-shaped areas of pinhead size (**19.27a**). Each acinus is made up of plates or sheets of **hepatocytes** with intervening blood spaces – the **liver sinusoids**. At two opposite corners of the diamond, small branches of the hepatic artery and portal vein and a biliary duct form a **portal triad**, from which blood enters the sinusoids. At each of the other two corners of the diamond is a vein into which the sinusoidal blood drains;

these are the **central veins** (although they are at *corners* of the acini, ***not*** their centres; the name is derived from the old concept of liver structure – the *lobule* – where the vein was considered the central feature with the portal triads at the edges). In the sinusoids, the arterial and portal blood become mixed (**19.27b**); it flows through the sinusoids into the central veins which eventually merge to form the hepatic veins that enter the inferior vena cava. While passing through the sinusoids, solutes in the blood plasma (the fluid part of the blood without the blood cells) diffuse through the walls of the sinusoids to become taken up by the hepatocytes; this is the way oxygen from the arterial blood and digested substances from the portal blood enter the liver cells, and is also the way that most products from the liver cells (except bile, p.276) enter the blood.

Like any other blood vessels, the liver sinusoids are lined by endothelial cells, but some of them (the **Kupffer cells**) are *phagocytic* and therefore capable of ingesting bacteria and taking part in immune responses (p.69).

FUNCTION

The liver is involved in many of the body's biochemical activities, and its principal functions can be summarized as in *Table* **19.1**.

EXAMINATION

The normal liver may just be *palpable* at the right costal margin (**19.3a**), especially if the patient is asked to take a deep breath (which moves the liver down as the diaphragm contracts); when enlarged or hardened by disease it will be more obvious. Small specimens of liver tissue for microscopic examination may be obtained by biopsy (p.270).

Since the liver takes part in so many metabolic processes, there is no single, simple test of its function, and it must also be remembered that it can still cope with its normal activities when 90% of it has been destroyed by disease. Among the many possible tests of liver function, those most commonly used include estimations of **plasma bilirubin** levels (which is a test of the liver's *excretory* function), and **plasma albumin** and **prothrombin** (which are tests of its *secretory* function). One of the commonest clinical problems is to decide whether jaundice (see below) is hepatic or extrahepatic in origin.

DISEASES

Although *cancer **originating*** in the liver is rare, the liver is frequently the site of cancerous deposits (**liver metastases** or 'secondaries in the liver') which have spread to it by the bloodstream or lymphatics, not only from organs within the abdomen such as the stomach or colon but also from many other sites, including the breast, lung and vertebral column.

Jaundice (from the French for 'yellow') is a yellowish discoloration of the skin, whites of the eyes (the sclerae) and mucous membranes. It is not itself a disease (and has a

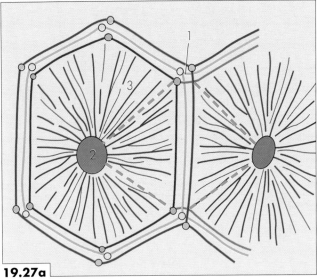

19.27a

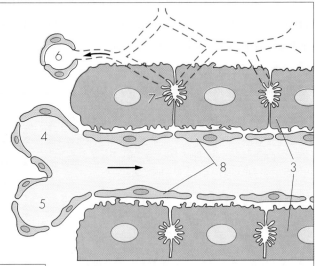

19.27b

Fig. 19.27 Diagrammatic representation of liver structure.
(a) Portal triads, with interconnecting vessels, and central veins. The region outlined by the interrupted green line is a diamond-shaped liver acinus, with central veins at one pair of opposite corners and portal triads at the other corners.
(b) The part of a sinusoid adjacent to a portal triad, with arrows indicating the direction of bloodflow towards the central vein, and bile towards a biliary duct.

1 Portal triad with branches of hepatic artery, portal vein and biliary ducts
2 Central vein
3 Cords of liver cells and sinusoids (see **b**)
4 Hepatic artery branch
5 Portal vein branch
6 Biliary duct
7 Bile canaliculus
8 Endothelium lining sinusoid

Table 19.1 Principal liver functions	
Digestion	Secretion of bile and the metabolism of bilirubin which is excreted in bile (p.276).
Protein metabolism	Manufacture of several plasma proteins, such as albumin, globulins, fibrinogen, and prothrombin (p.61) (but not the immunoglobulins of the immune response which are derived from plasma cells, p.69), and urea and uric acid (as the final stages of nitrogen metabolism, p.85).
Fat metabolism	Synthesis of fatty acids and cholesterol, and metabolism of steroids (p.85).
Carbohydrate metabolism	Manufacture of glycogen from monosaccharides (glycogenesis), synthesis of glucose from other substances such as pyruvate, lactate or amino acids (gluconeogenesis), and breakdown of stored glycogen to glucose (glycogenolysis) and its liberation into the bloodstream – probably the single most important function of the liver (p.84).
Storage	Glycogen, iron, vitamins A, D, E, K, B_{12} and folic acid.
Detoxication	Metabolism of foreign substances (including drugs) and hormones and their inactivation.

number of causes), but the fundamental reason is an increase in the amount of bilirubin in the blood (*hyperbilirubinaemia*). This may be due to excessive breakdown of red blood cells (*haemolytic jaundice*, see p.65), but is more commonly due to disease of the liver or biliary tract. Liver disease may so affect hepatocyte function that bilirubin is not removed from the bloodstream as it ought to be and so accumulates, giving rise to *hepatocellular* or *hepatic jaundice*. On the other hand, bilirubin may be produced normally by the liver but may be 'dammed back' by obstruction to the outflow of bile, as by a gallstone in the bile duct – this is *obstructive* or *cholestatic jaundice*.

Hepatitis is the general name for inflammatory and infectious disease of the liver, of which there are many causes. Among the most important infections are those due to viruses, especially the condition called *hepatitis B*. This, and other affections, may all cause varying degrees of hepatocellular jaundice. Hepatitis due to the type A virus (*hepatitis A*) is spread by faecal contamination because the virus lives in the alimentary tract. In contrast, hepatitis B is due to the type B virus which exists in the bloodstream and so can be spread by transfusions of infected blood or plasma, or through the use of contaminated needles (e.g. by drug addicts). This virus is also found in body fluids such as saliva and semen, so that spread by personal contact including sexual intercourse is another possibility.

Like jaundice, *cirrhosis* of the liver has many causes. The normal microscopic pattern of liver tissue is deranged by a characteristic mixture of excessive fibrous tissue formation and nodules of regenerating hepatocytes – all the response to prolonged and repeated liver-cell damage by the causal agents, of which the commonest are alcohol and hepatitis B. The distortion of the liver tissue disturbs the normal blood supply and so leads to further damage, and may cause such features as portal hypertension (with oesophageal varices, see p.273, and splenic enlargement, p.280), increasing liver failure, and *ascites* (the accumulation of fluid in the peritoneal cavity, which may occur not only with liver disease but in other conditions where there is increased venous pressure, such as congestive cardiac failure).

TRANSPLANTATION

Some patients with irreversible liver disease may be considered suitable for *liver transplantation*. The donor liver includes the gall bladder and suitable lengths of the inferior vena cava above and below the liver, of the bile duct, the portal vein and the hepatic artery, all of which are sutured to the cut ends of the appropriate structures after removal of the patient's own liver.

GALL BLADDER AND BILIARY TRACT

The sole liver product that does not normally enter the blood is **bile**. It assists fat digestion (see below) and is delivered to the duodenum from the liver by a system of channels – the **biliary tract** (also called the the **extrahepatic biliary system**, **19.28**). It consists of the **left** and **right hepatic ducts**, which leave the liver at the **porta hepatis** and join to form the **common hepatic duct** (about 4 cm long with a diameter of 4 mm). The common hepatic duct is joined by the **cystic duct** (about 3 cm long with a diameter of 3 mm) from the gall bladder to form the **bile duct** (formerly called the common bile duct and about 8 cm long with a diameter of 8 mm), which in turn opens into the second part of the **duodenum** (p.258).

The left hepatic duct drains bile from the left lobe and the caudate and quadrate lobes, and the right hepatic duct from the right lobe.

GALL BLADDER

The **gall bladder** (**19.16** and **19.28**) has the shape of a small, rather elongated pear about 7 cm (3 inches) long; it is slate-blue in colour and has a capacity of about 50 ml. The main part is the **body**, which adheres to the gall bladder bed on the liver. The peritoneum that forms the capsule for the liver

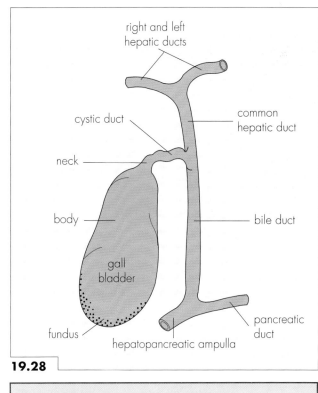

19.28

Fig. 19.28 Diagram of the biliary tract.

also encloses the gall bladder. At its upper end, the body narrows to a **neck** which in turn becomes the **cystic duct**, while the lower, broader end is the **fundus**. The fundus projects for about 1 cm below the lower border of the liver behind the anterior abdominal wall, at the level of the **ninth right costal cartilage**, where the lateral border of the rectus sheath meets the costal margin – one of the most important landmarks on the anterior abdominal wall (**19.3a**). The fundus is not normally palpable, but this area of the abdominal wall becomes tender on palpation when the gall bladder is the seat of inflammatory disease (*cholecystitis*, from the Latin for 'gall bladder'). The fundus normally overlies the junction of the first and second parts of the duodenum (hence the postmortem staining of the duodenum by bile that leaks through the gall bladder wall after death), and a high transverse colon may also be adjacent to the fundus.

HEPATIC DUCTS, CYSTIC DUCT AND BILE DUCT

The **right and left hepatic ducts** emerge from the porta hepatis and unite to form the **common hepatic duct** which, after a course of a centimeter or so, is joined just above the first part of the duodenum by the **cystic duct** from the gall bladder to form the **bile duct** (**19.14** and **19.28**). Running in the right free margin of the lesser omentum in front of the portal vein and towards its right side (p.270), the bile duct passes *behind* the first part of the duodenum and then runs in the groove between the head of the pancreas and the second part of the duodenum before penetrating the duodenal wall to unite with the end of the main pancreatic duct and open at the **major duodenal papilla** (**19.16**).

Circular smooth muscle fibres around the ends of the bile and pancreatic ducts and round the common channel (the **hepatopancreatic ampulla**) form the **ampullary sphincter** (the **sphincter of Oddi**). When the sphincter contracts to prevent bile entering the duodenum, bile flows along the cystic duct into the gall bladder. Although the wall of the gall bladder contains smooth muscle, the wall of the bile duct does not (except for the sphincter at the lower end).

BLOOD SUPPLY AND LYMPH DRAINAGE

The gall bladder receives small arteries through the gall bladder bed of the liver, but there is also a **cystic artery** which has a rather variable origin from some part of the hepatic artery (**19.13**). Veins drain directly into the bed on the liver; only rarely is there a **cystic vein** draining to the right branch of the portal vein.

Branches from the hepatic and gastroduodenal arteries supply the bile duct. Its vascularity is an important factor for successful liver transplantation (p.275).

Lymph from the biliary tract drains to nodes in the porta hepatis and to those associated with the head of the pancreas.

NERVE SUPPLY

Although both sympathetic and parasympathetic (vagal) nerve fibres supply the gall bladder, neural control is much less important than hormonal control by CCK (see below). However, the *sympathetic* supply is important because *pain* fibres from the gall bladder and the ducts run with the sympathetic nerves; they convey the pain of *biliary colic* (see below) into the spinal cord via the seventh to ninth thoracic nerves (p.273).

FUNCTION

Bile is a greenish-yellow mucoid fluid that is secreted constantly by hepatocytes at the rate of about 700 ml per day. It is collected into minute channels (**bile canaliculi**) between adjacent hepatocytes, and these drain into a system of ducts which eventually form the right and left hepatic ducts.

The purpose of bile is to aid the digestion of fat by acting as an emulsifying agent, so reducing surface tension and breaking down fat globules into smaller ones in order that lipase (from pancreatic juice, p.278) can act more effectively. Apart from water and some mineral salts, the constituents of bile are **cholesterol**, **bile pigments** (biliverdin and bilirubin – which give bile its colour and are breakdown products from the haemoglobin of old red cells destroyed by the liver), and **bile salts** (the sodium and potassium salts of the cholic and chenodeoxycholic acids secreted by the liver and which are the emulsifying agents).

The gall bladder acts as a contractile *storage* and *concentrating* organ. There is 'two way traffic' along the cystic duct: bile can flow along it into the gall bladder (which absorbs water and so concentrates the bile), and under the stimulus of the hormone **CCK** (which is released by small intestinal epithelium under the influence of fat in the duodenum, p.263), the gall bladder contracts to direct bile along the cystic duct into the bile duct and so into the duodenum.

EXAMINATION

The investigation of gall bladder function and disease is *radiological*. Pain and tenderness in the region of the right ninth costal cartilage (perhaps radiating round to the back) suggest gall bladder disease, but no part of the biliary tract is normally palpable, though the fundus may be if distended.

Modern *scanning* techniques, especially ultrasound, are often used in preference to long-standing radiological methods. A plain film of the abdomen may show gallstones, but not all gallstones are radio-opaque. The gall bladder and the duct system can be outlined by giving the patient an iodine-containing contrast medium (either orally or intravenously) which is taken up by the liver and excreted in the bile (outlining the gall bladder – *cholecystography*; outlining the duct system – *cholangiography*). The characteristic radiological position for the gall bladder is in the angle between the twelfth rib and the upper lumbar vertebrae. The patency or otherwise of the duct system can be assessed, e.g. the site and extent of obstruction by stone or tumour, and gall bladder function can be gauged by whether it can take up and concentrate the contrast medium, and whether it has contracted half an hour or so after taking a fatty meal. The duct system can also be outlined by injecting medium directly into a duct at operation (*operative cholangiography*), and, in the most recently developed investigative method, by cannulating the tip of the bile duct through the duodenal papilla via an endoscope passed through the mouth into the stomach and then the duodenum (the pancreatic duct can also be entered in this way – *ERCP, endoscopic retrograde cholangiopancreatography*).

DISEASES

For reasons that are not yet clear, some biliary constituents may precipitate in the gall bladder to form gallstones (*cholelithiasis*, **19.29**). They may be single or multiple, small or large, and may be formed from cholesterol or from other bile constituents. If small, they may pass through the cystic duct into the bile duct and so get discharged into the duodenum. As many as 10% of the population may have some kind of gallstones which may not cause any symptoms. Often they obstruct the cystic or bile ducts, giving rise to the painful spasms called *biliary colic* as biliary pressure tries to force the stone onwards. They are also the commonest cause of inflammatory disease of the gall bladder (*cholecystitis*). The gall bladder or bile duct may have to be opened surgically to remove the stone(s), or the gall bladder itself can be removed (opening the gall bladder – *cholecystostomy*; opening the bile duct – *choledochotomy*; removing the gall bladder – *cholecystectomy*).

Digestion can proceed quite normally after the removal of the gall bladder, despite the lack of bile storage. In time, the bile duct becomes rather dilated due to the prolonged accumulation of bile.

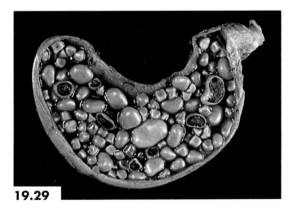

19.29

Fig. 19.29 Gallstones completely filling a gall bladder.

Cancer of the gall bladder is very uncommon, but it does occur occasionally in the elderly who have had gallstones for many years.

Complete and prolonged obstruction of the bile duct is one of the causes of *cholestatic jaundice* (p.275), and is most commonly due to a gallstone or carcinoma of the head of the pancreas.

PANCREAS

The **pancreas** is an abdominal gland whose **exocrine secretions** affect the digestion of protein, fat and carbohydrate, but which also contains **endocrine cells** that are involved principally in carbohydrate metabolism. It lies transversely behind the peritoneum, in the upper part of the abdomen (**19.15** and **19.16**). It is about 15 cm (6 inches) long, and is shaped rather like a thick hook or a short, stout walking-stick, with the crook or handle of the stick (the **head of the pancreas**) hanging downwards and lying within the 'C'-shaped curve of the duodenum, and the opposite end (the **tail of the pancreas**) overlying the hilum of the left kidney. Between these two ends is the the **body of the pancreas**, and the region where the body joins the head is known (appropriately) as the **neck of the pancreas**.

Behind the body is the splenic vein, a very straight vessel that joins the superior mesenteric vein behind the neck to form the portal vein. The splenic artery, in contrast to the vein, is a very tortuous vessel and runs along the upper border of the pancreas. The inferior vena cava, with the two renal veins joining it, is behind the head, with the aorta on the left side of the vena cava (**19.30**).

The bile duct runs behind the head of the pancreas, in the groove between it and the second part of the duodenum. The lowest part of the head is the **uncinate process** (**19.15**), which passes to the left behind the superior mesenteric vein and artery. These two large vessels bear the same relationship to one another as the vena cava does to the aorta: the vein is to the right of the artery.

The body is roughly triangular on cross section, and the duodenojejunal flexure of the small intestine is tucked up below the body at the left edge of the uncinate process. The transverse mesocolon – the fold of peritoneum that supports the transverse colon – hangs down from the lower border of the pancreas.

The exocrine secretions of the pancreas are delivered to the duodenum by the main and accessory pancreatic ducts (**19.15** and **19.16**). The **main pancreatic duct**, which has an internal diameter at its duodenal end of 3 mm, opens into the **hepatopancreatic ampulla** in common with the bile duct on the posteromedial surface of the second part of the duodenum. The **accessory pancreatic duct**, which is much smaller (and in fact is not even always present), opens on its own small papilla about 2 cm nearer the pylorus.

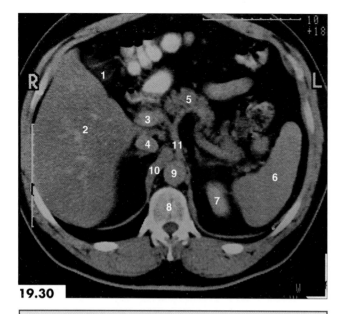

Fig. 19.30 CT scan of the upper abdomen, looking from below towards the head (the conventional view for scans of the trunk), showing the liver, spleen and pancreas, and various unlabelled parts of intestine. Compare with **19.14** and **19.15**.

1 Gall bladder
2 Liver
3 Portal vein
4 Inferior vena cava
5 Pancreas
6 Spleen
7 Upper part of left kidney
8 L1 vertebra
9 Aorta
10 Right crus of diaphragm
11 Coeliac trunk, here longer than usual and dividing like a Y into the common hepatic artery passing towards the liver (2) and the splenic artery running behind the pancreas (5) towards the spleen (6)

BLOOD SUPPLY AND LYMPH DRAINAGE

The blood supply comes mainly from the **splenic artery**, but the head receives branches from the **superior and inferior pancreaticoduodenal vessels** which lie between the pancreas and duodenum. Veins correspond to the arteries and drain into the portal system.

Lymph drains to any locally adjacent nodes.

STRUCTURE AND FUNCTION

Most of the gland (98% of it) is concerned with producing the **exocrine secretions**, which are derived from (microscopic) grape-like clusters of cells (called **acini**), rather like those of the parotid gland. The secretory products enter the duct system. The **endocrine secretions** come from a million or more rounded groups of cells, the **islets of Langerhans**, which are scattered among the exocrine acini and make up no more than 2% of the gland. Because the venous drainage of the pancreas is to the portal system, the hormonal products pass through the liver before entering the systemic circulation.

Although normally playing a part in the digestion of all three main foodstuffs – protein, fat and carbohydrate – the exocrine pancreas is not essential to life. The enzymes of the stomach and small intestine are capable of carrying out the functions of pancreatic juice, but the presence of a normal pancreas makes digestion more rapid and efficient. When malfunctioning, it is the effect on fat digestion that is most obvious.

Pancreatic juice is *alkaline* and therefore helps to neutralize the acid gastric contents that pass into the duodenum; pancreatic enzymes require an alkaline environment in which to act effectively – hence the high bicarbonate content of pancreatic secretions. The other main products of the exocrine pancreas are **lipase** which breaks down fats; **trypsin** and related enzymes which break down proteins; and **amylase** and **maltase** which break down carbohydrates.

The main stimulus to pancreatic exocrine secretion is hormonal. **Secretin** and **CCK** are released from intestinal endocrine cells when acid and foodstuffs, respectively, come into contact with small intestinal mucosa (p.263).

The principal endocrine secretions are **insulin** (from beta cells of the islets) and **glucagon** (from alpha cells); both these hormones are concerned with the control of blood sugar (p.84). Other cells produce **somatostatin** (*Table* 11.2, p.80).

EXAMINATION

Being so deeply placed, the pancreas cannot normally be palpated; by the time tumours become palpable, they will usually have made their presence felt in other ways, e.g. cancer of the head of the pancreas obstructing the bile duct and causing jaundice. The duct system can be examined radiologically by ERCP (p.277), and pancreatic juice can be collected for analysis by a nasogastric tube passed into the duodenum (though it will, of course, be contaminated by other secretions); the amounts of lipase, amylase, trypsin and bicarbonate can be determined. The commonest tests of exocrine function involve estimations of the **serum amylase** and **lipase**.

DISEASES

In pancreatic disease, the lack of lipase is the most obvious enzyme deficiency, and leads to *steatorrhoea* (excess fat in the faeces) that is due to inadequate fat **breakdown**. This type of steatorrhoea must be distinguished from that due to inadequate **absorption** of fat, which is an intestinal rather than a pancreatic defect (p.263). In inflammatory disease (*pancreatitis*) secretion may be dammed back in the duct system and lead to dangerous episodes of pancreatic autodigestion, with increased blood levels of lipase and amylase.

Pancreatic pain is felt in the upper abdomen and may radiate to the back, in the distribution of T8 to L1 dermatomes. It can be one of the most severe types of abdominal pain. The pain fibres, as from most viscera, run with the sympathetic nerves of the organ's blood vessels.

Carcinoma of the head of the pancreas may eventually cause cholestatic jaundice (p.277) due to pressure on the bile duct. Some uncommon pancreatic tumours are due to growths of the islet tissues, and cause symptoms according to the type of cells involved, e.g. beta-cell insulinomas cause excessive secretion of insulin.

The commonest disorder involving the pancreas is *diabetes mellitus* (from the Greek meaning 'sweet-water syphon', since an obvious symptom is excessive production of urine that contains sugar, p.286). This disease involves the endocrine part of the pancreas – the islets – rather than its exocrine part, and may be due to various causes. For example, the islet cells may secrete **insufficient** insulin (for unknown reasons): since insulin lowers blood-sugar levels, a reduction in insulin will lead to abnormally high blood glucose (*hyperglycaemia*). Such patients require insulin treatment (this is *Type I, insulin-dependent diabetes*), and must learn to test their own urine for glucose concentration and give themselves subcutaneous injections of insulin. (The hormone must be administered by injection rather than orally since it is broken down in the stomach.) Some patients can take tablets of a drug (*sulphonylurea*) that stimulates the islets to produce more insulin, but this is only effective if the islets are capable of responding.

In contrast to these diabetics, another group of people are diabetic because of *low responsiveness* to insulin: their islets can secrete normally, but the 'target cells' for insulin do not respond properly (perhaps due to insufficient insulin receptors, or to some abnormality in events inside the cells after receptor activation). Such patients may not, therefore, require insulin treatment but may be able to control their diabetes through dietary manipulation alone (this is *Type II, non-insulin dependent diabetes*).

In all cases of diabetes, proper control by some means or other is essential, not just to keep blood and urine levels of glucose near normal and to prevent ketosis and coma (p.85), but to diminish the risk of vascular and neural complications. The incidence of peripheral vascular diseases (which may lead to gangrene), and diseases of the retinal vessels and of peripheral nerves, is much higher in diabetics than in other people.

SPLEEN

The **spleen**, the largest of the **lymphoid organs** (p.68), is a highly vascular, purplish-red structure at the back of the left hypochondrial region of the abdomen (**19.11**, **19.15** and **19.33a**), and behind the midaxillary line. Some of its features are conveniently remembered by the odd numbers 1–11: it is 1 inch (2.5 cm) thick, 3 inches (7.5 cm) broad, 5 inches (12.5 cm) long, weighs 7 oz (200 g), and lies between the 9th and the 11th ribs. It is tucked away, well under cover of the costal margin, against the diaphragm and the upper part of the left kidney, and behind the stomach. These organs make concave impressions on it, and the middle of the region between these impressions is the **hilum**, where the vessels enter and leave. The anterior margin of the spleen usually shows one or more notches.

The spleen is surrounded by peritoneum that forms two 'pedicles' attaching it to the kidney and stomach. Between the two peritoneal layers of one of these supports, the **lienorenal ligament** ('lien' is Greek for spleen), the splenic vessels enter and leave.

BLOOD SUPPLY AND LYMPH DRAINAGE
The characteristically tortuous **splenic artery** (from the coeliac trunk) runs along the upper border of the pancreas to the hilum (**19.15**), while the **splenic vein**, a very straight vessel, runs behind the pancreas to join the superior mesenteric vein and so form the portal vein. Apart from producing lymphocytes that are discharged into the bloodstream (see below), the spleen has its own lymphatic drainage by vessels which leave the hilum and run beside the blood vessels to drain into coeliac nodes.

STRUCTURE AND FUNCTION
Underneath a capsule of connective tissue, the spleen can be regarded as a fine-textured sponge full of blood (up to about 200 ml) and containing lymphoid follicles. The spaces of the sponge are the **sinusoids**, which collectively form the 'red pulp'. The **lymphoid follicles**, which collectively form the 'white pulp', have small **arterioles** running through them – a feature unique to the spleen which immediately distinguishes it from other lymphoid organs (**9.2c**).

The spleen is not essential to life, and if it has to be removed due to injury or disease the patient suffers no ill effects. As in other lymphoid tissues, the follicles produce B and T lymphocytes as part of the immune response (p.69). Phagocytic cells, both in the walls of and outside the sinusoids, are concerned with removing old or damaged erythrocytes from the circulation. The spleen is thus a filter for blood and a lymphocyte producer, although much about its function and the need for its existence is obscure.

EXAMINATION

The normal spleen is not palpable; before it becomes so it usually has to be at least twice the normal size. When it enlarges (**19.35**) it moves round behind the anterior abdominal wall in the direction of the umbilicus (towards the right iliac fossa, in contrast to an enlarging left kidney which tends to move down towards the left iliac fossa). There are no specific tests for splenic function.

DISEASE AND INJURY

Lower thoracic and upper abdominal trauma may *rupture* the spleen, and, because of the resulting haemorrhage, this is a serious condition requiring emergency surgery. The possibility of rupture must be particularly remembered in children, because the thoracic cage in a child is more pliable than in an adult and therefore less protective. The organ is removed (in a *splenectomy*), since it is too difficult to stitch up a 'ruptured sponge'.

Enlargement of the spleen (*splenomegaly*) is frequently associated with disorders of red and white blood-cell formation, especially certain types of anaemia, leukaemia, lymphoma (including Hodgkin's disease) and thrombocytopenia (deficiency of blood platelets). It is also common in tropical climates as a result of infections such as malaria and kala-azar (*leishmaniasis*). Splenectomy may be required as part of the treatment.

ADRENAL GLANDS

There are two **adrenal glands** (also known as **suprarenal glands**) which are approximately triangular in shape and about 4 cm high, lying beside the upper end of each kidney in front of the lower part of the diaphragm (**19.15** and **19.31**). The one on the right is partly overlapped by the liver and inferior vena cava; the left adrenal is behind the stomach,

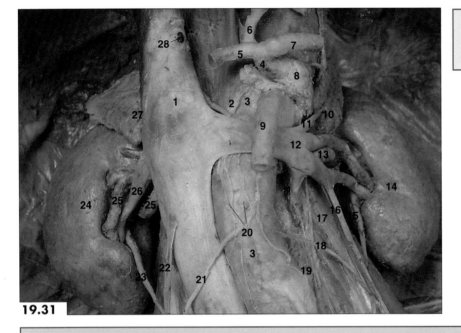

Fig. 19.31 Kidneys and adrenal glands, after removal of other abdominal viscera.

19.31

1 Inferior vena cava
2 Right crus of diaphragm and margin of aortic opening
3 Abdominal aorta
4 Coeliac trunk, dividing into common hepatic (5), left gastric (6) and splenic (7) arteries
5 Common hepatic artery
6 Left gastric artery
7 Splenic artery
8 Coeliac ganglia
9 Superior mesenteric artery
10 Left adrenal gland
11 Left adrenal vein, draining to the left renal vein (12)
12 Left renal vein, crossing the aorta (3) below the origin of the superior mesenteric artery (9). (When in position the splenic vein crosses above the superior mesenteric origin)
13 Left renal artery
14 Left kidney
15 Left ureter
16 Left gonadal vein, draining to the left renal vein (12)
17 Psoas major
18 Left gonadal artery
19 Left sympathetic trunk, at the left margin of the aorta. (The right sympathetic trunk is under cover of the right margin of the inferior vena cava, 1)
20 Aortic plexus
21 Right gonadal artery
22 Right gonadal vein, draining to the inferior vena cava (1)
23 Right ureter
24 Right kidney
25 Right renal artery
26 Right renal vein
27 Right adrenal gland, labelled where its own very short vein (obscured) drains into the inferior vena cava (1)
28 A hepatic vein

with its lower tip just being overlapped by the pancreas. Each has a very *profuse blood supply*, with numerous small branches coming from the aorta and from the renal and inferior phrenic arteries of its own side. In contrast, there is usually only *one vein on each side*; the right adrenal vein is very short and drains directly into the inferior vena cava, while the left one is longer and drains to the left renal vein. Being rather small and tucked away at the top of the kidneys, the normal adrenal glands cannot be felt on abdominal examination.

STRUCTURE AND FUNCTION

Each gland consists of two parts (**19.32**) that are functionally quite different. The outer part is the **adrenal cortex**, which secretes a variety of steroid hormones (principally aldosterone, cortisol and sex hormones), and the inner part is the **adrenal medulla**, which secretes two amine hormones (adrenaline and noradrenaline) and is closely associated with the sympathetic nervous system.

Adrenal Cortex

The outermost layer (the **zona glomerulosa**) of the adrenal cortex secretes **mineralocorticoids**, so called because they help to maintain the mineral balance of the body. The most important is **aldosterone** which acts on the kidneys to decrease the amount of sodium (salt) in the urine, so helping the body to retain salt; at the same time it increases potassium excretion in the urine and hence lowers blood potassium. A large amount of sweating, for example, which results in a loss of salt, causes an increase of aldosterone secretion to prevent further salt depletion. The secretion of aldosterone is controlled by the **renin–angiotensin mechanism of the kidney** (p.286), and *not* by pituitary ACTH.

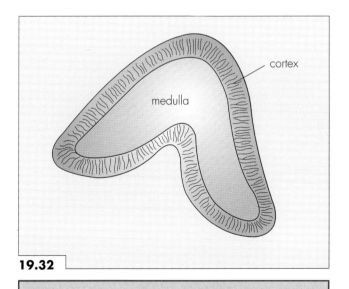

19.32

Fig. 19.32 Structure of the adrenal gland (as seen in cross-section), consisting of a continuous outer cortex surrounding a central medulla.

The middle layer (the **zona fasciculata**) secretes **glucocorticoids**, so called because of their role in glucose metabolism (although they also influence many other metabolic activities). The most important is **cortisol** (**hydrocortisone**). In particular, it stimulates gluconeogenesis (p.84) and the body's reaction to stress, whether caused by injury or infection. It is used as an anti-inflammatory and immunosuppressive agent. Cortisol secretion is normally under the control of **ACTH** from the anterior pituitary (p.140) which in turn is influenced by the hypothalamus responding to nervous and chemical messages from other parts of the brain and the affected parts of the body.

The level of cortisol in the blood also affects the amount of ACTH provided by the pituitary. If the cortisol level falls, more ACTH is released to restore the cortisol level to normal; if the cortisol level is high, ACTH secretion is depressed (this is an example of a 'feedback mechanism'). Since there are synthetic corticosteroids that closely resemble cortisol in their action, patients who are being treated with them are at risk of depriving their adrenals of their usual stimulation because the drugs give artificially high blood levels of cortisol-like substances which depress the amount of ACTH from the pituitary; the drugs have 'fooled' the pituitary that there is enough cortisol around and that no more ACTH is needed.

The third or innermost layer of the adrenal cortex (the **zona reticularis**) produces sex hormones (mainly androgens – male-type hormones) but in amounts that are usually insignificant unless affected by diease.

Adrenal Medulla

Cells of the **adrenal medulla** are quite different from those of the cortex. They resemble sympathetic nerve cells (and are derived embryologically from the same tissue). Upon stimulation by sympathetic preganglionic nerve fibres, they secrete two hormones into the circulation, **adrenaline** and **noradrenaline** (**epinephrine** and **norepinephrine**) which prepare the body for 'flight or fight' reactions. Thus they augment the actions of the sympathetic nervous system (p.47).

EXAMINATION

Being small and deeply placed, the adrenals are well out of reach on palpation of the abdomen. Scanning methods can define their position and size, but most adrenal investigations depend upon the analysis of the blood levels of its hormones.

DISEASES

Disease may affect the whole gland or just one of its parts or layers, and the effects will obviously vary according to whether there is overproduction (*hypersecretion*) or underproduction (*hyposecretion*) of the hormones concerned.

Excessive secretion of aldosterone (*hyperaldosteronism*) may be due to adrenal tumours (as in Conn's syndrome – *primary aldosteronism*) but may also be caused by kidney disturbances (*secondary aldosteronism*). The patient's symptoms include hypertension and muscle weakness (due to the loss of potassium). Single tumours can be removed intact but frequently the tumours are multiple so that the whole gland may have to be removed (*adrenalectomy*). If both glands are involved, *bilateral adrenalectomy* (removing both of them) may have to be carried out, in which case the patient must have replacement drug therapy throughout life.

Excessive cortisol secretion may be caused by tumours of the adrenal itself, or by tumours of the pituitary (and hence, excessive production of ACTH). This condition (*Cushing's syndrome*) is rare but is most common in females, and results in fatness and various metabolic disturbances, with hypertension, muscle weakness and often excessive hair growth. The patient develops the same type of rounded 'moon face' as those who have been on prolonged corticosteroid therapy. Strangely, some tumours of the lungs in males can also produce large amounts of ACTH. Treatment depends on the cause; adrenal or pituitary tumours may have to be removed, or the pituitary may have to be treated by radiation.

Too little secretion by the adrenal cortex occurs in *Addison's disease*, another rare condition, due to an autoimmune degeneration of the cortex (although some cases are due to tuberculosis). The principal features are due to lack of aldosterone and cortisol, and, although the disease is very slowly progressive, there may be sudden life-threatening crises from, say, a very minor infection because the adrenals cannot respond to stress in the usual way. There is loss of salt in the urine and low blood pressure, often with hypoglycaemia. One of the characteristic features is an increase of skin pigmentation, like suntan in those with fair skins, and pigmented spots often appear in the mucous membrane of the cheeks. Treatment with hydrocortisone is required, often intravenously if the patient is very ill.

Excessive secretion of androgens causes *adrenal virilism*, a rare condition that usually occurs in females and causes them to develop masculine features such as increased hairiness (hirsutism), deepening of the voice, reduction in breast size and an increase in skeletal muscularity.

Like the adrenal cortex, disease of the adrenal medulla is rare, but a special kind of tumour can occur (a *phaeochromocytoma*) which causes excessive secretion of adrenaline and therefore hypertension. In any surgery on the adrenal, the gland must be handled with delicacy because squeezing it will cause a sudden discharge of adrenaline into the bloodstream with undesirable surges in blood pressure. If the gland is being removed, the adrenal vein is tied off *before* the arteries to prevent this happening; usually when organs (such as the kidneys) are being removed, the arteries are tied off first.

KIDNEYS

The two **kidneys** lie in similar positions behind the peritoneum (i.e. they are both retroperitoneal) on each side of the posterior abdominal wall (**19.15** and **19.31**). The lowest part of the diaphragm is behind the uppermost part of each kidney, and the rest of the organ lies in front of the psoas major and quadratus lumborum muscles. The left kidney is at a slightly higher level than the right because of the bulk of the liver on the right; the top of the left kidney is level with the eleventh rib but the right one only rises as high as the twelfth rib. Behind the diaphragm, which is attached to the twelfth rib, is the lowest part of the pleural cavity. The **pleura** is the most important structure related to the back of the kidney, because many surgical operations on the kidney are carried out through an incision at the back below the last rib, so that the organ can be exposed retroperitoneally without entering the peritoneal cavity (so avoiding the possibility of introducing infection into the cavity).

Because of the forward bulge of the lumbar part of the vertebral column, the kidneys do not lie flat on the posterior abdominal wall but are tilted at an angle of about 45° (**19.33**), with the **hilum** (where the vessels and ureter enter or leave) in the middle of the medial border. Apart from being surrounded by its own **capsule**, which is an integral part of the organ, the kidney is surrounded by a variable amount of fat (**perinephric or perirenal fat**). The fat, in turn, lies inside a connective tissue covering – the **renal fascia**. The fat and the renal fascia, together with the overlying peritoneum, all help to keep the kidney in its normal position.

In front of the left kidney, a triangle of structures overlaps its upper part (**19.15**): the pancreas transversely across the hilum, the adrenal gland along its medial border, and the spleen along its lateral border. In front of all three, and with the transverse mesocolon hanging down from the pancreas, is the stomach with the lesser sac of peritoneum (p.243) intervening. Part of the colon in the region of the splenic flexure and a coil of small intestine overlap the lower pole.

On the right, the second part of the duodenum overlaps the hilum. The adrenal gland is at the top of the upper pole which is covered by the part of the peritoneum that forms the hepatorenal pouch (p.270). The upper pole is therefore adjacent to, but not actually in contact with (because peritoneum intervenes), the right lobe of the liver. The transverse mesocolon and colon cross the middle of the kidney lateral to the duodenum, and coils of small intestine overlie the lower pole.

The **renal pelvis** (**19.34**) emerges from the hilum; this is the collecting reservoir for urine, and it soon becomes narrow and changes its name to the **ureter** (p.288). (*Pelvis* is the Latin for 'basin', but from the Greek is derived *pyelitis*, meaning 'inflammatory disease of the renal pelvis'). In front

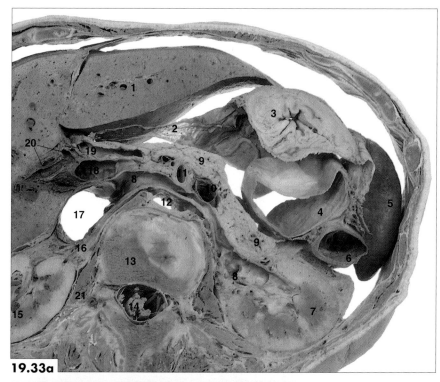

19.33a

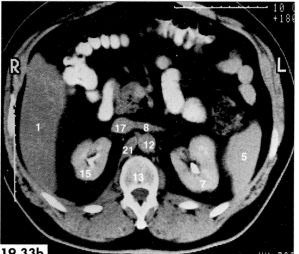

19.33b

Fig. 19.33 Horizontal sections through the upper abdomen.
(a) Section, seen from below looking towards the head (like the CT scan in **b**).
(b) CT scan, at a similar level to **(a)**, with various unlabelled parts of intestine.

1 Liver
2 Lesser omentum
3 Stomach
4 Transverse colon
5 Spleen
6 Descending colon
7 Left kidney
8 Left renal vein
9 Pancreas
10 Splenic vein
11 Superior mesenteric artery
12 Aorta
13 Body of L1 vertebra
14 Conus medullaris of spinal cord and nerve roots of cauda equina
15 Right kidney
16 Right renal artery
17 Inferior vena cava
18 Portal vein
19 Hepatic artery
20 Hepatic ducts
21 Right crus of diaphragm

of the renal pelvis is the renal artery, and in front of the artery lies the renal vein (see below). So, the general order of structures in the hilum of a kidney is remembered as vein, artery, ureter from front to back (**19.31**); this is the standard pattern, but occasional branches of the vessels may be out of order.

BLOOD SUPPLY AND LYMPH DRAINAGE

The paired **renal arteries** arise at right angles from each side of the aorta (**19.31**) at about the level of L1 vertebra. Although the way each artery divides as it enters the kidney is rather variable, the end result is always five principal branches which each supply a **segment** of renal tissue, i.e. there are five segments in each kidney. Each segment is a self-contained unit with no arterial anastomosis between segments, but the corresponding veins do make good connections between segments.

The single **renal vein** from each kidney lies *in front* of the corresponding artery, and drains directly into the inferior vena cava. The right vein is only about 2.5 cm (1 inch) long and has no tributaries, but the left one is 7.5. cm (3 inches) long, having farther to go to reach the vena cava, and it receives the left gonadal vein (whether testicular or ovarian) and the left adrenal vein. On the right, these veins drain directly to the vena cava.

Lymph drains to nodes beside the aorta.

STRUCTURE

As seen in a longitudinal section through the hilum (**19.34**), the outer part of the kidney is the **cortex**, which has projections, the **renal columns**, lying between darker areas, the **pyramids**, which collectively form the **medulla**. The tip of each pyramid projects as a **renal papilla** into a **minor calyx**, and the ten or so minor calyces unite to form two or three **major calyces**. These, in turn, join to form the **renal pelvis** that leaves the hilum to become the **ureter**. In general, the cortex contains the glomeruli and the convoluted parts of the nephrons, while the medulla contains the straight parts of the nephrons and collecting ducts, but no glomeruli (p.89).

FUNCTION: FORMATION OF URINE

The kidneys exist to control the *fluid* (i.e. water) and *electrolyte* (chiefly sodium) composition of the body within the narrow limits required by cells and tissues in order to function properly. They do this by producing a watery solution, **urine**, containing minerals and waste products. The kidneys also have an unexpected role in blood formation by secreting the hormone **erythropoietin** (p.64).

Body Water

The body obtains **water** (*Table* **19.2**) from the water contained in food (up to 1 litre per day), drunk as fluid (about 1.5 litres), and as a product of the body's own metabolism (about 500 ml). The body loses fluid from the lungs in the expired air (400 ml), in sweat (900 ml of insensible sweat, see p.18, and perhaps several litres depending on exercise, temperature and humidity), in the faeces (200 ml), and in the urine (1.5 litres per day). The intake of water is controlled by thirst, and the output of urine mainly by the pituitary hormone ADH (p.135 and below).

Certain specialized **receptor cells in the hypothalamus** of the brain are affected by slight changes in the water concentration in blood, and can increase or diminish the feeling of *thirst* – the need to drink. True thirst is satisfied by drinking, and must be distinguished from mere dryness of the mouth (from mouth breathing or too much talking!) which is cured by simply wetting the mouth.

The total amount of water in an adult male (*Table* **19.2**) is about 40 litres – roughly 60% of body weight. About two-thirds of it is within cells as the **intracellular fluid** (25 litres), and the rest (15 litres) is **extracellular fluid**, divided between **blood plasma** (3 litres in the vascular system or **intravascular compartment**), and **interstitial fluid** (12 litres) forming the **extravascular compartment**, within the tissues but outside the cells and the vascular system. The intracellular fluid contains relatively high concentrations of potassium (K^+, as in nerve cells, where its importance in nerve impulses has been

described on p.47), while in extracellular fluid the main ion is sodium (Na^+). The metabolic activity of cells is necessary for maintaining this distinction, and changes in the fluid in the various 'compartments' are linked to changes in ionic

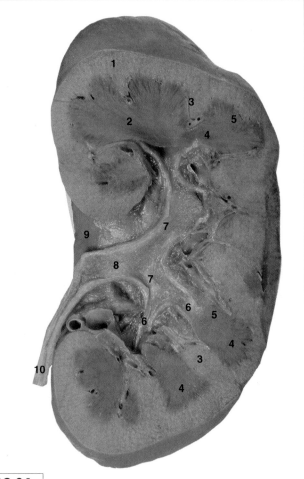

19.34

Fig. 19.34 Structure of the kidney, seen in a vertical section through the hilum but with most vessels removed to give a clear view of the renal pelvis.

1 Cortex
2 Medulla
3 Renal column, a projection of cortex between medullary pyramids (5)
4 Renal papilla, where collecting tubules open into a minor calyx (6)
5 Medullary pyramid
6 Minor calyx
7 Major calyx, receiving minor calyces
8 Renal pelvis, receiving major calyces
9 Hilum
10 Ureter

concentration: more Na⁺ leads to more extracellular fluid, and more K⁺ leads to more intracellular fluid. Two common clinical examples of changes in fluid volumes are an excess of extracellular fluid giving rise to oedema (p.119), and a fall in plasma volume causing shock (p.58).

In *starvation*, a certain minimal amount of water (about 700 ml) is needed every day for the excretion of the waste products of the body's cellular activity. If no water is drunk, death may be expected in about a week, but if water is taken survival for several weeks is possible.

Sodium is obtained from the diet in variable amounts, and is lost in sweat, in faeces (negligible, unless there is diarrhoea), and in the urine, whose sodium content is controlled by glomerular filtration (see below), by the adrenal hormone aldosterone (see below) and perhaps surprisingly by the recently discovered hormone from the right atrium of the heart (**atrial natriuretic hormone, atriopeptin**).

Table 19.2 Body Water (volumes in litres)	
Interstitial fluid	12.0
Plasma volume	3.0
Total extracellular fluid	**15.0**
Intracellular fluid	25.0
TOTAL BODY WATER:	**40.0**
DAILY LOSSES:	
Urine	1.5
Sweat	0.9
Lungs	0.4
Faeces	0.2
Total daily output	**3.0**
DAILY INTAKE:	
Fluid drunk	1.5
Fluid in food	1.0
Metabolic water	0.5
Total daily intake	**3.0**

Glomerular Filtration and Tubular Reabsorption

The functional unit of the kidney is the **nephron** (with about 1 million being present in each kidney); the different parts of a nephron are illustrated in **12.2**. Urine is produced mainly by *glomerular filtration* and *tubular reabsorption*: filtration of blood plasma through the glomerular capillaries into the space of Bowman's capsule, and reabsorption of substances from this filtered fluid when it is in the various parts of the tubule. There is also a small amount of *tubular secretion* (sometimes called *tubular* **excretion**), where substances are added to the filtrate in the tubules.

When a kidney is cut in half longitudinally (**19.34**), the renal pelvis can be followed inwards to the major and minor calyces. Urine flows into the minor calyces because the collecting ducts, which are the ends of the tubules of the nephrons, congregate in the medullary papillae and open into the calyces.

The formation of the **glomerular filtrate** depends on an adequate blood pressure in the capillaries of the glomeruli. A huge quantity of glomerular filtrate is produced every day – about 180 litres – but since the amount of urine produced in a day is only about 1.5 litres, most of the filtrate is reabsorbed. About 160 litres of filtrate (with its contained sodium chloride and other minerals) is reabsorbed by the proximal tubules of the nephrons and passes out into the surrounding capillaries and so into the bloodstream. The rest of the water is reabsorbed primarily by the distal tubules and collecting ducts. This part of the water absorption is under the control of ADH, the antidiuretic hormone of the posterior pituitary (p.135).

The loops of Henle, which extend into the papillae of the medulla of the kidney, are concerned with establishing a *gradient in osmolarity* (i.e. a gradient in solute concentration) of the interstitium in the medulla: the osmolarity of the interstitial fluid at the outer boundary of the medulla is similar to that of plasma, but it increases progressively towards the tips of the papillae. This increase in interstitial fluid osmolarity, from medullary boundary to tip, is essential for *concentrating* the urine during its final passage through the collecting ducts – a process to be described below. The mechanism for establishing the gradient involves a *countercurrent multiplier system* in the medulla (for details of which the reader is referred to specialized texts).

The amount of **sodium** reabsorbed by the **renal tubules** is under the influence of **aldosterone** secreted by the adrenal cortex. Aldosterone increases sodium reabsorption and so decreases the amount lost in the urine (it also decreases the amount lost in sweat, p.18). The control of aldosterone secretion occurs in a rather roundabout way. When the concentration of sodium in blood plasma falls (*hyponatraemia*, from *natrium* – the Latin for sodium), the kidney is

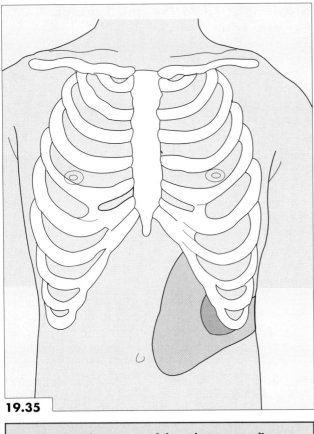

19.35

Fig. 19.35 Enlargement of the spleen, extending progressively downwards and inwards towards the umbilicus.

surrounding tissue. The extent to which this happens is controlled by **ADH** from the posterior pituitary. If there is ADH in the area (delivered by the bloodstream), the collecting ducts become permeable to water (but not salt), which leaves the urine, thus reducing its volume and making it more concentrated (and therefore reducing the tendency to diuresis). If there is no ADH, the ducts do not become permeable and so the amount of urine is not reduced. ADH also acts on the distal tubules in the same way.

What controls the amount of ADH released by the pituitary? There are certain nerve receptors in the hypothalamus which detect very small changes in the water concentration of the blood (p.284). If the water intake is low, the blood becomes slightly more concentrated (i.e. its osmotic pressure rises), and this stimulates these **osmoreceptors** which in turn stimulate the hypothalamic cells that manufacture and store ADH to secrete it into the bloodstream.

By the time fluid (i.e. urine) leaves the collecting ducts to enter the minor calyces, it has reached its final composition and osmolarity; the calyces, renal pelves, ureters and bladder do not modify it further in any way.

In order to illustrate the way in which the kidneys function, the above outline has mentioned only water and sodium chloride; of course, many other substances are in the watery solution that is processed by the kidneys. Some are completely reabsorbed, others not at all. Among those that are most important, **glucose** is normally completely reabsorbed (in the proximal tubules), but if the blood glucose level becomes unusually high, as in diabetes (p.279), the excess will appear in the urine. Many waste products of protein metabolism such as **creatinine** are not reabsorbed at all. **Potassium** usually moves in and out of tubules in the opposite direction to sodium. The maintenance of the **pH of the blood** is another important renal function; hydrogen ions which enter the tubules from the blood can combine with other ions and so be eliminated as salts in the urine.

In summary, *urine formation* is mainly the product of *glomerular filtration* (which depends on blood pressure) and *tubular reabsorption* (which includes the countercurrent multiplier system and the effect of ADH on distal tubules and collecting ducts). A third factor, *tubular secretion*, also plays a role in modifying urine composition. It follows that interference with any one, or more, of these mechanisms will lead to malfunction, i.e. varying degrees of renal failure.

EXAMINATION

The lower end of a normal kidney may just be *palpable* on bimanual examination: one hand is placed on the back below the rib margin, and the other on the anterior abdominal wall below the rib margin; when the patient takes a deep breath (which lowers the diaphragm) and the hands are pushed gently together, the lower edge of the kidney may be felt. An enlarged kidney will be relatively easy to feel through the

stimulated to increase the secretion of its own enzyme **renin**, which is derived from certain cells of the afferent arterioles adjacent to the distal convoluted tubules – the **juxta-glomerular** or **JG cells**, so called because these vessels and tubules lie beside the glomerulus. The renin released into the blood acts on a plasma protein, **angiotensinogen** (produced like other plasma proteins by the liver), splitting a smaller molecule, **angiotensin I**, away from it. After further modification (to **angiotensin II**) it is able to stimulate the adrenal cortex to secrete more aldosterone. As aldosterone concentration rises, more sodium is retained by the kidney tubules and the sodium levels then rise in the bloodstream and in body tissues in general. With *hypernatraemia* (increased plasma sodium), the renin–angiotensin system is suppressed, and so sodium is allowed to be lost in the urine.

Now consider the **collecting ducts**; before opening on to the tip of a papilla into a minor calyx, they have to pass through the papillary tissue with the high salt concentration. Since the urine in the collecting ducts is dilute (with a low osmotic pressure) and the tissue surrounding the lower end of the duct has a high salt concentration (with a high osmotic pressure), water will tend to leave the ducts and enter the anterior abdominal wall, and on the left must be distinguished from an enlarged spleen (p.280 and 19.35).

Tests carried out on urine (*urinalysis*) and blood plasma (*serum studies*) are designed to detect substances that are not normally present and those that are present but are at abnormal concentrations.

The simplest test of renal function is the determination of the *specific gravity* of the urine; this indicates the **concentrating power** of the kidney. Values less than 1.010 are abnormally low. Measurement of the total *volume* of urine voided over 24 hours is an index of the kidneys' **excretory capacity**.

Other simple and common tests are those for protein, glucose and ketone bodies, and all can be carried out using chemically impregnated paper strips that are dipped into the urine and which change colour to indicate particular concentrations of those substances. Protein in the urine (*proteinuria*) suggests a defect of glomerular filtration, but the presence of glucose (*glucosuria*) indicates a 'spill-over' from a high concentration in blood plasma rather than a renal defect. Ketone bodies in the urine (*ketonuria*) indicate a disturbance in the effect of insulin on fat metabolism (p.85). Many more complex laboratory tests can be used to measure such features as the glomerular filtration rate, and blood concentrations of creatinine, urea and other substances.

Radiology and modern scanning methods are essential tools for renal examination. Straight X-rays of the abdomen usually show faint outlines of the kidneys; stones (*calculi*) usually show as opacities. Contrast medium given intravenously (*intravenous pyelogram* or *urogram, IVP* or *IVU*) is concentrated by normally functioning kidneys and gives a radiographic outline of the renal calyces and ureters. A non-functioning kidney will not concentrate the medium and so the pattern of the calyces will not show up on the X-ray film. Scanning will indicate whether the kidneys are of normal size, shape and position, or whether they are distorted, e.g. by tumours.

DISEASES

Apart from infections (*pyelonephritis*) that may involve other parts of the urinary tract, the common diseases of the kidney are acute renal failure (*uraemia*), various types of nephritis, tumours and stones.

Acute renal failure (*acute tubular necrosis*) follows damage to the renal tubules from the decreased renal bloodflow after such conditions as the shock, haemorrhage and dehydration of severe accidents, or other renal or vascular diseases (such as hypertension). *Nephritis*, properly called *glomerulonephritis* (or *Bright's disease*), can be acute or chronic; it may be an immune reaction to streptococcal infection (such as a severe sore throat) but often the cause is not clear. Various types are described but all involve malfunction of the glomeruli.

Kidney tumours are of varying degrees of malignancy; the commonest is the *hypernephroma*, and while they may

eventually cause renal malfunction they may also spread dangerously to other organs such as the liver, lung and bones by the venous or lymphatic systems.

Any of the above conditions may give rise to a group of signs and symptoms including oedema, excessive urinary protein (*proteinuria*) and low serum albumin (*hypoalbuminaemia*) which collectively form the *nephrotic syndrome*. Frequent analysis of urine and blood is necessary to monitor progress and the effects of treatment, which is not usually curative but designed to minimize progressive disease.

Renal stones (*calculi*) collecting in the calyces and renal pelvis may cause intermittent pain (*renal colic*) and haemorrhage, leading to blood-stained urine (*haematuria*). Many stones are precipitates of various calcium salts, but there are other varieties including those derived from uric acid. Very small ones may pass down the ureter into the bladder and out through the urethra with the urine, but for larger ones surgical removal may be required. Successful dissolution by ultrasound without the need for surgery is a recent development.

Artificial Kidney

To maintain life in the presence of increasing renal failure and in the absence of a suitable renal transplant, it may be necessary to use an *artificial kidney*. The patient's blood (taken via a cannula inserted into the radial artery) is led into the kidney machine, which is designed to bring the blood into contact with a *semipermeable membrane* (in the form of a coiled tube immersed in a bath of fluid). This allows water, salts and products of the body's metabolism to diffuse freely through the membrane, but keeps blood cells and plasma proteins in the blood. The composition of the fluid on the other side of the membrane is carefully controlled so that waste products diffuse rapidly into it but leave the concentration of the normal electrolytes of the blood plasma essentially unchanged. The blood is then returned to the patient, through a cannula into the cephalic or other suitable forearm vein. The blood has thus been 'cleared' of unwanted substances, the process being known as *haemodialysis*; the fluid into which they diffuse is the *dialysate*. Alternatively, in *continuous ambulatory peritoneal dialysis* (CAPD), patients themselves can learn to pour dialysate into, and pump it out of, the peritoneal cavity three or four times a day through a tube placed permanently in the anterior abdominal wall; the peritoneum acts as the semipermeable membrane.

Renal Transplantation

In certain cases where renal disease is irreversible, a normal kidney from a donor, either living or recently deceased, can be *transplanted* to take over the function of the faulty organs. The donor kidney is usually placed in the lower abdomen above the pelvic brim; the renal artery and vein are anastomosed to the iliac vessels, and the ureter is joined to the top of the bladder. (The patient's own kidneys are not removed.) To minimize the problems of immunosuppression (p.70), tissue-typing must ensure that the new kidney is suitably compatible.

URETERS

Each **ureter** is a tube of smooth muscle about 25 cm (10 inches) long with a mucous membrane lined by **transitional epithelium** – a type of stratified epithelium about six layers thick which is characteristic of the urinary tract and does not allow absorption of urine. The ureter runs down behind the peritoneum of the posterior abdominal wall over the psoas major muscle (**19.10**). When filled with contrast medium in a radiograph, its normal position is seen to be over the transverse processes of the lumbar vertebrae. At the division of the common iliac artery into internal and external iliac branches, the ureter enters the pelvis and runs down the side wall in front of the internal iliac artery (**19.37**) where, in the female, the ovary lies just in front of it (**19.38**). On the left it lies beneath the apex of the sigmoid mesocolon (**19.26b**; p.265). When it reaches the pelvic floor it turns medially and forwards to enter the bladder; as it does so in the male it is crossed by the ductus deferens (**19.38**), while in the female it is crossed by the uterine artery (**19.40b**) and the base of the broad ligament of the uterus. The ureter in the female pelvis has been described as 'the gynaecologist's nightmare'; every care must be taken to avoid accidental damage to it during gynaecological operations, especially when disease alters its expected position.

As it lies on the posterior abdominal wall, the ureter adheres to the overlying peritoneum; if at operation the adjacent peritoneum is picked up by forceps, the ureter comes up with it. The ureter can be distinguished from blood vessels in the living body as a whitish cord-like structure that does not pulsate (as an artery would) and which can be made to show peristaltic movements by gently pinching it with forceps.

BLOOD SUPPLY AND LYMPH DRAINAGE
The ureter gets its blood supply by small branches from adjacent vessels, such as the **renal**, **gonadal** and **iliac arteries**. The vessels form an anastomotic network in the connective tissue on its outer surface, and at operation, when dissecting out a ureter, it is important not to strip loose tissue from its surface to make a nice 'clean' dissection; this destroys the blood supply.

Lymph drains to adjacent abdominal or pelvic nodes.

NERVE SUPPLY
Although receiving sympathetic and parasympathetic fibres, the pumping action of the ureter (see below) does not depend on this supply. The stimulus for ureteral *pain* is tension in the wall (see below), and, as with most other viscera, the pain fibres run with the **sympathetic** nerves; they enter the spinal cord via the last two thoracic and first two lumbar nerves.

FUNCTION
The ureter makes periodic *peristaltic movements* to pump urine down towards the bladder. They begin from certain specialized muscle cells in the walls of the minor calyces within the kidney, and the contractions then spread through the renal pelvis into the muscle of the ureteral wall. Peristalsis does *not* depend on the external nerve supply (see above).

EXAMINATION
Very rarely, a stone in the lower part of the ureter may be detected on rectal or vaginal examination (pp.268 and 300), but normally the ureters cannot be felt, and, apart from the possibility of seeing and feeling them during abdominal operations, *radiography* is the usual method of examination. *Urography* and other imaging methods (p.287) may reveal stones or other obstructions (termed *strictures*, e.g. following infections or pressure from adjacent structures). The openings of the ureters into the bladder can be seen on *cystoscopy* (p.295), and ureteral catheters can be introduced for retrograde injection of contrast medium. On a standard anteroposterior radiograph, the ureters should normally be seen to lie over the tips of the transverse processes of the lumbar vertebrae, and they can be identified on *CT scans*, especially when containing contrast medium.

DISEASES
The ureter itself is not commonly the site of disease. The commonest condition to affect it is a small stone in the kidney (a *renal calculus*, p.287), which moves into the renal pelvis and then down the ureter, causing bouts of pain which may be intense (i.e. *renal colic* – still so called even if the pain is ureteric rather than renal in origin). The stone may become 'stuck' at the places where the ureter is constricted: at its junction with the renal pelvis, where it crosses the pelvic brim, and at the ureteric orifice in the bladder (the narrowest part of all).

Such conditions as *congenital strictures of the ureter* or pressure from adjacent tumours may cause dilatation of the ureter (*hydroureter*) and of the renal pelvis and calyces (*hydronephrosis*). Excessive back pressure may interfere with renal function.

PELVIC CAVITY AND PERINEUM

The part of the abdominal cavity below the pelvic brim (p.243) is the **pelvic cavity**. Its posterior wall is formed by the sacrum and coccyx, with the overlying piriformis and coccygeus muscles. At the side lie the parts of the hip bone below the pelvic brim, with much of the bone covered by the obturator internus muscle. The lower boundary of the pelvis (the **pelvic floor** or **pelvic diaphragm**), is formed by the levator ani and coccygeus muscles of both sides (**19.22** and **19.36**). Thus, the region above the pelvic diaphragm is the **pelvis** (or **pelvic cavity**); the small remaining part of the trunk of the body below the pelvic diaphragm is the **perineum**. The peritoneum of the abdominal cavity extends down into the pelvis to cover at least part of its contents (**19.1c**), but does not reach the perineum. The lowest part of the peritoneal cavity is the **rectovesical pouch** in the male (**19.38**) or the **rectouterine pouch** (the **pouch of Douglas**) in the female (**19.40a**) – both are highly important because they are within reach during rectal and vaginal examination (pp.268 and 302; **19.23a**, **19.23b** and **19.44**).

Of the pelvic and perineal viscera, the rectum and anal canal have already been described (p.265); the remainder are considered below.

JOINTS AND LIGAMENTS OF THE PELVIS

The small **sacrococcygeal joint** attaches the coccyx to the apex of the sacrum, but the main joints of the pelvis are the two sacroiliac joints at the back and the single midline pubic symphysis at the front (see **4.1a**). The sacrotuberous and sacrospinous ligaments convert the greater and lesser sciatic notches of the hip bone into foramina.

The **sacroiliac joint** is synovial (p.31), but is unusual for this type of joint because there is virtually no movement; however, in the pregnant mother it does relax somewhat under the influence of the hormone **relaxin** (produced by the corpus luteum and placenta, p.303) to assist in childbirth. The joint surfaces of the sacrum and ilium are not smooth, but are thrown into rough projections to assist in the normal stability of the joint. There is a **capsule** which is reinforced on the outside by ligaments, especially at the back where the **interosseous sacroiliac ligament** binds the bones very firmly together; it is one of the strongest ligaments in the body, preventing the body weight from forcing the sacrum down into the pelvic cavity.

The **pubic symphysis** (see **5.2a**) is rather like the joint between the bodies of two vertebrae: there is a disc of fibrocartilage that unites with hyaline cartilage on the surfaces of the pubic bones. Small ligaments reinforce the joint above and below and help to hold the bones firmly together, though, as with the sacroiliac joint, there is some relaxation for childbirth.

The **sacrotuberous ligament** (see **20.4**) runs from the side of the sacrum to the ischial tuberosity. It is a very strong fibrous band, not because part of the large gluteus maximus muscle arises from it, but because (in the normal upright

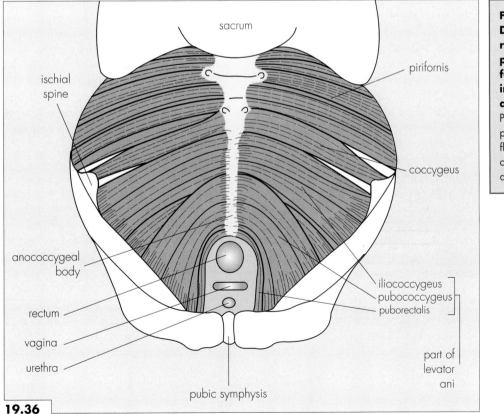

Fig. 19.36 Diagrammatic representation of the pelvic floor in the female, looking down into the pelvis from above.
Piriformis is seen on the posterior pelvic wall, and the floor is formed by the two coccygeus and the two levator ani muscles.

Labels in figure: sacrum, ischial spine, piriformis, coccygeus, anococcygeal body, rectum, vagina, urethra, iliococcygeus, pubococcygeus, puborectalis, part of levator ani, pubic symphysis

19.36

position of the body) it has to prevent the sacrum from tilting forwards at the sacroiliac joint.

The much smaller **sacrospinous ligament** runs from the side of the lower sacrum and coccyx to the ischial spine. It is really the posterior, fibrous part of the coccygeus muscle (see below).

MUSCLES OF THE PELVIS

The **piriformis** and **obturator internus muscles** (**20.4**) pass out from the pelvis through the greater and lesser sciatic foramina respectively, to become attached to the greater tuberosity of the femur; they therefore belong to the lower limb as well as to the pelvis. The nerves that form the sacral plexus (p.42 and **7.6**) are on the posterior pelvic wall, mostly in front of the piriformis muscle. **Coccygeus** (**19.36**) is the muscular part of the sacrospinous ligament (see above), and with its fellow of the opposite side forms the posterior part of the pelvic diaphragm; the larger and much more important anterior part is formed by the **levator ani muscles**.

Levator Ani

The **levator ani muscles** (**19.36**) are rather thin and sheet-like, but are of great importance: they not only play a major role in rectal continence but in the female they help to maintain the position of the uterus and vagina, as well as assisting in urinary continence.

The muscle on each side arises from the back of the pubic bone and from the front of the ischial spine, while between these two bony points it arises from fascia covering the obturator internus muscle. At the front there is a gap between the two muscles through which pass the urethra and rectum in the male or the urethra, vagina and rectum in the female. Some of the fibres from the muscles on each side unite behind the junction of the rectum and anal canal to form a muscular sling (**puborectalis, 19.36**) which is important in maintaining rectal continence (p.266). Other fibres at the medial edges of each muscle in the female (**pubo-vaginalis**) lie on either side of the urethra and assist the sphincter urethrae (see below) in maintaining urinary continence (p.291). The corresponding fibres in the male form the **levator prostatae** (p.308). The remaining fibres become attached to the dense midline tissue in front of and behind the anal canal and are known as the **perineal body** and the **anococcygeal body** (see below). It is this attachment to the central region of the perineum that gives stability to the vagina and uterus (see below and p.299).

PELVIC VESSELS AND URETERS

The **external iliac artery** (from the common iliac) runs along the pelvic brim with its companion vein, but the **internal iliac artery** runs down into the pelvis on the posterior wall and gives off numerous branches to pelvic structures (**19.37** and **19.38**).

The **ureter** also enters the pelvis by passing down immediately in front of the internal iliac artery, before turning forwards to reach the bladder (p.293). In the female it has to run beneath the broad ligament of the uterus which becomes attached to the side wall of the pelvis (p.297). In the male the ductus deferens (vas deferens) runs down the side wall well in front of the ureter but then crosses the ureter before passing down behind the bladder to join the duct from the seminal vesicle to form the ejaculatory duct (p.309).

The vessels supplying the pelvic part of the gut (from the inferior mesenteric) have already been described (p.266).

PELVIC NERVES

The anterior rami of the first four sacral nerves emerge from the anterior sacral foramina on the posterior pelvic wall. The lumbosacral trunk from the lumbar plexus (**7.5**) joins the first sacral nerve, and all of these nerves form the **sacral plexus** (see **7.6**) which lies in front of piriformis, with the internal iliac artery and its branches lying in front of the nerves.

The largest branch of the plexus, the **sciatic nerve**, passes backwards below piriformis to enter the gluteal region (see **20.4**), and other smaller branches take a similar course; these include the **inferior gluteal nerve** (supplying gluteus maximus), the **posterior femoral cutaneous nerve** (the posterior cutaneous nerve of the thigh, supplying a long strip of skin on the back of the thigh and leg), and the **pudendal nerve**, which hooks round the ischial spine to enter the perineum (see below) as its main motor and sensory nerve. The **superior gluteal nerve** leaves above piriformis to run between gluteus medius and minimus and supply them.

The **pelvic splanchnic nerves** (**nervi erigentes**) – the parasympathetic branches of the plexus – arise from the front of S2–S4 rami and run to supply pelvic organs and the blood vessels of the erectile tissue of the penis or clitoris. On the left side, some of the fibres pass upwards behind the peritoneum of the posterior abdominal wall to reach the splenic flexure of the colon, to supply the large intestine from this part down to the anal canal (the part of the gut supplied by the inferior mesenteric artery).

PERINEUM

This is the lowest part of the trunk of the body, below the pelvic diaphragm (see above). The anal canal is in its back part, while in front are the external genitalia (**19.39**). On either side of the anal canal is a large fat-filled space, the **ischiorectal fossa** (now properly called the **ischioanal fossa**), which allows for the expansion of the anal canal during defaecation but, more importantly, for the much larger expansion of the vagina during childbirth. The levator ani muscle forms the sloping roof of each fossa (**19.22** and **19.39**). The anal canal has already been described (p.266).

When looking at the bony pelvis from below, it can be seen that the bony boundaries of the perineum form a diamond-shaped area, with the pubic symphysis at the front, the ischiopubic rami and ischial tuberosities at the sides, and the coccyx at the back. The anal canal opens at the anus, well in front of the tip of the coccyx, in the part of the perineum known as the **anal region**. All the area in front of the anus is the **urogenital region**, known in the female as the **vulva** (p.301; **19.43**).

Perineal Membrane and Urogenital Diaphragm

In both sexes, a small but tough sheet of fibrous tissue stretches between the pubic rami of both sides. It is commonly called the **perineal membrane (19.39)** but is known more precisely as the **inferior fascia of the urogenital diaphragm**. Immediately above (deep to) this sheet, which is perforated centrally in the female by the vagina and urethra

and in the male by the urethra, is a small mass of skeletal muscle, the **urogenital diaphragm** (hence the proper name just mentioned for the perineal membrane). The main component of this muscular tissue is the **sphincter urethrae (19.37** and **19.38)**, often called the **external urethral sphincter**; it is the principal structure that maintains urinary continence.

The central area in front of the anus and behind the perineal membrane consists of a mass of tissue forming (in both sexes) the **perineal body** (recently renamed as the **central perineal tendon, 19.39**). It is important to note that obstetricians and gynaecologists use the word 'perineum' in a very restricted sense to mean the perineal body only, and not the whole diamond-shaped area described above.

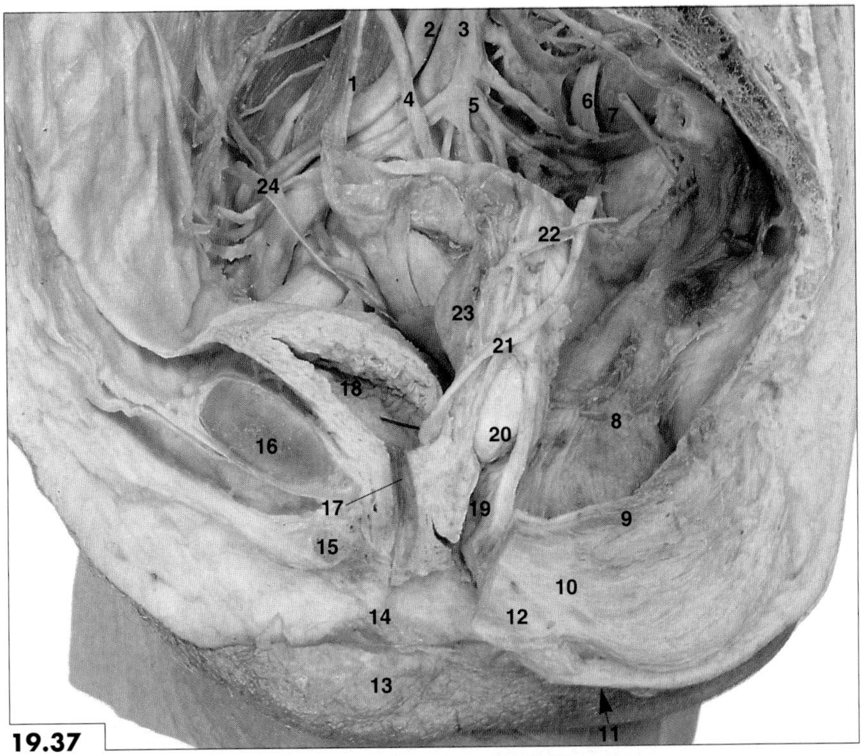

19.37

Fig. 19.37 Female pelvic vessels and viscera, seen on the right side in a sagittal section, after removal of most of the peritoneum.
The section is mostly in the midline, but the whole of the anal canal and the lower part of the left levator ani muscle have been preserved to show the external anal sphincter.

1 Ovarian vessels	13 Labium majus
2 External iliac artery	14 Labium minus
3 External iliac vein	15 Clitoris
4 Ureter, crossing the external iliac vessels (2 and 3) and running down the side wall of the pelvis in front of the internal iliac vessels (5)	16 Pubic symphysis
	17 Urethra, surrounded by sphincter urethrae
	18 Bladder, with bristle in opening of right ureter
5 Internal iliac vessels and branches	19 Vagina
6 Anterior ramus of S1 nerve	20 Cervix of uterus
7 Piriformis	21 Left ureter crossing lateral fornix of vagina
8 Rectum	22 Left uterine artery, crossing superficial to the ureter (21)
9 Cut edge of left levator ani	23 Body of uterus
10 External anal sphincter over anal canal	24 Round ligament of uterus, labelled as it hooks round the inferior epigastric vessels to enter the inguinal canal at the deep inguinal ring
11 Anus, just above arrowhead	
12 Perineal body (central perineal tendon)	

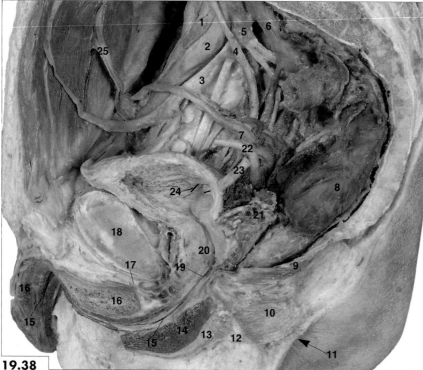

19.38

Fig. 19.38 Male pelvic viscera and vessels, seen on the right side in a sagittal section.
The section is mostly in the midline but the whole of the anal canal and the lower part of the left levator ani muscle have been preserved to show the external anal sphincter (as in the female section in **19.37**).

1 External iliac artery
2 External iliac vein
3 Superior vesical artery, continuing up on to the anterior abdominal wall as the medial umbilical ligament (obliterated umbilical artery)
4 Ureter, crossing the external iliac vessels (1 and 2) and running down the side wall of the pelvis in front of the internal iliac vessels (5 and 6)
5 Internal iliac artery
6 Internal iliac vein
7 Ductus deferens, labelled as it crosses superficial to the ureter after passing down the side wall of the pelvis from the inguinal canal
8 Rectum
9 Cut ledge of left levator ani
10 External anal sphincter, covering anal canal
11 Anus, just above arrowhead

12 Perineal body
13 Bulbospongiosus overlying corpus spongiosum
14 Corpus spongiosum, the part of the penis containing the urethra
15 Spongy part of urethra, within the corpus spongiosum (14)
16 Corpus cavernosum of penis
17 Deep dorsal vein of penis, draining back to the vesicoprostatic venous plexus, the spongelike tissue sectioned here in front of the prostate (20)
18 Pubic symphysis
19 Membranous part of urethra, surrounded by sphincter urethrae
20 Prostate and prostatic part of urethra
21 Left seminal vesicle, cut in section
22 Left ductus deferens
23 Left ureter
24 Bladder, with bristles in ureteral openings
25 Inferior epigastric vessels

In the female, the perineal membrane has a large slit through which the vagina passes, with a smaller perforation just in front for the urethra. On either side of the vagina it supports the **bulbs of the vestibule** and the very small **corpora cavernosa** of the clitoris (for these parts of the vulva, see p.302).

In the male, the perineal membrane forms the support for the base of the penis (see opposite; **19.39**). The **corpus spongiosum** (through which the urethra runs) is attached to the central part, and here there is a central perforation in the membrane so that the urethra can pass through it. This part of the corpus spongiosum is covered by the thin pair of **bulbospongiosus muscles** (of skeletal muscle, **19.39**), which are part of the mechanism of ejaculation. The ducts of the pair of tiny **bulbourethral glands**, which lie just deep to the membrane, pierce it near the urethra and run forward to open into the beginning of the part of the urethra that is within the corpus spongiosum (the spongy part of the urethra, p.295). At each side of the membrane, where it is attached to the pubic ramus, is the base of the **corpus cavernosum**,

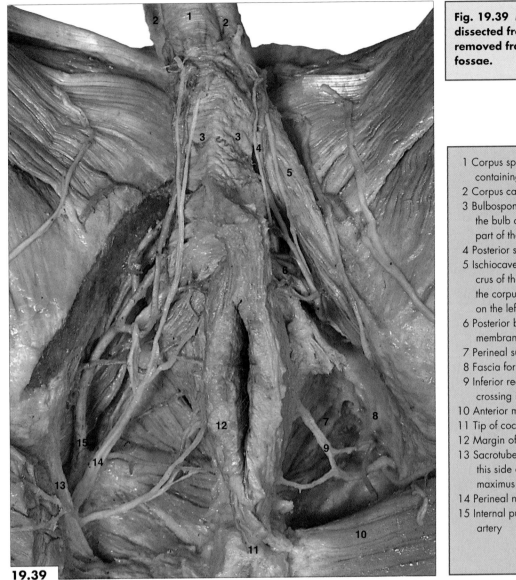

19.39

1 Corpus spongiosum of penis, the part containing the urethra
2 Corpus cavernosum
3 Bulbospongiosum muscle, overlying the bulb of the penis (the posterior part of the corpus spongiosum, 1)
4 Posterior scrotal vessels and nerves
5 Ischiocavernosus muscle, overlying the crus of the penis (the posterior part of the corpus cavernosum (2), removed on the left
6 Posterior border of perineal membrane
7 Perineal surface of levator ani
8 Fascia forming pudendal canal
9 Inferior rectal vessels and nerve, crossing ischiorectal fossa
10 Anterior margin of gluteus maximus
11 Tip of coccyx and anococcygeal body
12 Margin of anus
13 Sacrotuberous ligament, displayed on this side after removal of gluteus maximus
14 Perineal nerve } displayed here
15 Internal pudendal artery } after removal of fascia forming pudendal canal

which is covered by the small **ischiocavernosus muscle** (**19.42**).

Perineal Vessels and Nerves

In the lateral wall of the ischiorectal fossa is a canal of fibrous tissue, the **pudendal canal** (**19.39**), which adheres to the inner side of the ischial tuberosity. The main vessels and nerves of the perineum, the **internal pudendal artery** and **vein** and the **pudendal nerve** (from sacral nerves, **7.6**), run through this canal, giving off branches as they go. Among the first to be given off are the **inferior rectal vessels** and **nerve**, which cross the fossa to reach the anal canal, where the inferior rectal nerve provides the supply for the external anal sphincter. Towards the front of the fossa the **perineal**

nerve, another branch of the pudendal, supplies the small perineal muscles including the urethral sphincter. Further branches include the **dorsal nerve of penis** (or **clitoris**) which runs forward to supply penile (or clitoral) skin, and the **posterior scrotal** (or **labial**) vessels and nerves that supply the skin of most, but not all, of the scrotum or vulva. The front part of the scrotum or vulva is supplied instead by the **ilioinguinal nerve** (from the first lumbar nerve, see **7.5**).

During childbirth it may be desirable to anaesthetize the vulva. A *pudendal nerve block* will anaesthetize most of the area (via the posterior labial branches of the pudendal nerve), but, because of its separate innervation from L1, additional local injection is necessary to anaesthetize the front part of the vulva. A pudendal nerve block can be achieved by injection of anaesthetic solution through a needle inserted through the fornix of the vagina and directing it to the ischial spine where the pudendal nerve leaves the pelvis.

Disease and Injury

Diseases of the individual pelvic organs are described with the structures concerned. The term *pelvic inflammatory disease* (*PID*) most commonly refers to conditions affecting the uterine tubes (*salpingitis*, see p.301) or other female pelvic organs.

Perineal tears are a hazard of childbirth when the tissues do not stretch sufficiently as the fetal head emerges, and can lead to faecal incontinence if the tear spreads to involve the external anal sphincter. The operation of *episiotomy* is surgical incision of the 'obstetric perineum', cutting through it with scissors from the back of the vaginal opening towards the anal canal and so preventing an uncontrolled tearing of tissues which may be more difficult to stitch up than a deliberate incision.

Weakness of the female pelvic floor after childbirth, due to stretching of the levator ani muscles, may lead to *momentary incontinence of urine* when coughing, sneezing or laughing, because of the sudden increase in abdominal pressure overcoming the now rather poor sphincteric action of the pubovaginalis part of levator ani (p.290). With more severe weakness or displacements, there may be *uterine prolapse* (p.301) and greater degrees of urinary or even faecal incontinence. A frequent gynaecological operation is the 'perineal repair' (properly called *colpoperineorrhaphy*, from the Greek meaning 'suturing the vagina and perineum'), where part of the posterior vaginal wall is removed and suitable stitching of the levator ani muscles carried out, to 'tighten up the slack'.

URINARY BLADDER AND URETHRA

The **urinary bladder** (usually called simply the **bladder**) is the collecting organ for urine, which is stored until a convenient time for emptying through the urethra (micturition, voiding, 'passing water'). With more than about 250 ml (half a pint) of urine, bladder distension begins to become uncomfortable. The organ is really a muscular bag (smooth muscle) with an internal mucous membrane lined like the ureter by urine-proof transitional epithelium.

BLADDER

In both sexes the **bladder** is situated in the front of the pelvis, behind the pubic symphysis (**19.37** and **19.38**), and, when empty or only slightly filled, it remains entirely within the pelvis; when it is more distended it rises up behind the lower anterior abdominal wall, pushing the peritoneum away from the wall. This is a particularly important anatomical feature in the male, in whom prostatic enlargement may make emptying difficult; it means that a needle or drainage tube

can be inserted into the bladder through the abdominal wall without entering the peritoneal cavity. A full bladder above the level of the pubic symphysis can be detected by palpation and percussion. In pelvic operations through the lower abdominal wall, the bladder must be empty to avoid the risk of accidental injury when making the abdominal incision. It has been truly said that many a mistake has been made over a full bladder, both in the patient and the doctor: in the patient because the large bladder may be mistaken for some other 'tumour' (especially a pregnant uterus), and in the doctor because a full bladder can cause a certain loss of concentration! Due to the relatively small size of the pelvis in the infant, even the empty bladder before the age of 2–3 years extends normally above the pubic symphysis.

From the apex of the bladder, which is the uppermost anterior part, a fibrous cord (the remains of the **urachus** – an embryological tube) extends up behind the peritoneum of the anterior abdominal wall to the umbilicus. At the back (called the **base**), the bladder lies in front of the rectum in the male and the vagina in the female. In the male, the lower end of the ductus deferens and the seminal vesicle unite at the junction of the bladder and the prostate to form the ejaculatory duct which enters the prostate (**19.47**).

The lower part of the base is the **trigone of the bladder** (**19.46**), where the openings of the two ureters and the internal urethral meatus (at the upper end of the urethra) are situated. The region of the internal meatus at the lowest part of the trigone is the **neck of the bladder**. In the relaxed bladder, the mucous membrane is wrinkled into folds which obviously tend to disappear as the organ fills up; the trigone is an area where the mucosa is always smooth, even in the empty bladder. The openings of the urethra and the two ureters make the points of a triangle whose sides are all 2.5 cm (1 inch) long, but in a full bladder the ureteral orifices come to lie 5 cm (2 inches) apart.

The upper surface and the sides of the bladder are adjacent to coils of intestine, but, in the female, the body of the uterus normally lies over the top of the bladder (**19.37**), rising and falling with it as it fills and empties.

Blood Supply and Lymph Drainage

The blood supply is from the superior and inferior vesical branches of the **internal iliac artery**, with veins joining others on the pelvic floor to drain back to the **internal iliac veins**.

Lymphatic vessels run with the blood vessels to iliac and para-aortic nodes.

Nerve Supply – see Micturition (below)

FEMALE URETHRA

The **internal urethral meatus** in the neck of the bladder opens into the **urethra** which, in the female, is a straight tube 4 cm (1.5 inches) long lying immediately in front of the vagina (**19.37**); indeed, the urethra lies so close that the lower part is usually considered to be embedded within the connective tissue of the outside of the vaginal wall. The urethra is lined by the usual urine-proof transitional epithelium, and has longitudinal smooth-muscle fibres in its wall which are directly continuous with the muscle of the bladder. There are a few very small mucous glands in the mucous membrane (**paraurethral glands of Skene**) that are of interest because they are the female counterpart of the male prostate. The lower opening (the **external urethral meatus**) is in the vestibule of the vagina, in front of the vaginal opening and 2.5 cm (1 inch) behind the clitoris (**19.43**).

The shortness of the urethra makes it easy for organisms to ascend into the bladder and cause *cystitis*. It also makes catheterization easy compared with the male (see below), but the displacement of adjacent organs by the pregnant uterus may stretch the urethra considerably and in a full-term female it may be necessary to introduce a catheter for as much as 15 cm (6 inches) before the bladder is reached. The whole length of the urethra is surrounded by a rather pear-shaped mass of skeletal muscle forming the **external urethral sphincter** (the **sphincter urethrae**). This, together with some assistance from the most medial parts of the levator ani muscles (**pubovaginalis**, p.290) which support the lowest part of the bladder, maintains urinary continence.

MALE URETHRA

The urethra in the male consists of *three parts*: prostatic, membranous and spongy. The part into which the bladder opens at the internal urethral meatus is the **prostatic part**; it runs through the prostate (p.308) for 3 cm (just over 1 inch).

Leaving the prostate (**19.38**), the urethra passes through the external urethral sphincter (**sphincter urethrae**) as the **membranous part** (about 1.5. cm long). Immediately below the sphincter is the tough layer of connective tissue described above as the perineal membrane (**19.39**), and upon going through this, the urethra becomes the **spongy part**; this runs through the middle of the corpus spongiosum of the penis (p.309), to open at the **external urethral meatus** at the tip of the glans penis. Just before this meatus there is a slight dilatation, the **navicular fossa**. Apart from the bulbourethral glands (p.310) which open into the beginning of the spongy urethra, a few small mucous glands open into the pendulous (penile) part of the spongy urethra, and account for any mucus found in the urine; neither the kidneys, ureters nor bladder normally produce mucus.

When passing a catheter or other instrument such as a cystoscope into the bladder through the penis, it is of the greatest importance to remember that the spongy urethra takes a right angled turn to pass through the perineal membrane into the membranous part (**19.38**); the membranous part is likely to be the *most constricted* part of the urethra. Other sites of slight constriction are the external meatus, the

beginning of the navicular fossa just inside the external meatus, and the internal meatus at the bladder neck.

FUNCTION: MICTURITION

The smooth muscle of the bladder is a network of muscle fibres running in all directions, and not arranged in layers like those of the intestine. However, at the bladder neck in the male, there is a collection of circular fibres forming the **internal urethral sphincter**. Their purpose is ***not*** to control the flow of urine but to prevent the regurgitation of seminal fluid into the bladder during ejaculation (p.311). In the female there is no internal sphincter (despite statements to the contrary in many books).

Urine can accumulate in the bladder without at first causing any increase in tension in the bladder wall, but there comes a time when the tension does increase. This causes afferent impulses to travel along the pelvic splanchnic (parasympathetic) nerves to the sacral segments of the spinal cord, and so stimulate parasympathetic motor (lateral horn) cells whose fibres pass back to the bladder muscle in the same nerves to cause contraction. This **autonomic stretch reflex** with automatic filling and emptying is typical of the infant; with training, control by the brain (specifically the cerebral cortex) overrides this spinal activity and keeps the external sphincter closed so that the appropriate time for micturition can be chosen. The external sphincter (composed of skeletal muscle), which relaxes when the bladder muscle contracts, is supplied by the perineal branch of the pudendal nerve whose fibres arise from anterior horn cells in the same spinal cord segments (S2, S3 and S4) that gave rise to the para-sympathetic fibres. The conscious feeling that the bladder is full is conveyed by the afferent fibres of the parasympathetic nerves to the spinal cord, and up the cord to the brain by way of the gracile tract (part of the posterior column, p.208).

The loss of bladder control that may occur in senility indicates a reversion to the infantile pattern: cerebral cortical control is lost because of cerebral vascular disease. In spinal cord injuries where the cord is damaged above the sacral level, the afferent impulses indicating a full bladder cannot reach consciousness, so cortical control is again lost and relaxation of the external sphincter cannot be prevented; the bladder empties automatically when it becomes distended. If the sacral segments themselves are destroyed, the bladder muscle itself is paralysed and the bladder becomes abnormally distended, resulting in *overflow incontinence*, with frequent dripping away of small amounts of urine. Bladders that never empty properly and need prolonged or frequent catheterization are liable to infection – a major hazard of spinal cord injuries.

EXAMINATION

The empty bladder is too small to be palpable, but, when considerably distended, the upper part can be felt as a rounded swelling above the pubic symphysis (and not to be confused with the pregnant uterus or ovarian cysts).

The interior of the bladder can be examined visually through a *cystoscope* which has been passed through the urethra. With the bladder distended with saline, the openings of the ureters and the mucous membrane of the bladder wall can be inspected and the sites of tumours, haemorrhage, etc., detected. Fine catheters can be inserted into the ureters and injected with contrast medium for radiological examination to outline not only the ureter but the renal pelvis and calyces (*retrograde pyelogram*). Straight X-rays of the pelvis may show a faint outline of the bladder; stones (calculi) usually show as opacities. A more specialized radiological investigation for bladder function is the *voiding cystourethrogram*; contrast medium is injected through a cystoscope and films are taken before, during and after the act of voiding.

DISEASES

Infections of the urethra (*urethritis*) ascending to the bladder (*cystitis*) are common, especially so in females due to the shortness of the urethra. The commonest infection in both sexes is *non-specific urethritis* (*NSU*), sometimes called *non-gonococcal urethritis* (*NGU*). Some are due to the bacterium *Chlamydia trachomatis*, now the commonest cause of *sexually transmitted disease* (*STD*), but in about half the cases no specific cause can be found and it may not be associated with sexual activity. The predominant symptoms are pain and frequency of micturition, perhaps with blood-stained urine (*haematuria*); some infections are mild and unrecognized, however, and are therefore untreated and a possible reservoir for the spread of infection. *Gonorrhoea* and *other STDs* are other causes, and each has its own antibiotic therapy.

Carcinoma of the bladder is not common, but is often associated with those working in certain occupations such as the dye and rubber industries; presumably some substance enters the body by the respiratory or alimentary tracts and is eventually excreted by the kidney, to enter the urine where it acts as a carcinogenic irritant to the bladder wall.

PELVIC AND PERINEAL FEMALE ORGANS

The female internal genital organs (which are contained within the pelvis) consist of the paired ovaries and uterine tubes, and the single uterus and vagina (**19.37** and **19.40a**). The female external genitalia (in the perineum, **19.43**) include the mons pubis, labia majora, labia minora, clitoris, bulb of the vestibule, greater vestibular glands, and the vestibule of the vagina.

OVARY

Each **ovary** (**19.40b**) is an almond-shaped structure about 3 cm long, which lies near the side wall of the pelvis, suspended from the back of the broad ligament of the uterus (p.299) in a fold of peritoneum called the **mesovarium**. The ovary is usually below the external iliac vessels that run along the pelvic brim, and in front of the ureter which runs down to the pelvic floor. Its blood supply is from the **ovarian artery**, which arises from the abdominal aorta high up near the renal artery (this is because, early in fetal life, the ovary develops high up on the posterior abdominal wall, and then migrates down to the pelvis, retaining its original blood supply).

Ovulation and Ovarian Hormones

A female's reproductive years begin at about 13 years of age, when menstruation begins, and end at about 50 years, when menstruation ceases. During these years, once a month, an **ovum** is released from one of the two ovaries – a process known as *ovulation*. (Whether ovum release alternates between the two ovaries each month is not clear.) All ova begin their development in embryonic life; no new ova are formed after birth, so all that exist in adult life have been held, as it were, 'in suspended animation' for many years. Some of these will then come to maturity and be discharged from the ovaries on a monthly basis, while others will simply die where they are without coming to anything (see below).

Each ovum is a large cell which is surrounded by a number of smaller cells, the whole forming an **ovarian follicle**; these follicles are scattered in the peripheral part of the ovary (**19.41b**). By the middle of fetal life, there are about seven million follicles in the two ovaries, but most degenerate and disappear so that by birth there are only about two million. Most of these also degenerate, and a total of only 400–450 (one every month for about 35 years) come to maturity to liberate their ova. It is not known what determines which particular follicles are destined to survive and eventually to ovulate.

The stimulus for follicular growth preparatory to ovulation is the hormone **FSH** (**follicle-stimulating hormone**) – one of the two gonadotrophins secreted by the anterior pituitary (p.140). Although several follicles begin to develop each month under its influence, only one normally completes its maturation and the rest degenerate. The developing follicles and, later, the single 'dominant follicle', secrete the steroid hormone **oestrogen**. Once the concentration of oestrogen in the bloodstream reaches a critical level, it triggers the outpouring of **LH** (**luteinizing hormone**) – the second gonadotrophin of the anterior pituitary.

This 'LH surge', as it is called, is necessary to bring about the rupture of the mature follicle and the release of the ovum (*ovulation*, **19.41b**). It also causes the transformation of the ruptured follicle into a **corpus luteum** (hence the name 'luteinizing' hormone). The corpus luteum is, in effect, a

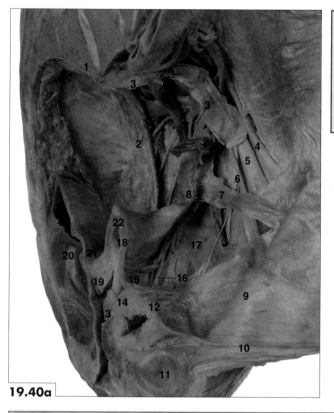

19.40a

Fig. 19.40 Female pelvic viscera.
(a) Left half of the female pelvis, viewed from above and in front and slightly obliquely so that the cut surfaces of the viscera can be seen, with most of the peritoneum removed and the vesicouterine pouch opened up by turning the uterus backwards.
(b) Uterus and ovaries, seen when looking straight down into the pelvis from above.

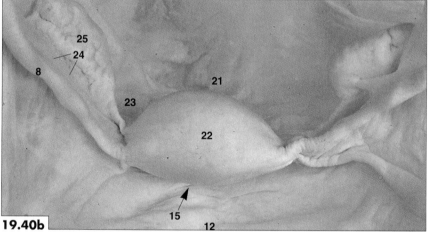

19.40b

1 Promontory of sacrum	12 Bladder, much contracted with a thick wall in **(a)** and overlying peritoneum
2 Uterosacral ligament, condensed retroperitoneal tissue passing from the lower uterus and upper vagina to the sacrum	13 Vagina
3 Root of sigmoid mesocolon	14 Fornix of vagina
4 External iliac artery	15 Vesicouterine pouch of peritoneum
5 External iliac vein	16 Ureter, labelled as it lies beside the vaginal fornix (14)
6 Obturator nerve	17 Uterine artery, passing superficial to the ureter (16)
7 Peritoneum containing round ligament of uterus, passing forwards to the inguinal canal	18 Body of uterus
8 Uterine tube, within its fold of peritoneum	19 Cervix of uterus
9 Posterior surface of anterior abdominal wall, turned forwards	20 Rectum
10 Median umbilical ligament, the obliterated remains of the urachus, running from the apex of the bladder (12) to the umbilicus	21 Rectouterine pouch of peritoneum
	22 Fundus of uterus
	23 Posterior surface of broad ligament
	24 Mesovarium, the peritoneal fold supporting the ovary (25)
11 Pubic symphysis	25 Ovary

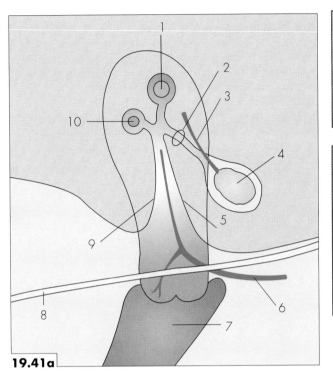

19.41a

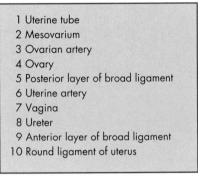

Fig. 19.41 Diagrammatic representation of the uterus and its peritoneal attachments, and events of the menstrual cycle.
(a) Uterus, from the left side.
(b) Ovarian follicles, blood levels of oestrogen and progesterone, and endometrial changes.

1 Uterine tube
2 Mesovarium
3 Ovarian artery
4 Ovary
5 Posterior layer of broad ligament
6 Uterine artery
7 Vagina
8 Ureter
9 Anterior layer of broad ligament
10 Round ligament of uterus

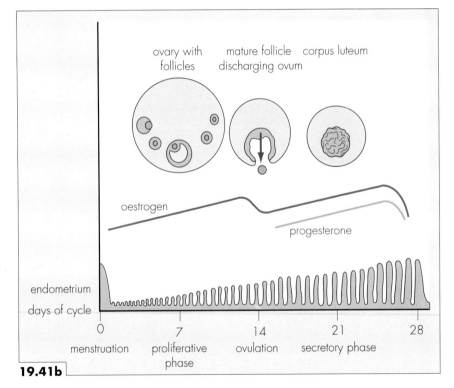

19.41b

small endocrine gland (reaching up to 2 cm in diameter) which secretes **progesterone**, as well as oestrogen, for about 12 days. These two hormones act on the lining of the uterus (the endometrium, see p.299) to prepare it for the possible reception of a fertilized ovum. If there is no fertilized ovum, the corpus luteum degenerates; the endometrium, being dependent upon the oestrogen and progesterone secreted by the corpus luteum, breaks down and menstruation ensues (see below). Another crop of follicles now becomes stimulated to prepare for ovulation, and so the cycle is repeated. If a fertilized ovum *does* implant in the endometrium, the corpus luteum persists and increases in size, continuing to secrete progesterone and oestrogen and so preventing endometrial breakdown.

The ovaries thus produce the main female sex hormones, oestrogen and progesterone, which are responsible for the cyclic changes described above. Oestrogen is also responsible for the further development of the external genitalia, increasing breast size, the appearance of axillary and pubic hair and general female body form – characteristics of the time of adolescent life known as puberty.

The fluid of ovarian follicles contains another hormone, **inhibin**, which, like the same hormone from the testis (p.308), appears to inhibit FSH secretion by the anterior pituitary; the role of this hormone in both sexes is still under investigation.

Examination

On vaginal examination (p.302) the ovaries may often be felt towards the lateral sides of the pelvis but it is not always possible to detect them. They can of course be directly examined during abdominal and pelvic operations and at laparoscopy (p.246), but they are not palpable on abdominal examination unless enlarged.

About one third of all cases of infertility are accounted for by some kind of ovarian dysfunction. Investigations include measurements of body temperature (p.306) and progesterone levels in the blood.

Diseases

Apart from biochemical defects which affect ovulation, the ovaries are subject to the formation of *tumours* and *cysts*. The vast majority of enlargements are benign, but the cancerous varieties can spread to the peritoneum and other pelvic organs, and give metastases to bones and lungs. Ovarian cysts may grow to large sizes before the patient seeks advice, perhaps because of pressure effects on neighbouring organs such as the bladder, but they may suddenly become painful due to internal haemorrhage or torsion (twisting on a pedicle). All tumours require surgical removal (*ovariectomy*).

UTERUS

The **uterus** (**womb**) is a muscular organ (composed of smooth muscle) which is shaped like a rather flattened pear (about 7.5 cm long, 5 cm wide and 2.5 cm thick – $3 \times 2 \times 1$ inches). It usually lies above the bladder and with its lower end, the **cervix** (the narrow end of the 'pear'), opening into the upper end of the vagina (**19.37** and **19.40b**). The main part of the uterus is the **body**, and its broad upper end is the **fundus**; at each side the **uterine tube** (the **Fallopian tube**, often called the oviduct in animals) joins the 'corner' of the body and fundus. The body is usually bent forwards to make a slight angle with the cervix (the *angle of anteflexion*), and the cervix makes a similar angle with the vagina (the *angle of anteversion*). Thus, the uterus is normally said to be *anteflexed* and *anteverted*. Sometimes, especially after childbirth, the uterus becomes bent backwards rather than forwards (*retroverted* and/or *retroflexed*).

The uterus is suspended from each side of the pelvis by a double fold of peritoneum – the **broad ligament** (**19.41a**). The upper edge of this fold encloses the uterine tube, which is a muscular extension from the upper angle of the uterus and about 10 cm (4 inches) long. Its lateral end, which possesses a number of finger-like projections (**fimbriae**) at the fimbriated end, is open and lies near the side wall of the pelvis below the ovary, so that at ovulation the ovum can migrate into the tube.

Just below and in front of the attachment of the tube to the uterus, a cord-like solid band of tissue, the **round ligament** (**19.40** and **19.41a**), runs within its own fold of peritoneum to enter the inguinal canal. It passes through the canal (like the spermatic cord in the male), and eventually disappears by merging with the tissue of the labium majus. Just below and behind the tubal attachment is a much shorter and smaller band, the **ligament of the ovary**, attaching one end of the ovary to the uterus and enclosed, like the ovary, in the mesovarium.

Uterine Supports

The broad ligaments and round ligaments are rather lax structures, and while they help to a certain extent to hold the uterus in its normal position, the most important structures in this respect are some **condensations of connective tissue** under the peritoneum in the region of the cervix of the uterus and the fornix of the vagina (p.301). Those condensations passing laterally beneath the broad ligament to the side wall of the pelvis are variously known as the **lateral ligaments**, **cervical ligaments**, **cardinal ligaments** or **ligaments of Mackendrodt**, while those passing backwards on either side of the rectum to the front of the sacrum are the **uterosacral ligaments** (**19.40a**). Unfortunately, these so-called ligaments are difficult to define in most embalmed cadavers of the dissecting room, but in the living body there is no doubt of their prime importance as uterine supports (together with the attachments of the levator ani muscles to the perineal body, see p.291). Their undue stretching in childbirth or by other pelvic conditions may lead to various kinds of uterine displacements. One such displacement is *prolapse of the uterus*, where it 'slides down' inside the vagina; the cervix may even appear in the vaginal opening.

Function

The bulk of the uterine wall consists of masses of smooth muscle fibres, and is known as the **myometrium**. The organ is lined internally by a mucous membrane, the **endometrium**, which is composed of connective tissue (the **endometrial stroma**) containing long tubular glands in continuity with the surface epithelium. The uterus increases vastly in size during pregnancy to accommodate the growing embryo and fetus, and the myometrium is responsible for the expulsive force that causes the child to be born.

During reproductive life, the endometrium of the body

and the fundus of the uterus undergoes *shedding* (sloughing) and subsequent regeneration during each menstrual cycle, under the influenece of the ovarian hormones oestrogen and progesterone. While the cervix and uterine tubes do not shed and renew their linings, like the body and fundus, they do participate in cyclical changes. Glands in the cervical lining, for example, secrete a mucus that is thinner and more abundant at the time of ovulation than at any other time of the menstrual cycle – a possible guide to whether ovulation has occurred.

Menstrual Cycle

The **menstrual cycle** (**19.41b**) consists of a series of events that occur within the female reproductive organs on a cyclical basis; on average, the cycle is 28 days' long. The main events of each cycle occur in the ovaries and uterus, but smaller changes occur in several other organs as well, including the uterine tubes, vagina and breasts. All these events are controlled and orchestrated by hormones – the gonadotrophins – causing changes in the ovaries, and the ovarian hormones in turn causing changes in the uterus and other organs.

The most obvious external manifestation of the cycle is the regular occurrence of *menstrual bleeding* (the *menstrual period*), and, by convention, the cycle is dated from the first day of the menstrual flow. This bleeding is caused by the breakdown of the endometrium following the withdrawal of the influence of the corpus luteum (p.296). Blood and endometrial debris flow through the cervix and vagina to the exterior. The breakdown involves all but the very bases of the endometrial glands, whose remaining cells can then proliferate to regenerate the glands and the surface epithelium, with the accompanying regeneration of endometrial stroma.

The menstrual flow lasts for the first 4–5 days of the cycle. During this time follicles are beginning to grow in the ovaries, and regeneration of the endometrium begins under the influence of oestrogen from these follicles. By day 14 or so, a mature follicle is ready to ovulate, and the endometrium has grown considerably. After ovulation and the formation of the corpus luteum (p.296), the endometrium continues to thicken (under the influence of oestrogen), but also becomes *secretory*; that is, its glands begin to synthesize a glycogen-rich secretion that will nourish an implanting embryo, should fertilization have occurred. This secretory function is promoted by progesterone, the other hormone of the corpus luteum. If fertilization does not occur, the corpus luteum ceases to function after about 12 days (i.e. on about day 26 of the cycle) and its hormones are promptly removed from the circulation. Withdrawal of these hormones undermines the hormonal support of the endometrium, and in a couple of days, therefore, it breaks down. The cycle begins anew with another episode of menstrual bleeding.

The menstrual cycle is often divided into phases, named according to the major events taking place in the endometrium. They are the *menstrual phase*, or *menses* (days 1–5), the *proliferative phase* (days 6–14), the *secretory phase* (days 15–26), and the *ischaemic phase* (days 27–28; 'ischaemic' means having reduced blood supply, and in this context refers to the reduction in blood supply to the upper endometrium, leading to tissue breakdown). Note that all the times given are approximate and variable. Alternative names for parts of the cycle reflect events in the ovary rather than the uterus: the *follicular phase* (days 1–14), for example, and the *luteal phase* (days 15–28).

In the last few days of the cycle, some females develop emotional and other upsets, collectively called *premenstrual tension* (*PMT*) or the *premenstrual syndrome* (*PMS*). The exact cause has not been defined; it does not appear to be related to fluctuating hormone levels, and treatment (often hormonal – see below) is very much on an individual basis.

Menarche and Menopause

Menstruation begins about the age of 13 years (the *menarche* – Greek for 'beginning'), and, because the increased production of the necessary hormones by the ovary only occurs slowly, it may take some months before a regular pattern is established.

At the opposite end of reproductive life, the *menopause* (the cessation of menstruation, sometimes called the 'change of life') occurs at about 50, and is usually not a sudden event; the menstrual flow gradually becomes shorter in duration and lower in quantity over perhaps many months. The changes are due to the waning endocrine function of the ovary, and the withdrawal of oestrogen may lead to a variety of symptoms, among which disturbances of the autonomic nervous system are often common and include 'hot flushes' with sweating. *Hormone replacement therapy* (*HRT*) with some kind of synthetic oestrogen may be required.

Disturbances of Menstruation

Dysmenorrhoea refers to pelvic pain during menstruation, and mild or severe degrees may occur in perhaps a third of all females. It is frequently alleviated by the combined contraceptive pill (p.306).

Amenorrhoea is failure to menstruate, and is called *primary* in young females who have never menstruated, and *secondary* in older females who have previously done so (excluding pregnancy and lactation, and the normal menopause). The cause may be complicated, involving ovaries, pituitary or hypothalamus.

Menorrhagia is the excessive and prolonged loss of blood at menstruation. There are many causes, including fibroids (see below).

Examination

Vaginal examination (p.302 and **19.44**) enables the cervix of the uterus to be palpated, and, when combined with the other hand on the lower abdomen (*bimanual examination*), the upper part of the body of the uterus may be felt. Visual examination of the vagina and cervix (*colposcopy*, p.302) is carried out through a vaginal speculum.

Specimens of endometrium can be obtained for microscopic examination by the operation commonly called *D and C* (*dilatation and curettage*) – dilating the canal of the cervix so that an instrument (i.e. a curette) can be introduced into the body of the uterus to scrape off the endometrium. Apart from diagnosis, D and C is the method of treatment for many endometrial disorders.

The injection of contrast medium into the uterus enables the uterine tubes to be outlined radiographically; this is to establish whether they are patent and, therefore, capable of allowing ovum and sperm to meet.

Diseases

Many uterine disorders are related to menstruation and have been mentioned above, together with uterine prolapse (p.299).

Fibroids (**19.42**) are the commonest of all body tumours. They are benign, multiple growths of uterine smooth muscle, varying in size from pinhead to football. Many are undetected during life but their principal symptoms are pain and menorrhagia, and they can cause sterility and abortion. Small fibroids can be 'shelled out' at operation, but, for large tumours, removal of the uterus (*hysterectomy*) is necessary.

The uterus is one of the commonest sites for *carcinoma*, which can occur in either the body or the cervix, and each has its distinct features. Carcinoma of the cervix is three times as common as that of the body of the uterus; it can occur at any age, and its characteristic feature is irregular bleeding. It is the type of cancer which, if discovered early, can be completely cured, using, for example, *diathermy* or *laser treatments*, or 'cone biopsy' (removal of a cone-shaped area of the cervix). In many communities, cervical screening programmes are designed to detect the condition early. A

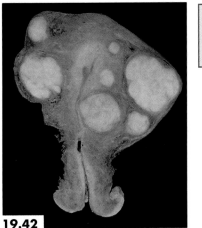

Fig. 19.42 Fibroids of the uterus.

19.42

swab introduced into the fornix of the vagina collects cells that have accumulated in the mucous secretion from the cervix, and a smear from the swab is made on a microscope slide so that it can be examined to see if any abnormal cells are present. (This was often called the 'Pap test', from the Greek Dr Papanicolaou who first described the method.)

Carcinoma of the body of the uterus (often called *endometrial carcinoma*) is commonest after the menopause, and its characteristic features are postmenopausal bleeding and pain (due to attempts by the uterine muscle to expel the mass). Lymphatic spread includes involvement of the palpable inguinal nodes (p.247) (to which the cervix does not drain). Curettage is necessary for proper diagnosis, and hysterectomy must be carried out, followed perhaps by radiotherapy.

Infection of the uterus (*endometritis*) or uterine tubes (*salpingitis*) is usually due to infection ascending from the vagina, and is commonest after childbirth or abortion. The lumen may become blocked, causing sterility, and if the whole thickness of the wall becomes involved, adhesions may form to surrounding organs such as the bladder, ovary and small intestine.

Endometritis must not be confused with *endometriosis*, which is not something to do with the uterus itself but a condition where bits of endometrium have become displaced into other organs such as the ovary or the peritoneum (probably by passing along the uterine tubes at menstruation instead of down into the vagina). The tissue often forms cysts which give rise to pain and haemorrhage, and it may have to be treated by hormones or surgery.

VAGINA AND VULVA

The **vagina**, the female organ of copulation, is a muscular tube (of smooth muscle, but with some skeletal muscle fibres at its lower end) about 10 cm (4.5 in) long, lying in front of the rectum and anal canal and behind the pubic symphysis, urinary bladder and urethra (**19.37**). Menstrual products are discharged into it from the uterus. It is easily distended – during sexual intercourse, for example, and especially during childbirth. Its lining mucous membrane consists of stratified squamous epithelium and an underlying connective tissue stroma devoid of glands. A variable amount of secretion, formed by a transudation of fluid through the vaginal wall as well as from mucous glands in the cervix of the uterus and from the greater vestibular glands (see below), occurs normally during sexual excitement. The urethra is embedded in the lower part of the anterior vaginal wall, and its opening (the external urethral meatus) is in the front of the vestibule of the vagina (see below).

The upper end of the vagina, into which the cervix of the uterus projects, is the **fornix**. The posterior part of the fornix (but not the anterior) is covered on the pelvic cavity side by peritoneum; instruments that are meant to be passed into the cervix but are misdirected and perforate the posterior fornix (as by amateur abortionists), enter the peritoneal cavity and cause serious risk of peritonitis.

The lower end of the vagina (the **vestibule of the vagina,** the vaginal opening or **introitus**) opens into the **vulva (19.43)** – the region of the perineum containing the external genitalia (p.291). The features of this region include the mons pubis, the labia (both majora and minora), the clitoris, the bulbs of the vestibule, and the greater vestibular glands.

The **mons pubis** is the mound of hairy skin and subcutaneous fat in front of the pubic symphysis and pubic bones; it continues backwards on either side as the fatty cutaneous folds that form the **labia majora** (singular – labium majus).

The **labia minora** (singular – labium minus) are cutaneous folds, without fat, lying internal to the labia majora and forming the boundary of the vestibule of the vagina. Just inside the vaginal orifice, a fold of mucous membrane – the **hymen**, of variable size and thickness – may partly obstruct the opening, and may be stretched or ruptured at the first attempt at sexual intercourse. If particularly thick it may need to be incised surgically.

The **clitoris** lies at the front ends of the labia minora. Although it is the female counterpart of the penis, it is not associated with the urethra as in the male. It is formed by two small **corpora cavernosa**, and its tip or glans is at the front end of the two **bulbs of the vestibule,** which are elongated masses of erectile tissue (corresponding in the male

to the single corpus spongiosum) at the side of the vaginal orifice and covered by the bulbospongiosus muscles.

The pea-like, mucus-secreting **greater vestibular (Bartholin's) glands** lie under cover of the back part of the bulbs of the vestibule, and each has a duct about 2 cm long opening into the vagina just above the back part of a labium minus.

Blood Supply and Lymph Drainage

Various branches of the **internal iliac artery** supply the vagina, with veins passing back over the pelvic floor to internal iliac veins. Lymphatics mostly pass to **iliac nodes,** but those from the lowest part of the vagina and adjacent parts of the vulva (like those from the lowest part of the anal canal) run to **inguinal nodes.**

Nerve Supply

Most of the vagina is supplied by *autonomic* fibres, but the lower end and adjacent parts of the vulva receive fibres from the **ilioinguinal nerves** at the front, and branches from the **pudendal nerves** at the back. This means that pudendal nerve block will not anaesthetize the *whole* of the vulva (p.293).

Vaginal Examination

As part of the surface of the body, the vulva can be inspected, and the interior of the vagina (with the uterine cervix projecting into it) can be examined through a speculum (during a *colposcopy,* derived from the Greek for vagina, which is itself a Latin word).

The term *vaginal examination* refers to digital examination, usually with the index and middle fingers (**19.44**). The cervix is easily felt at the upper end, with the rectum behind, and at the sides it may be possible to palpate the ovaries and uterine tubes. It is highly important to note that the lowest part of the peritoneal cavity, the rectouterine pouch (the pouch of Douglas, p.289), is within reach of the tips of the examining fingers, and cancerous deposits that have gravitated there may be palpable.

Diseases

Irritation of the vulva causing itching (*pruritus vulvae*) is a common and embarrassing condition with many causes (and therefore many possible treatments). Causes range from skin diseases that affect other parts of the body to vaginal discharges (see below) and other vulval conditions such as *leukoplakia* (whitened patches of thickened skin), *carcinoma,* and *sexually transmitted diseases* (*STD,* formerly called *venereal diseases,* after Venus, the goddess of love). Pruritis can also be of *psychogenic origin.*

Although the products of menstruation pass through the vagina, the term *vaginal discharge* is used for those not associated with menstruation. Abnormal discharges are usually caused by infections of the vagina and uterus. The commonest is due to the yeast *Candida albicans* (*candidiasis*

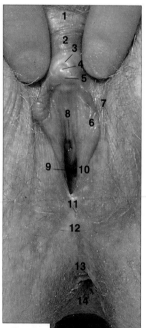

19.43

Fig. 19.43 Vulva, with labia minora held apart, to show the vaginal and urethral openings.

1 Mons pubis
2 Anterior commissure
3 Prepuce of clitoris
4 Clitoris
5 Frenulum of clitoris
6 Labium minus
7 Labium majus
8 External urethral orifice
9 Position of orifice of duct of greater vestibular (Bartholin's) gland
10 Margin of vaginal orifice
11 Posterior commissure
12 Skin over perineal body, the region often called 'the perineum' by obstetricians and gynaecologists
13 Margin of anus
14 Anococcygeal body

or *thrush*), and others may be caused by bacteria (e.g. *gonorrhoea*), or protozoa (e.g. *trichomoniasis*). Among the rarer causes are tumours and various kinds of fistulas – abnormal communications between viscera such as the bladder and vagina (*vesicovaginal fistula*) or rectum and vagina (*rectovaginal fistula*), occurring because a tumour of one organ invades the other and causes the communication.

Infection sometimes affects a Bartholin's gland, giving rise to a painful abscess (*Bartholinitis*) near the back of the vaginal opening that makes sitting and walking difficult. Surgical incision is needed to drain out the pus.

PREGNANCY AND CONTRACEPTION

Fertilization (conception), the fusion of the ovum with a single sperm, occurs in the upper (or ovarian) portion of the uterine tube, and the resulting single cell is called a **zygote**. Because each male and female gamete contains *half* the normal number of chromosomes (p.8), the zygote contains the *full* number, i.e. 22 pairs of autosomes plus one pair of sex chromsomes. If the zygote contains *two X chromosomes*, the offspring will be *female*; with *one X and one Y* it will be *male*. A woman is considered to be pregnant when a zygote has become implanted (embedded) in the endometrium, i.e. about one week after fertilization.

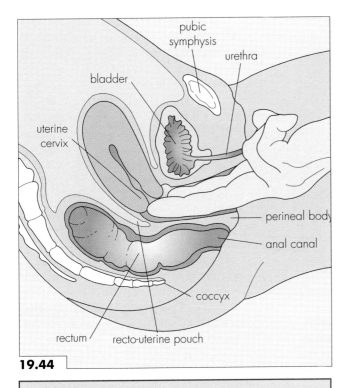

19.44

Fig. 19.44 Vaginal examination. Compare with rectal examination (19.23).

Growth of the Zygote, Embryonic Layers and Placenta Formation

The zygote undergoes several cell divisions to form a ball of cells, the **morula**. Since there is little cell growth between succeeding divisions, the 16-cell morula (at three days) is no bigger than the original zygote. By further growth and cell division it now increases in size. Fluid begins to accumulate here and there between the cells and, as these fluid accumulations coalesce, a fluid-filled cavity appears. The whole structure, which is now called a **blastocyst**, consists of a single layer of flattened cells, the **trophoblast**, surrounding the cavity, and a small knob of rounded cells, the **inner cell mass**, on one side of the cavity (**19.45a**). The term *conceptus* is often used to denote the products of conception, that is, the zygote, and later, the blastocyst and all its derivatives. It is only the inner cell mass that gives rise to the embryo itself; the trophoblast develops into extra-embryonic membranes and the placenta (p.304).

Just before the blastocyst implants (i.e. attaches to the lining of the uterus), changes occur in the region of the inner cell mass. A flat, circular plate of cells, the **embryonic disc**, appears with a bubble-like space, the **amniotic cavity**, above it, and a similar space, the **yolk sac**, below it (**19.45a**). In longitudinal section, the whole structure looks rather like a figure-of-eight, with the embryonic disc sandwiched between the two cavities. When first formed, the embryonic disc is a two-layered structure; its upper layer, the **epiblast**, will soon give rise to the *three* **embryonic germ layers** from which all the tissues and organs of the body develop. These layers are the **ectoderm, mesoderm** and **endoderm**. Although each layer gives rise to specific items (see below), normal development depends on the way these three elements react with and influence each other; they do not act entirely independently. Essentially, in brief and simplified terms, ectoderm forms the surface covering the body and the nervous system, endoderm forms most of the epithelial lining of the alimentary and respiratory tracts, and mesoderm forms connective tissues, muscle and genitourinary organs. Without becoming involved in complex embryological details which are available in specialist texts for those who need them, the following paragraphs summarize the derivatives of these layers.

Derivatives of ectoderm

- The epidermis and associated structures – hairs, nails, sweat glands, sebaceous glands and mammary glands.
- The epithelium of the mouth, salivary glands and palate, of the lower part of the anal canal, and of the terminal parts of the urinary and genital tracts.
- The enamel of the teeth (but not the dentine and pulp, which are mesodermal).
- The corneal epithelium and the lens, and the smooth muscle of the iris.
- The neurons and neuroglial cells of the nervous system (central and peripheral, except the microglial cells, which

are mesodermal), the pituitary gland (the posterior part as an outgrowth from the brain, and the anterior part from the primitive pharynx), the arachnoid and pia mater, the notochord (a primitive backbone which disappears except where it becomes the nucleus pulposus of intervertebral discs), and the cells of the medulla of the adrenal gland.

Derivatives of endoderm

- The epithelium of the digestive system (except at the upper and lower ends, which are ectodermal) and of the liver, biliary tract and pancreas.
- The thyroid and parathyroid glands, and the thymus (all derived from the primitive pharynx).
- The epithelium of the larynx and bronchial tree, and of the middle ear and auditory tube.
- The epithelium of most of the bladder and urethra, and of the lower part of the vagina.

Derivatives of mesoderm

- Connective tissues of organs, bone, teeth (except enamel, which is ectodermal), cartilage, synovial membranes, pleura, pericardium, peritoneum, and all types of muscle (except the smooth muscle of the iris, which is ectodermal).
- The heart (beginning as a tube which eventually becomes divided into the four chambers) and the rest of the vascular and lymphatic systems (including blood cells but excluding the thymus, which is endodermal).
- The cortex of the adrenal gland.
- The dura mater and microglial cells.
- The urinary and genital organs and tracts (except the terminal parts, which are ectodermal).

By one week after fertilization, the **conceptus** has travelled along the uterine tube, entered the uterus, and completed its development into a blastocyst. Implantation now begins: the trophoblast burrows into the endometrium, usually on the upper posterior part of the uterine wall. Part of the trophoblast develops into the **placenta**, which is connected to the embryo by the **umbilical cord** containing the umbilical arteries and veins. The placenta (often called the 'afterbirth' since it must be discharged from the uterus after the child is born) is a disc-shaped organ and has masses of finger-like processes (**chorionic villi**) which penetrate into the uterine wall and come into contact with maternal blood. Nutritive substances and waste products can therefore be exchanged between the placenta, which contains the blood of the developing child, and the uterus, which contains the mother's blood; the two circulations do not join one another. The non-placental part of the trophoblast forms the fetal membranes that surround the developing embryo and fetus, and contain it within a bag of fluid (**amniotic fluid**).

The trophoblast and, later, the placenta, secrete a hormone, **human chorionic gonadotropin** (**HCG**) which stimulates the corpus luteum of the ovary and prevents its normal demise. (In the absence of conception, the corpus luteum stops functioning about 12 days after it is formed, i.e. about 12 days after ovulation, p.296.) HCG causes significant growth of the corpus luteum and thus ensures an outpouring of the luteal hormones, oestrogen and progesterone, to maintain the endometrium and the implanted conceptus. Since the corpus luteum continues to function, the endometrium does not break down and menstrual bleeding does not occur. It is the detection of HCG, which is present in blood and urine, that is the basis for most pregnancy tests. The test becomes positive about two weeks after fertilization, i.e. about the time of the first missed period.

The placenta (like the corpus luteum) also appears to secrete the hormone relaxin, which relaxes pelvic joints and assists in dilating the uterine cervix at birth.

Embryo and Fetus

For the first seven weeks after conception the developing human is an **embryo**; from eight weeks until birth it is a **fetus**.

The early embryo bulges up into the **amniotic cavity** (p.303) and becomes folded into a 'C'-shaped curve, with a headfold and tailfold (**19.45b**). Embryos can be dated approximately by measuring a straight line between the extremities of the curve – the **crown–rump** length (CR length). As examples, a CR length of 1.5 mm indicates an embryo 2.5 weeks old, and it grows to 5 mm long at 4 weeks, 12 mm at 6 weeks and 40 mm at 10 weeks.

In the very early stages, the embryo exhibits the segmented pattern of more primitive vertebrates; evidence of this segmentation persists most obviously in the thorax with its regular segmental arrangement of intercostal muscles, vessels and nerves. The head end of the embryo becomes greatly enlarged, and, with the formation of the headfold, comes to lie adjacent to the mesodermal structures of the future thorax. This accounts for the nerve supply of the diaphragm from cervical nerves (p.101); structures retain their developmental nerve supply no matter how they migrate later. This principle is also well illustrated by the head and neck strucures that develop from the **pharyngeal arches** of the sides of the primitive mouth cavity. These arched formations are covered on the outside with ectoderm and on the inside with endoderm, and each has its own cartilage, muscle, nerve and blood vessels. The derivatives of these arches provide such structures in the head and neck such as the mandible and its muscles, the tongue and the larynx, and their different nerve supplies reflect their origins from different arches. The thymus and the thyroid and parathyroid glands are other important derivatives from the pharyngeal arches (which are sometimes called **branchial arches**).

Most organs are formed during the embryonic period; subsequent growth is mainly enlargement of structures already formed. Most, but not all, errors of development (*congenital defects*) have their origins in the embryonic period, perhaps before the female is even sure she is pregnant.

Stages of Pregnancy

A normal pregnancy extends over a period of approximately 40 weeks (about 280 days or nine months). The first sign of pregnancy is failure to menstruate at the expected time – the first 'missed period'. It is customary to date pregnancies in weeks from the first day of the last menstrual period; assuming that ovulation and fertilization occur on day 14 of a 28-day cycle, the embryo and fetus will be two weeks younger than this calculated time (i.e. a 284-day pregnancy implies a fetus 270 days old). Clinically, it is convenient to divide pregnancy into three periods of three months – the three *trimesters*. Each has its own characteristics with regard to fetal growth and possible complications.

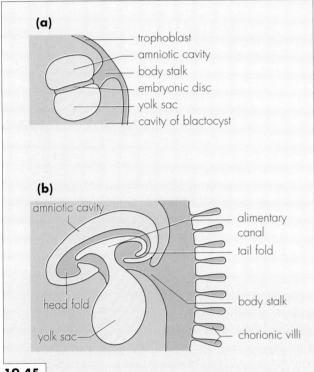

(a)
trophoblast
amniotic cavity
body stalk
embryonic disc
yolk sac
cavity of blactocyst

(b)
amniotic cavity
alimentary canal
tail fold
head fold
yolk sac
body stalk
chorionic villi

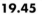
19.45

Fig. 19.45 Early embryonic development.
(a) A section of the derivatives of the inner cell mass at one side of the blastocyst, showing the embryonic disc with the cavities of the amnion and yolk sac on either side.
(b) Section of the early embryo, bulging into the amniotic cavity and developing a headfold and tailfold. The future alimentary canal can be recognised in continuity with the yolk sac.

In the *first trimester*, the uterus becomes about three times its normal size, filling the pelvis and becoming palpable just above the pubic symphysis. The fetus attains a length of about 7.5 cm (3 inches). The nausea and vomiting ('morning sickness') which may occur, especially in the early weeks, appear to be due to the increased secretions of HCG and oestrogen.

Abdominal pain and vaginal haemorrhage during this period suggest some kind of maldevelopment, and the embryo or fetus may be expelled (*spontaneous abortion* or *miscarriage*) or may have to be removed (*induced abortion*). More than 10% of pregnancies spontaneously abort, and many of these embryos have been shown to have abnormalities. Sometimes, the fertilized ovum remains in the uterine tube (*tubal pregnancy* or *ectopic pregnancy*) without passing on into the uterus; the embryo may die and the tube burst with serious haemorrhage. The tube must be surgically removed, but normal pregnancies may still occur via the remaining tube. An abnormal but rare cystic overgrowth of the **chorion** (a membrane around the embryo, developed from the trophoblast) produces a *hydatidiform mole*, with death of the embryo; the abnormal tissue must be removed, and the patient must be carefully followed up since a cancerous growth (*choriocarcinoma*) may ensue.

In the *second trimester*, the fetus grows to a weight of about 1 kg (2 lb 2 oz) and the uterus enlarges to the level of the mother's umbilicus. From about 16 weeks, the mother may become conscious of fetal movements. Premature birth may occur at any time, and is still called abortion or miscarriage; a fetus less than 28 weeks old is not usually considered viable, though it may survive if in the care of a specialized centre.

In the *third trimester*, the fetus grows to reach about 3.5 kg (over 7 lb) and the uterus seems to fill the abdomen. Haemorrhage during this time (*antepartum haemorrhage – APH*) indicates placental bleeding, and may occur from a placenta in a normal site (*accidental haemorrhage*), or from one situated at the cervix (*placenta praevia*). Both conditions require immediate bed rest and obstetrical care, since continued bleeding puts the life of the fetus at great risk. If the bleeding does not stop, labour must be induced or a *Caesarian operation* performed (delivery of the child by opening the abdomen and incising the uterus).

The occurrence of increasing hypertension, albuminuria and the accumulation of excess body fluid (oedema, as first evidenced by 'swelling of the ankles') constitutes *toxaemia of pregnancy*, and in its most severe form is known as *eclampsia*. Patients must be carefully watched, and labour may have to be induced to prevent continuing illness in the mother and possible fetal damage.

Labour and Birth

The term **labour**, in the obstetrical sense, means the series of rhythmical contractions of the uterus that lead to the **birth** of a baby (i.e. delivery or parturition). Although slight and fleeting at first, the contractions become gradually more frequent and powerful. The exact stimulus for the onset of labour is not known, though it appears to depend on oxytocin from the posterior pituitary (p.135). It is normal (in 96% of cases) for the child to be born head first (a *cranial presentation*); the head is the heavier end of the fetus, and so when floating in amniotic fluid tends to lie in the lower part of the uterus. If during the later stages of pregnancy the fetal buttocks are recognized as occupying this position (*breech presentation*), the obstetrician tries to turn the fetus round by manual pressure on the mother's abdominal wall. Breech deliveries are difficult because the relatively rigid head may become stuck in the birth canal after the rest of the body has passed through.

Labour is usually divided into three stages. The *first stage* is from the time rhythmic contractions begin to the time the cervix becomes fully dilated, i.e. wide enough for the passage of the fetal head; in a first pregnancy this lasts something like eight hours. It includes the escape of a slight blood-stained discharge, the **show**, due to some tearing away of fetal membranes from the uterine wall as the membranes (with the contained amniotic fluid, the 'bag of waters') project down into the canal of the cervix in advance of the fetal head and so help to dilate the canal.

The *second stage* is from cervical dilatation to the birth of the baby (usually about an hour), and the uterine contractions are usually assisted by the mother 'bearing down' – contracting her abdominal muscles to help in the expulsion. At about the time the cervix becomes fully dilated, the membranes rupture, allowing the escape of amniotic fluid (the 'breaking of the waters'), and the bare head of the child is seen stretching the tissues of the vulva. To prevent uncontrolled tearing of tissues, it may be necessary to perform episiotomy (p.294). There is a further gush of amniotic fluid ('residual waters') as the child's body is born.

In the *third stage*, the placenta is delivered; the sudden reduction of uterine size severs the placenta from its adherence to the uterine wall, and it should be expelled through the vagina within 10 minutes or so. The contraction of the uterus stops bleeding from the placental site.

Puerperium

The **puerperium** is the period of *six weeks* following delivery. A small amount of blood and tissue fluid (**lochia**) escapes from the uterus for the first week or two. By the end of a fortnight the uterus has contracted down into the pelvis and is not palpable above the pubic symphysis; by six weeks it has returned to its non-pregnant size.

Infection of the mother's genital tract during this time (*puerperal infection* or *puerperal fever*) is a particular danger, and in former years was a common cause of maternal death; this is now rare, owing to better understanding of the causes of infection and the use of antibiotics.

Contraception

Contraception is usually defined as the prevention of fertilization, but as will be seen below this is not always strictly correct. The methods used can be classified as 'natural' methods, barrier methods, chemical methods, and sterilization.

The commonest method in the West is the use of the *hormonal contraceptive pill* ('the pill'), which is usually a combination of **oestrogen** and **progesterone**. Under normal conditions these two hormones are secreted by the ovary in a cyclical manner; the blood levels of each hormone at any one time of the menstrual cycle are precisely controlled, such that the overall pattern of secretion promotes fertility. Relatively small changes in the secretory pattern interfere with fertility – a fact that is exploited in the dosage pattern (or *regimen*) of the oral contraceptive. Although most types of oral contraceptive actually prevent ovulation, others may not always do so, but they have other antifertility effects that are equally effective.

The pills must be taken on the appropriate days of the cycle, so there is always the risk of human error and forgetfulness; this risk may be diminished by the development of long-acting pills. The pill is not suitable for everyone because of various *side effects*, which include depression and vascular disorders, but some conditions such as acne and premenstrual tension improve, and the breasts may increase in size. Other conditions are positive *contraindications* for taking the pill, especially vascular diseases like myocardial infarction and deep venous thrombosis. When on the pill, *smoking*, and especially heavy smoking, greatly increases the risk of heart disease.

The *natural methods* include complete abstinence from sexual intercourse (the only absolutely certain method) or reliance on the so-called *safe period*. Since in each menstrual cycle the ovum remains capable of being fertilized for only three days (or less) after ovulation, abstinence is theoretically only necessary during this time, and the rest of the cycle is 'safe'. The problem is how to determine when ovulation has occurred. The basal body temperature rises by 0.5° C at ovulation, and, if the temperature is taken every morning before getting up, for a period of several weeks, this pattern of temperature rise should become apparent. However, cycles are not always regular (p.300), and experience has shown that ovulation can occur on any day, even during menstruation; the 'safe period' is therefore far from safe. (The temperature rise can be used by those who wish to have a family but who have not yet been able to conceive; it should indicate when intercourse is most likely to lead to conception, without of course guaranteeing it.)

Barrier methods include the use of the *condom*, a rubber

sheath that is rolled on to the erect penis and prevents the escape of seminal fluid at ejaculation. Condoms have the advantage of preventing direct contact between partners and therefore help greatly in preventing the spread of sexually transmitted diseases. These diseases includes AIDS (p.70), whose virus can gain entry into the body through the minutest gaps in skin or mucous membranes.

Diaphragms and *cervical caps* are designed to be inserted in the vagina to cover over the cervix and prevent semen progressing into the uterus. They should always be used with some kind of *spermicidal jelly*.

Intra-uterine contraceptive devices (*IUCDs*, *IUDs* or 'coils') are made of polythene rod (sometimes with a component of copper) and are inserted into the uterus through the cervical canal. They are believed to act by preventing implantation of the fertilized ovum, rather than by preventing conception. They can be kept in the uterus for many months or even some years. They usually cause the menstrual periods to be heavier.

Sterilization can be carried out in the female or male. In the female, this involves cutting or obstructing the lumen of the uterine tubes (e.g. by applying clips or using diathermy) so that ova and sperm cannot meet. In the male the operation is *vasectomy* (see below). In both sexes the procedures should be regarded as irreversible, although it is sometimes possible to re-unite the appropriate tubes to restore the lumen; the success rate of this reversal is low.

PELVIC AND PERINEAL MALE ORGANS

Of the male *external genitalia* (p.92), the scrotum has already been described with the anterior abdominal wall, in view of its possible involvement in inguinal hernia (p.248). Here the testis, with the epididymis and ductus deferens, and the penis are considered, together with the pelvic or *internal genital organs* – the prostateand its associated structures.

TESTIS

The **testis** is a roughly oval or egg-shaped structure about 4 cm long which is suspended in the **scrotum** (p.252) at the lower end of the **spermatic cord** (**19.47b** and **19.47c**). The left testis usually hangs at a slightly lower level than the right. Each is almost completely surrounded by an empty, closed sac (the **tunica vaginalis**) derived during early development from the abdominal peritoneum. In the early fetus the testes are on the posterior abdominal wall but, by the time of birth, they should have migrated through the inguinal canal (**descent of the testis**) to reach the scrotum (p.248).

EPIDIDYMIS

Each **epididymis** (**19.47b** and **19.47c**) is attached to the *back* of its own testis – an important point to remember when trying to distinguish whether a swelling in this region belongs to one or the other. The testis and epididymis together are sometimes collectively called the **testicle**. The epididymis is approximately 'C'-shaped and lies almost vertically with a rather larger upper end (**head**) and a smaller lower end (**tail**) which becomes continuous with the **ductus deferens**.

The epididymis is really a single, immensely coiled tube (about 6 m or 20 feet long if stretched out) receiving several ducts from the seminiferous tubules of the testis. It serves not only as a *storage organ* for sperm but as a site where they can *mature* and become capable of fertilization; sperm newly formed by the testis are not able to fertilize an ovum. The epididymis produces only a very small amount of seminal fluid. It is not often the site of disease but may become involved with testicular inflammation (*epididymitis*).

DUCTUS DEFERENS

The **ductus deferens** (**19.47b**), still often called by its old name **vas deferens**, is the continuation of the epididymis, and is a narrow, rather thick-walled muscular tube (of smooth muscle) about 25 cm (10 inches) long, running from the *lower* end (tail) of the epididymis to the ejaculatory duct in the prostate. With the testicular blood vessels it forms one of the main constituents of the **spermatic cord** which runs through the inguinal canal (p.248), and it can be palpated through the skin and distinguished from other cord constituents at the top of the scrotum. This is where the incision is made for *vasectomy* – cutting the duct (on both sides) and removing a length of it to produce male sterilization.

Having reached the abdomen through the inguinal canal, the ductus runs down the side wall of the pelvis (**19.38** and **19.46**) and then crosses the pelvic floor (under cover of the peritoneum) to reach the back of the prostate where it is joined by the **duct of the seminal vesicle** to form the **ejaculatory duct** (**19.47a** and **19.47b**).

BLOOD SUPPLY AND LYMPH DRAINAGE

The testis (with the epididymis) has its main blood supply from the **testicular artery** (**19.10**), a branch from the abdominal aorta just below the renal artery. It runs down on the posterior abdominal wall behind the peritoneum but superficial to the ureter, to enter the inguinal canal as part of the spermatic cord. The long course of the artery reflects the migration of the testis from the posterior abdominal wall to the scrotum during fetal development. The accompanying **testicular vein** drains on the left side into the renal vein but on the right into the inferior vena cava.

Lymph drainage from the testis is to paraaortic nodes; it is important to note that the testis does not drain to inguinal lymph nodes, although the overlying skin of the scrotum does.

STRUCTURE AND FUNCTION

The testis (**19.47c** and **19.47d**) has a tough connective tissue capsule (the **tunica albuginea**) from which more delicate partitions penetrate the organ dividing it up into 200–300 compartments. Each compartment contains up to four **seminiferous tubules**, which are microscopic thread-like structures which, if stretched out, would each be about 75 cm long. At puberty, the primitive **germ cells** within the tubules undergo various proliferative and maturational changes to form **spermatozoa** (**sperm**). The age of puberty is variable, say between 12 and 13, and delayed puberty does not imply any lack of later development. The whole process of producing spermatozoa from spermatogonia (*spermatogenesis*) takes 65–70 days. Different tubules, and different parts of the same tubule, have germ cells in varying stages of development, so that some mature sperm are always available for transport from the testis into the epididymis, the storage organ which is continuous with the ductus deferens. The sperm are carried in **semen** (see below).

Certain large cells in the seminiferous tubules (**Sertoli cells** – scattered among the developing germ cells) provide the supporting framework for spermatogenesis and also secrete the hormone **inhibin**, which inhibits the production of pituitary FSH.

However, the *principal* endocrine cells of the testis, the **interstitial cells of Leydig** (which are scattered in the connective tissue *outside* the seminiferous tubules), produce the male sex hormone **testosterone**, which is not only essential for the normal production of **spermatozoa** but is also responsible for the male characteristics of *puberty* which begin to change a boy into a man – growth of the beard and body hair, enlargement of the penis and scrotum, growth of body musculature, enlargement of the larynx with the male type of voice changes ('breaking of the voice'), and an interest in sex. Testosterone secretion (which, like any other endocrine secretion enters the blood stream, not the semen) is in turn dependent on the anterior pituitary's **LH** (p.140).

DISEASES

In the fetus, the migration of the testis from the abdomen to the scrotum may be delayed, giving an undescended testis (*crytorchidism*, from the Greek for 'hidden testis'). The testis may remain in the abdomen or become 'stuck' in some part of the inguinal canal, where it may be felt as a small swelling. Undescended (*cryptorchid*) testes do not manufacture sperm in the normal way; the slightly lower temperature of the scrotum compared with the inside of the abdomen is necessary for normal spermatogenesis. Hormone treatment or operation may be required to get them into the scrotum, but many such testes never function normally. In those that remain undescended, the incidence of cancerous change is 50 times greater than in normal testes.

In infants with the *congenital type of inguinal hernia* (p.248), the tunica vaginalis remains in open continuity with the peritoneal cavity and so forms the sac in which the coil of gut lies. In injury or disease, but often from no known cause, fluid may collect in the sac, forming a *hydrocele* – the commonest scrotal swelling. The fluid is just tissue fluid, not semen, for the sac has no connection with the sperm-forming system. The fluid may be aspirated with a needle and syringe, but sometimes surgery is necessary to turn the sac inside out and prevent the accumulation of further fluid.

Testicular tumours are characterized by occurring in young men before the age of 40, and many are sensitive to radiotherapy. *Orchitis* (inflammation of the testis) can be a complication of some sexually transmitted diseases; it can also be an unexpected and uncomfortable complication of mumps in young men, but it has no long-term adverse effects.

The term *hypogonadism* refers to the failure of the testis to produce testosterone (also called *androgen deficiency*) or to produce spermatozoa. Androgen deficiency **before puberty** leads to *eunuchoidism*, with lack of body hair, small sexual organs, poor muscle development, unusual tallness (due to lack of fusion of epiphyses), no breaking of the voice, and lack of sexual interest (lack of libido); in an **adult**, similar deficiency leads to loss of some body hair, decreased libido and impotence. In either case the fault may be in the testis itself (*primary hypogonadism*) or in the pituitary gland or hypothalamus (*secondary hypogonadism*). Treatment is by the administration of testosterone, either by injection or the implantation of hormone pellets, to restore the deficiency.

PROSTATE

The **prostate** (whose proper name is simply 'prostate', not 'prostate gland') is a glandular organ situated in the lowest part of the pelvis below the bladder and surrounding the first 3 cm of the urethra (**19.38** and **19.47a**). It is usually described as having the size and shape of a chestnut, and is approximately 4 cm wide, 3 cm long and 2 cm deep. It rests on the levator ani muscles (the pelvic floor – levator prostatae part, p.290), and being just in front of the rectum its back surface can be felt on rectal examination (**19.23a**).

The prostate consists of small **glands** embedded in a mixture of **fibrous tissue** and **smooth muscle**. The glands contribute about 30% of the seminal fluid; they have nothing to do with manufacturing spermatozoa which come only from the testes. The prostate is very small before puberty but then it enlarges under the influence of the **testosterone** secreted by the testes and quickly reaches adult size. As part of *ejaculation* (see below), the smooth muscle within the prostate contracts and causes the secretion of the glands to be discharged into the prostatic urethra through about 12 minute ducts.

The gland gets its blood supply from the **prostatic branch of the inferior vesical artery** or sometimes from the **middle rectal artery**. The veins do not accompany the arteries; they form a plexus in the groove between the bladder and prostate (the **vesicoprostatic venous plexus**), draining back to the internal iliac veins. The lymphatic drainage is likewise backwards to various pelvic nodes.

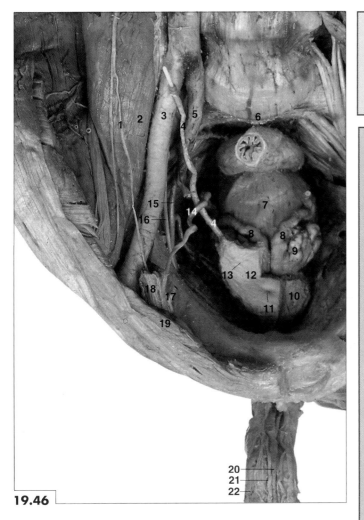

19.46

1 Genital branch of genitofemoral nerve, passing down to enter the spermatic cord (18)
2 Psoas major
3 External iliac artery
4 Ureter, running down into the pelvis in front of the internal iliac artery (5)
5 Internal iliac artery
6 Promontory of sacrum
7 Rectum
8 Lower end of ductus deferens, lying medial to the seminal vesicle (9)
9 Left seminal vesicle
10 Base (upper surface) of prostate
11 Internal urethral meatus
12 Trigone of bladder, the lower part of the base (posterior surface)
13 Right ureteral opening
14 Ductus deferens, passing down into the pelvis (after emerging from the spermatic cord, 18); its lower end is shown at 8
15 Obturator artery
16 Obturator nerve
17 Inferior epigastric artery
18 Spermatic cord, displaced backwards from the deep inguinal ring lateral to the inferior epigastric artery (17)
19 Cut margin of anterior abdominal wall
20 Deep dorsal vein of penis, the single midline vessel
21 Dorsal artery
22 Dorsal nerve

SEMINAL VESICLE AND EJACULATORY DUCT

The **seminal vesicles** are a pair of coiled structures with smooth muscle in their walls, usually 4–5 cm (2 inches) long but 15 cm (6 inches) long if unravelled. Each seminal vesicle lies below the ureter on its own side against the back of the bladder (**19.47a**) and in front of the rectum, on the outer side of the lower end of the ductus deferens, which has run down the side wall of the pelvis from the inguinal canal (p.307) and crossed over the ureter. Unless diseased, which is rare, the seminal vesicles are *not* usually palpable on rectal examination (p.268). Their function is to produce most of the *seminal fluid* in the ejaculate (see below).

The **ejaculatory duct**, the result of the union of the **duct** of the **seminal vesicle** with the **ductus deferens** (**19.47b**), is about 2 cm long and runs through the back of the prostate to open into the prostatic part of the urethra. Here, the genital tracts of each side join the urinary tract, so that the urethra from this point on serves as a common channel for urine and semen.

PENIS

The **penis** is the male organ of *copulation* (*sexual intercourse*) and also contains the longest section of the urethra, known in this location as the **spongy urethra** (p.295). The penis is composed of three elongated columns of spongy tissue (**19.39**): a central part, the **corpus spongiosum**, through which the urethra runs, and on each side a **corpus cavernosum** (plural – **corpora cavernosa**). The urethra opens on the **glans penis**, the expanded end of the corpus spongiosum. The corpora cavernosa, after running alongside the corpus spongiosum, terminate just behind the glans, which is covered by a retractable fold of skin, the **prepuce** (**foreskin**). Sometimes the fold is excessively tight (*phimosis*) and may interfere with micturition or erection, in which case it must be removed – the operation of *circumcision*, which is also carried out as part of religious or racial custom.

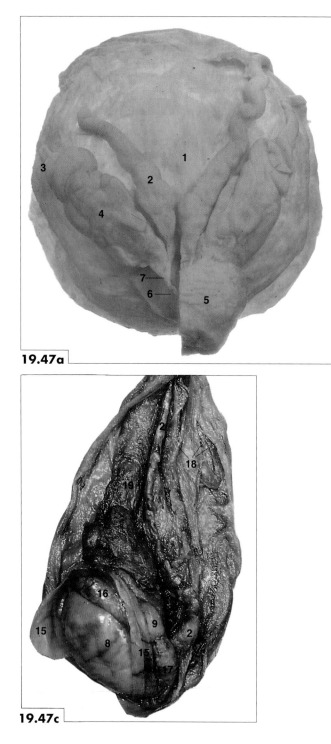

19.47a

19.47c

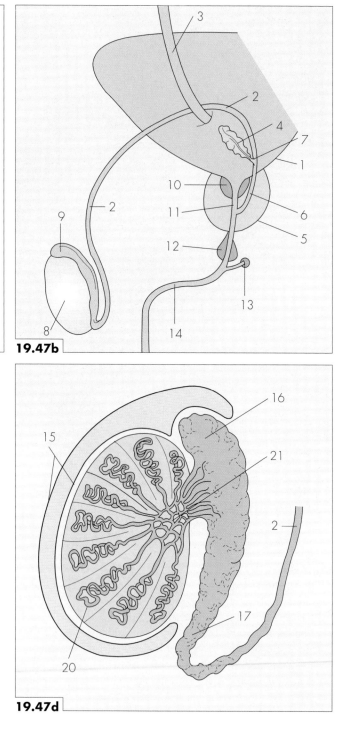

19.47b

19.47d

The beginning of the spongy part of the urethra receives the ducts of the **bulbourethral glands** (**19.41b**), which are small pea-like structures below the prostate. The bases of all three corpora lie in the perineum (p.292).

SEMEN, ERECTION AND EJACULATION

Semen (or, the **ejaculate**) consists of a large number of

spermatozoa suspended in a **fluid** produced mainly by the seminal vesicles and prostate. Roughly 60% of the fluid comes from the seminal vesicles, 30% from the prostate, and very small amounts from the bulbourethral glands and the ductus deferens on each side. (The ductus deferens fluid, while small in volume, contains the densely packed spermatozoa.) Semen is the opaque, slightly sticky, whitish fluid

Fig. 19.47 Bladder and genitalia in the male.
(a) Bladder and prostate, from behind, with most of the left half of the prostate removed, to show the left ejaculatory duct.
(b) Diagram of bladder and genitalia, from the left.
(c) Testis and lower end of spermatic cord, removed from the scrotum and with the coverings opened up to show the epididymis and ductus deferens.
(d) Diagrammatic representation of the structure of the testis.

1 Base (posterior surface) of bladder
2 Ductus deferens
3 Lower end of ureter, entering the bladder above the tip of the seminal vesicle (4)
4 Seminal vesicle
5 Posterior surface of prostate
6 Ejaculatory duct, formed by the lower end of the ductus (2) and the duct of the seminal vesicle (7)
7 Duct of seminal vesicle
8 Testis
9 Epididymis
10 Internal urethral sphincter (smooth muscle), which prevents regurgitation of seminal fluid into the bladder during ejaculation
11 Prostatic urethra
12 External urethral sphincter (skeletal muscle), pear-shaped, surrounding the membranous part of the urethra
13 Bulbourethral gland
14 Penile part of urethra
15 Cut edge of tunica vaginalis, turned back in **(c)** to expose the testis (8) and the head of the epididymis (16)
16 Head of epididymis, its upper end
17 Tail of epididymis, which becomes continuous with the beginning of the ductus deferens (2)
18 Incised margins of coverings of spermatic cord
19 Bundle of testicular vessels
20 Seminiferous tubule
21 Rete testis, a network of ducts from the seminiferous tubules and opening into the epididymis

which is deposited in the vagina during sexual intercourse.

Sexual excitement causes *erection* of the penis, which is due to *parasympathetic* activity dilating the **arteries** that supply the corpora cavernosa and corpus spongiosum and causing the sponge-like blood spaces to become engorged. At a later stage, the **smooth muscle** of the prostate, seminal vesicles and ductus deferens contracts due to *sympathetic* nerve activity, and causes semen to enter the urethra (*emission*). At the same time, smooth muscle at the base of the bladder contracts to stop the semen from passing back into the bladder. Then, as the climax of the sexual act, the *skeletal muscles* overlying the corpus spongiosum (**bulbospongiosus, 19.39**) contract rhythmically for a few seconds to cause *ejaculation* of semen from the penis.

A single specimen of ejaculate consists of 1–5 ml of fluid, containing perhaps **250 *million sperm***, only a ***single one*** of which is necessary to fertilize an ovum. After being deposited in the vagina, some sperm may enter the uterus but most seminal fluid becomes lost in the vaginal secretions, and the sperm die in a day or two. Sperm that enter the cervix take about an hour to travel through the cervix and body of the uterus to the end of the uterine tube where they may meet an ovum (p.303). Semen has no function or physiological effects other than to act as a vehicle for sperm.

DISEASES

After about the age of 50 the prostate may decrease in size, but frequently it undergoes enlargement (*hypertrophy*, 'enlarged prostate'), for reasons that are not yet understood but are probably hormonal. This is a benign (non-cancerous) change, affecting almost all males but causing significant symptoms in about 25%, of whom half may eventually need a surgical operation. The enlargement affects not the whole gland but part of it, often the region at the back between the urethra and the two ejaculatory ducts (the middle lobe of the prostate). The effect of this enlargement may be to obstruct the urethra and so interfere with micturition, particularly causing *nocturnal frequency* (having to get up several times in the night to pass urine) with difficulty both in starting the flow and ending it without dribbling. *Obstruction* may suddenly become complete, requiring the passage of a catheter through the urethra into the bladder in order to relieve it. In prostatic hypertrophy hormone treatment is not effective. Most prostatic operations are nowadays carried out through an instrument (*resectoscope*) introduced through the urethra, without the need to open the abdomen and the bladder, though this may be necessary in some cases.

Cancer of the prostate is the second commonest male cancer (after that of the lung). If detected early, treatment with female hormones is often very successful in controlling (but not curing) the disease, but if there has been local or more distant spread, surgery and/or radiotherapy may be necessary. Because of the way pelvic veins communicate with the venous plexuses of the vertebral column, metastatic spread to the spine, ribs or hip bones is common.

The penis may be affected by the various *sexually transmitted diseases* (*STDs*), several of which cause *urethral discharges* similar to those affecting the vagina (p.302), or rashes and ulceration. Infection by STDs may spread up the urethra to any of the genital organs, e.g. gonorrhoea, apart from causing urethral discharge, may cause *prostatitis* and *epididymitis*.

Carcinoma of the penis can occur, and is commoner in those who have not been circumcised.

Impotence is the inability to have an erection for successful sexual intercourse. The cause is frequently psychogenic, but it is a well-recognized complication of diabetes, alcoholism and some endocrine disorders.

CHAPTER 20

LOWER LIMB

PRINCIPAL FEATURES

Bones and joints (see *Table* **20.1**)

Important muscles (see *Table* **20.2**)

Important nerves (see *Table* **20.3**)

Important arteries (see *Table* **20.4**)

Important superficial veins (see *Table* **20.5**)

THIGH

The **thigh** is the upper part of the lower limb. The *front* of the thigh is continuous with the **inguinal region of the abdomen**, while the *back* of the thigh is below the **gluteal region** or **buttock**, which is at the back of the pelvis and the **hip joint**. This joint, between the head of the femur and the hip bone (**20.1** and **20.3**), is described later (p.321), after the gluteal region has been considered.

The **sacroiliac joints** (p.289) unite the two hip bones with the sacral part of the vertebral column (**20.1** and **20.3**). They

Table 20.1 Bones and joints of the lower limb		
Pelvic girdle	Ilium, ischium and pubis	The three bones are fused together and firmly united at the back with the sacrum of the axial skeleton (at the almost immobile sacroiliac joint), and at the front with the opposite hip bone at the pubic symphysis.
Bone of the thigh	Femur or os femoris	The longest bone in the body, with a rounded head at the upper end forming the hip joint with the acetabulum of the hip bone, and with two curved condyles at the lower end forming the knee joint with the tibia and the patella.
Bones of the leg	Tibia and fibula	The two flat condyles at the upper end of the tibia take part in the knee joint, and there is a separate (unimportant) superior tibiofibular joint between the upper ends of the two bones. The lower ends are held together at the fibrous inferior tibiofibular joint, below which the bones form a socket with the uppermost bone of the foot, the talus, making the ankle joint.
Bones of the foot	Seven tarsal bones, five metatarsal bones, two phalanges for the great toe and three phalanges for each of the other toes.	The largest tarsal bone, the calcaneus, forms the heel, with the talus above it. The joints beneath the talus are important for the movements of inversion and eversion of the foot. The metatarsals and phalanges correspond to the metacarpals and phalanges of the hand.

Table 20.2 Important muscles of the upper limb

Gluteus maximus	The muscle of the buttock, located behind the hip and important for extension of the hip in running and climbing stairs.
Gluteus medius and minimus	The muscles at the side of the hip, important in walking for preventing the pelvis from tilting to the opposite side when the opposite foot is off the ground.
Psoas major and iliacus	These pass from the lumbar part of the vertebral column and the iliac fossa within the abdomen, and are important as flexors of the hip.
Quadriceps femoris	Formed by the four muscles on the front of the thigh, uniting to a common tendon, and acting as important extensors of the knee.
Hamstrings	Three muscles at the back of the thigh, important for extending the thigh in walking.
Tibialis anterior	The muscle on the front of the leg, important for keeping the foot off the ground during the swing phase of walking, for maintaining the arch of the foot, and for inversion of the foot.
Tibialis posterior	A calf muscle that is important for maintaining the arch of the foot, for plantarflexion of the ankle and inversion of the foot.
Flexor hallucis longus	A calf muscle, important for the push-off by the great toe in walking.
Gastrocnemius	A calf muscle, important for plantarflexion of the foot.
Soleus	A calf muscle, important for maintaining balance when standing upright.
Peroneus longus	A muscle of the lateral side of the leg, it passes under the sole and is important for eversion of the foot and in helping to maintain the arch of the foot.

Table 20.3 Important nerves of the lower limb

Sciatic nerve	The largest nerve in the body, supplying the hamstrings at the back of the thigh and dividing into tibial and common peroneal branches.
Tibial nerve	The nerve of the back of the leg, supplying the calf and sole.
Common peroneal nerve	The nerve of the front and lateral side of the leg. (The adjective 'fibular' (Latin) is now replacing 'peroneal' (Greek) for some nerves and vessels; the older, more familiar term is used in this book.)
Superior gluteal nerve	Supplies gluteus medius and minimus.
Inferior gluteal nerve	Supplies gluteus maximus.
Femoral nerve	The nerve of the front of the thigh.
Obturator nerve	The nerve of the medial (adductor) compartment of the thigh.

Table 20.4 Important arteries of the lower limb

Femoral artery	The main artery of the lower limb, entering the thigh beneath the inguinal ligament as the continuation of the external iliac artery in the abdomen, and giving off the profunda femoris artery which is the main supply for the thigh muscles.
Popliteal artery	The continuation of the femoral artery behind the knee, dividing into anterior and posterior tibial arteries.
Anterior tibial artery	The artery of the anterior compartment of the leg, continuing on to the dorsum of the foot as the dorsalis pedis artery.
Posterior tibial artery	The artery of the posterior compartment of the leg, continuing into the sole as the medial and lateral plantar arteries.

Table 20.5 Important superficial veins of the lower limb	
Great saphenous vein	The longest vein in the body and the main superficial vein on the medial side of the limb; it drains from the foot to the femoral vein near the inguinal ligament. Some lower tributaries are the common site of 'varicose veins'.
Small saphenous vein	A superficial vein starting on the lateral side of the foot and draining to the popliteal vein behind the knee.

are classified as joints of the pelvis, as is also the **pubic symphysis** (p.289), where the two hip bones unite with each other at the front. The hip bones themselves are each the result of the fusion of three bones – ilium, ischium and pubis – collectively forming the **pelvic girdle**. Being a solid mass of bone, the pelvic girdle is very different from the jointed clavicle and scapula that form the shoulder girdle (p.213).

The main artery of the limb, the **femoral artery**, comes in at the front of the thigh; it is the continuation of the external iliac in the lower abdomen (**8.3**). The largest of all nerves, the **sciatic**, enters the gluteal region from the pelvis to run down the back of the thigh (**7.3b**).

BONE

The **shaft** of the **femur** or thigh bone (now properly called the os femoris, meaning, literally 'the bone of the thigh') is buried deeply within the surrounding muscles; only the lower end of the bone (**20.7**) which takes part in the knee joint (p.324) and the greater trochanter at its upper end (**20.1**) are palpable. The **head** of the femur articulates with the hip bone to make the hip joint (p.321). Severe trauma can fracture the shaft, and because the attached muscles exert a longitudinal pull on the lower fragment, leading to shortening of the limb, some kind of traction must be applied to bring the bone ends into apposition. (Such a procedure often requires the insertion of a steel pin through the upper end of the tibia, to which weights can be slung, to induce the contracting muscles to lengthen.)

FASCIA LATA

The deep fascia of the thigh, the **fascia lata**, forms a tough connective tissue 'stocking' surrounding the muscles. The part of the fascia on the outer aspect of the thigh is known as the **iliotibial tract** (**20.11**), since it extends from the iliac crest to the lateral condyle of the tibia. Its attachment to the

condyle is to the front rather than the side – an arrangement that gives the iliotibial tract an important role in helping to maintain the knee in the fully extended position (p.327). If there is not too much subcutaneous fat, the tract can be felt easily as a longitudinal band on the outer side of the thigh, especially when standing with the weight mostly on the limb being examined.

The **saphenous opening** (**19.5**) is a gap in the fascia lata, situated about 4 cm below and lateral to the (palpable) pubic tubercle, through which the great saphenous vein (see below) passes to enter the femoral vein.

MUSCLES

The **muscles** of the thigh (**6.1** and **6.2**) fall into three compartments or groups: the **anterior** or **extensor group** (supplied by the femoral nerve), the **medial** or **adductor group** (supplied by the obturator nerve) and the **posterior** or **hamstring group** (supplied by the sciatic nerve).

Anterior Compartment (Extensor Muscles)

The large muscle mass on the front of the thigh (see **6.1a**) is the **quadriceps femoris**. It is composed of four muscles: **rectus femoris** and the three **vastus muscles (medialis, intermedius and lateralis)**. All are supplied by the **femoral nerve** (**20.2a**, **7.3** and **19.5**), and all converge to be inserted into the patella. The patella in turn is attached to the tuberosity of the tibia by the **patellar ligament**, and through this attachment the quadriceps extends the knee (p.327). The vastus muscles all arise from the femur, but rectus femoris has origins from the hip bone above the acetabulum and so can act as a flexor of the hip as well as an extensor of the knee.

Sartorius (**6.1a**), the muscle with the longest fibres in the body, crosses the front of the thigh obliquely from the anterior superior iliac spine laterally to the upper medial side of the tibia.

The upper, outer part of the thigh is a safe site for *intramuscular injections*, since there are no major vessels or nerves here (**20.6**). A needle inserted into vastus lateralis is well out of the way of the femoral nerve and vessels which are on the front of the thigh, and of the sciatic nerve and profunda femoris vessels which are at the back.

Medial Compartment (Adductor Muscles)

The inner aspect of the thigh (the medial compartment) is occupied by the **adductor group** of muscles (**6.1**), all of which are supplied by the **obturator nerve** (**7.3a**), whose branches are deeply placed among the muscles. Horseriders rely on the adductor muscles for gripping the saddle, and they occasionally suffer from painful ossification at the origin of the adductor longus muscle from the pubis (*myositis ossificans*).

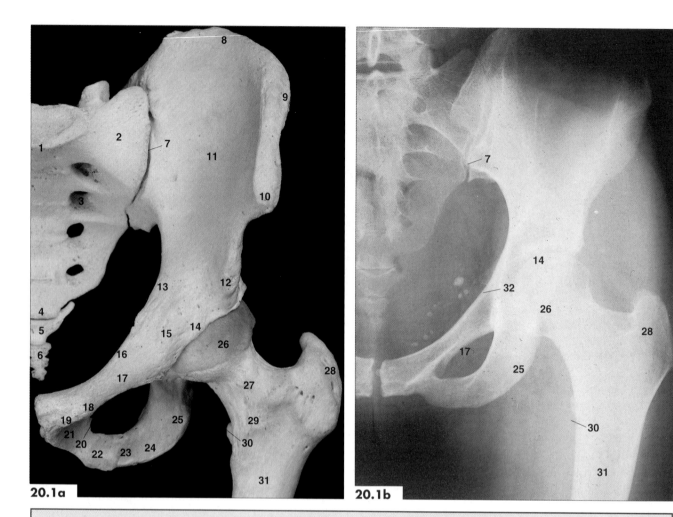

20.1a

20.1b

Fig. 20.1 Left hip bone and femur, with sacrum and coocyx.

(a) From the front

(b) Radiograph (the translucent areas are gas shadows in the large intestine).

1 Sacral promontory
2 Ala of sacrum
3 Second anterior sacral foramen, for anterior ramus of S2 nerve
4 Apex of sacrum
5 First coccygeal vertebra, with transverse process
6 Fused coccygeal vertebrae
7 Sacroiliac joint
8 Iliac crest, palpable throughout its whole length, and a possible site (like the sternum) for bone marrow biopsy
9 Tubercle of iliac crest
10 Anterior superior iliac spine, for inguinal ligament and sartorius
11 Iliac fossa, a term also applied to the lower lateral region of the anterior abdominal wall (**19.2**)
12 Anterior inferior iliac spine, for part of rectus femoris
13 Arcuate line of ilium, forming part of the pelvic brim
14 Rim of acetabulum, the socket for the head of the femur (26)
15 Iliopubic eminence, site of union between ilium and superior ramus of the pubis (12)

16 Pectineal line (pecten) of pubis
17 Superior ramus of pubis
18 Pubic tubercle, a palpable landmark
19 Pubic crest, for rectus abdominis
20 Obturator foramen
21 Body of pubis
22 Inferior ramus of pubis
23 Site of union of pubic and ischial rami (22 and 24)
24 Ramus of ischium
25 Ischial tuberosity, best seen from behind (**20.3**)
26 Head of femur
27 Neck, the part of the femur most commonly fractured
28 Greater tronchanter. Gluteus medius and minimus are attached to its front and lateral side
29 Intertrochanteric line, for the capsule of the hip joint and not to be confused with the intertrochanteric crest on the back of the bone (**20.3**)
30 Tip of lesser trochanter, best seen from behind (**20.3**)
31 Shaft of femur
32 Ischial spine

Posterior Compartment (Hamstring Muscles)

The **hamstring muscles** (6.2a) occupy the posterior compartment of the thigh, and are supplied by the **sciatic** nerve (**20.4**, **20.6** and **7.3b**) which runs down the middle under cover of the muscles. Since they cross both the hip joint and the knee joint, these muscles can affect both joints, acting as extensors of the hip (as in walking, p.340) and as

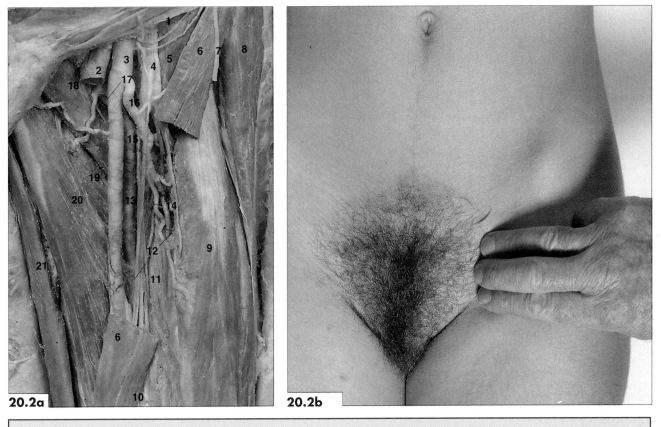

20.2a   20.2b

Fig. 20.2 Left femoral region.
(a) With part of sartorius removed, together with most of the femoral vein and its tributaries.

(b) Palpation of the femoral pulse, below the inguinal ligament and midway between the anterior superior iliac spine and the pubic symphysis.

---

1 Inguinal ligament
2 Femoral vein
3 Femoral artery. From its pulsation, the position of the femoral vein on its medial side (2) and the femoral nerve on its lateral side (4) can be gauged. The tendon of psoas is behind the upper part of the artery, separating the artery from the hip joint.
4 Femoral nerve, dividing into its various branches as soon as it passes under the inguinal ligament (1)
5 Iliacus, separating the femoral nerve (4) from the hip joint
6 Sartorius
7 Lateral femoral cutaneous nerve
8 Tensor fasciae latae
9 Rectus femoris, part of quadriceps femoris (with the three vastus muscles)
10 Vastus medialis

11 Vastus intermedius, the deepest of the three vasti
12 Muscular branches of femoral nerve
13 Profunda femoris artery, the main vessel for thigh muscles
14 Branches of lateral circumflex femoral artery
15 Saphenous nerve, which will become the only branch of the femoral nerve to extend as far as the foot
16 Lateral circumflex femoral artery, here arising from the femoral artery (3), a common variation from its usual origin from the profunda femoris artery
17 Medial circumflex femoral artery, passing backwards between psoas and pectineus to the gluteal region
18 Pectineus, separating the femoral vein from the hip joint
19 Adductor brevis and the anterior division of the obturator nerve
20 Adductor longus
21 Gracilis, the most medial of the adductor muscles

flexors of the knee (p.327). On the lower, outer side of the thigh, **biceps femoris** (the outer hamstring) and **vastus lateralis** (part of the quadriceps) lie adjacent. Here, there is a groove between these two muscles (**20.11**), caused by a septum of connective tissue passing from the fascia lata to the femur; when sitting with the knee at a right angle, the groove is seen and felt between the biceps tendon (running towards the head of the fibula) and the iliotibial tract in front. On the lower medial side, the other two hamstrings can be felt – the tendon of **semitendinosus** overlies the **semimembranosus** (**20.10** and **6.2a**).

FEMORAL TRIANGLE

The term **femoral triangle** describes a region at the front of the upper thigh, just below the inguinal ligament. One side of the triangle is formed by the inguinal ligament itself, while the other two sides are formed by adductor longus (medially) and sartorius (laterally)(**20.2a**). The contents of the triangle are (in order, from medial to lateral): the **femoral canal**, **femoral vein**, **femoral artery** and **femoral nerve**. The vein and artery, together with the femoral canal, are enclosed in a connective tissue sleeve, the **femoral sheath**.

The contents of the femoral triangle are separated from the more deeply lying hip joint by muscles: medially is **pectineus** (intervening between the joint and the femoral vein), while laterally is **iliacus** (underneath the femoral nerve). In the middle, and level with the middle of the head of the femur, is **psoas major**, here becoming tendinous and separating the femoral artery from the capsule of the joint. The upper ends of these femoral structures are described with the inguinal region (p.248 and **19.5**).

FEMORAL ARTERY

The **femoral artery** (**20.2a** and **8.3**), the main arterial supply for the lower limb, enters the thigh beneath the inguinal ligament and runs through the femoral triangle. At the lower end (the apex) of the triangle, it continues downwards under cover of sartorius, in the region of the thigh known as the **adductor canal**. In the lower part of the thigh it passes through an opening in adductor magnus on the medial side of the femur to reach the popliteal fossa at the back of the knee, where it changes its name to the **popliteal artery**. While for most of its course the femoral artery is in the extensor compartment of the thigh, it actually provides arterial supply to muscles in all three compartments via its principal branch, the **profunda femoris artery**.

The *pulsation* of the femoral artery (**20.2b**) can be felt just below the inguinal ligament, midway between the anterior superior iliac spine and pubic symphysis. This is where it can be cannulated for arteriography and cardiac catheterization (p.118 and **15.24**).

FEMORAL NERVE

The **femoral nerve** (**20.2a** and **7.3a**) is the main nerve of the anterior compartment of the thigh. As soon as it passes under the inguinal ligament from the abdomen it breaks up into a number of cutaneous and muscular branches, mainly for the quadriceps femoris. The nerve is rarely injured, but it may be affected by stab wounds of the lower abdomen.

GREAT SAPHENOUS VEIN

The **great saphenous vein**, the longest vein in the body (**8.4**), begins on the medial side of the foot (p.332). It passes up the medial side of the limb in the subcutaneous tissues (superficial to the deep fascia), and eventually passes through the saphenous opening in the fascia lata to drain into the femoral vein (**19.5**) as its only large and obvious tributary. The saphenous vein itself receives several small tributaries – a distinction from the femoral vein.

GLUTEAL REGION

The **gluteal region**, commonly called the **buttock**, extends from the iliac crest to the gluteal fold (the fold of the buttock, **20.4b**), and from the midline over the sacrum to the greater trochanter of the femur; it includes the area at the back of the hip joint. The subcutaneous tissue contains a large amount of fat which, together with the gluteal muscles, helps to give the area its characteristic prominence. The skin over the sacrum is the commonest site for *pressure sores* in the bedridden, and the region of the greater trochanter is another danger area (p.60).

GLUTEUS MAXIMUS

The large **gluteus maximus** muscle overlies other muscles that are above and behind the hip joint (**6.2a**). The fibres of gluteus maximus run obliquely downwards and laterally from the sacrum towards the femur but only one quarter of the muscle is actually attached to the femur (to the gluteal tuberosity on the back of the bone, **20.3**), the rest being inserted into the iliotibial tract – the lateral part of the fascia lata of the thigh (p.315 and **6.1a**).

Supplied by the **inferior gluteal nerve** (**20.4a**), gluteus maximus is a powerful *extensor of the hip* as in running or climbing stairs, but because of its attachment to the iliotibial tract which is inserted into the front of the tibia just below the knee, the muscle also helps to hold the **knee** in its fully *extended* (straight) position. Note that the gluteal fold of fatty skin does not correspond to the lower border of gluteus maximus; the fold is essentially a skin crease associated with movement of the hip joint.

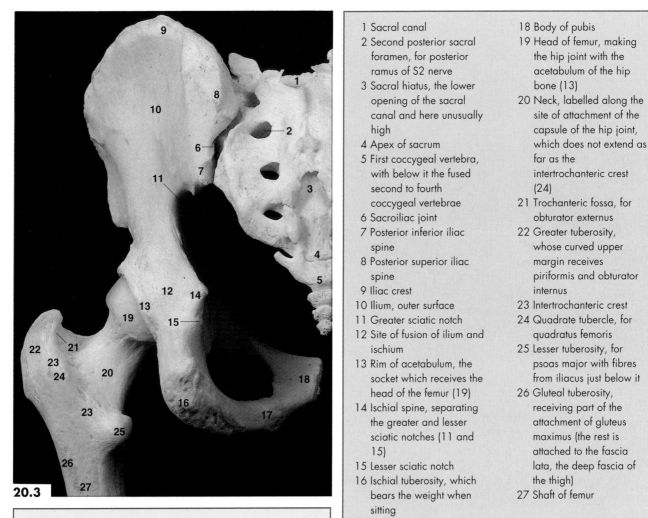

1 Sacral canal
2 Second posterior sacral foramen, for posterior ramus of S2 nerve
3 Sacral hiatus, the lower opening of the sacral canal and here unusually high
4 Apex of sacrum
5 First coccygeal vertebra, with below it the fused second to fourth coccygeal vertebrae
6 Sacroiliac joint
7 Posterior inferior iliac spine
8 Posterior superior iliac spine
9 Iliac crest
10 Ilium, outer surface
11 Greater sciatic notch
12 Site of fusion of ilium and ischium
13 Rim of acetabulum, the socket which receives the head of the femur (19)
14 Ischial spine, separating the greater and lesser sciatic notches (11 and 15)
15 Lesser sciatic notch
16 Ischial tuberosity, which bears the weight when sitting
17 Ramus of ischium joining inferior ramus of pubis

18 Body of pubis
19 Head of femur, making the hip joint with the acetabulum of the hip bone (13)
20 Neck, labelled along the site of attachment of the capsule of the hip joint, which does not extend as far as the intertrochanteric crest (24)
21 Trochanteric fossa, for obturator externus
22 Greater tuberosity, whose curved upper margin receives piriformis and obturator internus
23 Intertrochanteric crest
24 Quadrate tubercle, for quadratus femoris
25 Lesser tuberosity, for psoas major with fibres from iliacus just below it
26 Gluteal tuberosity, receiving part of the attachment of gluteus maximus (the rest is attached to the fascia lata, the deep fascia of the thigh)
27 Shaft of femur

Fig. 20.3 Left hip bone and femur, with sacrum and coccyx, from behind.

OTHER GLUTEAL MUSCLES

Gluteus medius and **gluteus minimus** pass from the outer surface of the hip bone to the greater trochanter (**20.4a** and **6.2**). Supplied by the **superior gluteal nerve**, they act together as abductors of the hip joint. Their more important role, however, is to *prevent adduction* – keeping the pelvis level during walking (as described on p.323).

Tensor fasciae latae is a smaller muscle arising from the outer, front part of the iliac crest (**6.1a**), to be inserted into the iliotibial tract of the fascia lata (p.315). By this attachment it assists gluteus maximus in extension of the knee (see above).

Below the lower borders of gluteus medius and minimus lie (in order from above downwards) **piriformis, obturator externus** with the **gemelli** at its upper and lower borders, and **quadratus femoris** (**20.4a**). The **sciatic nerve** and most other structures that leave the pelvis to enter the gluteal region do so by passing under the lower border of piriformis

– a key landmark in the gluteal region. By converging on to the greater trochanter, these small muscles act as *lateral rotators* of the femur (p.323).

SCIATIC NERVE

The most important structure in the gluteal region is the **sciatic nerve** – the largest nerve in the body (**7.3b**). It enters the gluteal region from the pelvis by emerging *below* piriformis (**20.4a**) to lie under cover of gluteus maximus before running down the back of the thigh deep to the hamstrings (**20.6**). Its surface marking as it leaves the gluteal region to pass into the thigh is midway between the ischial tuberosity and the greater trochanter.

The commonest cause of sciatic nerve *injury* is (regrettably) misplaced gluteal injections (see below). It may also be damaged by posterior dislocations of the hip, as in motor vehicle accidents where contact with the flexed knee forces the femur backwards. A complete sciatic nerve lesion

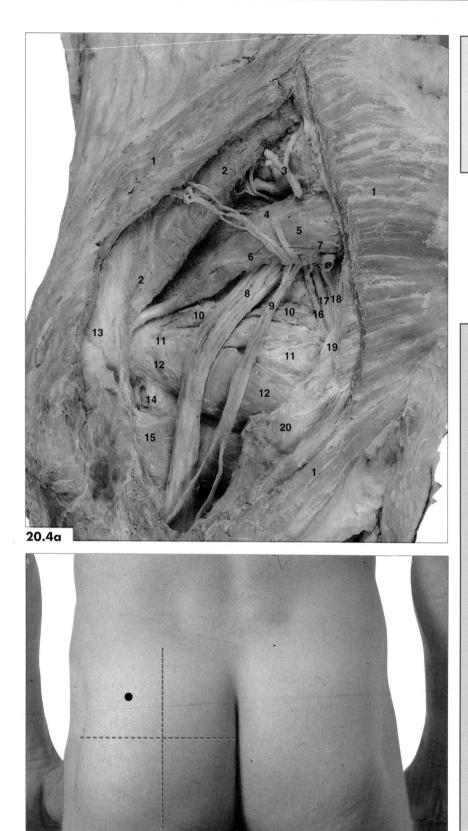

20.4a

20.4b

Fig. 20.4 Left gluteal region.
(a) After most of gluteus maximus and all veins have been removed
(b) Site for intramuscular injection (well away from the sciatic nerve) in the upper outer quadrant of the four quadrants described in the text and indicated here by the interrupted lines

1 Gluteus maximus
2 Gluteus medius
3 Superior gluteal artery, emerging with the nerve (4) above piriformis (5)
4 Superior gluteal nerve, supplying gluteus medius and minimus (under cover of medius) and tensor fasciae latae (on the outer side of the upper thigh)
5 Piriformis, the main landmark of the gluteal region, passing out of the greater sciatic foramen with the sciatic nerve (8) emerging below it
6 Inferior gluteal nerve, supplying gluteus maximus
7 Inferior gluteal artery
8 Sciatic nerve, emerging below piriformis (5) to pass down the thigh deep to the hamstrings
9 Posterior femoral cutaneous nerve, passing down the thigh superficial to the hamstrings
10 Superior gemellus
11 Obturator internus, passing out of the lesser sciatic foramen
12 Inferior gemellus
13 Greater trochanter
14 Obturator externus
15 Quadratus femoris
16 Nerve to obturator internus (11)
17 Internal pudendal artery. With the pudendal nerve (18) it passes out of the greater sciatic foramen into the lesser sciatic foramen to reach the perineum
18 Pudendal nerve
19 Sacrotuberous ligament
20 Ischial tuberosity

paralyzes the hamstrings and all the muscles below the knee. There is also anaesthesia of the skin below the knee except on the medial side where the supply is by the saphenous branch of the femoral nerve. There is no thigh anaesthesia because the sciatic nerve does not supply any skin here; any anaesthesia on the back of the thigh must be due to simultaneous damage to the posterior femoral cutaneous nerve which is just behind the sciatic and liable to be injured with it.

GLUTEAL INTRAMUSCULAR INJECTION

The bulky gluteus maximus with gluteus medius underneath it is a possible site for *intramuscular injections*, but it is of course absolutely vital to choose the correct position for injection in order to avoid damaging the sciatic nerve. The proper site is usually described as the *upper outer quadrant* of the gluteal region (**20.4b**). In estimating the four quadrants by vertical and horizontal lines through the midpoint of the region, it must be remembered that the *upper* boundary of the region is the *iliac crest*, not the most prominent part of the bulge of the buttock or a suntanned bikini line, which are both far too low. Only by choosing the properly defined quadrant can injury to the sciatic nerve be avoided. The needle should enter either gluteus maximus or the adjacent part of gluteus medius.

HIP JOINT

The **hip joint** is formed by the articulation of the **head of the femur** with the **acetabulum of the hip bone** (**20.1** and **4.1a**). It is deeply surrounded by muscles and is not directly palpable. However, the greater trochanter of the femur forms a palpable knob at the side of the region, where its subcutaneous position makes that area a possible site for pressure sores (**4.1c**).

At the front of the thigh, just below the inguinal ligament, at the top of the femoral triangle (p.318), the centre of the joint is crossed by the psoas tendon with the femoral artery in front of the tendon (**20.2a**). Medial to the tendon is pectineus (with the femoral vein and canal in front of it), while lateral to the tendon is iliacus (with the femoral nerve in front). Gluteus minimus is the immediate cover for the upper part of the joint, and winding below it from front to back is obturator externus. At the back, piriformis is immediately behind the joint (**20.4a**), with obturator internus and the gemelli and quadratus femoris lower down.

BONES

The shape of the head of the femur (it is rounded) and the acetabulum (which is cup-like) make this an excellent example of a *ball-and-socket joint* (**20.1**). The acetabulum is made even deeper by a rim of fibrocartilage (the **acetabular labrum, 20.5**), and this alone without the capsule of the joint

would be sufficient to hold the head of the femur into the acetabulum. The bony deficiency at the lower part of the acetabulum (the **acetabular notch**) is made good by a band of fibrous tissue (the **transverse ligament**), and, from this, a rounded ligament (the **ligamentum teres** or **ligament of the head of the femur**) passes upwards inside the joint to be attached to the pit or fovea in the head. In the very young, this ligament contains an artery which helps to supply the head, but by the age of 7 years or so it has usually become obliterated and plays no significant part in supplying the adult head.

LIGAMENTS

The joint is surrounded by a tough **capsule**; at the front of the femur it is attached to the intertrochanteric *line* (**20.1a**) but at the back it does ***not*** extend as far as the intertrochanteric *crest* – only to halfway along the neck of the femur (**20.3**). Thus, at the back, part of the neck is inside the capsule (*intracapsular*) and part is outside (*extracapsular*).

The outside of the capsule is reinforced by ligaments. The most important is the **iliofemoral ligament**, which blends with the front of the capsule (**20.5b**). It is in the shape of an inverted 'Y' or 'V', passing from the anterior inferior iliac spine to each end of the intertrochanteric line. It is one of the strongest ligaments in the body, and is important because, when standing in the normal upright position, the body's centre of gravity lies just behind the hip joint so that there is a constant tendency for the trunk to fall backwards; the iliofemoral ligament helps to prevent this.

The ligaments inside the capsule (the acetabular labrum, the transverse ligament, and the ligament of the head of the femur) have already been mentioned (see above).

MOVEMENTS

Movements of the hip joint are in some respects similar to those of the shoulder joint, but are more limited in range because of the tight fit between the head of the femur and acetabulum, and also because the hip bone (pelvic girdle) is virtually immobile, being firmly fixed to the sacrum at the sacroiliac joint and to the opposite hip bone at the pubic symphysis (see **4.1a**). *Flexion* and *extension* (bending forwards and backwards) and *abduction* and *adduction* (moving sideways outwards and inwards) are relatively easy movements to understand, but *medial* and *lateral rotation* of the femur at the hip requires some explanation (see below).

With the knee bent (flexed), the hip can be flexed to bring the thigh almost into contact with the anterior abdominal wall, but when the knee is straight the amount of flexion is limited because of tension in the hamstrings at the back of the thigh (p.318 and **6.2**) (though, with training, as in the athlete's or dancer's high kick, the hamstrings can be stretched). The main *flexors* of the hip are psoas major, iliacus and rectus femoris (**6.1**). *Extension* is usually limited to about 20° by tension in the iliofemoral ligament and the flexor

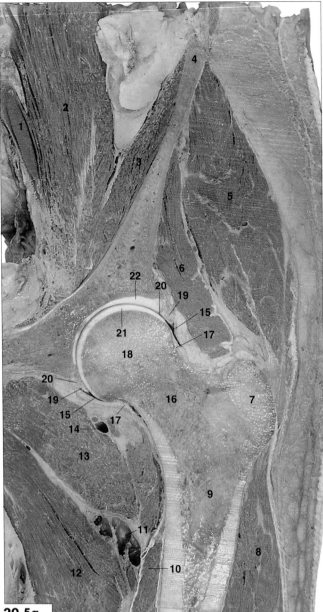

20.5a

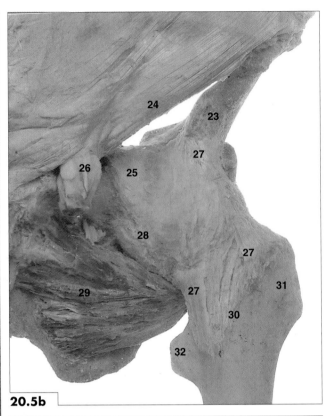

20.5b

Fig. 20.5 Left hip joint.
(a) Coronal section, looking from the front towards the back.
(b) Joint capsule, from the front, with all surrounding muscles removed except for obturator externus.

1 External iliac artery, which continues into the front of the thigh to become the femoral artery
2 Psoas major, whose tendon passes down in front of the hip joint and then curves backwards to reach the lesser trochanter on the back of the femur
3 Iliacus
4 Iliac crest
5 Gluteus medius
6 Gluteus minimus, converging on to the greater trochanter (7) with gluteus medius (5). During walking, contraction of these two muscles prevents the pelvis from tilting to the opposite side when the opposite leg is off the ground
7 Greater trochanter
8 Vastus lateralis
9 Shaft of femur
10 Vastus medialis
11 Profunda femoris vessels

12 Adductor longus
13 Pectineus
14 Medial circumflex femoral vessels
15 Capsule of hip joint, the thickest of all joint capsules
16 Neck of femur
17 Zona orbicularis, circular fibres of the capsule, helping to keep the capsule close to the neck of the femur
18 Head of femur, forming the hip joint with the acetabulum of the hip bone
19 Acetabular labrum, fibrocartilage deepening the socket of the acetabulum
20 Rim of acetabulum
21 Hyaline cartilage of head
22 Hyaline cartilage of acetabulum
23 Anterior inferior iliac spine
24 Inguinal ligament
25 Iliopubic eminence
26 Spermatic cord
27 Iliofemoral ligament, like an inverted V, reinforcing and blending with the front of the capsule
28 Pubofemoral ligament, reinforcing and blending with the more medial part of the capsule
29 Obturator externus
30 Intertrochanteric line
31 Greater trochanter
32 Lesser trochanter

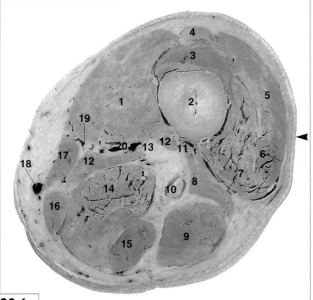

20.6

Fig. 20.6 Cross section of the left lower thigh, looking upwards from the knee to the hip.
The arrow indicates the site for intramuscular injection.

1 Vastus medialis
2 Femur
3 Vastus intermedius, wrapping round much of the femur (2) and blending with vastus lateralis (5)
4 Rectus femoris
5 Vastus lateralis, with the arrow indicating the site for intramuscular injection, well away from major vessels and nerves (10, 11 and 20)
6 Iliotibial tract of fascia lata
7 Lateral intermuscular septum
8 Short head of biceps
9 Long head of biceps, the hamstring passing down the back of the lateral side of the thigh
10 Sciatic nerve, deeply placed under cover of the hamstrings (9, 14 and 15)
11 Profunda femoris vessels, adjacent to the back of the femur
12 Adductor magnus
13 Opening in adductor magnus, through which at a slightly lower level the femoral vessels pass backwards to become the popliteal vessels
14 Semimembranosus
15 Semitendinosus, with semimembranosus (14), the hamstrings passing down the medial side of the back of the thigh
16 Gracilis, the most medial muscle of the thigh
17 Sartorius
18 Great saphenous vein
19 Saphenous nerve, the large cutaneous branch of the femoral nerve that will reach the medial side of the foot
20 Femoral vessels, just before passing through the opening in adductor magnus (13)

muscles, and is brought about by the hamstrings and gluteus maximus (**6.2**). In the small amount of extension involved in walking, it is the hamstrings which are responsible, and there is very little activity in gluteus maximus. It is only in the more extreme range of extension that gluteus maximus comes into play (as in running, for example), or when extending from the flexed position (as in rising from the sitting position or walking upstairs).

Crossing one leg over the other when sitting down is an everyday example of *adduction of the hip*, and is carried out by the adductor group of muscles. In *abduction* the limbs are 'opened wide' by gluteus medius and minimus, but these muscles are actually far more important in **preventing adduction** rather than in abducting, because this is how they act in walking: when say the right leg is off the ground, the left gluteus medius and minimus contract to prevent the pelvis tilting down to the right.

To understand *medial* and *lateral rotation* of the femur at the hip (**1.2e**), it is necessary to remember that the neck and shaft of the femur lie at an angle to one another (of about 120°), and that the axis about which rotation movements take place is **not** along the line of the **shaft** of the femur but along a line drawn from the **head** of the femur to the lower end of the bone **between the condyles**. In the normal position, the greater trochanter (which is at the upper end of the shaft) is thus situated well lateral to the axis, and it is the way the greater trochanter moves that must be considered. The head, neck and greater trochanter are often described as resembling a gate, with the hinged end of the gate corresponding to the head of the femur and the opening end of the gate corresponding to the greater trochanter. When the trochanter moves **forwards** (like the gate opening forwards), the femur rotates **medially**, and when the trochanter moves **backwards** (like the gate opening backwards) the femur rotates **laterally**.

Although it was formerly believed that psoas major and iliacus were medial rotators of the hip joint (because of the way they passed across the front of the joint to become attached to the lesser trochanter which is on the back of the femur, so pulling the lesser trochanter forwards), electromyographic studies do not support this concept; *medial rotation* is produced by the anterior fibres of gluteus medius and minimus. This can only be understood if it is remembered that in the normal anatomical position the pelvis is tilted well forwards, with these anterior fibres arising from the hip bone at a level in front of their attachment to the greater trochanter. The *lateral rotators* are the small muscles at the back of the joint such as piriformis, obturator internus and quadratus femoris (p.319 and **20.4a**); gluteus maximus can also assist.

INJURIES

Fracture of the *neck of the femur* is a common injury in the elderly, when a seemingly trivial accident such as tripping over the edge of a carpet can lead to a fall which breaks the bone. The patient is typically seen lying on the back with the affected limb *laterally rotated* (with the foot turned well out); this is because psoas and iliacus have rotated the shaft of the femur laterally since, with its neck broken, the normal axis of rotation is altered and the femur is free to rotate in the long axis of the shaft (like a humerus, p.217). Bed rest with the limb held in traction may be sufficient to keep the bone ends in position while healing occurs, but often some kind of metal pin passing through the greater trochanter and neck into the head may have to be used to keep the head in a proper alignment.

A fractured neck of femur may seriously interfere with the blood supply of the femoral head, since small arteries reach it by running along the surface of the neck within the joint, under cover of the synovial membrane. Usually new vessels grow in across the fracture line to link up with the old ones in the head, but if sufficient blood supply is not restored, bone death will occur (*ischaemic necrosis*) and the head will have to be removed and replaced by an artificial one.

The hip joint is one of the common sites for arthritic disease (whether *rheumatoid arthritis* or *osteoarthritis*), leading to varying degrees of pain and limitation of movement. Total hip replacement with an artifical acetabulum and head of femur may become necessary.

KNEE AND POPLITEAL FOSSA

In the region of the **knee** (**20.7** and **20.11**) much of the lower end of the **femur** and upper end of the **tibia**, the **patella** and the upper end of the **fibula** are all readily palpable. The fibula here makes a small synovial joint with the outer side of the tibia – the **superior tibiofibular joint** – but it is of little importance compared with the knee joint, from which it is quite separate. The area at the back of the knee is the **popliteal fossa**, containing the popliteal vessels and the sciatic nerve dividing into the tibial and common peroneal nerves.

KNEE JOINT

The **knee joint** (**20.7–20.9**) is the synovial joint between the two **condyles of the femur** and the two **condyles of the tibia**. The **patella** also participates in the knee joint, since it articulates with the femoral condyles (but not with the tibia). A **capsule** lined by synovial membrane covers all aspects of the joint except at the front, where its place is taken by the patella and the patellar ligament (see below). Although at first sight the joint may appear to be involved only in simple hinge movements, it is geometrically and mechanically an extremely complex structure, which makes the design and function of artificial knee joints more difficult than those for the hip.

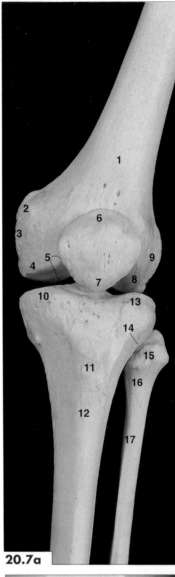

20.7a

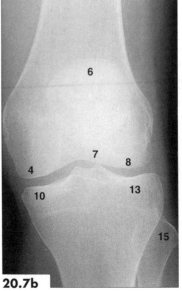

20.7b

Fig. 20.7 Left knee, from the front.
(a) Femur, patella, tibia and fibula
(b) Radiograph

1 Shaft of femur
2 Adductor tubercle, for the adductor magnus tendon which is palpable just above the bone on the medial side of the knee
3 Medial epicondyle, the most prominent medial part of the bone
4 Medial condyle, with the lower surface cartilage–covered
5 Knee joint
6 Base of patella
7 Apex of patella, for the patellar ligament
8 Lateral condyle, with the lower surface cartilage–covered
9 Lateral epicondyle, the most prominent lateral part of the bone
10 Medial condyle of tibia, with the upper surface cartilage–covered
11 Tuberosity of tibia
12 Shaft of tibia
13 Lateral condyle, with the upper surface cartilage–covered
14 Superior tibiofibular joint, separate from the knee joint
15 Head of fibula
16 Neck, against whose lateral side the common peroneal nerve can be palpated
17 Shaft

Ligaments

The main factors holding the femur and tibia together are the **anterior** and **posterior cruciate ligaments** inside the joint and the **medial** and **lateral ligaments** outside the capsule.

The **cruciate ligaments** (**20.8b** and **20.9b**) are strong bands which, when viewed from the side, cross each other in the shape of an 'X' (hence their name), passing from the inside surfaces of the femoral condyles to the central intercondylar area on the upper surface of the tibia; they are named **anterior** and **posterior** from their tibial attachments. Synovial membrane covers the side and front of the cruciate ligaments but not the back of them (as though they had been pushed into the 'synovial balloon' from behind). In the common type of knee joint dislocation, as in a motor vehicle accident, where, with the knee flexed to a right angle, the tibia is forced backwards, the posterior cruciate ligament is torn.

The **medial ligament** (**20.8b** and **20.9b**), properly called the **tibial collateral ligament**, is a broad flat band about 12 cm long running from the medial epicondyle of the femur to the upper part of the medial surface of the tibia. The **lateral ligament** (**20.8a** and **20.9b**), properly called the **fibular collateral ligament**, is a rounded structure like a short, very thin pencil about 5 cm long, passing from the lateral epicondyle of the femur to the apex of the head of the fibula.

Lying on the top of the articular surfaces on the tibia are the **medial** and **lateral menisci** (formerly known as the **semilunar cartilages** and still commonly called the 'cartilages of the knee', **20.9c**). They are approximately 'C'-shaped, and are composed of fibrocartilage which is thick at the periphery and very thin towards the centre. They are not covered by synovial membrane. The ends or prongs of the 'C' are the **horns** of the menisci and attach them to the intercondylar

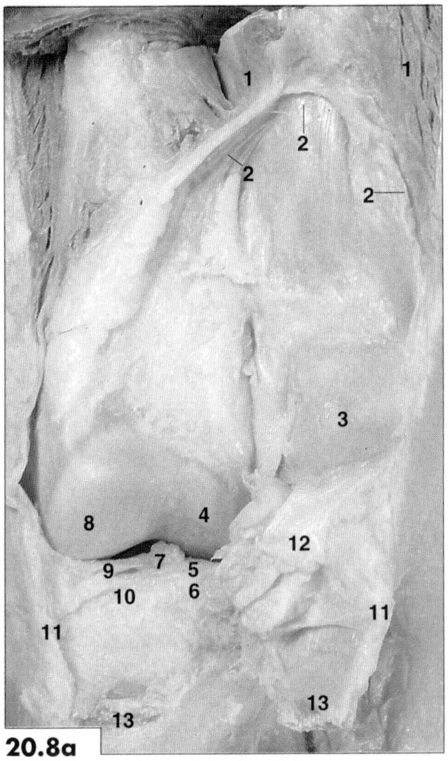

20.8a

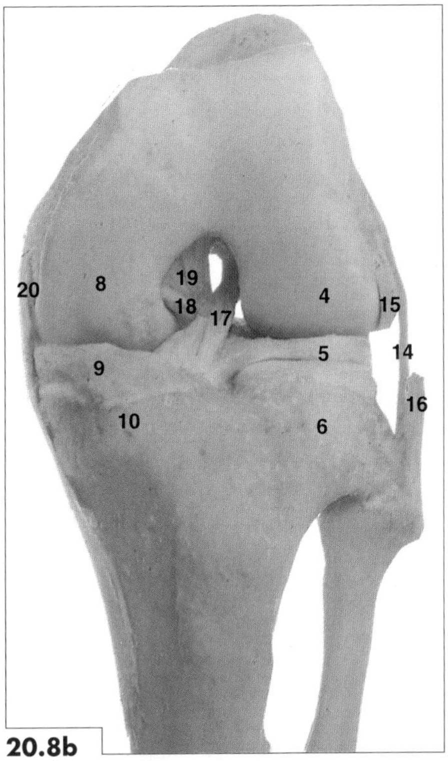

20.8b

Fig. 20.8 Left knee joint.
(a) Opened up from the front by cutting the quadriceps muscle and patellar tendon and turning the flap outwards, preserving the margin of the suprapatellar bursa.
(b) Ligaments, from the front. Compare with the back view in **20.9b** where more details of the ligaments are given.

1 Quadriceps muscle
2 Margin of suprapatellar bursa, which is always in continuity with the knee joint cavity and extends for about 5 cm above the patella
3 Posterior surface of patella
4 Lateral condyle of femur
5 Lateral meniscus
6 Lateral condyle of tibia
7 Cut end of mucosal ligament, the attachment of the infrapatellar fat pad to the intercondylar area of the femur
8 Medial condyle of femur
9 Medial meniscus
10 Medial condyle of tibia
11 Capsule
12 Synovial membrane covering infrapatellar fat pad, which when in place obliterates the space in front of the condyles
13 Patellar ligament
14 Lateral ligament
15 Popliteus tendon, passing backwards
16 Biceps tendon, attached to the head of the fibula
17 Anterior cruciate ligament
18 Anterior meniscofemoral ligament
19 Posterior cruciate ligament
20 Medial ligament

area of the tibia near the cruciate ligaments. The medial meniscus is also firmly attached to the medial ligament (**20.9b**), but the lateral meniscus is *not* attached to the lateral ligament (although it does have an attachment to the tendon of popliteus – see below). They fill up space between the curved femoral condyles and the flat articular surfaces of the

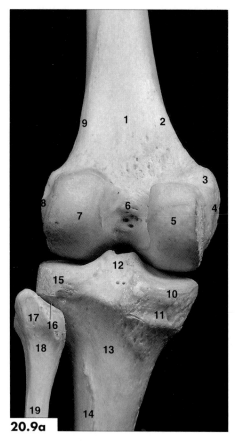

20.9a

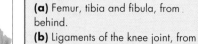

20.9c

> **Fig. 20.9 Left knee.**
> **(a)** Femur, tibia and fibula, from behind.
> **(b)** Ligaments of the knee joint, from behind, after removal of the capsule.
> **(c)** Ligaments of the knee joint attached to the upper end of the tibia, looking down on the tibia from above, after removal of the capsule and the femur.

20.9b

1 Popliteal surface of femur
2 Medial supracondylar line
3 Adductor tubercle, for attachment of the tendon of adductor magnus
4 Medial epicondyle, for attachment of the medial ligament (20)
5 Medial condyle
6 Intercondylar fossa, the gap between the condyles (5 and 7)
7 Lateral condyle
8 Lateral epicondyle, for attachment of the lateral ligament (26)
9 Lateral supracondylar line
10 Medial condyle of tibia
11 Groove for semimembranosus insertion
12 Intercondylar area, for attachments of cruciate ligaments and menisci (c), and intercondylar eminence with tubercles
13 Posterior surface, for attachment of popliteus
14 Soleal line on shaft, for attachment of part of soleus
15 Lateral condyle
16 Superior tibiofibular joint (with capsule in (b), a small synovial joint which is quite separate from the knee joint
17 Head of fibula, for attachment of the lateral ligament (26) and the tendon of biceps (28)
18 Neck
19 Shaft
20 Medial ligament, with attachment to medial meniscus (21)

21 Medial meniscus
22 Posterior cruciate ligament, passing forwards and medially to the lateral side of the medial condyle (5)
23 Posterior meniscofemoral ligament, passing from the lateral meniscus (25) behind the posterior cruciate ligament (22) to the medial condyle of the femur (5)
24 Anterior cruciate ligament, passing upwards and laterally to the medial side of the lateral condyle (7)
25 Lateral meniscus, which is not attached to the lateral ligament (26), with marker under its thin inner margin in (c)
26 Lateral ligament, passing from the lateral epicondyle of the femur (8) to the head of the fibula (17)
27 Popliteus tendon, whose muscle fibres are attached to the posterior surface of the tibia (13) above the soleal line (14)
28 Biceps tendon
29 Anterior meniscofemoral ligament, passing from the lateral meniscus (25) in front of the posterior cruciate ligament (22) to the medial condyle of the femur (5)
30 Attachment of popliteus tendon to lateral meniscus (25), important for pulling the meniscus backwards and preventing it getting trapped between tibia and femur when flexing the knee

tibia, and help to spread synovial fluid over the moving bones. They act as shock absorbers, bearing over half the weight transmitted across the joint.

The **patella** is a sesamoid bone (p.29) in the quadriceps tendon and is kept at a constant distance from the upper surface of the tibia by the **patellar ligament** which fixes it to the tuberosity of the tibia (**20.11** and **6.1a**). As the knee joint bends, the back of the patella slides over the femoral condyles but never comes into contact with the tibia.

A pad of fat (the **infrapatellar fat pad, 20.8a**) pushes the synovial membrane backwards below the patella to fill up the gap between the fronts of the condyles.

Movements

Flexion (bending) and *extension* (straightening) are obvious movements at the knee joint, with the curved condyles of the femur moving on the almost flat condyles of the tibia. The main flexors are the hamstrings (p.317), with assistance from gastrocnemius (p.332), sartorius and gracilis, while extension is produced by quadriceps femoris (p.315). What is not so obvious is that at the end of extension and the beginning of flexion there is a small amount of *rotation* of one bone on the other. When the knee is fully extended (straight), it is said to be in the 'locked' position. To visualize what happens when flexion begins, imagine that the tibia is fixed (with the foot on the ground). Before flexion can begin, the joint has to be 'unlocked' by **popliteus** (p.332) which, acting from its attachment to the back of the tibia (**6.2b**), causes the femur to rotate laterally on the tibia by pulling the lateral condyle backwards. Popliteus is also attached to the back of the lateral meniscus and pulls it back slightly, so actively making space for the femoral condyle to move backwards. After this unlocking, the hamstrings can now carry on with flexion. Similarly when the flexed knee is being extended (again imagining the tibia to be fixed), the femur rotates medially on the tibia at the very end of extension. This rotation occurs because of the geometry of the joint surfaces and the way the cruciate and collateral ligaments are attached to the two bones. If the femur is the fixed bone, it is the tibia which rotates.

The bulge at the upper, inner side of the patella is due to the *lowest* fibres of **vastus medialis** overlying the lower end of the femur (**6.1a**). These fibres are particularly important, not only in helping to keep the patella in its normal position on the front of the femur but also because they are *essential* for obtaining *complete extension* of the knee joint. If these fibres become wasted, e.g. from paralysis or, more commonly, by prolonged rest in bed with lack of normal activity, the knee cannot be fully extended and the patient feels 'weak at the knees' when trying to walk again – the typical feeling after any prolonged lack of use of the limbs. Even a few days in bed causes a measurable loss of bulk in the quadriceps muscle; this is why quadriceps exercises are so important in patients with lower limb injuries.

The locking and unlocking movements involving slight rotation of one bone upon the other when the leg is nearly straight must be distinguished from the rotations occurring when the knee is flexed and which depend on the action of different muscles. Assuming, for example, that the knee is flexed to a right angle and the femur is fixed, biceps on the outer side can laterally rotate the tibia on the femur, and semitendinosus and semimembranosus on the inner side can medially rotate it. With the tibia fixed, the femur rotates on the tibia.

Injuries

Any knee joint damage can result in an excessive *effusion* of fluid into the synovial cavity – 'water on the knee'. The amount of synovial fluid in a normal knee joint (the largest synovial joint in the body) is less than 0.5 ml – merely a capillary film to lubricate the moving surfaces – but injury can stimulate the accumulation of 100 ml or more. A large bursa above the patella under the quadriceps tendon (**suprapatellar bursa, 20.8a**) always communicates with the synovial cavity, so that any effusion spreads into the bursa and helps to alter the normal contours on either side of the patella. Fluid can be removed from the joint through a needle inserted at the upper outer border of the patella.

Sudden twisting movements of the knee may trap the *menisci* between tibia and femur and cause them to be *torn*; this is a common injury in footballers. The medial meniscus is damaged twenty times more commonly than the lateral, because the medial is anchored by its attachment to the medial ligament; the lateral meniscus is more mobile and so 'gets out of the way', since it is not attached to the lateral ligament and can be pulled back slightly because of its attachment to the tendon of popliteus. A damaged meniscus can be wholly or partly removed surgically, without any resulting disability.

Direct trauma may *fracture* the condyles of the tibia more often than those of the femur. A fractured patella may be difficult to heal because of the strong pull of the quadriceps muscle. The bone fragments may have to be wired together, but sometimes the whole bone has to be removed, with remarkably little resulting disability.

The knee joint is among the commonest to be affected by *arthritic changes*, leading to pain and diminished movement.

BICEPS TENDON

The **tendon of biceps** (**20.11**) is easily felt (especially with the knee bent) running down on the outer side of the thigh behind the knee, to be inserted into the head of the fibula. 'Pulling' the biceps tendon is a common athletic injury; some of the tendon fibres themselves may be torn or they may be detached from the bone, in both cases with accompanying pain and tenderness.

COMMON PERONEAL AND TIBIAL NERVES

The **common peroneal nerve**, the only palpable major nerve of the lower limb, is one of the two major divisions of the sciatic nerve at the top of the popliteal fossa (**20.10a**). It runs downwards and laterally, behind the tendon of biceps, and turns forwards round the neck of the fibula where it is subcutaneous and can be rolled against the bone (**20.11** and **7.3a**). This exposed position renders it liable not only to accidental injury but to pressure from plaster casts applied to the limb for treating fractures. Casts must be carefully padded to prevent nerve injury. Damage to the nerve here causes 'drop foot', due to paralysis of the extensor (dorsiflexor) muscles of the foot (p.338), and anaesthesia over the lateral side of the leg and dorsum of the foot.

The **tibial nerve** is the most superficial of the large structures in the popliteal fossa. It appears to be the direct continuation of the sciatic nerve, running straight down the middle of the fossa (**20.10a**) to enter the posterior compartment of the leg (p.332).

POPLITEAL ARTERY

The **popliteal artery** is the deepest of the large neurovascular structures in the fossa (**20.10a**). Its companion vein lies between the artery and the tibial nerve. Although a large vessel, the *popliteal pulse* is rather difficult to feel; it is best palpated (**20.10b**) with the knee slightly flexed, using the fingertips of both hands which are pressed forwards into the fossa, with the thumbs on either side of the patella.

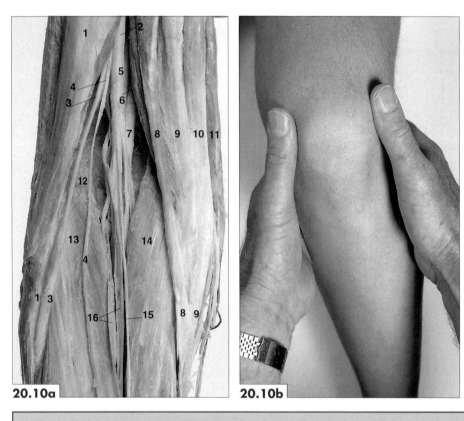

20.10a

20.10b

Fig. 20.10 Right popliteal fossa and popliteal pulse.
(**a**) Dissection of the popliteal fossa, after removal of deep fascia and fat.
(**b**) Palpation of the popliteal pulse. Because the popliteal artery is the deepest structure in the fossa, it is best felt from the front by pressing the fingertips of both hands into the middle of the fossa at the back.

1 Biceps, forming the upper lateral boundary of the fossa
2 Sciatic nerve, dividing at the top of the fossa into the tibial and common peroneal nerves (5 and 3)
3 Common peroneal nerve, branching from the sciatic nerve (2) to run down along the posterior border of biceps (1) to reach the lateral side of the neck of the fibula where it divides into the superficial and deep peroneal nerves
4 Lateral cutaneous nerve of calf, from the common peroneal nerve (3)
5 Tibial nerve, the continuation of the sciatic nerve (2) and the most superficial of the neurovascular structures in the fossa
6 Popliteal vein, deep to the tibial nerve (5)
7 Popliteal artery, deep to the vein (6) and the deepest of the neurovascular structures in the fossa
8 Semitendinosus. Do not confuse the long tendon of this muscle

on the medial side of the fossa with the common peroneal nerve (3) on the lateral side
9 Semimembranosus, with the overlying semitendinosus (8) forming the upper medial boundary of the fossa
10 Gracilis
11 Sartorius
12 Plantaris, forming with the lateral head of gastrocnemius (13) the lower lateral boundary of the fossa
13 Lateral head of gastrocnemius
14 Medial head of gastrocnemius, forming the lower medial boundary of the fossa
15 Sural nerve, a cutaneous branch of the tibial nerve (5)
16 Small saphenous vein (here double), accompanying the sural nerve (15) on the back of the calf and joining the popliteal vein (6)

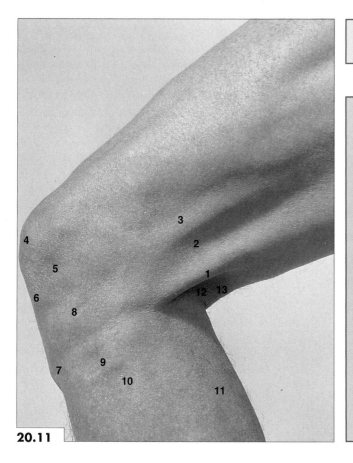

20.11

1 Biceps tendon, at the lateral boundary of the popliteal fossa
   and passing to the head of the fibula (9)
2 Furrow between biceps (1) and iliotibial tract (3), due to
   attachment of the lateral intermuscular septum to the fascia
   lata
3 Iliotibial tract, the thickened band of the fascia lata passing
   down to be attached to the front of the tibia below the lateral
   condyle (8)
4 Patella
5 Lateral condyle of femur
6 Patellar ligament, attaching the apex of the patella to the
   tibial tuberosity (7)
7 Tuberosity of tibia
8 Lateral condyle of tibia
9 Head of fibula
10 Common peroneal nerve, easily felt as it crosses the neck of
   the fibula, and because of its superficial position the nerve
   most commonly injured in the lower limb
11 Lateral head of gastrocnemius
12 Popliteal fossa
13 Semitendinosus and semimembranosus, at the medial
   boundary of the popliteal fossa

LEG

The word **leg** is used by anatomists to denote only the portion of the lower limb between the knee and the ankle – not the entire limb, as in common parlance.

BONES

The **bones** of the leg are the **tibia** (the shin bone) and the **fibula**, on the outer side of the tibia (**4.1**). The rather sharp anterior border of the tibia is the part struck when 'barking the shins'. The flat **medial surface of the tibia** is **subcutaneous** (**20.16b**) and is easily felt throughout its length, right down to the medial malleolus. The subcutaneous position of so much of this bone means that *fractures* of it are liable to break the skin, so converting what might have been a 'closed' fracture (with intact skin) into an 'open' one which is more liable to infection and other complications. It is commonly believed that fractures of the lower third of the tibia often heal poorly because the bone here has a poor blood supply, being surrounded by skin and tendons rather than by muscle attachments which are a good source of blood for bone.

The long thin **fibula** can be broken by direct violence to the outer side of the leg, but its upper or lower thirds can also be fractured by injuries of the ankle joint (p.336).

The tibia and fibula are joined over much of their length by the **interosseous membrane** (**20.16b**) which divides the muscles of the leg into two main compartments – an **anterior** or **extensor compartment** and a **posterior** or **flexor compartment**. A smaller compartment on the outer side of the fibula is the **peroneal compartment**.

MUSCLES OF THE ANTERIOR COMPARTMENT

The largest muscle of the anterior compartment (see **6.1**) is **tibialis anterior**, which forms most of the bulge in the upper part of the leg on the outer side of the sharp anterior border of the tibia. Lateral to this muscle are **extensor hallucis longus, extensor digitorum longus** and **peroneus tertius**. The tendons of all these muscles cross in front of the ankle joint to enter the foot (**20.13a**) where they act as extensors (dorsiflexors) of the ankle and foot (p.338).

The **nerve supply** of this group of muscles is from the **deep peroneal nerve** (from the common peroneal branch of the sciatic, **7.3a**), and the main **artery** is the **anterior tibial** (from the popliteal artery, **8.3**). Narrowing of this vessel by

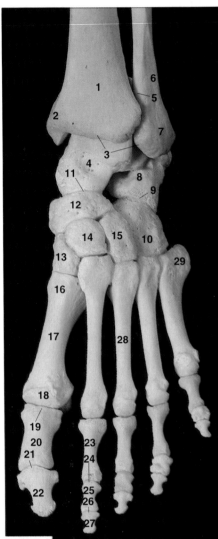

20.12a

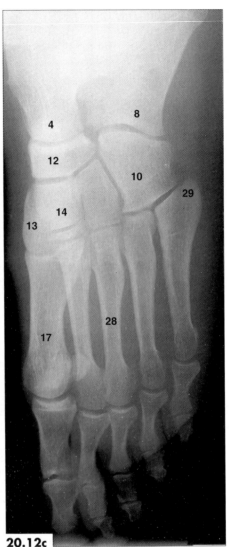

20.12c

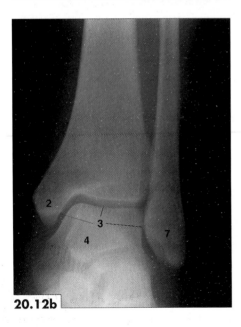

20.12b

Fig. 20.12 Bones of the left ankle and foot.
(a) From above and in front
(b) Radiograph, from the front
(c) Radiograph, from above

1 Lower end of tibia
2 Medial malleolus of tibia
3 Ankle joint, between the tibia, fibula and talus
4 Talus
5 Inferior tibiofibular joint, a fibrous joint, not synovial, and separate from the ankle joint
6 Subcutaneous surface of fibula
7 Lateral malleolus of fibula
8 Calcaneus, the largest tarsal bone forming the heel at the back
9 Calcaneocuboid joint
10 Cuboid bone
11 Talonavicular joint, forming with the calcaneocuboid joint (9) the midtarsal joint
12 Naviocular bone

13 Medial ⎫
14 Intermediate ⎬ cuneiform bone
15 Lateral ⎭
16 Base ⎫
17 Shaft ⎬ of first metatarsal bone
18 Head ⎭
19 Metatarsosphalangeal (MP) joint of great toe
20 Proximal phalanx
21 Interphalangeal (IP) joint
22 Distal phalanx
23 Proximal phalanx of second toe
24 Proximal interphalangeal (IP) joint
25 Middle phalanx
26 Distal interphalangeal (IP) joint
27 Distal phalanx
28 Third metatarsal bone
29 Tuberosity of base of fifth metatarsal bone

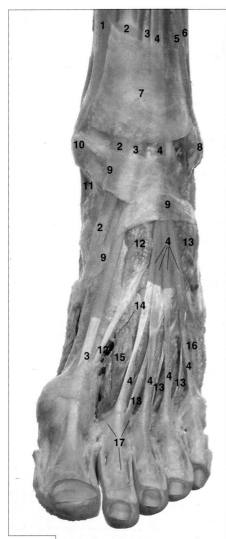

20.13a

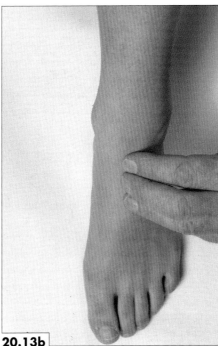

20.13b

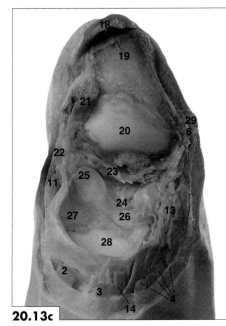

20.13c

Fig. 20.13 Left leg and foot.
(a) Superficial dissection of the lower leg and foot, from the front, with synovial sheaths emphasized by blue tissue.
(b) Palpation of the dorsalis pedis pulse, on a line from midway between the malleoli towards the first toe cleft.
(c) Joints beneath the talus, looking down on the foot from above after removal of the talus.

1 Lower end of tibia
2 Tibialis anterior
3 Extensor hallucis longus, for the great toe
4 Extensor digitorum longus, for the other four toes
5 Subcutaneous surface of fibula
6 Peroneus brevis
7 Superior extensor retinaculum, a broad transverse band
8 Lateral malleolus
9 Inferior extensor retinaculum, a Y-shaped band
10 Medial malleolus
11 Tibialis posterior
12 Extensor hallucis brevis, the part of extensor digitorum brevis (13) going to the big toe
13 Extensor digitorum brevis, for the second, third and fourth toes (but not the little toe)
14 Dorsalis pedis artery, labelled in **(a)** where its pulse is palpated **(b)** lateral to the tendon of extensor hallucis longus (3)
15 First dorsal interosseus
16 Peroneus tertius
17 Extensor expansion of the second toe
18 Tendo calcaneus (Achilles' tendon)
19 Bursa deep to Achilles" tendon (18)
20 Posterior articular surface of calcaneus, for the talocalcanean joint

21 Flexor hallucis longus
22 Flexor digitorum longus
23 Interosseous talocalcanean ligament, passing between the grooves on the upper surface of the calcaneus and lower surface of the talus
24 Cervical ligament, passing between the calcaneus and the neck of the talus
25 Middle } articular surface of
             } calcaneus, for the
             } talocalcanean part of the
             } talocalcaneonavicular
26 Anterior } joint
27 Cartilageon upper surface of spring ligament, supporting part of the head of the talus
28 Posterior articular surface of navicular bone, for the talonavicular part of the talocalcaneonavicular joint
29 Peroneus longus

arterial disease (e.g. *arteriosclerosis*) may lead to pain in these anterior compartment muscles with exercise (*intermittent claudication*); the patient may have to stop walking for a while until the pain wears off before being able to continue. Athletes, especially long distance runners, may get a different kind of pain in these muscles (*anterior tibial syndrome*), due to tension in the anterior compartment from the increased blood supply; the deep fascia forms a tough and inextensible 'stocking' round the limb and cannot expand to allow for the increased bulk of fluid.

MUSCLES OF THE POSTERIOR COMPARTMENT

The muscles of the posterior compartment (the **calf**) are **gastrocnemius** and **soleus** (which form the subcutaneous calf muscles, 6.2), with, at a deeper level, **tibialis posterior**, **flexor hallucis longus** and **flexor digitorum longus**. In muscular individuals, the two parts of gastrocnemius are easily seen under the skin of the calf; the medial head of the muscle extends to a slightly lower level than the lateral head. All the tendons pass behind the ankle joint into the foot to act as plantarflexors (**20.15b** and **20.16c**, p.338); the tendons of gastrocnemius and soleus unite to form the large **Achilles' tendon** (**tendo calcaneus**, **20.16a**) at the back of the ankle. Note that the two heads of gastrocnemius come from the lower end of the femur (**6.2a**), so the muscle can help to flex the knee, but that soleus has a lower origin, from the back of the tibia and fibula, and so cannot act on the knee joint.

There is one other deep muscle in the upper part of the calf – **popliteus** (**6.2b**), which has already been mentioned as the muscle that 'unlocks' the knee joint at the beginning of flexion (p.327). Rather triangular in shape, it passes up from the back of the upper tibia to the outer side of the knee, where its tendon enters the knee joint within a sleeve of synovial membrane and becomes attached to the femur just below the lateral epicondyle.

The muscles are all supplied by the **tibial nerve** (from the sciatic, **20.10a** and **7.3b**), and the **arteries** of this compartment are the **posterior tibial** (from the popliteal), which runs down behind the tibia, and its **peroneal branch** which runs down behind the fibula (**20.16b** and **8.3a**). The *pulsation* of the **posterior tibial artery** can be felt behind the medial malleolus and 2.5 cm (1 inch) in front of the medial border of the Achilles' tendon (**20.15c**)

Soleus and Gastrocnemius

Soleus (see **6.2a**) is particularly important as a *postural* muscle, helping to keep the body upright when standing. In the upright position, the centre of gravity of the body is slightly in front of the axis of movement of the knee joint, so there is a constant tendency for the body to tilt forwards at the ankle. Soleus counteracts this by intermittent bursts of activity in varying groups of its fibres (so that the same fibres are not used all of the time). Because of the repeated

contractile activity required, many of its muscle fibres are of the 'slow-twitch' variety which is less subject to fatigue than the commoner 'fast-twitch' type. **Gastrocnemius**, by contrast, contains a preponderance of 'fast-twitch' fibres because it is used in more *active* plantarflexion movements of the ankle, such as lifting the heel off the ground in walking and running.

Soleus has further importance because, within and around it and its neighbouring muscles are many **dilated venous channels** which drain into the veins accompanying the main arteries (**20.16b**). In patients who are lying in bed, especially if prolonged pressure on the calves is allowed, *deep venous thrombosis* (*DVT*, or *thrombophlebitis*; p.63) may occur due to sluggish venous circulation, especially after operations. Fragments of the clot (*emboli*) may pass from the leg into the inferior vena cava and thence, via the heart and the pulmonary artery, to the lungs – here they may lodge as *pulmonary emboli*. If large, such emboli can cause sudden death. Although DVT may be accompanied by pain and tenderness in the calf, it must be remembered that it can also occur without any symptoms and the first indication of its presence may be a pulmonary embolus. *Prevention* is therefore of the utmost importance. The period up to about 10 days after any operation is the most dangerous time for thrombus formation, hence the need wherever possible to get patients up out of bed quickly and restore good circulation by walking (not just getting up to sit in a chair). If early ambulation is not possible, leg exercises must be carried out in bed. Antithrombotic agents such as heparin form the basis of DVT therapy, but thrombolytic therapy using streptokinase may be required. In those who are continually throwing off emboli it may be necessary to ligate the inferior vena cava (below the level of the renal veins, **19.31**) to prevent them reaching the heart. Blood from the lower part of the body must then reach the heart through the *superior* vena cava, by means of the many small anastomoses (in the skin and abdominal wall) between the territories drained by the two venae cavae (p.57).

MUSCLES OF THE PERONEAL COMPARTMENT

In the peroneal compartment of the outer side of the leg are the **peroneus longus** and **peroneus brevis** muscles (**20.16**). They are supplied by the **superficial peroneal** branch of the common peroneal nerve, and they act as *plantarflexors* and *evertors* of the foot (p.338).

GREAT SAPHENOUS VEIN

The largest superficial vein of the lower limb, the **long** or **great saphenous vein** (**8.4**), begins as the continuation of the medial marginal vein of the foot and lies immediately *in front* of the **medial malleolus** where it can be seen and felt (**20.15a**). From here, it runs upwards and slightly backwards over the lower medial part of the tibia and then over the side of soleus and gastrocnemius until, at the level of the knee joint, it lies a handsbreadth behind the medial border of the patella. (For its course in the thigh see p318.) The vein has a number of **valves** (up to 20 in its whole length) to prevent backflow down the leg. In the lower leg, the vein has no superficial tributaries but is joined some way below the knee by the **posterior arch vein**. This vessel communicates with deep veins by means of **perforating veins** which penetrate the deep fascia (**20.15a**); they lie immediately behind the tibia and their number is variable, but there is usually one just below and one just above the medial malleolus and another a few centimeters higher. The perforating veins have valves which ensure that blood flows *from superficial to deep*, so that when the calf muscles pump blood up the leg in the deep veins the pressure of blood in the superficial veins is reduced.

Varicose Veins

If the valves in the perforating veins and the great saphenous itself become *incompetent* (probably due to a congenital defect in vein structure) and allow backflow, pressure in the superficial veins increases and eventually leads to localized dilatations – *varicosities* or *varicose veins* (**20.15d**). The increased venous pressure in the skin and superficial tissues can lead to poor circulation and tissue breakdown from lack of adequate nutrition, so causing *venous (varicose) ulcers*.

Varicose veins are often symptomless, in which case there is no call for treatment, but they can lead to aching pain, especially with prolonged standing, and to cramplike pain at night. Suitably supportive stockings may relieve the symptoms but operation may be required; this includes 'stripping out' the great saphenous vein and ligating some of the perforating veins. Many of the small remaining venous channels will enlarge to compensate for the vessels removed.

FOOT

The **foot** is joined to the **leg** at the **ankle joint**. The word 'ankle' usually means the ankle joint, but it is also used to mean the lower part of the leg just above the foot – the part with the obvious bony prominences, the **medial malleolus of the tibia** and the **lateral malleolus of the fibula** (**4.1**). The lower ends of the tibia and fibula are bound together firmly by the **interosseous tibiofibular ligament**, constituting the (fibrous) **inferior tibiofibular joint**.

The **skin of the dorsum** (i.e. the upper surface) of the foot is thin, but that of the **sole** is thick, especially over the heel and at the base of the great toe (the ball of the foot). It is firmly bound to the underlying connective tissue and to the **plantar aponeurosis** (a sheet of tissue covering the muscles of the sole), forming multiple small pockets of fatty tissue (**20.18**) which are designed to withstand weightbearing and other frictional stresses on the sole.

As in the hand, the foot has its own **small muscles** (the intrinsic muscles of the foot), as well as long tendons extending into it from the leg. Many are illustrated in the dissections here but are not individually described further since they are generally less important than those of the hand.

BONES

The numerous **bones** of the foot (7 **tarsal bones**, 5 **metatarsal bones** and 14 **phalanges**) (**20.12**, **20.14a** and **20.14b**) are held together in such a way that rigidity is combined with elasticity, so enabling the foot to function effectively as a supporting, propulsive or shock-absorbing mechanism, as and when required. The bodyweight is normally borne by the **calcaneus** (the heel bone – the largest of the tarsal bones) at the back, and by the heads of the metatarsals at the front. The tarsal and metatarsal bones form

---

1 Medial malleolus of tibia
2 Ankle joint
3 Talus
4 Talocalcanean joint
5 Calcaneus, forming the heel
6 Sustentaculum tali, the shelf-like projection from the medial side of the calcaneus (5), supsporting part of the head of the talus (7)
7 Head of talus
8 Talocalcanean part ⎫ of talocalcaneo-
9 Talonavicular part ⎭ navicular joint
10 Navicular bone
11 Tuberosity of navicular bone, for attachment of tibialis posterior (in **c**)
12 Cuboid (on lateral side of foot)
13 Tuberosity of base of fifth metatarsal (on lateral side of foot)

14 Medial cuneiform, whose lower part adjacent to the first metatarsal bone (17) receives the tendon of tibialis anterior
15 Intermediate cuneiform
16 First tarsometatarsal (cuneometatarsal) joint
17 Base ⎫
18 Shaft ⎬ of first metatarsal bone
19 Head ⎭
20 First metatarsophalangeal (MP) joint
21 Sesamoid bones
22 Proximal phalanx
23 Interphalangeal (IP) joint of big toe
24 Distal phalanx
25 Shadow of lateral malleolus of fibula overlying tibia and talus
26 Tarsal sinus
27 Calcaneocuboid joint (on the lateral

side)
28 Medial ligament of ankle joint
29 Cut tendon of tibialis posterior
30 Long plantar ligament on the sole (item 22 in **20.19b**)
31 Talonavicular ligament
32 Lateral malleolus of fibula
33 Calcaneofibular ligament, in this view obscuring the posterior talofibular ligament
34 Anterior talofibular ligament
35 Lateral end of tarsal sinus, the gap between the grooves of the talus and calcaneus
36 Cervical ligament, passing from the calcaneus to the neck of the talus (and shown transected as 25 in **20.13**)

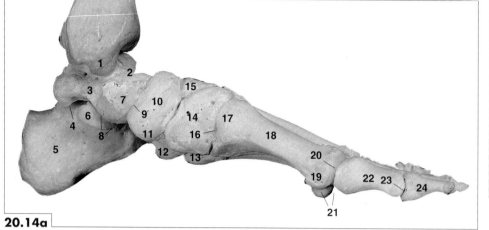

20.14a

Fig. 20.14 Bones and ligaments of the left ankle and foot.
(a) Lower end of tibia and the foot bones, from the medial side
(b) Medial ligament of the ankle joint and other features
(c) Radiograph, from the side.
(d) Lateral ligaments of the ankle joint
For key see p.333

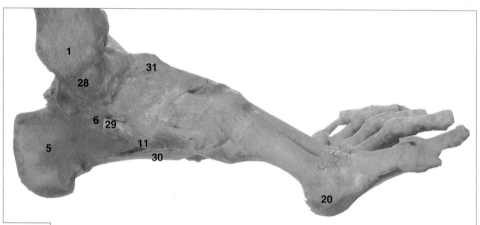

20.14b

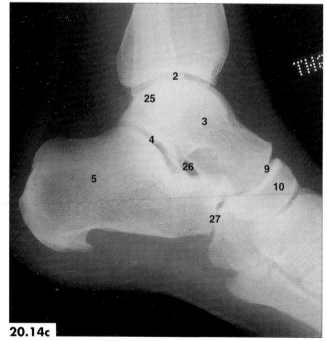

20.14c

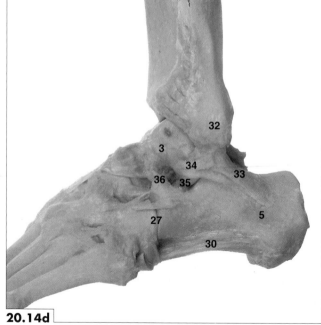

20.14d

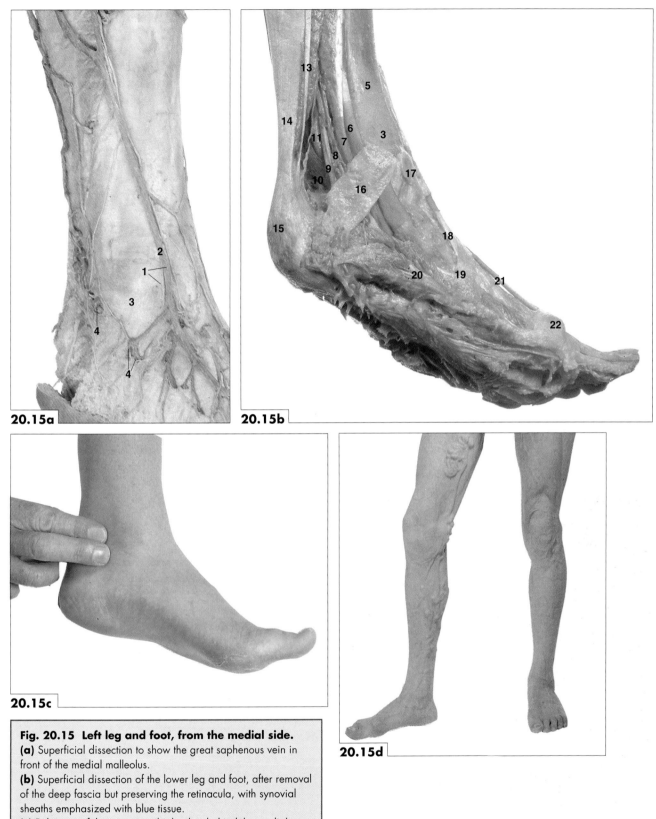

20.15a

20.15b

20.15c

20.15d

Fig. 20.15 Left leg and foot, from the medial side.
(a) Superficial dissection to show the great saphenous vein in front of the medial malleolus.
(b) Superficial dissection of the lower leg and foot, after removal of the deep fascia but preserving the retinacula, with synovial sheaths emphasized with blue tissue.
(c) Palpation of the posterior tibial pulse, behind the medial malleolus and 2.5 cm in front of the Achilles' tendon.
(d) Varicose veins of both legs, most prominent on the right.
For key see p.336

1 Branches of saphenous nerve
2 Great saphenous vein, passing upwards in front of the medial malleolus
3 Medial malleolus
4 Perforating veins, emerging from below the deep fascia
5 Subcutaneous (medial) surface of tibia
6 Tibialis posterior, the tendon adjacent to the medial malleolus (3)
7 Flexor digitorum longus, immediately behind tibialis posterior (6)
8 Posterior tibial artery and venae comitantes
9 Tibial nerve, behind the posterior tibial vessels (8) and about to divide into the medial and lateral plantar nerves
10 Flexor hallucis longus, whose tendon lies in a groove on the back of the talus
11 Medial calcanean branch of tibial nerve
12 Lowest fibres of soleus
13 Plantaris tendon
14 Tendo calcaneus (Achilles' tendon)
15 Posterior surface of calcaneus
16 Flexor retinaculum
17 Upper band of inferior extensor retinaculum (9 in **20.13a**)
18 Tibialis anterior
19 Lower band of inferior extensor retinaculum 9 in **20.13a**)
20 Abductor hallucis
21 Extensor hallucis longus
22 Tarsometatarsal joint of big toe

the longitudinal and transverse arches of the foot, as described on p.338.

TENDONS AT THE ANKLE

The **long tendons** of the leg muscles that pass over the ankle joint into the foot are kept in place by fascial thickenings (**retinacula**), which form compartments for vessels and nerves as well as tendons. It is important to identify the structures in their correct order; many of them can be seen and/or felt. Passing *in front* of the ankle joint from the medial to the lateral side (**20.13a**) are: tibialis anterior, extensor hallucis longus, anterior tibial vessels, the deep peroneal nerve, extensor digitorum longus and peroneus tertius. *Behind* the *medial* malleolus from front to back (**20.15b** and **20.16c**) are: tibialis posterior, flexor digitorum longus, posterior tibial vessels, the tibial nerve and flexor hallucis longus. *Behind* the *lateral* malleolus (**20.16a** and **20.16c**) are the tendons of peroneus brevis and peroneus longus. As they pass under their respective retinacula the tendons are each surrounded by their own **synovial sheaths** which help to prevent friction as the tendons move. As at the wrist, damage to tendon sheaths (e.g. from a kick on the ankle) may cause pain and swelling with limitation of movement (*tenosynovitis*).

The **Achilles' tendon** (**tendo calcaneus, 20.16a** andf **6.2**), the thickest tendon in the body, receives the muscle fibres of soleus and gastrocnemius, and is inserted into the middle (not the top) of the back surface of the calcaneus. A bursa separates it from the upper margin of the bone (**20.20**). The tendon, just above the bone, is the site for testing the *ankle jerk* (p.50 and **7.13d**). The tendon has to cope with varying degrees of tension, ranging from the small amount when soleus is acting as a postural muscle to help keep the body upright when standing, to the much greater stress involved when gastrocnemius and soleus are supporting the whole bodyweight, as in lifting the heel off the ground during walking, running and jumping. Despite its toughness, it can be torn right across, an inch or two above its insertion, giving a palpable gap. It is commonly a sports injury, giving rise to sudden pain with the patient feeling as though hit in the back of the leg; surgical repair is usually required.

ANKLE JOINT

The **ankle joint** is the joint between the **talus** (the uppermost bone of the foot) and the lower ends of the **tibia** and **fibula** (**20.14** and **4.1**). The two leg bones form a socket which fits the slightly curved upper surface of the talus and at the same time prevents the talus from slipping sideways (because of the downward projection of the two malleoli).

Ligaments

Apart from the **capsule**, the main ligaments of the ankle joint are those on the medial and lateral sides. The **medial ligament** (**20.14b**), running downwards from the medial malleolus to the calcaneus (including the sustentaculum tali) and navicular bone, is usually called the **deltoid ligament** because of its triangular shape (like a capital Greek letter delta: Δ), and is such a tough structure that, in ankle injuries, the medial malleolus can be broken off from the tibia (*Pott's fracture*) without tearing the ligament. On the *lateral* side (**20.14d**), instead of a single ligament, there are three small ones; two pass between the fibula and talus (the **anterior** and **posterior talofibular ligaments**) and the third runs downwards and backwards from the fibula to the calcaneus (the **calcaneofibular ligament**). In a 'sprained ankle' where the foot is forcibly turned inwards, these ligaments are stretched or torn (especially the anterior one) and there is pain and swelling in the surrounding tissues.

Movements

Since the talus is gripped between the two malleoli, the only movements possible at the ankle joint are *extension* and *flexion*. Extension is commonly called *dorsiflexion* because it involves moving the upper surface or dorsum of the foot upwards towards the front of the leg; flexion is often called *plantarflexion* because it involves movement of the sole or plantar surface of the foot in a downward direction. From the neutral or right-angle position of the foot in relation to

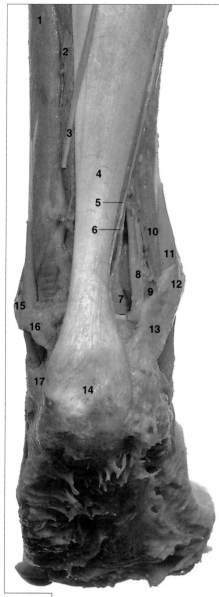

20.16a

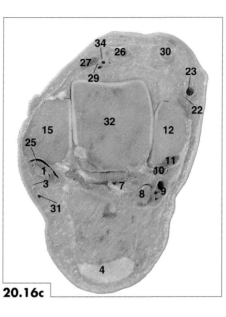

20.16c

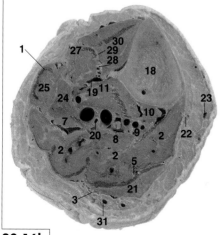

20.16b

Fig. 20.16 Left leg and foot.
(a) Dissection of the lower leg and foot, from behind, with synovial sheaths emphasized by blue tissue.
(b) Cross section of the middle of the leg, viewed from above looking towards the foot.
(c) Cross section of the ankle, viewed from above looking towards the heel.

1 Peroneus longus, with its tendon in a synovial sheath (with peroneus brevis) behind the lateral malleolus (15)
2 Soleus, showing within it and adjacent to it in (b) many large veins which can become the site of dangerous deep venous thrombosis, making (b) one of the most important pictures in the whole book
3 Sural nerve, in (a) cut short and with the adjacent small saphenous vein removed but shown (31) in (b) and (c)
4 Tendo calcaneus (Achilles' tendon)
5 Plantaris tendon, on the medial side of the tendo calcaneus (4) and in (b) between soleus (2) and gastrocnemius (21)
6 Medial calcanean nerve, a cutaneous branch of the tibial nerve
7 Flexor hallucis longus, in (c) the most medial of the flexor tendons
8 Tibial nerve
9 Posterior tibial artery and venae comitantes
10 Flexor digitorum longus, in (a) and (c) behind the tibialis posterior tendon (11)
11 Tibialis posterior, whose tendon lies adjacent to the medial malleolus (12) (seen best in c)
12 Medial malleolus
13 Flexor retinaculum
14 Posterior surface of calcaneus
15 Lateral malleolus of fibula, with the

tendon of peroneus brevis (25) in contact with it in (c)
16 Superior peroneal retinaculum
17 Inferior peroneal retinaculum
18 Tibia
19 Interosseous membrane
20 Peroneal artery and large venae comitantes. Note the adjacent large veins within soleus (2)
21 Gastrocnemius
22 Saphenous nerve
23 Great saphenous vein, at this level on the medial side of the leg but at the ankle in front of the medial malleolus (c, 12)
24 Fibula
25 Peroneus brevis, in (c) in contact with the lateral malleolus (15)
26 Extensor hallucis longus
27 Extensor digitorum longus
28 Anterior tibial vessels
29 Deep peroneal nerve
30 Tibialis anterior
31 Small saphenous vein, at this level at the back of the calf but in (c) passing up behind the lateral malleolus (15), in contrast to the great saphenous vein (23) which runs up in front of the medial malleolus (12)
32 Talus
33 Posterior talofibular ligament
34 Dorsalis pedis artery, lateral to the tendon of extensor hallucis longus

the leg, the range of dorsiflexion is more limited than that of plantarflexion because the front of the articulating surface of the talus is wider than the back part, and, after about 20° or so of dorsiflexion, the talus becomes so tightly squeezed between the two malleoli that it cannot move any further. In contrast the amount of plantarflexion possible is about 40°.

The *dorsiflexors* are the muscles passing in front of the ankle joint, principally tibialis anterior assisted by the toe extensors (**20.13a**). *Plantarflexion* is produced by any of the muscles behind the ankle, mainly gastrocnemius and soleus through their attachment to the Achilles' tendon, assisted by the flexor muscles on the medial side and the peroneal muscles on the lateral side (**20.16a** and **20.16c**).

ARCHES OF THE FOOT

There are two longitudinal arches in the foot. The larger, the **medial longitudinal arch**, consists of the calcaneus, talus, navicular, the cuneiforms and the medial three metatarsals, while the smaller **lateral longitudinal arch** is composed of the calcaneus, cuboid and the two lateral metatarsals (**20.12a** and **20.14a**). Note that the calcaneus does not lie flat but is tilted upwards, with only the back part in contact with the ground, so forming the back part of the arches. It not only takes the strain of the normal body weight but bears the brunt of any heavy falls on to the feet (such as falling off a ladder) when it may be fractured.

The **transverse arch** is really only half an arch in each foot, and consists of the bases of the five metatarsals and the adjacent cuboid and cuneiform bones.

The arches exist because of the *shapes* of the participating bones, but the *maintenance* of the arched form depends not only on the *ligaments* that hold the bones together but also on *muscular activity* (because muscles are capable of contracting and 'taking up slack' but ligaments cannot). When standing still, however, there is negligible muscle activity, and the ligaments of the sole of the foot have to take the strain of holding the bones together, with little muscular help. For this reason, they are dense structures, much denser than the ligaments on the dorsum. The most important are the **long** and **short plantar ligaments**, the **spring ligament** (i.e. the **plantar calcaneonavicular ligament**) and the **plantar aponeurosis** (**20.18–20.20**). With activity such as walking, the arches become somewhat accentuated, owing to the action of both the intrinsic muscles and those of the long tendons from the leg. **Tibialis anterior** is particularly important in holding up the medial longitudinal arch, and **peroneus longus**, whose tendon runs under the foot from the lateral side, supports the lateral arch. The tendon of **flexor hallucis longus** acts as a mobile 'tie-beam' on the medial side of the sole (**20.19b**).

People with high transverse and medial longitudinal arches are said to have a 'high instep', and those with low arches have *flatfoot*, although there is no precise definition – it is simply a general appearance. Such variations from the so-called normal are usually without significance, and, contrary to popular opinion, any symptoms attributed to flat feet are almost invariably due to factors other than flatness.

SUBTALAR JOINTS

Between the talus and calcaneus there are two joints (**20.13c**): at the back, the **talocalcanean joint** (also known anatomically as the **subtalar joint**), and, in front of it, the **talocalcaneonavicular joint** (between the under surface of the head of the talus, the upper surface of the sustentaculum tali of the calcaneus, the back of the navicular, and the upper surface of the spring ligament). Clinicians often call these two joints collectively the **subtalar joint**, which serves to emphasize that the whole of the rest of the foot can swing inwards and outwards underneath the talus (*inversion* and *eversion* – see below). Each joint has its own **capsule**, and there are two other ligaments helping to hold the talus and calcaneus together (**20.13c**): the **interosseous talocalcanean ligament** which occupies the grooves (i.e. the sulci) on the adjacent surfaces of the two bones, and more laterally the **cervical ligament**, so called because it runs to the under surface of the *neck* of the talus from the upper surface of the calcaneus.

One other joint must be mentioned as being involved in inversion and eversion: the **midtarsal** or **transverse tarsal joint** (**20.12a** and **20.17**). This is the collective name for the calcaneocuboid joint and the talonavicular part of the talocalcaneonavicular joint, and forms a transverse separation between the talus and calcaneus at the back and the rest of the foot (the forefoot) in front.

Movements

The movements of **inversion** and **eversion** of the foot (turning the sole inwards and outwards respectively, **1.2q**) take place essentially at the two joints underneath the talus, with some initial movement at the midtarsal joint; note that there is **no** inverting or everting movement at the **ankle** joint. A very small amount of gliding movement takes place between any other tarsal and metatarsal bones that are adjacent to one another, but it is negligible compared with the amount occurring at the main joints mentioned.

The main muscles producing *inversion* are the two tibialis muscles, anterior and posterior, while the *evertors* are the two peroneal muscles, longus and brevis. The tendons of all these muscles have their insertions to bones *in front of the midtarsal joint line* (**20.19b**), so that at the very beginning of inversion and eversion there is a very small amount of gliding and rotatory movement at this midtarsal joint. However, the available range of movement here is soon exhausted, which is why most of inversion and eversion occurs at the joints underneath the talus. The interosseous ligament becomes tightest in eversion and the cervical ligament tightest in inversion; they assist the joint capsules in limiting these movements.

The purpose of all these movements is to enable the foot

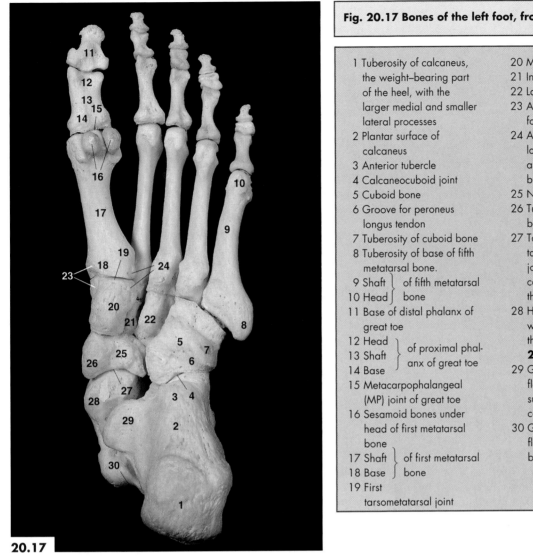

Fig. 20.17 Bones of the left foot, from below.

1 Tuberosity of calcaneus, the weight–bearing part of the heel, with the larger medial and smaller lateral processes
2 Plantar surface of calcaneus
3 Anterior tubercle
4 Calcaneocuboid joint
5 Cuboid bone
6 Groove for peroneus longus tendon
7 Tuberosity of cuboid bone
8 Tuberosity of base of fifth metatarsal bone.
9 Shaft ⎱ of fifth metatarsal
10 Head ⎰ bone
11 Base of distal phalanx of great toe
12 Head ⎱
13 Shaft ⎬ of proximal phalanx of great toe
14 Base ⎰
15 Metacarpophalangeal (MP) joint of great toe
16 Sesamoid bones under head of first metatarsal bone
17 Shaft ⎱ of first metatarsal
18 Base ⎰ bone
19 First tarsometatarsal joint

20 Medial
21 Intermediate ⎱
22 Lateral ⎬ cuneiform bone
23 Attachment ⎰ for tibialis anterior
24 Attachment for peroneus longus, to the same bones as tibialis anterior (23) but at the opposite side
25 Navicular bone
26 Tuberosity of navicular bone, for tibialis posterior
27 Talonavicular part of talocalcaneonavicular joint, making with the calcaneocuboid joint (4) the midtarsal joint
28 Head of talus, labelled where it is supported by the spring ligament (27 in **20.13c**)
29 Groove for tendon of flexor hallucis longus on sustentaculum tali of calcaneus (2)
30 Groove for tendon of flexor hallucis longus on back of talus

to adjust itself to whatever surface is in contact with the sole. In walking across the side of a steep hill, for example, one foot will be inverted and one everted.

PULSES IN THE FOOT

The *pulsation* of the **posterior tibial artery** (**20.15c**) can be felt behind the medial malleolus, 2.5 cm in front of the medial border of the Achilles' tendon.

The *pulsation* of the **dorsalis pedis artery** (**20.13b**) can be felt on the dorsum of the foot, along a line from the midpoint between the two malleoli (just lateral to the tendon of extensor hallucis longus) towards the first toe cleft. Both this and the posterior tibial pulse are occasionally absent, even in normal feet.

TOES

The general structure of **toes** is similar to that of fingers, with **phalanges** and their **joints, extensor tendons** and **expansions** on their dorsal surfaces (**20.13a**), and **flexor tendons** and their **sheaths** on the plantar surfaces (**20.19a**). As in the hand, the action of **interosseus** and **lumbrical muscles** (p.238) is important in extending the smaller toes – keeping them straight and preventing the formation of 'hammer toes' where there is persistent flexion of the proximal interphalangeal joints which project up and rub against the shoe. The baseline for *abduction* and *adduction* of the toes, which is very limited compared with those of the fingers, is the *second* toe (the second digit, compared with the *third* digit or middle finger in the hand). The **great toe** has particular importance in walking, with flexor hallucis

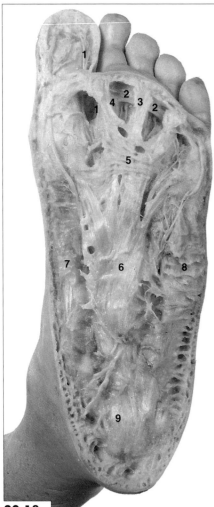

20.18

Fig. 20.18 Superficial dissection of the left sole, to show the plantar aponeurosis.
Note that its surface is not smooth but has many fibrous attachments to anchor the tough overlying subcutaneous tissues and skin (see also the part of the sole visible in **20.16a**).

1 A plantar digital nerve
2 Superficial transverse metatarsal ligament
3 Superficial layer of digital band, attached to skin
4 Deep layer of digital band, which becomes attached to the metatarsophalangeal joint capsule and the deep transverse metatarsal ligament (16 in **20.19**)
5 Transverse fibres of aponeurosis
6 Central part of aponeurosis, overlying flexor digitorum brevis
7 Medial part of aponeurosis, overlying abductor hallucis
8 Lateral part of aponeurosis, overlying abductor digiti minimi
9 Medial process of tuberosity of calcaneus

longus providing much of the propulsive force (see below); the metatarsophalangeal joint is dorsiflexed against the resistance of the ground while the interphalangeal joint is kept straight.

The main vessels of the toes are the **digital arteries**; a pair run up the sides of each toe, one of each pair being derived from the dorsal metatarsal arteries (from the dorsalis pedis artery on the dorsum of the foot) and the other from the plantar metatarsal branches of the plantar arch deep in the sole (**8.3a**). The digital vessels supply not only the skin but also all other tissues including the pulps of the toe pads (similar in structure to finger pulps, p.236).

STANDING, WALKING AND RUNNING

When *standing* in the normal upright position, the centre of gravity of the body passes just **behind the hip joint** but **in front of the knee and ankle joints**, roughly along the line of the anterior border of the tibia. Slight contraction of the soleus muscles (the postural part of the soleus–gastrocnemius partnership) counteracts the tendency to fall forwards.

In *walking*, one or other foot is always on the ground (with a short time when both are), but in *running* there are periods when both feet are off the ground. The movements of a whole lower limb in walking (the *gait cycle*) are usually described as beginning from the point where one heel hits the ground (*heel-strike*) and then continuing through phases of *stance*, *toe-off* and *swing*. There are obviously varying degrees of flexion and extension at the hip, knee and ankle, with some rotation at the hip and stabilization of the pelvis, but muscle actions are modified by the effect of gravity and the forward momentum imparted to the limb and the body as a whole. There are further compensatory movements of the trunk and swinging of the upper limbs, all adding up to a highly coordinated and complicated mechanism. Comment is made here on only some major muscle activities.

From heel-strike to toe-off, the hip joint moves from flexion to extension, the knee joint moves from full extension to flexion and then to full extension again, and the ankle joint moves into plantarflexion and then to dorsiflexion at toe-off. The stance phase occupies about 60% of a single cycle and the swing phase 40%. In ordinary walking there is a period when both limbs are on the ground (about 15% of a whole cycle), and this period becomes shorter the more rapid the walking; when running this 'double support' period disappears.

As the heel comes to the ground, tibialis anterior and other dorsiflexors are important in controlling the lowering of the rest of the foot; without this action the foot would 'flop down'. They come into action again at the beginning of the swing phase, as the foot is moving forward, to prevent scraping the toes along the ground.

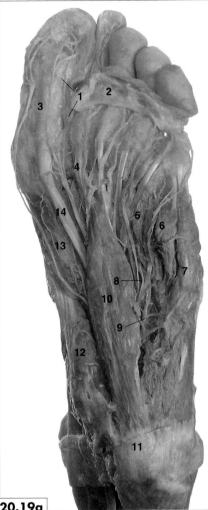

20.19a

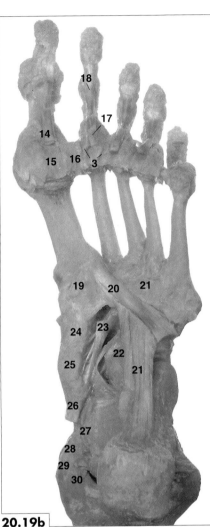

20.19b

Fig. 20.19 Sole of the left foot.
(a) Superficial dissection, after removal of the plantar aponeurosis.
(b) Deep dissection, leaving only some ligaments and tendons.

1 Plantar digital nerves
2 Superficial transverse metatarsal ligament
3 Fibrous flexor sheath, cut open in the second toe in **(b)**
4 A lumbrical muscle
5 An interosseous muscle
6 Flexor digiti minimi brevis
7 Abductor digiti minimi
8 Deep branch of lateral plantar nerve, supplying most of the small foot muscles
9 Lateral plantar artery
10 Flexor digitorum brevis
11 Cut edge of plantar aponeurosis
12 Abductor hallucis
13 Flexor hallucis brevis
14 Flexor hallucis longus
15 Plantar ligament of first metatarsophalangeal (MP) joint
16 Deep transverse metatarsal ligament, joining the plantar ligaments (15) of the MP joints and preventing spreading of the toes
17 Flexor digitorum brevis tendon, passing forwards to reach the middle phalanx and splitting to allow the flexor digitorum longus tendon (18) to pass through

18 Flexor digitorum longus tendon
19 Plantar tarsometatarsal ligament
20 Peroneus longus tendon, displayed by removing part of the long plantar ligament (21), and passing to its insertion into the medial cuneiform and the base of the first metatarsal
21 Long plantar ligament
22 Short plantar ligament (plantar calcaneocuboid ligament)
23 Slip from tibialis posterior
24 Plantar cuneonavicular ligament
25 Tuberosity of navicular, receiving tibialis posterior insertion
26 Tibialis posterior
27 Spring ligament (plantar calcaneonavicular ligament), passing from the sustenaculum tali (30) to the navicular, supported by the tendon of tibialis posterior (26) and supporting on its upper surface part of the head of the talus (27 in **20.13c**)
28 Medial (deltoid) ligament of ankle joint, fusing with the spring ligament (27)
29 Medial malleolus of tibia
30 Sustenaculum tali of calcaneus, with groove for the tendon of flexor hallucis longus

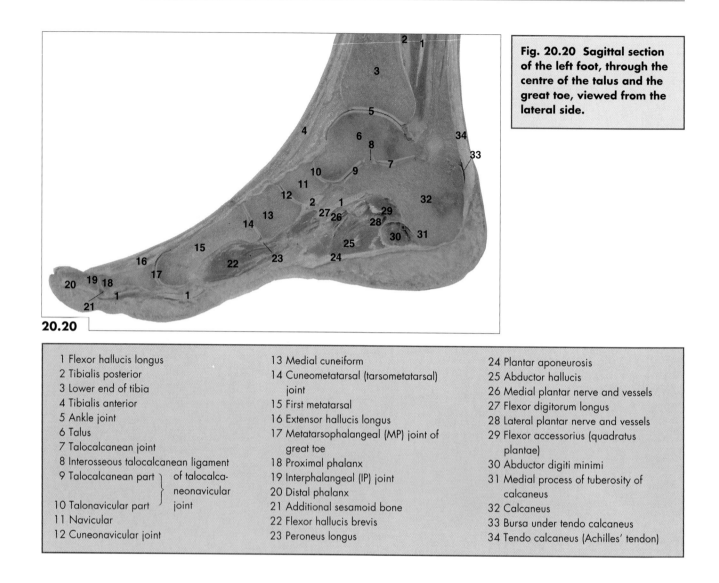

20.20

1 Flexor hallucis longus	13 Medial cuneiform	24 Plantar aponeurosis
2 Tibialis posterior	14 Cuneometatarsal (tarsometatarsal) joint	25 Abductor hallucis
3 Lower end of tibia	15 First metatarsal	26 Medial plantar nerve and vessels
4 Tibialis anterior	16 Extensor hallucis longus	27 Flexor digitorum longus
5 Ankle joint	17 Metatarsophalangeal (MP) joint of great toe	28 Lateral plantar nerve and vessels
6 Talus	18 Proximal phalanx	29 Flexor accessorius (quadratus plantae)
7 Talocalcanean joint	19 Interphalangeal (IP) joint	30 Abductor digiti minimi
8 Interosseous talocalcanean ligament	20 Distal phalanx	31 Medial process of tuberosity of calcaneus
9 Talocalcanean part ⎱ of talocalca-	21 Additional sesamoid bone	32 Calcaneus
10 Talonavicular part ⎰ neonavicular joint	22 Flexor hallucis brevis	33 Bursa under tendo calcaneus
11 Navicular	23 Peroneus longus	34 Tendo calcaneus (Achilles' tendon)
12 Cuneonavicular joint		

Soleus and gastrocnemius become active towards the end of the stance phase to prepare for toe-off, where the action of flexor pollicis longus in particular assists in the propulsion. Quadriceps femoris keeps the knee extended at heel-strike and toe-off, and helps to control the small amount of flexion just after heel-strike.

The hamstrings extend the hip at heel-strike; there is less activity in gluteus maximus than might be imagined in ordinary walking, but it is much more involved in the greater extension required for running.

Gluteus medius and minimus of one side are of major importance in keeping the pelvis from tilting down on the opposite side when the opposite limb is in the swing phase (off the ground), and in rotating the pelvis forwards.

MISCELLANEOUS FOOT CONDITIONS

In *congenital clubfoot* (*talipes equinovarus*) the infant foot is held in plantarflexion and inversion, and orthopaedic procedures such as the repeated application of casts as the foot grows may be necessary to correct the deformity.

The second metatarsal is the longest of the metatarsal bones, which may account for the fact that it is particularly subject to stress or *march fracture*, commonest in people who are 'on their feet all day' such as nurses and soldiers. There is pain but no significant deformity, and healing depends on suitable rest.

In many adults, the great toe does not remain in the same straight line as the first metatarsal bone but becomes deviated laterally, causing the condition known as *hallux valgus*. This deformity frequently develops in individuals who wear shoes with pointed toes for a prolonged period of time. The head of the first metatarsal becomes unduly prominent with excessive bone growth (*exostosis*) and presses on the side of the shoe, causing pain and swelling in the bursa and other soft tissues at the side of the first metatarsophalangeal joint. The whole projecting mass is commonly called a *bunion*. Not all cases of hallux valgus cause symptoms, but when they do surgery may be necessary to straighten out the toe. Possible procedures include trimming off the exostosis and removing part of the metatarsal or first phalanx to restore the normal alignment.

Being at the very end of the limb, blood circulation in the toes can be readily affected by cold as well as by arterial disease. Severe vasoconstriction as from prolonged exposure to extreme cold (*frostbite*) may lead to tissue death of the tips of the toes, which may drop off or require surgical removal. A similar but more slowly progressive condition can result from arterial disease (*arteriosclerosis*) narrowing the lumen of the vessels; this is a common complication of diabetes (*diabetic gangrene*).

A *callus* is a localized thickening of the uppermost keratinized layer of the skin (*hyperkeratosis*) caused by repeated pressure or friction, often over a bony prominence; in the feet, footware is the usual cause. A small rounded area of hyperkeratosis is a *corn*. Corns are common on prominent parts of the toes (*hard corns*), especially over hammer toes (see above). They may also occur between toes (*soft corns*). They may be tender on pressure and the hard keratin may have to be pared off – one of the commonest activities of the podiatrist or chiropodist.

There are more *sweat glands* in the sole of the foot than any other part of the body (over 600 per square cm), and this, coupled with the wearing of socks or stockings and shoes, accounts for the fact that many people complain of excessively sweaty feet. It is not a disease with a particular cause, and any antisocial effects can only be combated by constant attention to foot hygiene.

The clefts between the toes in which dead skin and sweat accumulate are the sites of *athlete's foot* (*tinea pedis*), a fungus infection which usually begins in the third and fourth clefts and may spread on to the sole. Careful foot hygiene with frequent washing and drying and the application of dusting powder and a fungicide are required to clear the condition.

An *ingrowing toenail*, usually in the great toe, causes discomfort at the sides of the nail where it grows downwards instead of forwards. The nail can be encouraged to grow forward by introducing cotton wool or lint between the edge of the nail and the nail fold. The nail should always be cut straight across without attempting to dig down into the corner; this simply predisposes to further ingrowth. Severe cases require excision of the nail fold and adjacent part of the nail.

MUSCLE ATTACHMENTS, ACTIONS AND NERVE SUPPLIES

The more important muscles have been described in the text. A brief synopsis of the attachments of these and other muscles is given here for reference if required. (A few of the smaller or less important muscles are mentioned only by name, since for most students detailed knowledge of them is not required.)

MUSCLES OF THE HEAD AND NECK

MUSCLES OF THE SCALP AND FACE

Occipitofrontalis – from highest nuchal line to epicranial aponeurosis (occipitalis) and from aponeurosis to blend with orbicularis oculi and skin (frontalis, which has no bony attachment)
Movement of scalp and wrinkling of forehead
Facial nerve

Orbicularis oculi – from frontal process of maxilla and anterior lacrimal crest of lacrimal bone (orbital part) and medial palpebral ligament (palpebral part), forming concentric loops in eyelids and round orbital margins
Closure and 'screwing up' of eyelids
Facial nerve

Orbicularis oris – circular fibres within lips, blending at sides with buccinator
Closure of lips
Facial nerve

Buccinator – from pterygomandibular raphe and maxilla and mandible opposite the three molar teeth, forward to blend with orbicularis oris
Compression of cheek against gums, keeping food in mouth cavity
Facial nerve

Procerus
Nasalis
Corrugator supercilii
Levator palpebrae superioris – *see* Muscles of the orbit
Levator labii superioris
Levator labii superioris alaeque nasi
Zygomaticus major
Zygomaticus minor
Levator anguli oris
Depressor anguli oris
Mentalis
Risorius

MUSCLES OF MASTICATION

Lateral pterygoid – from infratemporal surface of greater wing of sphenoid (upper head) and lateral surface of lateral pterygoid plate (lower head) to neck of mandible and capsule and disc of temporomandibular joint
Opening mouth wide and assisting side-to-side chewing movements
Mandibular nerve

Medial pterygoid – from medial surface of lateral pterygoid plate, pyramidal process of palatine and tuberosity of maxilla to lower part of medial surface of ramus and angle of mandible
Closure of mouth and assisting side-to-side chewing movements
Mandibular nerve

Temporalis – from temporal fossa and overlying fascia to coronoid process and anterior margin of ramus of mandible
Closure of mouth
Mandibular nerve

Masseter – from zygomatic arch to outer surface of ramus of mandible
Closure of mouth
Mandibular nerve

MUSCLES OF THE NECK

Platysma – fascia over upper pectoralis major to lower part of body of mandible and adjacent skin and facial muscles
Wrinkling skin of neck
Facial nerve

Sternocleidomastoid – from upper front part of manubrium of sternum (sternal head) and medial third of clavicle (clavicular head) to mastoid process of temporal bone and adjoining occipital bone
Tilting head and face upwards and to opposite side
Accessory nerve (spinal part)

Trapezius – *see* Muscles of the upper limb

Scalenus anterior – from transverse processes of vertebrae C3–6 to scalene tubercle of first rib
Elevation of first rib
Anterior rami of C4, 5, 6

Scalenus medius – from transverse processes of axis and vertebrae C3–7 to upper surface of first rib between scalene tubercle and groove for subclavian artery
Elevation of first rib
Anterior rami of C5, 6, 7, 8

Longus colli
Longus capitis
Rectus capitis anterior
Rectus capitis lateralis

Suprahyoid muscles

Digastric – digastric groove on medial side of mastoid process (posterior belly) and digastric fossa on inner surface of mandible (anterior belly); intermediate tendon held by fascial sling to lesser horn of hyoid
Depression of mandible and elevation of hyoid bone
Facial nerve (posterior belly) and nerve to mylohyoid (anterior belly)

Stylohyoid – from back of upper part of styloid process to base of greater horn of hyoid
Elevation of hyoid
Facial nerve

Mylohyoid – from mylohyoid line of mandible to anterior surface of body of hyoid and midline raphe
Elevation of tongue and hyoid
Own nerve from inferior alveolar

Geniohyoid – from inferior mental spine of mandible to upper border of body of hyoid
Elevation of hyoid
Hypoglossal nerve, by C1 fibres

Infrahyoid muscles

Sternohyoid – from back of manubrium to lower border of hyoid
Depression of hyoid and larynx
Ansa cervicalis, C1, 2, 3

Sternothyroid – from back of manubrium below sternohyoid to oblique line of thyroid cartilage
Depression of larynx
Ansa cervicalis, C2, 3

Omohyoid – from hyoid bone lateral to sternohyoid (superior belly) and transverse scapular ligament and upper border of scapula (inferior belly); intermediate tendon bound by fascial sling above clavicle
Depression of hyoid and larynx
Ansa cervicalis, C1, 2, 3

Thyrohyoid – from greater horn of hyoid bone to oblique line of thyroid cartilage above sternothyroid
Depression of hyoid or elevation of larynx
Hypoglossal nerve, by C1 fibres

MUSCLES OF THE PHARYNX

Superior constrictor – from medial pterygoid plate and hamulus, pterygomandibular raphe and adjacent mandible to pharyngeal raphe and tubercle
Peristaltic action in swallowing
Pharyngeal plexus

Middle constrictor – from stylohyoid ligament and lesser and greater horns of hyoid to pharyngeal raphe
Peristaltic action in swallowing
Pharyngeal plexus

Inferior constrictor – from thyroid and cricoid cartilages to pharyngeal raphe
Peristaltic action in swallowing and elevation of larynx
Pharyngeal plexus

Stylopharyngeus – from upper part of styloid process to back of thyroid lamina
Elevation of larynx
Glossopharyngeal nerve

Palatopharyngeus – from hard palate and palatine aponeurosis to back of thyroid lamina
Elevation of larynx and sphincteric action on oropharyngeal isthmus
Pharyngeal plexus

Salpingopharyngeus – from cartilage of auditory tube, passing down to blend with constrictors
Opening auditory tube
Pharyngeal plexus

MUSCLES OF THE SOFT PALATE

Palatopharyngeus – *see* above

Palatoglossus – from palatine aponeurosis to blend with styloglossus
Elevation of tongue
Hypoglossal nerve

Tensor veli palatini – from scaphoid fossa, lateral lamina of auditory tube and spine of sphenoid to palatine aponeurosis
Stabilization of palatine aponeurosis and opening of auditory tube
Nerve to medial pterygoid (mandibular nerve)

Levator veli palatini – from apex of petrous temporal to palatine aponeurosis
Elevation of palate
Pharyngeal plexus

Musculus uvulae – from posterior nasal spine to palatine aponeurosis
Elevation of uvula
Pharyngeal plexus

MUSCLES OF THE TONGUE

Genioglossus – from superior mental spine to body of hyoid
Protrusion and depression of tongue
Hypoglossal nerve

Hyoglossus – from body and greater horn of hyoid to side of tongue
Depression of tongue
Hypoglossal nerve

Styloglossus – from tip of styloid process and stylohyoid ligament to back and side of tongue
Elevation and retraction of tongue
Hypoglossal nerve

Palatoglossus – *see* soft palate, above

Intrinsic muscles – superior and inferior longitudinal, transverse and vertical, with no external attachment
Alteration of tongue shape
Hypoglossal nerve

MUSCLES OF THE LARYNX

Cricothyroid – from anterolateral part of cricoid cartilage to inferior horn and lower border of lamina of thyroid cartilage
Tensor of vocal folds
External laryngeal nerve

Posterior cricoarytenoid – from back of lamina of cricoid cartilage to muscular process of arytenoid cartilage
Abduction of vocal folds
Recurrent laryngeal nerve

Lateral cricoarytenoid – from upper border of cricoid cartilage to muscular process of arytenoid cartilage
Adduction of vocal folds
Recurrent laryngeal nerve

Transverse arytenoid – between the backs of both arytenoid cartilages
Adduction of vocal folds
Recurrent laryngeal nerve

Oblique arytenoid – from muscular process of one arytenoid cartilage to apex of the opposite arytenoid cartilage
Adduction of aryepiglottic folds
Recurrent laryngeal nerve

Thyroarytenoid – from lower part of front of lamina of thyroid cartilage and cricothyroid ligament to side of arytenoid cartilage. Lower fibres form vocalis muscle; uppermost fibres run to epiglottic cartilage as thyroepiglottic muscle
Relaxation and adduction of vocal folds
Recurrent laryngeal nerve

MUSCLES OF THE ORBIT

Levator palpebrae superioris – from inferior surface of lesser wing of sphenoid to tarsus and skin of upper eyelid
Elevation of upper eyelid
Oculomotor nerve, and sympathetic fibres

Superior rectus – from upper part of tendinous ring and sheath of optic nerve to upper part of sclera in front of coronal equator
Elevation and medial rotation of eye
Oculomotor nerve

Inferior rectus – from lower part of tendinous ring to inferior surface of sclera in front of coronal equator
Depression and medial rotation of eye
Oculomotor nerve

Medial rectus – from medial part of tendinous ring and sheath of optic nerve to medial surface of sclera in front of coronal equator
Medial rotation of eye
Oculomotor nerve

Lateral rectus – from lateral part of tendinous ring bridging superior orbital fissure to lateral surface of sclera in front of coronal equator
Lateral rotation of eye
Abducent nerve

Superior oblique – from body of sphenoid above and medial to optic canal and medial rectus to upper outer quadrant of sclera behind coronal equator
Depression and lateral rotation of eye
Trochlear nerve

Inferior oblique – from orbital surface of maxilla lateral to nasolacrimal groove to lower outer quadrant of sclera behind coronal equator
Elevation and lateral rotation of eye
Oculomotor nerve

MUSCLES OF THE UPPER LIMB

MUSCLES OF THE SHOULDER

Deltoid – from lateral third of clavicle, acromion and lower border of spine of scapula to deltoid tuberosity of humerus
Abduction, flexion and medial rotation (anterior fibres) and extension and lateral rotation (posterior fibres) of arm
Axillary nerve, C5, 6

Supraspinatus – supraspinous fossa of scapula to upper facet of greater tubercle of humerus
Abduction of arm and stabilization of shoulder joint
Suprascapular nerve, C5, 6

Infraspinatus – infraspinous fossa of scapula to middle facet of greater tubercle of humerus
Lateral rotation of arm and stabilization of shoulder joint
Suprascapular nerve, C5, 6

Teres minor – back of inferior angle of scapula to lower facet of greater tubercle of humerus
Lateral rotation of arm and stabilization of shoulder joint
Axillary nerve, C5, 6

Teres major – back of inferior angle of scapula to medial lip of intertubercular groove of humerus
Medial rotation, adduction and extension of arm
Lower subscapular nerve, C5, 6

Subscapularis – subscapular fossa of scapula to lesser tubercle of humerus
Medial rotation ofarm and stabilization of shoulder joint
Upper and lower subscapular nerves, C5, 6

MUSCLES OF THE SHOULDER GIRDLE

Connecting limb to the vertebral column

Trapezius – from occipital bone, nuchalligament and spines of C7–T12 vertebrae to lateral third of clavicle, acromion and upper lip of spine of scapula
Upper fibres: elevation and rotation of scapula; lower fibres: depression of scapula; middle fibres: retraction of scapula
Accessory nerve, spinal part, C1–6

Latissimus dorsi – from spines of T7–12 and all L vertebrae and lumbar fascia to floor of intertubercular groove of humerus
Adduction and medial rotation of arm, and extension (if flexed)
Thoracodorsal nerve, C6, 7, 8

Levator scapulae – from transverse processes of C1–4 vertebrae to vertebral border of scapula from base of spine to superior angle
Elevation of scapula
Nerves from C3, 4

Rhomboid minor – from spines of C7 and T1 vertebrae to vertebral border of scapula from base of spine to inferior angle
Retraction and elevation of scapula
Dorsal scapular nerve, C4, 5

Rhomboid major – from spines of T2–5 vertebrae to vertebral border of scapula from base of spine to inferior angle
Retraction and elevation of scapula
Dorsal scapular nerve, C4, 5

Connecting limb to the thoracic wall

Pectoralis major – from lateral half of clavicle, body of sternum and costal cartilages 1–7 to lateral lip of intertubercular groove of humerus
Adduction, medial rotation, flexion (clavicular head) and extension (sternal head) of arm
Medial and lateral pectoral nerves, C5–8, T1

Pectoralis minor – from ribs 3–5 near costal cartilages to coracoid process of scapula
Rotation and depression of scapula
Medial and lateral pectoral nerves, C6, 7, 8

Serratus anterior – from upper 8 ribs to vertebral border of scapula
Protraction and rotation of scapula
Long thoracic nerve, C5, 6, 7

Subclavius – from rib 1 and costal cartilage to groove on clavicle
Stabilizes clavicle
Own nerve, C5, 6

MUSCLES OF THE UPPER ARM

Biceps brachii – from supraglenoid tubercle of scapula (long head) and coracoid process of scapula (short head) to tuberosity of radius
Flexion and supination of forearm
Musculocutaneous nerve, C5, 6

Coracobrachialis – from coracoid process of scapula to shaft of humerus (medial border, half way down)
Flexion and adduction of arm
Musculocutaneous nerve, C5, 6, 7

Brachialis – from lower half of front of humerus to tuberosity of ulna (coronoid process)
Flexion of forearm
Musculocutaneous nerve, C5, 6

Triceps – from infraglenoid tubercle of scapula (long head) and posterior surface of shaft of humerus (lateral and medial heads) to posterior surface of olecranon of ulna
Extension of forearm
Radial nerve, C6, 7, 8

MUSCLES OF THE FOREARM

Anterior forearm muscles, superficial group

Pronator teres – from common flexor origin (medial epicondyle of humerus) and coronoid process of ulna to middle of lateral surface of radius
Pronation and flexion of forearm
Median nerve, C6, 7

Flexor carpi radialis – common flexor origin to bases of second and third metacarpals
Flexion and abduction of wrist, flexion and pronation of forearm
Median nerve, C6, 7

Palmaris longus – from common flexor origin to distal part of flexor retinaculum
Flexion of wrist
Median nerve, C7, 8

Flexor carpi ulnaris – from common flexor origin (humeral head) and posterior border of ulna (ulnar head) to pisiform bone and through it to pisohamate and pisometacarpal ligaments
Flexion and adduction of wrist
Ulnar nerve, C7, 8

Flexor digitorum superficialis – from common flexor origin and coronoid process of ulna (humero-ulnar head) and oblique line on anterior surface of radius (radial head) to sides of middle phalanges of fingers
Flexion of wrist, MP and proximal IP joints
Median nerve, C7, 8, T1

Anterior forearm muscles, deep group

Flexor pollicis longus – from anterior surface of radius and interosseous membrane to distal phalanx of thumb
Flexion of thumb joints and wrist
Median (anterior interosseous) nerve, C8, T1

Flexor digitorum profundus – from anterior and medial surfaces and posterior border of ulna and interosseous membrane to distal phalanx of fingers
Flexion of finger joints and wrist
Ulnar and median (anterior interosseous) nerves, C8, T1

Pronator quadratus – from lower anterior surface of ulna to lower anterior surface of radius
Pronation of forearm
Median (anterior interosseous) nerve, C8, T1

Posterior forearm muscles, superficial group

Brachioradialis – from lateral supracondylar ridge of humerus to radius above styloid process
Flexion and partial pronation of forearm
Radial nerve, C5, 6

Extensor carpi radialis longus – from lateral supracondylar ridge of humerus to base of second metacarpal
Extension and abduction of wrist
Radial nerve, C6, 7

Extensor carpi radialis brevis – from common extensor origin (lateral epicondyle of humerus) to bases of second and third metacarpals
Extension and abduction of wrist
Radial nerve, C7, 8

Extensor digitorum – from common extensor origin to dorsal digital expansions of fingers
Extension of wrist and MP joints
Radial nerve, C7, 8

Extensor digiti minimi – from common extensor origin to dorsal digital expansion of little finger
Extension of wrist and little finger
Radial nerve, C7, 8

Extensor carpi ulnaris – from common extensor origin and posterior border of ulna to tubercle of base of fifth metacarpal
Extension and adduction of wrist
Radial nerve, C7, 8

Anconeus – from posterior surface of lateral epicondyle to olecranon and upper posterior surface of ulna
Extension of forearm
Radial nerve, C7, 8

Posterior forearm muscles, deep group
Supinator – from lateral epicondyle of humerus, lateral and annular ligaments of elbow joint and supinator crest of ulna to upper lateral third of radius
Supination of forearm
Radial nerve (posterior interosseous), C5, 6

Abductor pollicis longus – from upper posterior surfaces of radius and ulna and interosseous membrane to base of first metacarpal and trapezium
Abduction and extension of thumb metacarpal
Radial nerve (posterior interosseous), C7, 8

Extensor pollicis brevis – from posterior surface of radius and interosseous membrane below abductor to base of proximal phalanx of thumb
Extension of thumb, flexion and abduction of wrist
Radial nerve (posterior interosseous), C7, 8

Extensor pollicis longus – from middle part of posterior surface of ulna and interosseous membrane to ulnar side of dorsal digital expansion of index finger
Extension of index finger and wrist
Radial nerve (posterior interosseous), C7, 8

Extensor indicis – from lower part of posterior surface of ulna and interosseous membrane to ulnar side of dorsal digital expansion of index finger
Extension of index finger and wrist
Radial nerve (posterior interosseous), C7, 8

MUSCLES OF THE HAND

Adductor pollicis – from capitate, bases of second and third metacarpals and shaft of third metacarpal to ulnar side of base of proximal phalanx of thumb
Adduction and opposition of thumb
Ulnar nerve, C8, T1

Lumbricals (4) – from tendons of flexor digitorum profundus in palm to radial sides of dorsal digital expansions of fingers
Flexion of MP joints and extension of IP joints of fingers (with interossei)
Median nerve (lateral two) and ulnar nerve (medial two), C8, T1

Dorsal interossei (4) – from shafts of adjacent metacarpals to dorsal digital expansions and bases of proximal phalanges (2 and 3 to radial and ulnar side of middle finger, 1 to radial side of index finger, and 4 to ulnar side of ring finger)
Flexion of MP joints and extension of IP joints of fingers (with lumbricals and palmar interossei); abduction of fingers from baseline through middle finger
Ulnar nerve, C8, T1

Palmar interossei (4) – from palmar surface of shafts of metacarpals (except third) to ulnar side of base of proximal phalanx of thumb (1), and dorsal digital expansions and bases of proximal phalanges (2 to ulnar side of index finger, 3 and 4 to radial sides of ring and little fingers)
Flexion of MP joints and extension of IP joints of fingers (with lumbricals and dorsal interossei); adduction of digits towards middle finger
Ulnar nerve, C8, T1

Thenar muscles
Abductor pollicis brevis – from flexor retinaculum, trapezium and scaphoid to radial side of base of first phalanx of thumb
Abduction and opposition of thumb
Median nerve, C8, T1

Opponens pollicis – from flexor retinaculum and trapezium to anterior surface of shaft of first metacarpal
Opposition of thumb
Median nerve, C8, T1

Flexor pollicis brevis – from flexor retinaculum and trapezium to radial border of proximal phalanx of thumb
Flexion and opposition of thumb
Median or ulnar nerve or both, C8, T1

Hypothenar muscles

Palmaris brevis – from palmar aponeurosis to skin of ulnar side of hypothenar eminence
Wrinkles skin of ulnar side of palm
Ulnar nerve, C8, T1

Abductor digiti minimi – from pisiform and piso-hamate ligament to ulnar side of base of proximal phalanx and dorsal digital expansion of little finger
Abduction of little finger
Ulnar nerve, C8, T1

Opponens digiti minimi – from flexor retinaculum and hook of hamate to ulnar border of fifth metacarpal
'Cupping' of hand
Ulnar nerve, C8, T1

Flexor digiti minimi brevis – from flexor retinaculum and hook of hamate to ulnar side of base of proximal phalanx of little finger
Flexion of MP joint of little finger
Ulnar nerve, C8, T1

MUSCLES OF THE TRUNK

SUBOCCIPITAL MUSCLES

Rectus capitis posterior major and minor
Obliquus capitis superior and inferior

DEEP MUSCLES OF THE BACK

Splenius – from spines of upper T vertebrae and lower ligamentum nuchae to superior nuchal line and mastoid process
Extension and rotation of head
Posterior rami of upper C nerves

Erector spinae – spinalis (medial part), longissimus (intermediate part) and iliocostalis (lateral part), with multiple attachments to vertebrae and adjacent parts of ribs
Extension of spine and maintenance of posture
Posterior rami of spinal nerves

Transversospinalis (semispinalis, multifidus, rotator)
Interspinal and intertransverse

MUSCLES OF THE THORAX

Diaphragm – lumbar part from crura (right, bodies of L1–L3 vertebrae and discs; left, bodies of L1 and L2 vertebrae and disc) and medial and lateral arcuate ligaments; costal part from lower six costal cartilages and adjacent ribs; sternal part from back of xiphoid process. All converging to central tendon, which has no bony attachment
Inspiration, abdominal straining
Phrenic nerve, C3, 4, 5

Intercostals – external: downwards and forwards between adjacent ribs; internal: downwards and backwards between adjacent ribs; innermost intercostals and subcostals: spanning more than one rib in lateral and some posterior parts of thoracic cage
Approximation of ribs
Intercostal nerves

Transversus thoracis – from body of sternum to costal cartilages 2–6
Approximation of ribs
Intercostal nerves

Levatores costarum – from transverse processes of C7–T11 vertebrae to rib below
Elevation of ribs
Posterior rami of spinal nerves

Serratus posterior superior – from spines of C6–T2 vertebrae to ribs 2–5
Elevation of upper ribs
Intercostal nerves

Serratus posterior inferior – from spines of T11–L2 vertebrae to lowest four ribs
Depression of lower ribs
Intercostal nerves

MUSCLES OF THE ABDOMEN

ANTEROLATERAL MUSCLES

Rectus abdominis – from pubic crest, and body of pubis of opposite side, to costal cartilages 5–7
Flexion of trunk, compression of abdomen
Intercostal nerves T7–12

External oblique – from lower eight ribs to aponeurosis fusing with front of rectus sheath and (lowest part) iliac crest, also forming inguinal ligament and lacunar ligament
Compression of abdomen, depression of ribs and flexion of trunk
Intercostal nerves T7–12

Internal oblique – from lateral part of inguinal ligament, iliac crest and lumbar fascia to lower four ribs, aponeurosis which splits to form rectus sheath, and (lowest fibres) conjoint tendon
Compression of abdomen, depression of ribs and flexion of trunk
Intercostal nerves T7–12, and iliohypogastric and ilio-inguinal nerves L1

Transversus abdominis – from lateral part of inguinal ligament, iliac crest and lumbar fascia to lower six costal cartilages, aponeurosis fusing with back of rectus sheath, and (lowest fibres) conjoint tendon
Compression of abdomen, depression of ribs and flexion of trunk
Intercostal nerves T7–12 and iliohypogastric and ilio-inguinal nerves L1

Cremaster – from internal oblique and transversus, spiralling down over spermatic cord and returning to internal oblique and pubic tubercle
Retraction of testis
Genital branch of genitofemoral nerve, L2

POSTERIOR MUSCLES

Iliacus – from iliac fossa to tendon of psoas major and lesser trochanter of femur
Flexion of thigh and (acting from below) flexion of trunk
Femoral nerve L2, 3

Psoas major – from sides of lumbar vertebrae and intervertebral discs to lesser trochanter of femur
Flexion of thigh and (acting from below) flexion of trunk
Nerves L1–3

Psoas minor – from sides of T12 and L1 vertebrae to iliopubic eminence
Flexion of lumbar spine
Nerve from L1

Quadratus lumborum – from iliolumbar ligament and adjacent iliac crest to medial part of twelfth rib and transverse processes of L1–L4 vertebrae
Stabilization and depression of twelfth rib and lateral flexion of lumbar spine
Nerves from T12 and L1–4

MUSCLES OF THE PELVIS

Piriformis – *see* Muscles of the gluteal region

Obturator internus – *see* Muscles of the gluteal region

Levator ani – from pelvic surface of body of pubis and anterior part of obturator fascia (pubococcygeus, forming puborectalis and levator prostatae or pubovaginalis) to central perineal tendon and anococcygeal ligament, and posterior part of obturator fascia and inner surface of ischial spine (iliococcygeus part) to anococcygeal body and coccyx
Pelvic floor, with puborectalis maintaining rectal continence
Perineal branches of S3, 4

Coccygeus – from ischial spine and sacrospinous ligament to coccyx and lowest piece of sacrum
Part of plevic floor
Perineal branches of S4, 5

MUSCLES OF THE PERINEUM

External anal sphincter – from tip of coccyx to central perineal tendon, with upper part blending with puborectalis part of levator ani, and lower part subcutaneous, curving inwards below internal sphincter (smooth muscle)
Maintenance of rectal continence
Inferior rectal branch of pudendal nerve, S3, 4

Sphincter urethrae – (male) fibres encircle membranous urethra within deep perineal pouch and extend round lower prostatic urethra, with some attachment to pubic rami; (female) fibres encircle urethra
Sphincteric action on urethra (external urethral sphincter)
Perineal branch of pudendal nerve, S3, 4

Bulbospongiosus – central perineal tendon and perineal membrane to midline raphe (male) or clitoris (female)
Expulsion of urine and semen from urethra (male) or constriction of vaginal orifice (female)
Perineal branch of pudendal nerve, S3, 4

Superficial transverse perineal
Ischiocavernosus
Deep transverse perineal

MUSCLES OF THE LOWER LIMB

MUSCLES OF THE GLUTEAL REGION

Gluteus maximus – from posterior gluteal line of hip bone, back of sacrum and sacrotuberous ligament to iliotibial tract and gluteal tuberosity of femur
Extension and lateral rotation of femur

Inferior gluteal nerve, L5, S1, 2
Gluteus medius – from ilium between anterior and posterior gluteal lines to greater trochanter of femur
Abduction and medial rotation of femur, and prevention of adduction
Superior gluteal nerve, L4, 5, S1

Gluteus minimus – from ilium between anterior and inferior gluteal lines to greater trochanter of femur
Abduction and medial rotation of femur, and prevention of adduction
Superior gluteal nerve, L4, 5, S1

Piriformis – from middle three pieces of sacrum to greater trochanter of femur
Abduction and lateral rotation of femur
Nerves from L5, S1, 2

Quadratus femoris – from ischial tuberosity to inter-trochanteric crest of femur
Lateral rotation of femur
Own nerve, L4, 5, S1

Obturator internus – from inner surface of obturator membrane to greater trochanter of femur
Lateral rotation of femur
Own nerve, L5, S1, 2

Gemellus superior and inferior – from ischial spine and upper part of ischial tuberosity respectively, to upper and lower parts of obturator internus
Assist obturator internus
Nerves to obturator internus and quadratus femoris respectively

Obturator externus – from outer surface of obturator membrane and adjacent rami of pubis and ischium to trochanteric fossa of femur
Lateral rotation of thigh
Obturator nerve, L3, 4

MUSCLES OF THE FRONT OF THE THIGH

Psoas major – *see* Muscles of the trunk

Iliacus – *see* Muscles of the trunk

Tensor fasciae latae – from anterior part of iliac crest to iliotibial tract
Extension and lateral rotation of leg
Superior gluteal nerve L4, 5, S1

Sartorius – from anterior superior iliac spine to upper medial surface of shaft of tibia in front of gracilis and semi-tendinosus
Flexion, abduction and lateral rotation of thigh
Femoral nerve, L2, 3

Rectus femoris – from anterior inferior iliac spine (straight head) and ilium above rim of acetabulum to base of patella
Flexion of thigh and extension of leg
Femoral nerve, L3, 4

Vastus lateralis – from upper part of intertrochanteric line, front of greater trochanter, gluteal tuberosity and upper linea aspera of femur to quadriceps tendon and patella
Extension of leg
Femoral nerve, L2, 3, 4

Vastus medialis – from lower part of intertrochanteric line, spiral line, linea aspera and medial supracondylar line of femur to quadriceps tendon and patella
Extension of leg
Femoral nerve, L2, 3, 4

Vastus intermedius – from anterior and lateral parts of upper two–thirds of shaft of femur to deep part of quadriceps tendon
Extension of leg
Femoral nerve, L2, 3, 4

Articularis genu – from lower anterior surface of shaft of femur to synovial membrane of knee joint
Retraction of synovial membrane
Femoral nerve, L2, 3

MUSCLES OF THE MEDIAL SIDE OF THE THIGH

Pectineus – from pectineal line of pubis to femur between lesser trochanter and linea aspera
Flexion, adduction and lateral rotation of thigh
Obturator nerve, L2, 3

Gracilis – from body of pubis and ischiopubic ramus to upper medial surface of shaft of femur between sartorius and semitendinosus
Flexion, adduction and medial rotation of thigh
Obturator nerve, L2, 3

Adductor brevis – from body and inferior ramus of pubis to shaft of femur between lesser trochanter and upper linea aspera
Adduction of thigh
Obturator nerve, L2, 3, 4

Adductor longus – from front of pubis to middle of linea aspera of femur
Adduction of thigh
Obturator nerve, L2, 3, 4

Adductor magnus – from lower lateral part of ischial tuberosity and ischiopubic ramus to linea aspera of femur from gluteal tuberosity down to medial supracondylar line and adductor tubercle
Adduction and lateral rotation of thigh
Obturator nerve, L2, 3, 4 and sciatic nerve, L4, 5, S1

MUSCLES OF THE BACK OF THE THIGH

Biceps femoris – from medial facet of ischial tuberosity (long head) and from linea aspera and lateral supracondylar line of femur (short head) to head of fibula
Flexion and lateral rotation of knee, and extension of hip
Sciatic nerve, L5, S1

Semitendinosus – from medial facet of ischial tuberosity (with long head of biceps) to upper part of subcutaneous surface of tibia, behind gracilis
Flexion and medial rotation of knee, and extension of hip
Sciatic nerve, L5, S1

Semimembranosus – from lateral facet of ischial tuberosity to groove on back of medial condyle of tibia, with expansions forming oblique popliteal ligament and fascia over popliteus
Flexion and medial rotation of knee, and extension of knee
Sciatic nerve, L5, S1

MUSCLES OF THE LEG AND FOOT

MUSCLES OF THE FRONT OF THE LEG AND DORSUM OF THE FOOT

Tibialis anterior – from upper two-thirds of lateral surface of tibia and interosseous membrane to medial surface of medial cuneiform and base of first metatarsal
Dorsiflexion and inversion of foot
Deep peroneal nerve, L4, 5

Extensor hallucis longus – from middle third of medial surface of fibula to base of distal phalanx of great toe
Extension of great toe and dorsiflexion of foot
Deep peroneal nerve, L5, S1

Extensor digitorum longus – from upper two-thirds of medial surface of fibula to middle and distal phalanges of lateral four toes
Extension of toes and dorsiflexion of foot
Deep peroneal nerve, L5, S1

Peroneus tertius – from lower third of medial surface of fibula to shaft of fifth metatarsal
Dorsiflexion and eversion of foot
Deep peroneal nerve, L5, S1

Extensor digitorum brevis – from upper surface of calcaneus to tendons of extensor hallucis longus and lateral three tendons of extensor digitorum longus
Extension of toes
Deep peroneal nerve, L5, S1

MUSCLES OF THE LATERAL SIDE OF THE LEG

Peroneus longus – from upper two-thirds of lateral surface of fibula to lateral side of medial cuneiform and base of first metatarsal
Plantarflexion and eversion of foot
Superfical peroneal nerve, L5, S1, 2
Peroneus brevis – from lower two-thirds of lateral surface of fibula to tuberosity of base of fifth metatarsal
Plantarflexion and eversion of foot
Deep peroneal nerve, L5, S1

MUSCLES OF THE BACK OF THE LEG AND SOLE OF THE FOOT

Muscles of the calf

Gastrocnemius – from upper posterior part of medial condyle of femur (medial head) and lateral surface of lateral condyle (lateral head) to middle of posterior surface of calcaneus (by Achilles' tendon with soleus)
Plantarflexion of foot and flexion of leg
Tibial nerve, S1, 2

Soleus – from soleal line of tibia, upper medial border of tibia and upper posterior surface of fibula to Achilles' tendon
Plantarflexion of foot
Tibial nerve, S1, 2

Plantaris – from lateral supracondylar line of femur to medial side of Achilles' tendon
Plantarflexion of foot and flexion of leg
Tibial nerve, S1, 2

Popliteus – from back of tibia above soleal line to outer surface of lateral epicondyle of femur
Lateral rotation of femur on fixed tibia (or vice versa)
Tibial nerve, L4, 5, S1

Tibialis posterior – from posterior surface of interosseous membrane and adjacent surfaces of tibia and fibula to tuberosity of navicular, with slips to other tarsal bones (except talus) and middle metatarsals
Plantarflexion and inversion of foot
Tibial nerve, L4, 5

Flexor hallucis longus – from lower two-thirds of posterior surface of fibula to base of distal phalanx of great toe
Plantarflexion of great toe and foot
Tibial nerve, S2, 3

Flexor digitorum longus – from medial part of posterior surface of tibia below soleal line to base of distal phalanges of four lateral toes
Plantarflexion of four lateral toes and foot
Tibial nerve, S2, 3

Muscles of the sole of the foot

First layer

Abductor hallucis – from medial process of calcanean tuberosity and plantar aponeurosis to medial side of proximal phalanx of great toe
Abduction and plantar flexion of great toe
Medial plantar nerve, S2, 3

Flexor digitorum brevis – from medial process of calcanean tuberosity and plantar aponeurosis to sides of middle phalanges of four lateral toes, splitting to allow tendons of flexor digitorum longus to pass through
Plantarflexion of toes
Medial plantar nerve, S2, 3

Abductor digiti minimi – from lateral and medial processes of calcanean tuberosity and plantar aponeurosis to lateral side of base of proximal phalanx of little toe
Abduction and plantarflexion of little toe
Lateral plantar nerve, S2, 3

Second layer

Flexor accessorius (quadratus plantae) – from medial and plantar surfaces of calcaneus to lateral side of flexor digitorum longus before it divides into tendons
Assists plantarflexion of four lateral toes
Lateral plantar nerve, S2, 3

Lumbricals – from tendons of flexor digitorum longus to medial sides of dorsal digital expansions
Plantarflexion of four lateral MP joints and extension of IP joints (with interossei)
Medial plantar nerve (first lumbrical) and lateral plantar nerve, S2, 3

Tendons of flexor digitorum longus and flexor hallucis longus

Third layer

Flexor hallucis brevis – from plantar surface of cuboid and lateral cuneiform to both sides of proximal phalanx of great toe
Plantarflexion of MP joint of great toe
Medial plantar nerve, S2, 3
Adductor hallucis – from bases of second, third and fourth metatarsals (oblique head) and plantar MP ligaments of three lateral toes (transverse head) to lateral side of base of proximal phalanx of great toe (with part of flexor hallucis brevis)
Adduction of great toe
Lateral plantar nerve, S2, 3

Flexor digiti minimi brevis – from plantar surface of base of fifth metatarsal to lateral side of base of proximal phalanx of little toe (with abductor digiti minimi)
Plantarflexion of MP joint of little toe
Lateral plantar nerve, S2, 3

Fourth layer

Dorsal interossei (4) – from adjacent sides of shafts of metatarsals to bases of proximal phalanges and dorsal digital expansions (1 and 2 to either side of second toe, 3 and 4 to lateral sides of third and fourth toes)
Plantarflexion of MP joints and extension of IP joints of second, third and fourth toes (with lumbricals and plantar interossei); abduction of toes from second toe axis
Lateral plantar nerve, S2, 3

Plantar interossei (3) – from bases of medial sides of third, fourth and fifth metatarsals to medial sides of bases of proximal phalanges of corresponding toes
Plantarflexion of MP joints and extension of IP joints of three lateral toes (with dorsal interossei and lumbricals); adduction of toes towards second toe
Lateral plantar nerve, S2, 3

Tendons of peroneus longus and tibialis posterior

INDEX

357